Pharmacist Services

Special Issue Editors

Jon C. Schommer
Anthony W. Olson

MDPI • Basel • Beijing • Wuhan • Barcelona • Belgrade

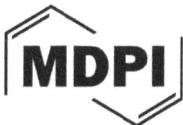

MDPI

Special Issue Editors
Jon C. Schommer
University of Minnesota
USA

Anthony W. Olson
University of Minnesota
USA

Editorial Office
MDPI
St. Alban-Anlage 66
4052 Basel, Switzerland

This is a reprint of articles from the Special Issue published online in the open access journal *Pharmacy* (ISSN 2226-4787) from 2018 to 2019 (available at: https://www.mdpi.com/journal/pharmacy/special_issues/Pharmacist_Services).

For citation purposes, cite each article independently as indicated on the article page online and as indicated below:

LastName, A.A.; LastName, B.B.; LastName, C.C. Article Title. *Journal Name* **Year**, *Article Number, Page Range.*

ISBN 978-3-03921-754-0 (Pbk)
ISBN 978-3-03921-755-7 (PDF)

Pharmacist Services

Contents

About the Special Issue Editors

Jon C. Schommer, R.Ph., PhD, is Professor at the University of Minnesota. He received his BS, MS, and PhD degrees from the University of Wisconsin–Madison. Since graduating with his PhD in 1992, he has devoted his career to teaching and research. His research is focused on information processing and decision making related to the provision, use, and evaluation of drug products and pharmacist services. He recently completed the National Consumer Survey on the Medication Experience—a study of over 36,000 individuals. Dr. Schommer has served as Peters Chair for Pharmacy Practice Innovation, President for the Academy of Pharmaceutical Research and Science, and Member of the American Pharmacists Association Board of Trustees. He holds a Distinguished Teaching Professor appointment and was inducted into the Academy of Distinguished Teachers at the University of Minnesota. In March 2019, he received the Academy of Pharmaceutical Research and Science Research Achievement Award. https://www.pharmacy.umn.edu/bio/cop-experts/jon-schommer.

Anthony W. Olson, M.Ed., Pharm.D., PhD candidate, is a graduate student at the University of Minnesota. He received his BA degree from St. Olaf College in Northfield, MN and his M.Ed. from George Mason University in Fairfax, VA. Anthony graduated with a Pharm.D. from the University of Minnesota College of Pharmacy in 2015 and entered the Social & Administrative PhD program shortly thereafter. His expected graduation date is in the spring of 2020, where after he will pursue a career in academic pharmacy. His research has focused on the theory and application of patient-centered care approaches as it relates to pharmacist practice and patient care services. The work is grounded in patient-centered care principles; health behavior theories; decision-making theories; and cognitive, social, and behavioral psychology. Dr. Olson has served as Speaker of the House for the Minnesota Pharmacists Association (MPhA) and Postgraduate Officer for the American Pharmacist Association. He has received the United States Public Health Service Excellence in Public Health Pharmacy Practice Award from the U.S. Deputy Surgeon General, Lilly Achievement Award, and Albert Wertheimer Leadership Fellowship. In October 2019, Dr. Olson was recognized as MPhA's Distinguished Young Pharmacist. https://www.pharmacy.umn.edu/bio/social-and-administrative-phar/anthony-olson.

Preface to "Pharmacist Services"

Welcome to the Special Issue "Pharmacist Services" of Pharmacy—an open access journal with a focus on pharmacy education and practice. Articles in this Special Issue reveal how pharmacist services can progress in (1) societal relevance, (2) innovative delivery, (3) integration into broader systems, (4) enhanced image to both payers and consumers, and (5) growth into new roles and markets. The articles reveal the overwhelming opportunities that pharmacists can embrace and fill, such as (1) medication optimization, (2) wellness and prevention, (3) chronic care management, (4) acute care management, (5) patient education, (6) care transitions, (7) population health, (8) emergency preparedness, (9) health informatics, and (10) patient-centered, living-in-place care.

We trust that you will find the articles in this Special Issue not only informative, but inspiring as well. We greatly appreciate the colleagues who worked to meet a short deadline and were willing to share their work with us. We also wish to thank the editorial staff who coordinated the review and publishing processes. Their professionalism is highly valued. Finally, we wish to thank you, the reader. Please apply the ideas in these articles to your work. Expand upon them. Challenge them. And, then, share your work with us.

Jon C. Schommer, Anthony W. Olson
Special Issue Editors

pharmacy **MDPI**

Editorial

Pharmacist Services

Jon C. Schommer [1],* and Anthony W. Olson [2],*

[1] College of Pharmacy, University of Minnesota-Twin Cities, Minneapolis, MN 55455, USA
[2] College of Pharmacy, University of Minnesota-Duluth, Duluth, MN 55812, USA
* Correspondence: schom010@umn.edu (J.C.S.); olso2001@umn.edu (A.W.O.)

Received: 29 September 2019; Accepted: 1 October 2019; Published: 10 October 2019

Welcome to the "Pharmacist Services" special issue in the journal Pharmacy, an open access journal with a focus on pharmacy education and practice. In 2018, an invitation was dispersed to scholars in the pharmacist services domain asking them to submit a manuscript to this special issue no later than 31 July 2019. We invited these colleagues to think about a full breadth of topics including, but not limited to: (1) The history and development of pharmacist services, (2) service settings, (3) service management, (4) service profitability, (5) service recovery, (6) service relationships, (7) service quality, (8) service tailoring, (9), service design and standards, (10) service performance, and (11) service evaluation. We sought manuscripts of all types including: (1) reviews, (2) commentaries, (3) idea papers, (4) case studies, (5) demonstration studies, and (6) research studies. The call for papers was delineated using ideas published by renowned experts in the services management and marketing domains including: Teresa Swartz, Dawn Iacobucci, Roland Rust, Richard Oliver, Valerie Zeithaml, and Mary Jo Bitner. With this foundational context described and the invitations sent, we waited to learn about what would be submitted in a timeframe of just several months.

We are pleased to report that over 30 articles have been published in this special issue and represent the work of about 100 scholars in this domain. To receive such a response from busy colleagues in such a short time-frame is incredible. The overall goal of this special issue on "Pharmacist Services" is to give the reader a state-of-the-art synopsis of the pharmacist services domain in the year 2019. To accomplish this goal, we sought papers that address the social, psychosocial, political, legal, historic, clinical, and economic factors that are associated with pharmacist services. Papers that translate concepts from other domains into the pharmacist services realm were welcomed. As we review the articles in this special issue, a great deal can be learned about (1) pharmacist professionalism, (2) pharmacist practice, and (3) pharmacist progression.

Pharmacist Professionalism

The articles reveal that pharmacist services vary by country, design, delivery environment, payment schemes, end-user, requisite training, regulatory standards, and more. As different as pharmacist services are, they are all linked by the individuals who provide them. Whether dispensing or immunizing, reconciling medication lists or performing medication management, pharmacists use their expertise related to medications to pursue excellent, affordable, and accessible healthcare for a common beneficiary: their patients. Pharmacist professionalism is a driving force for translating pharmacists' expertise into medication use, for helping people achieve medication experiences that are life enhancing.

Pharmacist Practice

Another emergent theme for pharmacist services described in this special issue is to view them through the Joint Commission of Pharmacy Practitioners (JCPP) Pharmacist Patient Care Process (PPCP), which was created and is supported by pharmacist organizations representing managed care, education, consultants, in-patient practice, outpatient practice, governmental regulatory bodies, and more. This model identifies a consistent process of care in the delivery of patient care services consisting of the following five steps: (1) Collect, (2) Assess, (3) Plan, (4) Implement, and (5) Follow-up: Monitor and Evaluate. The articles in this special issue give readers a state-of-the-art snapshot regarding the diversity of pharmacist services through the prism of the JCPP Pharmacist Patient Care Process.

Pharmacist Progression

Finally, many articles in this special issue reveal how pharmacist services can progress in (1) societal relevance, (2) innovative delivery, (3) integration into broader systems, (4) enhanced image to both payers and consumers, and (5) growth into new roles and markets. The articles reveal the overwhelming opportunities that pharmacists can embrace and fill such as: (1) Medication optimization, (2) wellness and prevention, (3) chronic care management, (4) acute care management, (5) patient education, (6) care transitions, (7) population health, (8) emergency preparedness, (9) health informatics, and (10) patient-centered, living-in-place care.

We trust that you will find the articles in this special issue not only informative, but inspiring as well. We greatly appreciate the colleagues who worked to meet a short deadline and were willing to share their work with us. We also wish to thank the editorial staff who coordinated the review and publishing processes. Their professionalism is highly valued. Finally, we wish to thank you, the reader. Please apply the ideas in these articles to your work. Expand upon them. Challenge them. And then, share your work with us.

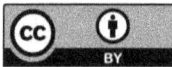

pharmacy

MDPI

Review

Towards a Greater Professional Standing: Evolution of Pharmacy Practice and Education, 1920–2020

Benjamin Y. Urick * and **Emily V. Meggs**

Eshelman School of Pharmacy, University of North Carolina, Chapel Hill, NC 27599, USA
* Correspondence: benurick@email.unc.edu

check for
updates

Received: 31 May 2019; Accepted: 18 July 2019; Published: 20 July 2019

Abstract: The history of community pharmacy in America since the 1920s is one of slow progress towards greater professional standing through changes in pharmacy education and practice. The history of American community pharmacy in the modern era can be divided into four periods: 1920–1949 (Soda Fountain Era), 1950–1979 (Lick, Stick, Pour and More Era), 1980–2009 (Pharmaceutical Care Era), and 2010–present (Post-Pharmaceutical Care Era). As traditional compounding has waned, leaders within community pharmacy have sought to shift focus from product to patient. Increasing degree requirements and postgraduate training have enhanced pharmacists' ability to provide patient care services not directly associated with medication dispensing. However, the realities of practice have often fallen short of ideal visions of patient-focused community pharmacy practice. Positive trends in the recognition of the impact of community pharmacists on healthcare value and the need for more optimal medication management suggest that opportunities for community pharmacists to provide patient care may expand through the 21st century.

Keywords: history of pharmacy; 20th century history; 21st century history; community pharmacy services; pharmacy education

1. Introduction

As long there has been a belief in the medicinal properties of natural substances, there have been people whose duty it was to transform these materia medica into medicines. By the 1800s, however, this traditional role of pharmacy had begun to change. The Industrial Revolution led to mass manufacture of medicinal products which once only the pharmacist could produce. Additionally, new medicines were being discovered which could not be easily derived from traditional materia medica. As traditional compounding began to wane and proprietary products began to replace those which the pharmacist used to make himself, merchandising in pharmacies began to increase. The erosion of traditional roles led to a crisis of professionalism within American community pharmacy, requiring the profession to rethink its role in society. It is with this backdrop that the modern era of community pharmacy in the United States begins.

For this narrative review, the history of American community pharmacy in the modern era can be divided into four periods: 1920–1949 (Soda Fountain Era), 1950–1979 (Lick, Stick, Pour and More Era), 1980–2009 (Pharmaceutical Care Era), and 2010–present (Post-Pharmaceutical Care Era). A slow march towards greater patient care and higher professional standing can be observed across each of these periods as the profession of pharmacy has struggled with what defines community pharmacy and how community pharmacy adds value to society.

2. 1920–1949: Soda Fountain Era

2.1. Education

By the time the modern era of pharmacy dawned in the 1920s, pharmacy education was rapidly adopting three and four-year degrees as the standard for education [1]. Old-fashioned short courses, designed as supplements to apprenticeship, were falling out of favor and would soon be made obsolete. Pharmacy education in the early part of the 20th century was guided by *The* Pharmaceutical Syllabus [1]. This detailed guide to pharmacy education, created by the American Association of Colleges of Pharmacy (AACP), helped to standardize degree programs as training became more formalized.

The first major study of pharmacy practice, Basic Material for a Pharmaceutical Curriculum, was published in 1927 [2]. This study sought to revise the curriculum contained in the Pharmaceutical Syllabus by developing a new curriculum based on the functional needs of the pharmacy profession [2]. Reflecting the makeup of the profession in the 1920s, the Pharmaceutical Curriculum was focused solely on the needs of pharmacists working in retail settings. The report focused on many areas of study deemed essential to pharmacy practice at the time, including basic sciences of chemistry and physics; medicine-related subjects such as pharmacognosy, botany, pharmacology, physiology, and public health; and practice-related subjects such as small-scale pharmaceutical manufacturing, prescription filling, and retail sales operations. The Pharmaceutical Curriculum did not, however, include any information on diagnosis and treatment of disease. While the authors acknowledged that a pharmacist has a duty to assist their "customers" who have questions on "the cure for an ailment," they were concerned that too much education would lead to counter-prescribing—dispensing pharmaceuticals to treat a disease without or contrary to a prescription from a physician.

Merchandising and commercial aspects of pharmacy practice were only begrudgingly included in the Pharmaceutical Curriculum. It was acknowledged that merchandising and commercial interests were rampant within the community pharmacy practice. However, one goal of creating a standardized curriculum was to raise professional standards and train more professionally-oriented graduates who were better able to engage with other healthcare practitioners [1]. As such, it was thought that inclusion of merchandising and commercial interests would undermine pharmacy's professionalism and these aspects of pharmacy practice were excluded from the Pharmaceutical Curriculum. Aided in educational transformation during the Soda Fountain Era was the founding of the Accreditation Council for Pharmaceutical Education (ACPE) in 1932. The ACPE established the first national standards for pharmacy degree program accreditation and, as a result, by 1941, 64 out of 67 colleges of pharmacy had adopted a four-year degree standard.

The educational change began in The Pharmaceutical Syllabus was furthered by the Pharmaceutical Survey which was commissioned by the American Council on Education in 1946 [3]. The Pharmaceutical Survey recognized the growing tension between pharmacists as distributors of mass manufactured products and pharmacists as healthcare professionals. The distribution and merchandising roles were seen as undermining pharmacy's professionalism. Additionally, the four-year degree was thought to be too short a course of study for the pharmacist to complete a general education as well as a pharmacy education [4], and did not "confer the status that is desired by pharmacists, particularly those who work in rather intimate professional association with physicians, dentists, and members of other health professions who hold professional doctor's degrees. [4]"

Therefore, to provide a complete education and firm the professional foundation of pharmacy practice, the report recommended the establishment of a six-year Doctor of Pharmacy program to afford "new opportunities for raising the level of preparation for the professional areas of pharmacy [5]." However, the recommendation to lengthen the curriculum was met with opposition by pharmacy educators, and the majority of pharmacy school deans at the time favored the status quo [4]. The debate within the American Association of Colleges of Pharmacy about degree standards would result in substantial changes to pharmacy education in the 1950s.

2.2. Practice

As compounding waned, pharmacy in the 1920s found itself questioning its own professional standing. This is reflected in practice as well as education. Concurrently, the enactment of national prohibition in 1919 was a boon to pharmacies' front-end commercial interest in two major ways [6]. First, the sale and consumption of "medicinal" alcohol was allowed and this created a legal loophole which many pharmacists and physicians exploited. Second, soda fountains became very popular destinations for those seeking alcohol-alternatives. Neither was considered a "professional" activity, but both were surely profitable.

Accordingly, traditional prescription compounding and dispensing became a minor part of pharmacy operations in the 1920s and 1930s. Although 75% of prescriptions still required some compounding [7], less than 1% of pharmacies of pharmacies had more than 50% of their sales from prescription drugs [8]. Even when drugs were dispensed, ethical standards at the time limited pharmacists' engagement with patients. For example, the 1922 American Pharmaceutical Association (APhA) Code of Ethics [9] stated that:

> *"[The pharmacist] should never discuss the therapeutic effect of a Physician's prescription with a patron nor disclose details of composition which the Physician has withheld, suggesting to the patient that such details can be properly discussed with the prescriber only".*

In the 1920s, the transition away from compounding and towards premanufactured proprietary products led to a crisis within the community pharmacy—pharmacy's traditional role was waning, and it was not clear what the role of a pharmacist was, if not, compounding. The answer, in many ways, was to increase front-end commercial interests through expanding soda fountains and other goods for purchase. Prescription dispensing was essential to the identity of the pharmacy, but was de-emphasized as a part of the pharmacy's business. This would change as advances in pharmaceutical research in the mid-20th century led to an explosion of new prescription drug products.

3. 1950–1979: Lick, Stick, Pour and More Era

As the patient care roles of the pharmacist and educational standards increased from the 1950s through the 1970s, the highest professional activity was no longer dispensing, as it was in the 1920s. The provision of patient care services replaced dispensing as the highest professional activity. This created a cultural shift within community pharmacy practice—and gave rise to the tension between dispensing and patient care which persists into the 21st century. Arguments over the degree needed to support this new version of professionalism were heated, and would not be ended until the 1980s.

3.1. Education

The recommendations of the Pharmaceutical Survey laid the foundation for changes to pharmacy education throughout the 1950s, 60s, and 70s. Leaders in pharmacy education acknowledged that the four-year degree was insufficient for the level of training needed to become a pharmacist. There was strong resistance, however, to a mandatory professional doctorate as the entry level practice degree. An uneasy compromise was made with the adoption of a five-year degree standard, despite specific recommendations against the degree from the Pharmaceutical Survey.

As clinical pharmacy and the desire for higher professional standing began to permeate throughout the profession in the 1960s and early 1970s, the movement towards a degree which provided the appropriate professional foundation for clinical pharmacy accelerated. The first pharmacy program to adopt an all-Doctor of Pharmacy (PharmD) standard was the University of Southern California in 1950 [10]. Other programs followed USC's lead, and by the mid-1970s there were 20 PharmD programs.

Through its emphasis on clinical education and experience, proponents of the PharmD redefined professionalism as not just an avoidance of merchandising or commercial endeavors, but also de-emphasized medication dispensing as a professional activity befitting a PharmD-trained pharmacist. Indeed, dispensing was called a "temporary obfuscation" of the clinical objective of the profession [10]. Educational changes associated with the clinical pharmacy movement also re-emphasized the practice component of pharmacy education, reducing educational focus on theory-based training in basic sciences [11].

3.2. Practice

By 1950, the percent of prescriptions which were compounded had fallen to 25% [7]. This percentage would decrease further to less than 5% by 1960 and 1% by 1970 [7]. Concurrent with decreases in traditional compounded prescriptions was a large increase in the number and diversity of premanufactured drug products. An explosion of newly discovered drugs led to an increase of over 50% in the number of drugs dispensed during the 1950s [6]. By the mid-1950s, pharmacists were stepping away from soda fountain and were back behind the pharmacy counter. However, the role had changed substantially from the 1920s. Pharmacists were primarily dispensing premanufactured capsules and tablets, and ethical standards at the time still prohibited them from discussing the contents of prescriptions with patients [12]. Prescription labels from that era commonly omitted the name of the product dispensed—with the idea that labeling the vial with the name of the drug would violate the physician-patient relationship. This was the origin of the modern "lick, stick, and pour" pharmacy practice.

This new version of pharmacy irked many patient care-oriented pharmacists at the time because they desired to do more than simply dispense a product. Eugene White, among the more well-known visionaries of what would become patient care-oriented community pharmacy practice, began working in 1950 at a typical retail-oriented pharmacy. He quickly became disillusioned with practice standards at the time, saying, "After five months of selling lawn seed and paint, cutting glass for window frames, and dispensing a few prescription orders in between, I could longer take it ... [13]" White purchased his own pharmacy in 1957 and in 1960 completely transformed his pharmacy into what he termed a "pharmaceutical center." Gone was the soda fountain and self-serve retail space for candy, stationary, billfolds, toys, and gifts. He added a record system to keep track of families' prescriptions. He hired a receptionist to greet patients when they entered and built a semi-private patient counseling area. His model even served as the basis for professional pharmacies promoted and designed by McKesson in the mid-1960s [14].

Also innovating during this era were pharmacists in community pharmacy practice settings like the Indian Health Service, which in 1966 required private patient counseling areas in all new pharmacies [15]. The 1960s also witnessed the birth of clinical pharmacy services, with major innovation stemming from experiments including the Ninth Floor Project led by University of California, San Francisco School of Pharmacy faculty [16]. This project revolutionized the provision of pharmacy services in hospitals by building a satellite pharmacy to dispense unit-dose medications specific to each order and to prepare admixtures by pharmacists instead of nurses, which at the time were radical advancements. In addition, the pharmacist was available for consultation on drug information and other clinical questions as they arose. This experiment spurred the development of similar clinically-focused pharmacy roles nationwide would substantially influence changes in pharmacy practice philosophy in the 1980s.

Eugene White and innovators like him replaced customers with patients, and through this they redefined how a professional community pharmacy operated. Combined with the growth in clinical pharmacy in hospitals during this same time, this transformation revolutionized how the profession saw itself. This was change was reflected in the 1969 revision to APhA's Code of Ethics [17] which referred to a pharmacist's duty to his patient in the first section:

> *A pharmacist should hold the health and safety of patients to be of first consideration; he should render to each patient the full measure of his ability as an essential health practitioner.*

Practice changes continued through the 1970s. Products became more diverse, and spillover from the clinical pharmacy movement began to expand the array of non-dispensing services provided in pharmacies. Additionally, the first computer systems in the 1970s expanded pharmacists' abilities to keep dispensing records and check for drug–drug interactions [6].

The period from the 1950s to 1970s was a pivotal time for American pharmacy. The emphasis on front-end merchandising and soda fountains waned as dispensing increased. A new version of professionalism had started to arise within community pharmacy—one focused not on dispensing alone but on dispensing as a part of care for a patient's medication-related needs. Education also witnessed a similar evolution, with new PharmD degree programs supporting the training needed to provide robust patient care services. Ethical standards likewise evolved, with the 1969 APhA Code of Ethics calling for pharmacists to engage in activity that would have been ethically suspect under previous codes. These changes built the foundation for changes in the 1980s that would further propel the notion that community pharmacists had an obligation to their patients which extended beyond simple dispensing of products.

4. 1980–2009: Pharmaceutical Care Era

4.1. Education

The final major change to pharmacy education in the last 100 years was the transition from the five-year, entry-level B.S. degree with the optional post-graduate PharmD training to the PharmD becoming the entry level degree. Echoing the Pharmaceutical Survey from nearly 40 years prior, the Final Report of the Task Force on Pharmacy Education, commissioned by the American Pharmaceutical Association (APhA) and released in 1984, called for a universal six-year PharmD degree [18]. Following this call, the universal PharmD degree was put to a vote in the American Association of College of Pharmacy (AACP) House of Delegates in 1985 but was defeated by a narrow margin. Nevertheless, major national conferences and academic papers throughout the end of the 1980s helped sway opinion towards a universal PharmD and acceptance of pharmacy as a clinical profession which needed a professional doctorate. In 1989, A Declaration of Intent was made by ACPE to adopt the PharmD as the universal standard for pharmacy education as soon as 2000 [19,20]. Through the early 1990s, APhA, the National Association of Retail Druggists, and the American Society of Hospital Pharmacists, the American College of Clinical Pharmacy, the National Association of Boards of Pharmacy, and AACP came to actively support the single degree standard but the organization representing chain pharmacies, the National Association of Chain Drug Stores, continued to oppose the concept [20–22]. On schedule, the last student to enter an accredited BSPharm program enrolled in 2000 and the transition to a universal PharmD was completed in 2005 [23].

The most evident education-related aspect of the patient care movement within community pharmacy was the development of the first community pharmacy residency programs in the mid-1980s. Training on the provision of clinical services was an explicit goal of these first community pharmacy residencies [24], and this focus has expanded over time [25]. Community pharmacy residency sites have often served as laboratories for advanced practice, requiring community pharmacists to engage in practice-based research and expanding the scope of services offered [26]. The development of formal postgraduate training focused on patient care in community pharmacy settings, combined with a universal PharmD, created a strong foundation for the expanded delivery of patient care services in community pharmacies.

4.2. Practice

The 1980s witnessed major change to the philosophy of practice as pharmacy leaders considered pharmacy's role in the 21st century. Many of these changes were, however, aspirational with some innovative pharmacies leading the way and most lagging behind. In many ways, the movement to bring clinical pharmacy into the community setting was seen as idealistic and out-of-touch with the busy community pharmacy work environment [27].

Nevertheless, the declaration of pharmacy as a clinical profession at the 1985 Hilton Head Conference [28] and the conceptualization of pharmacists' duties vis-à-vis pharmaceutical care in 1989 through a presentation at the Second Hilton Head Conference [29] and a seminal paper entitled "Opportunities and Responsibilities in Pharmaceutical Care" [30] were a boost to those seeking a greater patient care orientation for community pharmacy practice. Hepler and Strand's definition of pharmaceutical care placed patient care at the center of pharmacy practice:

> *Pharmaceutical care is the responsible provision of drug therapy for the purpose of achieving definite outcomes that improve a patient's quality of life. These outcomes are (1) cure of a disease, (2) elimination or reduction of a patient's symptomatology, (3) arresting or slowing of a disease process, or (4) preventing a disease or symptomatology.*

These changes to practice philosophy were boosted when the federal government in 1990 required prescription counseling as a part of the Medicaid program [31]. The combination of these elements enthusiastically propelled community pharmacy into the last decade of the 20th century. Several pilot projects in the 1990s demonstrated that pharmacists could provide and be remunerated for pharmaceutical care services, which would later be rebranded as medication therapy management (MTM) in the 2000s. The Minnesota Pharmaceutical Care Demonstration Project [32], private and public initiatives in Iowa [33], and the Asheville Project [34], for example, are well-known examples of projects which paid community pharmacists for non-dispensing related services. Training programs, like that of the Iowa Center for Pharmaceutical Care [33], were used nationally and internationally to prepare pharmacists to provide services tested through these demonstration projects. By the end of the 1990s, the market for pharmaceutical care services was sufficiently well-developed to support the launch of OutcomesMTM® in 1999.

The progress of pharmaceutical care era culminated in 2003 with the passing of the Medicare Prescription Drug, Improvement, and Modernization Act (MMA). This act created the Medicare Part D benefit, the first Medicare benefit for retail prescription drugs. The MMA required Part D plan sponsors to include MTM as a part of their benefit structure. Pharmacy viewed MTM as a major victory—finally, the federal government was recognizing the need for more optimal medication use and creating a payment mechanism for it. The enthusiasm was short-lived, however, as the benefit allowed a variety of non-pharmacist providers to deliver MTM, and many Part D plan sponsors sought cost-minimal ways to offer the mandatory benefit.

Also growing during the 1990s was the new role of pharmacists as immunizers. The first immunization training programs were developed by state and national pharmacy organizations in the mid-1990s [35]. By 2003, 34 states allowed pharmacists to provide immunizations but many restrictions were placed on pharmacists' immunization-related scope of practice [36], but by the end of the decade, all states allowed pharmacists at least some level of immunization authority, and many of the earlier restrictions had been lifted [37]. Pharmacists were critical vaccine distribution sites during the response to the 2009-10 H1N1 influenza pandemic [38] and research from the time suggests that this expanded role had a positive impact on public health [39]. Pharmacist-provided immunizations expanded the total number of patients who were vaccinated, not just shift sites of care from primary care offices to pharmacies.

Despite this momentum, the National Pharmacy Workforce Survey found that in 2004 only 5–10% of community pharmacists reported that their pharmacy provided MTM services [40]. Other services such as health screenings, immunizations, and smoking cessation were more common, but none of these enhanced services were provided at the majority of pharmacies where respondents worked. The 2009 National Pharmacy Workforce Survey, delivered after the full implementation of Medicare Part D, found slightly higher engagement in patient care services, but pharmacists still only spent 8–11% of their time providing patient care services and 70–78% of their time dispensing [41].

As the 21st century dawned, the long-awaited opportunity for community pharmacists to shift from dispensing to patient care services seemed nearly at hand. many hoped that the universal PharmD, evidence supporting the positive impact of pharmacist services, and the Part D MTM benefit would create new opportunities for pharmacists to transition from a product focus to a patient focus. However, the vast majority of community pharmacists still found themselves dispensing by the end of the 2000s. Substantial progress had been made since the 1980s, but the pace of change was slower than what pharmacy's leaders had hoped for.

5. 2010–Present: Post-Pharmaceutical Care Era

5.1. Education

By 2010, the all-PharmD requirement had been fully implemented for a decade. Instead of changes to degrees, the largest changes in pharmacist education occurred after graduation. Pursuit of residencies has increased steadily in the post-pharmaceutical care era, with the number of students pursuing residencies over this period more than doubling between 2009 and 2018 [42,43] and percent of students pursuing residencies increasing from 21.8% to 29.0% [42,43]. Residencies have become a prerequisite for entry-level clinical pharmacy jobs in inpatient settings, but community pharmacy residencies have not become the de facto standard for entry into community pharmacy practice. The number of sites remains small, and few graduating students pursue them. This may change in the future, but residencies for community pharmacists remain limited primarily to those pharmacists who intend to provide an exceptional amount of non-dispensing services [27].

5.2. Practice

Immunizations and patient care services have both increased in the 2010s. Community pharmacists' immunization-related scope of practice has continued to increase and pharmacies have become an accepted place to receive an immunization. The majority of patients report feeling comfortable receiving vaccines in pharmacy settings [44], and more than 22% of all people who got vaccinated for influenza during the 2014–15 flu having received their immunization from a pharmacy or store [45]. Evidence supports the role of the pharmacist in positively impacting vaccination rates for a variety of immunizations [46], and immunizations will remain a feature of community pharmacy practice for the foreseeable future.

Other non-dispensing services have increased throughout the second decade of the 2000s, but the rate of increase has been slow. More than 20 years after the publication of his landmark paper on the opportunities and responsibilities of pharmaceutical care, Dr. Hepler referred to the idea of pharmacy as a clinical profession as a "dream deferred" when giving the 2010 Whitney Lecture [47]. This frames well the state of pharmaceutical care services in the 2010s—not dead, but not as viable as pharmacy leaders in the 1980s and 1990s had hoped. Results of the most recent pharmacy workforce survey find that pharmacists in community settings spend about an hour of each day providing patient care services not associated with dispensing [48]. This is more than past workforce surveys, but more than two-thirds of community pharmacists' time remains spent dispensing [48], and dispensing remains the role patients perceive as most valuable [44].

Accordingly, the promise of MTM in Part D had lost some of its shine by 2010. Low beneficiary uptake and lackluster offerings resulted in the federal government efforts to strengthen requirements for offering MTM [49]. Additionally, the federal government began to include the comprehensive medication review (CMR) completion rate as a quality measure for the Medicare Stars Rating program [50]. Higher quality scores within this program result in greater marketing and revenue opportunities for Part D plan sponsors, and since the CMR completion rate measure was first introduced, completion rates have increased from 15.4% to 38.0% and 30.9% to 71.0% for standalone prescription drug plans and Medicare Advantage prescription drug plans respectively [51]. OutcomesMTM®, a major facilitator of pharmacist-provided MTM services, processed 2.4 million MTM claims in 2016 alone [52]. This was an increase over prior years [53], but was still less than a claim a week for the 50,000 pharmacists actively participating in the OutcomesMTM network.

One potential opportunity to expand services is through provider status in Medicare Part B Legislation that would expand billing opportunities for pharmacists in Medicare Part B was introduced during the 114th and 115th Congress but failed to pass [54]. This would create a sustainable source of revenue for non-dispensing services, but the passage of federal legislation is uncertain. More movement towards provider status has happened at the state level [55], but these efforts oftentimes expand privileges without expanding opportunities to bill insurers.

The brightest light for the post-pharmaceutical care area are the opportunities beginning to emerge for community pharmacies as partners with payers and care givers to improve medication-related quality measures and decrease total cost of care. These engagements have taken two general forms. The first is pharmacists being held to account on quality measures like medication adherence, and receiving upside and downside payment adjustment based on performance. Nearly all pharmacies in the US have the ability to support performance measurement for intermediate outcomes like medication adherence [44], and nearly 60% of 2019 Medicare beneficiaries are in a plan that has a performance-based pharmacy payment program related to quality measures [56]. The second type of engagement is contracting between community pharmacies and payers or other provider groups to share risk and provide enhanced services aimed deliberately at impacting cost and quality. These types of engagements are relatively new, but are being supported by groups such as CPESN USA [57] which brings together community pharmacies willing to provide enhanced services into clinically integrated networks able to manage populations of patients across groups of pharmacies. This approach is a step far beyond one-off pharmacy collaborations, and could finally establish a working business model for the professional service-oriented pharmacy.

6. Conclusions

Throughout the modern era, pharmacy has pursued higher professional standing. In the 1920s, this meant eschewing the soda fountain and front-end sales to focus on compounding and dispensing. By the 1950s, professional standing had begun to be defined more by patient care services than by simple dispensing. However, dispensing has remained stubbornly prominent in community pharmacy practice, and the opportunities to provide patient care services have not been as plentiful as hoped. Over the same period, there has been an interplay between education and practice, with education driving higher professional standing through the eventual adoption of the universal PharmD standard, and entrepreneurial pharmacists developing new, innovative practices focused on providing greater patient care services. Looking towards the future, it is hard to imagine a community pharmacist in the mid-21st century doing nothing but dispensing, but it is equally hard to imagine that dispensing would not be a part of how the average community pharmacist spends his or her day. Immunizations will almost certainly remain a common feature of pharmacy practice, as will some degree of patient care services not associated with dispensing. Evidence linking the provision of these services to reductions in healthcare spending and improvements in healthcare quality is growing. If community pharmacists can demonstrate that their services have a meaningful impact on healthcare value, it is likely their non-dispensing roles will continue to increase. Absent this evidence, one wonders how the community pharmacist in 2050 will spend their day. Nevertheless, developments in the last 100 years have created new opportunities for community pharmacists to provide patient care services not associated with dispensing, and as society evolves community pharmacy practice will continue to evolve alongside it.

Author Contributions: The authors shared work on this manuscript thusly: Conceptualization, B.Y.U. and E.V.M.; methodology, B.Y.U.; writing—original draft preparation, B.Y.U.; writing—review and editing, B.Y.U. and E.V.M.

Funding: This research received no external funding.

Conflicts of Interest: The authors declare no conflict of interest.

References

1.   Mrtek, R. An Interpretive Historical Essay of the Twentieth Century. *Am. J. Pharm. Educ.* **1976**, *40*, 339–365. [PubMed]
2.   Charters, W.W.; Lemon, A.B.; Monell, L.M. Section 1. Introduction to the Complete Report. In *Basic Material for a Pharmaceutical Curriculum*; McGraw-Hill Book Company Inc.: New York, NY, USA, 1927; pp. 1–14.
3.   Elliott, E.C. Part I: The Pharmaceutical Survey. In *The General Report of the Pharmaceutical Survey*; American Council on Education: Washington, DC, USA, 1950; pp. 1–14.

4.	Elliott, E.C. Part V: The Pharmaceutical Curriculum. In *The General Report of the Pharmaceutical Survey, 1946–1949*; American Council on Education: Washington, DC, USA, 1950; pp. 98–118.
5.	Elliott, E.C. Part X: Retail Pharmacy Projects. In *The General Report of the Pharmaceutical Survey, 1946–1949*; American Council on Education: Washington, DC, USA, 1950; pp. 198–209.
6.	Higby, G.J. Introduction to the History and Profession of American Pharmacy. In *The Pharmacist in Public Health: Education, Applications and Opportunities*; Truong, H.-A., Jill, B.J.L., Sellers, A., Eds.; American Pharmacists Association: Washington, DC, USA, 2010; pp. 31–55.
7.	Higby, G.J. Evolution of Pharmacy. In *Remingtonthe Science and Practice of Pharmacy*, 21st ed.; David, B., Troy, M.J.H., Eds.; Lippincott Williams & Wilkins: Baltimore, MD, USA, 2005; pp. 7–19.
8.	Sonnedecker, G. Economic and Structural Development. In *Kremers and Urdang's History of Pharmacy*, 4th ed.; Sonnedecker, G., Ed.; American Institute of the History of Pharmacy: Madison, WI, USA, 1976; pp. 290–338.
9.	Code of Ethics of the American Pharmaceutical Association. *J. Am. Pharm. Assoc.* **1922**, *11*, 728–729.
10.	Haskell, A.R.; Benedict, L.K. The universal Doctor of Pharmacy degree. *Am. J. Pharm. Educ.* **1975**, *39*, 425–427. [PubMed]
11.	Hepler, C.D. The third wave in pharmaceutical education: The clinical movement. *Am. J. Pharm. Educ.* **1987**, *51*, 369–385. [PubMed]
12.	American Pharmaceutical Association. *Code of Ethics of the American Pharmaceutical Association*; American Pharmaceutical Association: Washington, DC, USA, 1952.
13.	White, E.V. Behind the scenes of the pharmaceutical center. *J. Am. Pharm. Assoc.* **1965**, *5*, 532–535. [CrossRef]
14.	Apple, W.S. Reformation in Pharmaceutical Practice. *J. Am. Pharm. Assoc.* **1965**, *216*, 188–189. [CrossRef]
15.	Fisher, R. History of the Indian Health Service Model of Pharmacy Practice: Innovations in Pharmaceutical Care. *Pharm. Hist.* **1995**, *37*, 107–122.
16.	Day, R.L.; Goyan, J.E.; Herfindal, E.T.; Sorby, D.L. The origins of the Clinical Pharmacy Program at the University of California, San Francisco. *DICP* **1991**, *25*, 308–314. [CrossRef]
17.	American Pharmaceutical Association. APhA Code of Ethics. *J. Am. Pharm. Assoc.* **1969**, *NS9*, 552.
18.	American Pharmaceutical Association. *Final Report of the Task Force on Pharmacy Education*; American Pharmaceutical Association: Washington, DC, USA, 1984.
19.	Accreditation Council for Pharmacy Education. *Accreditation Standards and Guidelines for the Professional Program in Pharmacy Leading to the Doctor of Pharmacy Degree*; Accreditation Council for Pharmacy Education: Chicago, IL, USA, 14 June 1997.
20.	Martin, S. Uniting for One Degree. *Am. Pharm.* **1999**, *NS32*, 52–55.
21.	American College of Clinical Pharmacy. Pharmaceutical Education: A commentary from the American College of Clinical Pharmacy. *Pharmacotherapy* **1992**, *12*, 419–427.
22.	ASHP, APhA, NARD issue joint statement on entry-level Doctor of Pharmacy degree. *Am. J. Hosp. Pharm.* **1992**, *42*, 246–258.
23.	Accreditation Council for Pharmacy Education. *Accreditation Standards and Guidelines for the Professional Program in Pharmacy Leading to the Doctor of Pharmacy Degree*; Accreditation Council for Pharmacy Education: Chicago, IL, USA, 23 January 2011.
24.	American Pharmaceutical Association. APhA community pharmacy residency program: Programmatic essentials. *Am. Pharm.* **1986**, *NS26*, 34–43.
25.	Accreditation Council for Pharmacy Education. *Accreditation Standards and Key Elements for the Professional Program in Pharmacy Leading to the Doctor of Pharmacy Degree*; Accreditation Council for Pharmacy Education: Chicago, IL, USA, January 2015.
26.	Heaton, P.; Westrick, S.C. Community-based pharmacy residents: Transforming the health care landscape. *J. Am. Pharm. Assoc. (2003)* **2018**, *58*, S5–S6. [CrossRef]
27.	Reinsmith, W.A. Patient-centered community pharmacy: A mirage. *Am. Pharm.* **1985**, *NS25*, 6–8. [CrossRef]
28.	Hepler, C.D. Pharmacy as a Clinical Profession. *Am. J. Hosp. Pharm.* **1985**, *42*, 1298–1306. [CrossRef]
29.	Cocolas, G.H. Pharmacy in the 21st Century Conference: Executive Summary. *Am. J. Pharm. Educ.* **1989**, *53*, 1S–5S.
30.	Hepler, C.D.; Strand, L.M. Opportunities and Responsibilities in Pharmaceutical Care. *Am. J. Pharm. Educ.* **1989**, *53*, S7–S15. [CrossRef]

31. Schatz, R.; Belloto, R.J.; White, D.B., Jr.; Bachmann, K. Provision of drug information to patients by pharmacists: The impact of the Omnibus Budget Reconciliation Act of 1990 a decade later. *Am. J. Ther.* **2003**, *10*, 93–103. [CrossRef]
32. Isetts, B.J. Pharmaceutical care, MTM, & payment: The past, present, & future. *Ann. Pharmacother.* **2012**, *46*, S47–S56.
33. *Celebrating a Decade of Progress in Shaping a New Generation of Pharmacy Practice*; Iowa Center for Pharmaceutical Care: Des Moines, IA, USA, 1994.
34. Cranor, C.W.; Christensen, D.B. The Asheville Project: Short-term outcomes of a community pharmacy diabetes care program. *J. Am. Pharm. Assoc.* **2003**, *43*, 149–159. [CrossRef]
35. Hogue, M.D.; Grabenstein, J.D.; Foster, S.L.; Rothholz, M.C. Pharmacist involvement with immunizations: A decade of professional advancement. *J. Am. Pharm. Assoc. (2003)* **2006**, *46*, 168–179. [CrossRef]
36. Catizone, C.A. *Survey of Pharmacy Law-2003–2004*; National Association of Boards of Pharmacy: Park Ridge, IL, USA, December 2003.
37. Catizone, C.A. *Survey of Pharmacy Law-2010*; National Association of Boards of Pharmacy: Mount Prospect, IL, USA, 2009.
38. Association of State and Territorial Health Officials. Operational Framework for Partnering with Pharmacies for Administration of 2009 H1N1 Vaccine. Available online: http://www.astho.org/Infectious-Disease/Operational-Framework-for-Partnering-with-Pharmacies-for-Administration-of-2009-H1N1-Vaccine/ (accessed on 18 July 2019).
39. Steyer, T.E.; Ragucci, K.R.; Pearson, W.S.; Mainous, A.G., 3rd. The role of pharmacists in the delivery of influenza vaccinations. *Vaccine* **2004**, *22*, 1001–1006. [CrossRef] [PubMed]
40. Gaither, C.A.; Schommer, J.C.; Doucette, W.R.; Kreling, D.H.; Mott, D.A. Executive Summary of the Final Report of the 2014 National Sample Survey of the Pharmacist Workforce to Determine Contemporary Demographic and Practice Characteristics and Quality of Work-Life. Final Report of the National Sample Survey of the Pharmacist Workforce to Determine Contemporary Demographic and Practice Characteristics. Midwest Pharmacy Workforce Research Consortium, 1 September 2005. Available online: https://www.aacp.org/sites/default/files/executivesummaryfromthenationalpharmacistworkforcestudy2014.pdf (accessed on 18 July 2019).
41. Doucette, W.R.; Gaither, C.A.; Kreling, D.H.; Mott, D.A.; Schommer, J.C. 2009 National Pharmacist Workforce Survey. Available online: https://www.ncpanet.org/pdf/dose_2009_national_pharm_workforce_survey.pdf (accessed on 18 July 2019).
42. *Graduating Pharmacy Student Survey Summary Report-2009*; American Association of Colleges of Pharmacy: Arlington, VA, USA, 2009.
43. *Graduating Student Survey: 2018 National Summary Report*; American Association of Colleges of Pharmacy: Arlington, VA, USA, July 2018.
44. Sega, T. Industry Trend Report in Pharmacy Quality. Available online: http://www.pharmacyquality.com/2019/05/29/pqs-trend-report-reveals-consumer-perceptions-towards-pharmacist-roles-and-how-pharmacies-and-payers-may-respond/ (accessed on 18 July 2019).
45. Centers for Disease Control and Prevention. National and State-Level Place of Flu Vaccination among Vaccinated Adults in the United States, 2014–2015 Flu Season. 2018. Available online: https://www.cdc.gov/flu/fluvaxview/place-vaccination-2014-15.htm (accessed on 28 May 2019).
46. Baroy, J.; Chung, D.; Frisch, R.; Apgar, D.; Slack, M.K. The impact of pharmacist immunization programs on adult immunization rates: A systematic review and meta-analysis. *J. Am. Pharm. Assoc. (2003)* **2016**, *56*, 418–426. [CrossRef]
47. Hepler, C.D. A dream deferred. *Am. J. Health Syst. Pharm.* **2010**, *67*, 1319–1325. [CrossRef]
48. Doucette, W.R.G.C.; Kreling, D.H.; Mott, D.A.; Schommer, J.C. *Final Report of the 2014 National Sample Survey of the Pharmacist Workforce to Determine Contemporary Demographic Practice Characteristics and Quality or Work-Life*; Midwest Pharmacy Workforce Research Consortium: Minneapolis, MN, USA, 8 April 2015.
49. 2010 Medicare Part D Medication Therapy Management (MTM) Programs [press release]. CMS Web Site, 8 June 2010. Available online: https://www.cms.gov/Medicare/Prescription-Drug-Coverage/PrescriptionDrugCovContra/downloads/MTMFactSheet_2010_06-2010_final.pdf (accessed on 28 May 2019).

50. Request for Comments: Enhancements to the Star Ratings for 2016 and Beyond [press release]. CMs Web Site: Centers for Medicare and Medicaid Services, 21 November 2014. Available online: https://www.cms.gov/Medicare/Prescription-Drug-Coverage/PrescriptionDrugCovGenIn/Downl oads/2016-Request-for-Comments-v-11_25_2014.pdf (accessed on 28 May 2019).

51. Medicare 2019 Star Rating Threshold Update. Available online: https://www.pharmacyquality.com/wp-con tent/uploads/2018/10/2019StarRatingThreshold4.pdf (accessed on 18 July 2019).

52. OutcomesMTM. *MTM Trends Report*; OutcomesMTM: West Des Moines, IA, USA, 2016.

53. OutcomesMTM. *2015 MTM Trends Report*; OutcomesMTM: West Des Moines, IA, USA, 2015.

54. American Society of Health-System Pharmacists. ASHP Applauds Reintroduction of Pharmacy and Medically Underserved Areas Enhancement Act [press release]. 2017. Available online: https://www.pharmacytimes.com/association-news/ashp-applauds-reintroduction-of-pharmacy-and-medically-underserved-areas-enhancement-act (accessed on 29 May 2019).

55. Yap, D. State provider status advances in 2017. *Pharm. Today* **2018**, *24*. Available online: https://www.pharma cytoday.org/article/S1042-0991(18)30262-7/fulltext (accessed on 18 July 2019). [CrossRef]

56. Sega, T. Medicare 2019 Star Ratings Update. Quality Forum Webinar, 2018. Available online: https: //vimeo.com/299946946 (accessed on 10 December 2018).

57. CPESN Web Site. 2019. Available online: https://www.cpesn.com/ (accessed on 29 May 2019).

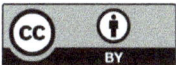

pharmacy

MDPI

Article

Gender and Age Variations in Pharmacists' Job Satisfaction in the United States

Manuel J. Carvajal [1,*], **Ioana Popovici** [1] **and Patrick C. Hardigan** [2]

[1] Department of Sociobehavioral and Administrative Pharmacy, College of Pharmacy, Nova Southeastern University, 3200 South University Drive, Fort Lauderdale, FL 33328-2018, USA; ip153@nova.edu

[2] College of Medicine, Nova Southeastern University, 3200 South University Drive, Fort Lauderdale, FL 33328-2018, USA; patrick@nova.edu

* Correspondence: cmanuel@nova.edu; Tel.: +1-954-262-1322; Fax: +1-954-262-2278

Received: 26 April 2019; Accepted: 13 May 2019; Published: 17 May 2019

check for updates

Abstract: While several studies have attested the presence of systematic gender and age variations in pharmacists' satisfaction with their jobs, only a few of them have considered both classifications simultaneously. None have done so while systematically examining multiple facets of practitioners' work. This article estimated U.S. pharmacists' satisfaction levels with various facets of their work, compared them simultaneously between genders and among age groups, and tested for the presence of gender–age interaction effects. The study was based on self-reported survey data collected from 701 pharmacists (31.0% response rate). Mean and standard deviation values for 18 indices related to pharmacists' work were calculated. When age groups were controlled, female pharmacists expressed overall higher levels of satisfaction with their job than male pharmacists; they also expressed greater satisfaction with multiple specific facets and with the profession, as well as greater workload and stress than male pharmacists. The findings revealed few significant differences among age groups and a limited gender–age interaction effect for pharmacists' satisfaction with key facets of their work. These findings should contribute to the development and refinement of rational criteria for increasing sources of satisfaction in pharmacy settings.

Keywords: age disparities; gender disparities; job satisfaction; job-related preferences; pharmacist workforce

---

1. Introduction

Organizational commitment issues (i.e., turnover, absenteeism, tardiness, theft, etc.) and quality of services rendered by pharmacists throughout the world have been linked to practitioners' levels of satisfaction and dissatisfaction with various facets of their work [1–15]. While intuitively most analysts would agree that it is in the best interests of employers to keep their pharmacist employees happy, satisfaction with one's work is an elusive concept pervaded by subjectivity and difficult to conceptualize and measure in an operational context. Not only is it interpreted differently by different persons that may experience a common set of conditions such as working in the same location or performing the same kind of work, but there are tradeoffs involved that often are perceived unequally. For example, the prospect of a higher paying job or a promotion may be a strong source of satisfaction for some practitioners, but the additional hours of work, stress, or possible relocation that the prospect entails may be even stronger sources of dissatisfaction for other practitioners. Further blurring the concept is a recent empirical finding of a weak association between pharmacists' overall job satisfaction responses and reported satisfaction with several facets that were hypothesized to configure job satisfaction [16].

2. Background

The existence of systematic gender and age variations in how the facets of pharmacists' jobs constitute sources of satisfaction or dissatisfaction, the tradeoffs among them, and their intensity is a commonly held platitude in the literature [17,18]. Work-related decisions usually are made within the context of household decision packages configured by the size and composition of the household, which are largely influenced by the gender-role ideology and age of the marital partners. Traditionally men and women experience socially defined, differentiated involvement with childcare and household responsibilities, with women picking up the brunt of the burden. Thus, compared to men, women are more likely to work part-time [19–22] and exhibit job-related preferences compatible with work-family balance such as hours of work, scheduling flexibility, and proximity of job site to home.

Work-related differences between men and women transcend family commitments and delve into intrinsic traits. Maier [23] argues that men primarily engage in competition to win and strive for success, subordinating other life activities to the pursuit of career goals, while women tend to search for equilibrium in life activities and are more interested than men in advancing others as well as themselves. He further argues that men use communication as a tool to solve problems, establish status, and convey independence while women use communication largely to establish connections. If these views are correct, one would expect male practitioners to be more motivated than their female counterparts by the adequacy of salaries and benefits, autonomy, and availability of advancement opportunities facets of their work, and female practitioners to be more motivated than their male peers by facets such as fairness in the workplace, job atmosphere, and relations with coworkers.

Age differences in pharmacists' satisfaction and dissatisfaction with various facets of their work also have been reported across the continents [1,4,5,10,11,15,24–31]. Invariably these studies have found that younger pharmacists are more dissatisfied with their job, or some part of it, than older pharmacists. Younger practitioners possess little workforce experience and may not be able to assess their working conditions accurately; the gap between expectations and reality may contribute to their dissatisfaction. As they grow older, their aspirations are reduced and they realize that they face limited choices in the workplace [32,33] and are likely to attach less importance to professional ambitions, acquiring more awareness of areas within the profession from which they derive greater levels of satisfaction.

Younger versus older worker comparisons have a deeper perspective that goes beyond mere age differences. This perspective focuses on the role that work plays in practitioners' lives. Baby boomers, who comprise the older segment of the pharmacist workforce, commonly are portrayed as a generation characterized by solid work ethics, with clearly defined professional goals, a drive for material success, and commitment to their employers. They frequently consider work as the most important part of their lives, and define themselves in terms of what they do. Conversely, pharmacists younger than baby boomers exhibit a preference for autonomy and flexible work schedules, express more interest in family and close friends than in material success, are motivated by the latest technologies, and view organizations with cynicism and contempt [34]. Younger pharmacists criticize baby boomers for being too competitive, overly cautious, and loyal to their organizations beyond reason, while baby boomers view younger pharmacists' emphasis on balancing work and leisure as lack of commitment and an erosion of work ethics. In short, their values and expectations are different, which probably translates into different sources of satisfaction and dissatisfaction with the various facets of their work.

Independently of their respective trends and influence on the configuration of job satisfaction patterns, gender and age may have some interaction effect. For example, younger women are prone to experience more work-family conflicts than other gender-age group combinations [35] for several reasons. Besides being in the family formation years, which makes them more susceptible to children's time intensive demands, their jobs are frequently viewed by themselves and others as a secondary income source, with needs and preferences of their own that may not coincide with the needs and preferences of older women or younger men. Their participation in the labor force tends to be countercyclical; when many men become unemployed or are forced to work fewer hours during a downturn of the business cycle, younger women tend to work more to compensate for the loss of household income [36,37]. Another asymmetry is found in the distribution of costs and benefits of family migration; younger women are less likely than their husbands to initiate moves, or resist moves initiated by their husbands, because their gains/losses from migration frequently are surpassed by their husbands' losses/gains [38].

At the other end of the spectrum, older workers continue to work more years than their predecessors partly because of their relatively better health and longevity. The trend away from defined benefit pension plans and toward defined contribution plans, plus the ability to receive full social security benefits beyond a certain age regardless of labor force participation, provide incentives to remain active in the workforce [39,40], oftentimes on a part-time basis [41]. Older male pharmacists experience issues that may be of little or no concern to younger male practitioners or older female practitioners, so their perceived sources of satisfaction or dissatisfaction at work may be different from those of other practitioners of the same gender and/or the same age group. Their motivating factors to seek part-time employment include, among others, avoiding depletion of savings, supplementing retirement benefits, fighting boredom, and validating their personal worth [42].

3. Objectives

Within the context of the background outlined in the previous section, this article sought to (1) estimate U.S. pharmacists' levels of satisfaction with various facets of their work, (2) compare simultaneously levels of satisfaction between genders and among age groups, and (3) test for the presence of a gender–age interaction effect. While many studies have addressed the influence of both gender and age on the configuration of pharmacists' job satisfaction patterns, only a few of them have taken into account both classifications at the same time and none has done so in examining systematically multiple facets of practitioners' work. It is important to analyze both classifications simultaneously in order to avoid attributing variation in satisfaction to one classification that should be attributed to the other classification or to the interaction of both. The study is important because a uniform set of job-related rewards and incentives (or disincentives) offered by employers to practitioners of both genders and all age groups may not be adequate if indeed significant differences are observed.

4. Methods

This study was based on self-reported survey data. Participants were asked to assess their satisfaction with key facets of their work as pharmacists using 0-to-10 intensity scales, with 10 denoting the greatest intensity. This procedure posed the advantage of response homogeneity, as practitioners were able to rate their experience with various facets of their work using a common measurement standard, with more room for discrimination in their responses than is normally provided by the traditional Likert scale. The rather narrow range of options ensured the adequacy of the mean as a measure of central tendency since there was no room for outliers. The indicator used here has been applied successfully in previous studies.

4.1. Indices

Eighteen assessment indices related to pharmacists' work were included in the analysis. Most of these had to do with important aspects of their job, but three were not job-related: assessment of satisfaction with the profession, own capability as a pharmacist, and own performance as a pharmacist. The other indices focused on adequacy of earnings and benefits, importance of earnings and benefits, amount of workload, stress, job security, availability of advancement opportunities, autonomy, scheduling flexibility, supervisor's support, relations with coworkers, fairness in the workplace, job atmosphere, importance of job to patients, importance of job to the organization, and job satisfaction in general.

Mean and standard deviation values for each index were calculated by gender and age group. The analysis was conducted for each gender-age group cell as well as for both genders within each age group and all age groups within each gender. The disaggregation by gender and age group took into consideration different values previously reported in the literature for male and female pharmacists [43,44] as well as for practitioners of different ages [34,45]. The disaggregation for both of these classifications is not commonly found for any other independent variable. As a general rule and consistently with earlier work [16], overall average index values under 3.00 were considered low, values ranging from 3.00 to 6.99 were considered moderate, and values 7.00 and above were considered high. The cutoff point for statistical significance was $p = 0.10$. In addition, mean and standard deviation values were calculated by gender and age group for the wages and salaries reported by the pharmacists in the sample to compare actual earnings with the adequacy perceived by respondents in the different categories.

4.2. Statistical Model

A two-way classification model with multiple replications was designed to probe the nature of differences in indices related to job satisfaction. One classification consisted of both genders ($i = 1, 2$). The other classification identified three age groups ($j = 1, ..., 3$): under 45 years old, 45–59 years old, and 60 years or older. Within each gender-age group cell, n_{ij} replications were observed. This design posed the advantage of allowing not only gender and age-group differences to be tested simultaneously and independently of each other, but also testing a gender–age group interaction effect. The model has been applied successfully in the analysis of variations in pharmacists' earnings and other variables [17].

The linear additive model for each index was as follows:

$$X_{ijk} = \mu + \gamma_i + \alpha_j + (\gamma\alpha)_{ij} + \varepsilon_{ijk} \qquad (1)$$

where

X_{ijk} was the index value reported by the *k*th pharmacist in the *j*th age group and the *i*th gender;
μ was the overall mean;
γ_i was the systematic effect of the *i*th gender;
α_j was the systematic effect of the *j*th age group;
$(\gamma\alpha)_{ij}$ was the gender-age group interaction effect;
ε_{ijk} was the stochastic disturbance (random error) term of the *k*th pharmacist in the *j*th age group and the *i*th gender;

and where

$i = 1$ for men and $i = 2$ for women;
$j = 1$ for pharmacists under 45 years of age, $j = 2$ for 45–59 year-old pharmacists, and $j = 3$ for pharmacists 60 years or older; and
n_{ij} was the number of pharmacists of the *i*th gender and the *j*th age group reporting their index value for each index assessing satisfaction with key facets of their work.

4.3. Data

The survey data were gathered from responses to a questionnaire sent by the authors to 2400 pharmacists practicing throughout the United States. These pharmacists were selected by Medical Marketing Services (MMS) using a simple random scheme. MMS is a leading provider of lists of pharmacists and other healthcare professionals. Its data depository includes pharmacists from all fields within the profession; approximately 90% of the estimated 281,560 U.S. registered pharmacists in 2012 [46] were included in the MMS data file.

The survey questionnaire, previously validated [16,17], was exclusively designed for this and other pharmacist workforce studies. It was mailed in March 2012 and a reminder was sent two weeks later. No major environmental or other factors affecting job satisfaction were anticipated since

2012. The sample size was chosen according to Cochran's formula developed for categorical and other outcomes [47], with a 5% sampling error. The research effort was supported solely by internal university funds, and institutional review board approval was secured to conduct the probe.

5. Results

Of the 2400 questionnaires mailed to potential participants, 139 packets were returned undelivered for various reasons. A total of 701 pharmacists participated in the study by providing answers to all relevant questions. The number of observations and the response rate (31.0%) compared favorably with those reported by similar undertakings [2,48–51]. Out of the total respondents, 403 pharmacists (57.5%) were men and 298 pharmacists (42.5%) were women; in terms of age, 27.0% were less than 45 years old, 45.6% were 45–59 years old, and 27.4% were 60 years or older. Reflecting the "womanization" of the profession and the demographics of the population from which they were drawn, male pharmacists were outnumbered by female pharmacists under 45 years of age, while the opposite occurred with older pharmacists.

5.1. Indices

The means and standard deviations of the 18 assessment indicators reported by pharmacists are presented in Table 1. All aggregate values, with the exception of perceived importance of job to patients, were in the moderate range; perceived importance of job to patients was slightly higher. Importance of job to patients, own capability as a pharmacist, and amount of workload were reported as the top three aggregate index values; availability of advancement opportunities, perceived support from one's supervisor, and scheduling flexibility were ranked, in that order, at the bottom of the scale.

Table 1. Means and standard deviations (in parentheses) of indices related to pharmacists' work by gender and age group.

Index and Statistical Significance	Age Group	Gender		
		Men ($i = 1$)	**Women ($i = 2$)**	**Both Genders**
Number of observations	Under 45 years old ($j = 1$)	71 (n_{11})	118 (n_{21})	189
	45–59 years old ($j = 2$)	173 (n_{12})	147 (n_{22})	320
	60 years or older ($j = 3$)	159 (n_{13})	33 (n_{21})	192
	All age groups	403	298	701
Adequacy of earnings and benefits Interaction effect ($p = 0.038$)	Under 45 years old ($j = 1$)	5.45 (3.12)	6.93 (2.60)	6.38 (2.88)
	45–59 years old ($j = 2$)	5.64 (3.00)	6.37 (2.70)	5.97 (2.88)
	60 years or older ($j = 3$)	7.27 (2.63)	6.29 (1.96)	7.08 (2.53)
	All age groups	6.21 (2.99)	6.58 (2.58)	6.37 (2.82)
Importance of earnings and benefits Between genders ($p = 0.038$)	Under 45 years old ($j = 1$)	6.03 (3.02)	7.11 (2.65)	6.70 (2.83)
	45–59 years old ($j = 2$)	5.73 (3.00)	7.17 (2.37)	6.37 (2.82)
	60 years or older ($j = 3$)	6.90 (2.83)	6.59 (2.37)	6.84 (2.74)
	All age groups	6.21 (2.99)	7.08 (2.47)	6.58 (2.80)
Amount of workload Between genders ($p = 0.015$)	Under 45 years old ($j = 1$)	6.01 (3.27)	7.03 (2.55)	6.65 (2.88)
	45–59 years old ($j = 2$)	6.83 (2.51)	7.39 (2.06)	7.09 (2.33)
	60 years or older ($j = 3$)	6.75 (2.37)	6.81 (2.25)	6.76 (2.34)
	All age groups	5.86 (3.30)	7.18 (2.29)	6.88 (2.50)
Stress Between genders ($p \leq 0.001$)	Under 45 years old ($j = 1$)	5.86 (3.30)	6.96 (2.56)	6.54 (2.90)
	45–59 years old ($j = 2$)	6.54 (2.74)	6.95 (2.50)	6.73 (2.64)
	60 years or older ($j = 3$)	5.78 (3.14)	6.81 (2.62)	5.95 (3.08)
	All age groups	6.12 (3.02)	6.94 (2.53)	6.47 (2.85)

Table 1. *Cont.*

Index and Statistical Significance	Age Group	Gender		
		Men ($i = 1$)	Women ($i = 2$)	Both Genders
Job security Between genders ($p = 0.043$)	Under 45 years old ($j = 1$)	5.54 (2.99)	6.84 (2.44)	6.34 (2.73)
	45–59 years old ($j = 2$)	5.70 (3.11)	6.13 (2.81)	5.90 (2.98)
	60 years or older ($j = 3$)	6.09 (3.30)	5.97 (2.86)	6.07 (3.22)
	All age groups	5.82 (3.16)	6.39 (2.69)	6.06 (2.98)
Availability of advancement opportunities	Under 45 years old ($j = 1$)	3.42 (2.68)	4.11 (3.15)	3.85 (2.99)
	45–59 years old ($j = 2$)	3.34 (2.86)	3.37 (3.03)	3.35 (2.93)
	60 years or older ($j = 3$)	3.10 (3.20)	3.61 (2.90)	3.19 (3.15)
	All age groups	3.26 (2.97)	3.69 (3.07)	3.44 (3.02)
Autonomy	Under 45 years old ($j = 1$)	5.55 (2.78)	6.27 (2.37)	5.99 (2.55)
	45–59 years old ($j = 2$)	5.80 (2.70)	6.14 (2.86)	5.96 (2.78)
	60 years or older ($j = 3$)	5.93 (2.96)	5.59 (2.01)	5.87 (2.82)
	All age groups	5.81 (2.82)	6.13 (2.60)	5.94 (2.73)
Scheduling flexibility Between genders ($p = 0.045$)	Under 45 years old ($j = 1$)	5.11 (3.02)	6.15 (3.15)	5.76 (3.14)
	45–59 years old ($j = 2$)	5.27 (3.22)	6.27 (3.09)	5.72 (3.20)
	60 years or older ($j = 3$)	5.88 (3.27)	5.55 (2.86)	5.82 (3.20)
	All age groups	5.48 (3.21)	6.14 (3.09)	5.76 (3.18)
Supervisor's support Between genders ($p = 0.005$)	Under 45 years old ($j = 1$)	5.07 (2.88)	6.00 (3.04)	5.65 (3.01)
	45–59 years old ($j = 2$)	5.00 (3.25)	5.92 (3.32)	5.42 (3.31)
	60 years or older ($j = 3$)	5.51 (3.62)	6.15 (2.68)	5.62 (3.48)
	All age groups	5.21 (3.34)	5.98 (3.13)	5.54 (3.27)
Relations with coworkers Between genders ($p = 0.009$)	Under 45 years old ($j = 1$)	6.01 (3.08)	7.27 (2.24)	6.79 (2.65)
	45–59 years old ($j = 2$)	6.25 (2.90)	6.86 (2.56)	6.53 (2.76)
	60 years or older ($j = 3$)	6.63 (2.92)	6.70 (2.67)	6.64 (2.87)
	All age groups	6.36 (2.94)	7.00 (2.45)	6.63 (2.76)
Fairness in the workplace	Under 45 years old ($j = 1$)	6.13 (2.73)	6.38 (2.51)	6.29 (2.59)
	45–59 years old ($j = 2$)	5.78 (2.88)	6.08 (2.88)	5.92 (2.88)
	60 years or older ($j = 3$)	6.18 (3.36)	5.94 (2.68)	6.14 (3.25)
	All age groups	6.00 (3.05)	6.19 (2.71)	6.08 (2.91)
Job atmosphere	Under 45 years old ($j = 1$)	5.92 (2.48)	6.53 (2.59)	6.30 (2.56)
	45–59 years old ($j = 2$)	5.70 (2.95)	6.39 (2.72)	6.02 (2.86)
	60 years or older ($j = 3$)	6.42 (3.07)	6.18 (2.40)	6.38 (2.96)
	All age groups	6.02 (2.93)	6.42 (2.63)	6.19 (2.81)
Importance of job to patients Between genders ($p = 0.001$) Among age groups ($p = 0.063$)	Under 45 years old ($j = 1$)	5.70 (3.71)	7.42 (2.64)	6.77 (3.18)
	45–59 years old ($j = 2$)	6.15 (3.49)	7.87 (2.54)	6.91 (3.21)
	60 years or older ($j = 3$)	7.62 (2.86)	7.94 (0.97)	7.68 (2.60)
	All age groups	6.62 (3.38)	7.70 (2.45)	7.08 (3.06)
Importance of job to the organization Between genders ($p = 0.016$) Interaction effect ($p = 0.002$)	Under 45 years old ($j = 1$)	5.15 (3.21)	7.64 (2.12)	6.70 (2.84)
	45–59 years old ($j = 2$)	5.99 (3.22)	7.18 (2.67)	6.51 (3.04)
	60 years or older ($j = 3$)	7.56 (2.81)	6.53 (2.72)	7.36 (2.80)
	All age groups	6.42 (3.19)	7.28 (2.48)	6.78 (2.94)
Overall job satisfaction Between genders ($p = 0.024$)	Under 45 years old ($j = 1$)	5.76 (2.91)	6.45 (2.48)	6.19 (2.66)
	45–59 years old ($j = 2$)	5.60 (3.19)	6.60 (2.72)	6.06 (3.02)
	60 years or older ($j = 3$)	6.14 (3.28)	6.24 (2.50)	6.16 (3.15)
	All age groups	5.84 (3.18)	6.50 (2.60)	6.12 (2.96)

Table 1. *Cont.*

Index and Statistical Significance	Age Group	Gender		
		Men ($i = 1$)	Women ($i = 2$)	Both Genders
Professional satisfaction Between genders ($p \leq 0.001$)	Under 45 years old ($j = 1$)	5.73 (2.69)	7.19 (1.96)	6.64 (2.37)
	45–59 years old ($j = 2$)	5.81 (3.00)	6.95 (2.76)	6.33 (2.94)
	60 years or older ($j = 3$)	6.28 (3.19)	6.67 (2.34)	6.35 (3.06)
	All age groups	5.98 (3.03)	7.01 (2.42)	6.42 (2.83)
Own capability as a pharmacist Between genders ($p = 0.093$)	Under 45 years old ($j = 1$)	6.18 (3.46)	7.31 (3.19)	6.89 (3.32)
	45–59 years old ($j = 2$)	6.22 (3.49)	7.72 (2.70)	6.88 (3.24)
	60 years or older ($j = 3$)	7.37 (2.96)	6.76 (2.80)	7.25 (2.93)
	All age groups	6.64 (3.33)	7.45 (2.91)	6.98 (3.18)
Own performance as a pharmacist Between genders ($p = 0.018$)	Under 45 years old ($j = 1$)	5.91 (3.80)	7.35 (2.96)	6.81 (3.36)
	45–59 years old ($j = 2$)	5.80 (3.75)	7.71 (3.01)	6.65 (3.56)
	60 years or older ($j = 3$)	7.23 (3.33)	6.94 (2.79)	7.17 (3.22)
	All age groups	6.35 (3.65)	7.48 (2.96)	6.83 (3.42)

The average index values of female pharmacists were consistently greater than the values reported by their male counterparts, and the differences were statistically significant except for adequacy of earnings and benefits, availability of advancement opportunities, autonomy, fairness in the workplace, and job atmosphere. Significant differences among age groups were detected only for the amount of workload and perceived job importance to patients, and the gender–age group interaction effect was significant only for perceived adequacy of earnings and benefits and perceived job importance to the organization.

5.2. *Wages and Salaries*

The empirical evidence showed significant differences in wages and salaries between genders (see Table 2). On average, male pharmacists in the sample earned 11.2% higher wages and salaries than their female counterparts for an estimated gap of 10.1%. This gender gap varied by age group: 10.8% for pharmacists under 45 years old, 19.0% for pharmacists 45–59 years old, and –2.0% for pharmacists 60 years or older; in other words, female older pharmacists earned, on average, 2.0% higher wages and salaries than their male peers. Yet the interaction effect was not statistically significant, nor were differences among age groups.

Table 2. Estimated means and standard deviations (in parentheses) of pharmacists' wages and salaries by gender and age group.

Age Group	Gender		
	Men	Women	Both Genders
Under 45 years old	121,463 (31,896)	108,395 (31,135)	113,388 (31,978)
45–59 years old	126,350 (108,660)	102,330 (33,390)	115,055 (83,087)
60 years or older	104,798 (67,700)	106,914 (20,238)	105,143 (62,432)
All age groups	116,951 (84,131)	105,177 (31,437)	111,923 (67,126)

Differences between genders are statistically significant ($p = 0.061$).

6. Discussion

Several findings are worth noting in this analysis of U.S. pharmacists' assessment of satisfaction with key facets of their work. The first is that when age groups were controlled, female pharmacists expressed overall higher levels of satisfaction with their job than male pharmacists; they also expressed greater satisfaction with multiple specific facets as well as with the profession. These findings accorded with those of other studies that did not account for variation in age [6,16,52,53]. Women's relatively greater overall job and professional satisfaction levels were observed in every age group, but the differences were wider for younger than older practitioners.

Women also reported consistently greater satisfaction than men in every age group when assessing the quality of their supervisor's support, relations with coworkers, and perceived importance of job to patients. These findings were in line with those of previous studies regarding women's perceived importance of supervision issues [54–56], interaction with fellow workers [57], and the nature of tasks performed [15,53]. In four other job facets in which gender differences were statistically significant—importance of earnings and benefits, job security, scheduling flexibility, and importance of job to the organization—female pharmacists' estimated response values were greater than the values of male pharmacists, but women 60 years or older actually registered lower values than the estimated values reported by men 60 years or older. Yet the gender–age group interaction effect was not statistically significant for any of the four indices.

Despite the relatively greater satisfaction experienced by female pharmacists regarding different facets of their work, they reported higher levels of workload and stress than male pharmacists, and the inequalities were observed at all ages. Usually an excessive workload constitutes a major source of dissatisfaction for pharmacists [1,2,6,10,14,15,51,58]. The incongruence was particularly confounding in light of the finding of a previous study whereby female practitioners actually worked fewer hours than male practitioners [16].

Another observed incongruence was the absence of a gender differential in perceived adequacy of salaries and benefits, especially when men in the sample earned 11.2% higher wages and salaries than women. This incongruence has been documented in the literature as the paradox of the contented female worker [54,59–61]. Several plausible explanations for this paradox have been postulated [18]. One is that women feel less pressure to exceed at work than men because of the traditional division of labor; men are primarily responsible for the household's financial well-being and women are primarily responsible for housework and childcare. Another plausible explanation may be that women have lower labor outcomes expectations than men, so their goals are more easily fulfilled. A third explanation suggests that additional earnings contribute more to the job satisfaction of men than to women's job satisfaction [62,63], which leads women to compensate for the foregone satisfaction of less pay with social aspects such as interaction with patients, good supervisors, congenial coworkers, and scheduling flexibility, all of which registered gender satisfaction differentials.

In any event, perceived adequacy of salaries and benefits exhibited a statistically significant gender–age group interaction effect: relatively more women than men under 60 years of age thought that their salaries and benefits were adequate, but the opposite was the case for practitioners 60 years or older. Although the interaction effect of reported wages and salaries lacked statistical significance, female practitioners under 60 years of age reported lower earnings than male pharmacists of the same age groups, and the opposite was true for practitioners 60 years or older. Thus, the evidence observed here points toward an even greater incongruence that may be more adequately termed "the paradox of the contented male and female pharmacists."

In general, pharmacists in the sample thought highly of their professional capability and performance. In both instances women reported higher scores than men, and the differences were significant. However, also in both instances, men 60 years or older reported higher satisfaction scores than women in the same age group. Perhaps further research may shed some light into why the satisfaction relationship between the genders is atypical for the 60 years or older group compared to younger practitioners.

Another important finding in this paper was the paucity of significant differences among age groups or an interaction effect when pharmacists assessed their satisfaction with key facets of their work. This paucity was contrary to commonly accepted platitudes found in the literature [18]. In the only two indices that were statistically significant for age-group differences, pharmacists 45–59 years old reported more dissatisfaction with their workload and gave higher ratings to the importance of their jobs to patients than did younger or older pharmacists. Notwithstanding the absence of statistically significant differences among age groups, a common pattern of women scoring higher values in the less than 60 years age group, but lower values among older pharmacists, in seven indices should not be ignored; it might not have occurred by chance alone.

7. Limitations

Job satisfaction is a subjective issue. Not only is it subject to different interpretations by different people, even when they share a common background and professional outlook, but its assessment by any one person may fluctuate over time, depending on the person's emotions and feelings. It is virtually impossible to fully standardize as a variable. This is the first constraint that limits the interpretation of the findings presented in this paper. A second limitation is that the study rested on a cross-sectional survey, so there was no measurement of whether or how practitioners' satisfaction with key facets of their work varied with time or was influenced by changing labor market conditions affecting the pharmacist workforce or the ongoing revamping of the healthcare system. Self-reported data were used, which opened the door to validity and reliability criticism even though the questionnaire was tested prior to being mailed to participants.

The study was limited to analyzing the influence of gender and age group on reported satisfaction. Other factors such as marital status, number of children, or the amount of outstanding student loans, not considered here, may affect pharmacists' satisfaction with key facets of their work independently of gender or age, may be gender or age selective, or may contribute to the interaction effect. This limitation may be addressed in a subsequent study.

Another limitation is that although the MMS data files utilized in configuring the sample were broad-based and included about 90% of pharmacists practicing in 2012, the sample might not have been representative of the other 10%. Furthermore, there was no way to ensure that the questionnaires were received or completed by the intended respondents, which was another limitation. In addition, some analysts might criticize the 31.0% response rate as relatively low. Information about earnings and satisfaction with different facets of one's work is considered by some people as of an intimate nature, so some practitioners might have been reluctant to share it. No incentives such as monetary remuneration or a chance to win a raffle prize were used to motivate participation, which might have altered the number of respondents. In any event, the sample consisted of 701 observations, a sizable data set whose volume compensated for a modest response rate.

8. Conclusions

Despite its limitations, this study was successful in estimating U.S. pharmacists' levels of satisfaction with various facets of their work, comparing simultaneously their levels of satisfaction between genders and among age groups, and testing for the presence of a gender–age interaction effect. It identified the facets in which practitioners scored highest and lowest satisfaction levels, and found that when age was controlled, female pharmacists were consistently more satisfied with most facets of their work than male pharmacists. Since men and women responded differently to multiple facets, a uniform set of job-related rewards and incentives (or disincentives) offered by employers to practitioners of both genders may not be adequate.

The seemingly atypical behavior exhibited by pharmacists 60 years or older (compared to younger pharmacists), whereby men's levels of satisfaction with several facets of their work were greater than those of their female counterparts, should be analyzed more thoroughly. A potentially significant trend along these lines, discovered in future research, might signal a need for further adjustment by employers in their efforts to keep their pharmacist employees happy and manage a diverse workforce more effectively. Perhaps the age-group boundaries in this study were not specified properly, and practitioners with heterogeneous needs and preferences were placed together, thereby weakening the statistical outcomes of the age-group classification and the gender-age interaction effect. The specification of different age groups might yield different results.

Finally, it is important to observe that while pharmacists' satisfaction with their work remains an elusive concept plagued with subjectivity, this study was successful in conceptualizing and applying a methodological framework that produced concrete results. The empirical evidence obtained here, and the conclusions derived from it, should be regarded as preliminary in nature, but, hopefully, they will contribute to the development and refinement of rational criteria for increasing sources of satisfaction in pharmacy settings.

Author Contributions: M.J.C., I.P., and P.C.H. contributed equally to the conceptualization, data collection, analysis, results interpretation, and writing of the manuscript.

Funding: This research received no external funding.

Conflicts of Interest: The authors declare no conflict of interest.

References

1. Ahmad, A.; Khan, M.U.; Elkalmi, R.M.; Jamshed, S.Q.; Nagappa, A.N.; Patel, I.; Balkrishnan, R. Job satisfaction among Indian pharmacists: An exploration of affecting variables and suggestions for improvement in pharmacist role. *Indian J. Pharm. Educ. Res.* **2016**, *50*, 9–16. [CrossRef]
2. Al Khalidi, D.; Wazaify, M. Assessment of pharmacists' job satisfaction and job related stress in Amman. *Int. J. Clin. Pharm.* **2013**, *35*, 821–828. [CrossRef] [PubMed]
3. Awalom, M.T.; Tesfa, A.F.; Kidane, M.E.; Ghebremedhin, M.R.; Teklesenbet, A.H. Eritrean pharmacists' job satisfaction and their attitude to re-professionalize pharmacy in to pharmaceutical care. *Int. J. Clin. Pharm.* **2015**, *37*, 335–341. [CrossRef] [PubMed]
4. Belay, Y.B. Job satisfaction among community pharmacy professionals in Mekelle city, Northern Ethiopia. *Adv. Med. Educ. Pract.* **2016**, *7*, 527–531. [CrossRef] [PubMed]
5. Calgan, Z.; Aslan, D.; Yegenoglu, S. Community pharmacists' burnout levels and related factors: An example from Turkey. *Int. J. Clin. Pharm.* **2011**, *33*, 92–100. [CrossRef] [PubMed]
6. Chua, G.N.; Yee, L.J.; Sim, B.A.; Tan, K.H.; Sin, N.K.; Hassali, M.A.; Shafie, A.A.; Ooi, G.S. Job satisfaction, organisation commitment and retention in the public workforce: A survey among pharmacists in Malaysia. *Int. J. Pharm. Pract.* **2014**, *22*, 265–274. [CrossRef]
7. Eslami, A.; Kouti, L.; Javadi, M.-R.; Assarian, M.; Eslami, K. An investigation of job stress and job burnout in Iranian clinical pharmacist. *J. Pharm. Care* **2016**, *3*, 21–25.
8. Ferguson, J.; Ashcroft, D.; Hassell, K. Qualitative insights into job satisfaction and dissatisfaction with management among community and hospital pharmacists. *Res. Soc. Adm. Pharm.* **2011**, *7*, 306–316. [CrossRef]
9. Fernandes, L.G.; Rodrigues, V.F.; Ribeiro, M.I.; Pinto, I.C. Work satisfaction within community pharmacy professionals. *Adv. Pharmacol. Pharm.* **2014**, *2*, 6–12.
10. Gaither, C.A.; Nadkarni, A.; Mott, D.A.; Schommer, J.C.; Doucette, W.R.; Kreling, D.H.; Pedersen, C.A. Should I stay or should I go? The influence of individual and organizational factors on pharmacists' future work plans. *J. Am. Pharm. Assoc.* **2007**, *47*, 165–173. [CrossRef]
11. Manan, M.M.; Azmi, Y.; Lim, Z.; Neoh, C.F.; Khan, T.M.; Ming, L.C. Predictors of job satisfaction amongst pharmacists in Malaysian public hospitals and healthcare clinics. *J. Pharm. Res.* **2015**, *45*, 404–411. [CrossRef]
12. Suleiman, A.K. Stress and job satisfaction among pharmacists in Riyadh, Saudi Arabia. *Saudi J. Med. Med. Sci.* **2015**, *3*, 213–219. [CrossRef]
13. Urbonas, G.; Kubilienė, L.; Kubilius, R.; Urbonienė, A. Assessing the effects of pharmacists' perceived organizational support, organizational commitment and turnover intention on provision of medication information at community pharmacies in Lithuania: A structural equation modeling approach. *BMC Health Serv. Res.* **2015**, *15*, 82. [CrossRef] [PubMed]

14. Willis, S.; Elvey, R.; Hassell, K. *What Is the Evidence That Workload Is Affecting Hospital Pharmacists' Performance and Patient Safety?* Centre for Workforce Intelligence: Manchester, UK, 2011.

15. Liu, C.S.; White, L. Key determinants of hospital pharmacy staff's job satisfaction. *Res. Soc. Adm. Pharm.* **2011**, *7*, 51–63. [CrossRef]

16. Carvajal, M.J.; Popovici, I.; Hardigan, P.C. Gender differences in the measurement of pharmacists' job satisfaction. *Hum. Resour. Health* **2018**, *16*, 33. [CrossRef]

17. Carvajal, M.J.; Popovici, I. Interaction of gender and age in pharmacists' labour outcomes. *J. Pharm. Health Serv. Res.* **2016**, *7*, 23–29. [CrossRef]

18. Carvajal, M.J.; Popovici, I. Gender, age, and pharmacists' job satisfaction. *Pharm. Pract.* **2018**, *16*, 1396. [CrossRef]

19. Cunningham, M. Influences of gender ideology and housework allocation on women's employment over the life course. *Soc. Sci. Res.* **2008**, *37*, 254–267. [CrossRef]

20. Fogli, A.; Veldkamp, L. *Nature Or Nurture? Learning and Female Labour Force Dynamics*; Centre for Economic Policy Research: London, UK, 2007.

21. Poeschl, G.; Pinto, I.; Múrias, C.; Silva, A.; Ribeiro, R. Representations of family practices, belief in sex differences, and sexism. *Sex Roles* **2006**, *55*, 111–121. [CrossRef]

22. Quesenberry, J.L.; Trauth, E.M.; Morgan, A.J. Understanding the "mommy tracks": A framework for analyzing work-family balance in the IT workforce. *Inf. Resour. Manag. J.* **2006**, *19*, 37–53. [CrossRef]

23. Maier, M. On the gendered substructure of organization: Dimensions and dilemmas of corporate masculinity. In *Handbook of Gender and Work*; Sage Publications Inc.: Thousand Oaks, CA, USA, 1999; pp. 69–94.

24. Cavaco, A.M.; Krookas, A.A. Community pharmacies automation: Any impact on counselling duration and job satisfaction? *Int. J. Clin. Pharm.* **2014**, *36*, 325–335. [CrossRef]

25. Foroughi Moghadam, M.J.; Peiravian, F.; Naderi, A.; Rajabzadeh, A.; Rasekh, H.R. An analysis of job satisfaction among Iranian pharmacists through various job characteristics. *Iran. J. Pharm. Res.* **2014**, *13*, 1087–1096.

26. Jacobs, S.; Hassell, K.; Ashcroft, D.; Johnson, S.; O'Connor, E. Workplace stress in community pharmacies in England: Associations with individual, organizational and job characteristics. *J. Health Serv. Res. Policy* **2014**, *19*, 27–33. [CrossRef]

27. Katoue, M.G.; Awad, A.I.; Schwinghammer, T.L.; Kombian, S.B. Pharmaceutical care in Kuwait: Hospital pharmacists' perspectives. *Int. J. Clin. Pharm.* **2014**, *36*, 1170–1178. [CrossRef]

28. Lau, W.M.; Pang, J.; Chui, W. Job satisfaction and the association with involvement in clinical activities among hospital pharmacists in Hong Kong. *Int. J. Pharm. Pract.* **2011**, *19*, 253–263. [CrossRef]

29. Majd, M.; Hashemian, F.; Sisi, F.Y.; Jalal, M.; Majd, Z. Quality of life and job satisfaction of dispensing pharmacists practicing in Tehran private-sector pharmacies. *Iran. J. Pharm. Res.* **2012**, *11*, 1039–1044.

30. Seston, E.; Hassell, K. British pharmacists' work-life balance–Is it a problem? *Int. J. Pharm. Pract.* **2014**, *22*, 135–145. [CrossRef]

31. Mak, V.S.; Clark, A.; March, G.; Gilbert, A.L. The Australian pharmacist workforce: Employment status, practice profile and job satisfaction. *Aust. Health Rev.* **2013**, *37*, 127–130. [CrossRef]

32. Schroder, R. Job satisfaction of employees at a Christian university. *J. Res. Christ. Educ.* **2008**, *17*, 225–246. [CrossRef]

33. Smerek, R.E.; Peterson, M. Examining Herzberg's theory: Improving job satisfaction among non-academic employees at a university. *Res. High Educ.* **2007**, *48*, 229–250. [CrossRef]

34. Carvajal, M.J.; Armayor, G.M. The generational effect on pharmacists' labour supply. *J. Pharm. Health Serv. Res.* **2015**, *6*, 11–18. [CrossRef]

35. Mott, D.A.; Doucette, W.R.; Gaither, C.A.; Pedersen, C.A.; Schommer, J.C. Pharmacists' attitudes toward worklife: Results from a national survey of pharmacists. *J. Am. Pharm. Assoc.* **2004**, *44*, 326–336. [CrossRef]

36. DiCecio, R.; Engemann, K.M.; Owyang, M.T.; Wheeler, C.H. Changing trends in the labor force: A survey. *Rev.-Fed. Reserve Bank St. Louis* **2008**, *90*, 47–62. [CrossRef]

37. Mosisa, A.; Hipple, S. Trends in labor force participation in the United States. *Mon. Labour Rev.* **2006**, *129*, 35–57.

38. Shauman, K.A.; Noonan, M.C. Family migration and labor force outcomes: Sex differences in occupational context. *Soc. Forces* **2007**, *85*, 1735–1764. [CrossRef]

39. Rix, S.E. Aging of the American Workforce, the. *Chic.-Kent Law Rev.* **2006**, *81*, 593–617.

40. Toossi, M. Labor force projections to 2016: More workers in their golden years. *Mon. Labor Rev.* **2010**, *130*, 33–52.
41. Knapp, K.K.; Cultice, J.M. New pharmacist supply projections: Lower separation rates and increased graduates boost supply estimates. *J. Am. Pharm. Assoc.* **2007**, *47*, 463–470. [CrossRef]
42. Teeter, D.S. Part-time pharmacists: A growing phenomenon. *US Pharm.* **2004**, *29*, 77–83.
43. Carvajal, M.J.; Armayor, G.M.; Deziel, L. The gender earnings gap among pharmacists. *Res. Soc. Adm. Pharm.* **2012**, *8*, 285–297. [CrossRef]
44. Carvajal, M.J.; Deziel, L.; Armayor, G.M. Labor supply functions of working male and female pharmacists: In search of the backward bend. *Res. Soc. Adm. Pharm.* **2012**, *8*, 552–566. [CrossRef]
45. Carvajal, M.J.; Armayor, G.M. The life-cycle argument: Age as a mediator of pharmacists' earnings. *Res. Soc. Adm. Pharm.* **2015**, *11*, 129–133. [CrossRef]
46. Bureau of Labor Statistics. Occupational Employment and Wages: Pharmacists 2014: 29–1051. Available online: http://www.bls.gov/oes/2012/may/oes291051.htm (accessed on 18 October 2018).
47. Cochran, W.G. *Sampling Techniques*, 2nd ed.; John Wiley & Sons: Hobiken, NJ, USA, 1963.
48. Lin, B.Y.-J.; Yeh, Y.-C.; Lin, W.-H. The influence of job characteristics on job outcomes of pharmacists in hospital, clinic, and community pharmacies. *J. Med. Syst.* **2007**, *31*, 224–229.
49. Polgreen, L.A.; Mott, D.A.; Doucette, W.R. An examination of pharmacists' labor supply and wages. *Res. Soc. Adm. Pharm.* **2011**, *7*, 406–414. [CrossRef]
50. Quiñones, A.C.; Pullin, R.F. Reexamining shift work pharmacists in Illinois. *Res. Soc. Adm. Pharm.* **2011**, *7*, 444–450. [CrossRef]
51. Murphy, S.M.; Friesner, D.L.; Scott, D.M. Do in-kind benefits influence pharmacists' labor supply decisions? *J. Reg. Anal. Policy* **2011**, *41*, 33–52.
52. Hassell, K.; Seston, E.; Shann, P. Measuring job satisfaction of UK pharmacists: A pilot study. *Int. J. Pharm. Pract.* **2007**, *15*, 259–264. [CrossRef]
53. Seston, E.; Hassell, K.; Ferguson, J.; Hann, M. Exploring the relationship between pharmacists' job satisfaction, intention to quit the profession, and actual quitting. *Res. Soc. Adm. Pharm.* **2009**, *5*, 121–132. [CrossRef]
54. Bilimoria, D.; Perry, S.R.; Liang, X.; Stoller, E.P.; Higgins, P.; Taylor, C. How do female and male faculty members construct job satisfaction? The roles of perceived institutional leadership and mentoring and their mediating processes. *J. Technol. Transf.* **2006**, *31*, 355–365. [CrossRef]
55. Carvajal, M.J.; Hardigan, P.C. Pharmacists' sources of job satisfaction: Inter-gender differences in response. *Am. J. Pharm. Educ.* **2000**, *64*, 420–425.
56. Kim, S. Gender differences in the job satisfaction of public employees: A study of Seoul Metropolitan Government, Korea. *Sex Roles* **2005**, *52*, 667–681. [CrossRef]
57. Hawthorne, N.; Anderson, C. The global pharmacy workforce: A systematic review of the literature. *Hum. Resour. Health* **2009**, *7*, 48. [CrossRef] [PubMed]
58. Rothmann, S.; Malan, M. Work-related well-being of South African hospital pharmacists. *S. Afr. J. Ind. Psychol.* **2011**, *37*, 1–11. [CrossRef]
59. Bender, K.A.; Heywood, J.S. Job satisfaction of the highly educated: The role of gender, academic tenure, and earnings. *Scot. J. Polit. Econ.* **2006**, *53*, 253–279. [CrossRef]
60. Kaiser, L.C. Gender-job satisfaction differences across Europe: An indicator for labour market modernization. *Int. J. Manpow.* **2007**, *28*, 75–94. [CrossRef]
61. Long, A. Happily ever after? A study of job satisfaction in Australia. *Econ. Rec.* **2005**, *81*, 303–321. [CrossRef]
62. Donohue, S.M.; Heywood, J.S. Job satisfaction and gender: An expanded specification from the NLSY. *Int. J. Manpow.* **2004**, *25*, 211–238. [CrossRef]
63. Sloane, P.J.; Williams, H. Job satisfaction, comparison earnings, and gender. *Labour* **2000**, *14*, 473–502. [CrossRef]

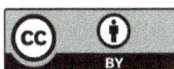

pharmacy

MDPI

Opinion

Alignment of Community Pharmacy Foundation Grant Funding and the Evolution of Pharmacy Practice in the United States of America

Brittany Hoffmann-Eubanks [1,*]**, Anne Marie Kondic** [2] **and Brian J. Isetts** [3]

1   Banner Medical LLC, Frankfort, IL 60423, USA
2   Community Pharmacy Foundation, Chicago, IL 60680, USA;
    amkondic@CommunityPharmacyFoundation.org
3   College of Pharmacy, University of Minnesota, 308 Harvard St., SE, Room WDH 7-125-c,
    Minneapolis, MN 55455, USA; isett001@umn.edu
*   Correspondence: bheubanks@bannermedicalwriting.com

Received: 1 May 2019; Accepted: 5 June 2019; Published: 14 June 2019

check for
updates

Abstract: The Community Pharmacy Foundation is a non-profit organization dedicated to the advancement of community pharmacy practice and patient care delivery through grant funding and resource sharing. Since 2002, CPF has awarded 191 grants and over $9,200,000 (US dollars) in research and project grants. The purpose of this manuscript is to highlight the evolution of pharmacy practice and pharmacy education in the United States through the presentation of exemplary cases of Community Pharmacy Foundation funding that is aligned with new care delivery models and approaches to the advancement of patient-centered pharmacy care. Pharmacy began in colonial America as the United States of America was just beginning to form with apothecary shops and druggists. Over time, the pharmacy industry would be revolutionized as America became urbanized, and drug products became commercially produced. The role of the pharmacist and their education evolved as direct patient care became a clear expectation of the general public. By the 1990s, the pharmacy profession had carved out a new path that focused on pharmacist-led, patient-centered pharmaceutical care and medication therapy management services. The Community Pharmacy Foundation grant funding has aligned with this evolution since its founding in 2000, and multiple exemplary grants are presented as support. As the role of pharmacists again transitions from a fee-for-service model to a value-based model, the Community Pharmacy Foundation continues to provide grant funding for research and projects that support the advancement of community pharmacy practice, education, and expanded training of pharmacists.

Keywords: community pharmacy; pharmaceutical care; medication therapy management; pharmacy practice; pharmacy education; grants

1. Introduction

The Community Pharmacy Foundation (CPF) is a non-profit organization founded in 2000 that is dedicated to the advancement of community pharmacy practice and patient care delivery through grant funding and resource sharing [1]. CPF was originally founded as part of a federal settlement on behalf of community pharmacies in the United States (US) from class action litigation against discriminatory drug pricing. As a result, CPF was originally governed by a court-appointed Board of Directors (BOD) that consisted of four community pharmacists and a retired judge of the United States District Court in Illinois. As part of the settlement, $18.6 million (US dollars) were awarded to establish the CPF to advance the profession of community pharmacy. In the first two years after

CPF was founded, the BOD established a formal process for the receipt, review, evaluation, awarding, and monitoring of grant dollars based upon submission of grant application requests [1].

The primary goals of CPF grant funding are:

1. The development, processing, and use of findings that affirm the value of community pharmacy practice in the healthcare delivery system.
2. The measurement, publication, and dissemination of findings documenting the value of professional services delivered to patients by community pharmacists.
3. Efforts that measure the impact of pharmacist interventions in achieving the targeted therapeutic goals set collaboratively by the patient, the pharmacist, and other members of the healthcare team.
4. Efforts that evaluate patient-specific outcomes with regard to the quality of care delivered by community pharmacists.

In January of 2002, CPF received its first grant submissions, and awarded its first two grants in May, 2002. Since 2002, CPF has awarded 191 grants and over $9,200,000 (US dollars) in research and project grants for the advancement of community pharmacy practice and patient care delivery improvement. The extent to which CPF grants have aligned with the primary goals of CPF has been reviewed in detail elsewhere [2,3]. In general, CPF grants in the early years (2002–2008) primarily focused on adding to the knowledge base of medical conditions and medications only, but have since (2009–2019) moved toward studies that affect health outcomes and change pharmacy practices [2]. This evolution of grant funding is in line with changes in the scope of practice of American pharmacy and pharmacists since its founding.

The purpose of this manuscript is to highlight the evolution of pharmacy practice and pharmacy education in the United States through the presentation of exemplary cases of the Community Pharmacy Foundation funding that is aligned with new care delivery models and approaches to the advancement of patient-centered pharmacy care.

2. Colonial America: The Roots of Pharmacy Practice in the United States

In Colonial America, there were very few standalone pharmacies. The first documented "pharmacist" was Bartholomew Browne of Salem in 1698 [4,5]. He operated a daily pharmacy and traded produce and merchandise in exchange for services. Still, Mr. Browne's pharmacy was not the norm, as most physicians had their own apothecary shops and only utilized the druggist to purchase the raw materials required for compounding medicines [4,5]. Similarly, the majority of drugs utilized for compounding were imported from England. It was not until the Revolutionary war that apothecaries became more common, due to a need for domestic sources of medicine [6]. The products that apothecaries stocked also became more standardized, and typically included drugs, medicines, surgical supplies, dyestuffs, essences, and chemicals [4].

Combined physician medical practice and apothecary shops had been widely debated in England and were considered a conflict of interest [5]. However, the idea of separating physician and apothecary practices in colonial American was not introduced until the late 18th century by John Morgan [5]. He proposed the idea after traveling to Europe where drug distribution and physician practices had been separated to avoid conflicts of interest [5]. This concept was not popular and was widely rejected, since drug distribution was a large part of physicians' livelihoods, and patients did not want the extra expense of seeing two practitioners [5]. It was not until the 19th century (after the war of 1812) that the preparation of medicine became the pharmacist's responsibility and physician drug shops were phased out; however, very few physicians actually gave up their dispensing practice [5].

Pharmacy education was also evolving as American apothecary shops began to pop up across the country. For example, the first diploma for apothecary practices was awarded in 1808 by the Legislature of the territory of Orleans, and in 1818, South Carolina was the first state to require a pharmaceutical examination before obtaining a pharmaceutical license [4]. In December of 1820, the first official print of the Pharmacopoeia of the United States of America was published in English and Latin [4].

Also, state-affiliated pharmacy schools were created, with the Philadelphia College of Pharmacy (1821) and the Massachusetts College of Pharmacy (1823) being the first two in America [6]. Furthermore, these state-affiliated colleges had legislative curriculum requirements to ensure quality [6].

In the 1840s, inferior drug products were being shipped from Europe that led to the Drug Importation Act of 1848 [6]. This act led to drug examiners being stationed at points of entry to verify the quality, purity, and fitness of drug products being imported to America. Due to political cronyism, incompetent drug inspectors led to the failure of the Drug Importation Act and calls for a national pharmacy organization began to grow [6]. As a result, a group of 21 pharmacists and non-credentialed apothecaries met to form the American Pharmaceutical Association now called the American Pharmacists Association (APhA) on 6 October 1852 [7]. By the 1880s, the practice of pharmacy was recognized as an important public service, serving as the foundation for modern pharmacy practice in the United States.

3. CPF Grant Funding Aligns with the Evolution of Pharmacy Practice in the United States

By the end of the 19th century, the practice of pharmacy was significantly changing. Parke, Davis, & Company created the first standardized pharmaceutical extract (Liquor Erogtae Purificatus) in 1879 that revolutionized the business of pharmacy [8]. Instead of pharmacists compounding medications, a growing list of chemical companies began quickly expanding their research and development programs to develop and commercialize standardized drug products and delivery systems. For example, gelatin capsules became commercially available in 1875 followed by tablets and enteric coated tablets in 1884 [8]. Therefore, the role of the pharmacist shifted from primarily being a medication preparer to dispenser of commercially prepared medication. The 20th century would again bring further changes as a result of several factors, including increased urbanization in America, expansion of the manufacturing of drug products, and the emergence of new pharmacy business models (Figure 1).

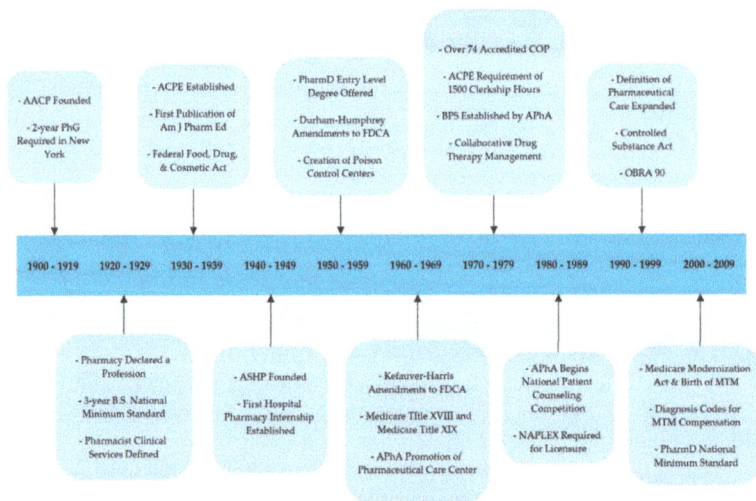

Figure 1. The Evolution of Modern Pharmacy Practice in the United States [4]. AACP: American Association of Colleges of Pharmacy; PhG: Pharmacy Graduate; B.S.: Bachelor of Science; COP: Colleges of Pharmacy; ACPE: American College of Pharmacy Education; Am J Pharm Ed: American Journal of Pharmacy Education; ASHP: American Society of Health System Pharmacists; PharmD: Doctor of Pharmacy; FDCA: Federal Food, Drug & Cosmetic Act; APhA: American Pharmacists Association; BPS: Board of Pharmacy Specialties; NAPLEX: National Association of Pharmacy Licensure Exam; OBRA: Omnibus Budget Reconciliation Act; MTM: Medicare Therapy Management.

As these changes were occurring, so too was the education of pharmacists within the United States. In the 1950s, the entry-level degree for pharmacists transitioned to a professional degree, which has been the standard since 2000 [4]. Furthermore, as the scope of practice for pharmacists began to evolve, so did the training required to meet those demands when pharmacists graduated and entered into practice. As such, the development of post-graduate hospital training programs was created in the early 1960s by the American Society of Health System Pharmacists (ASHP) [9]. Then in 1973, APhA established the Board of Pharmacy Specialties (BPS) which helped pave the way for post-graduate residency training in specialized practice areas [9]. For the next 20 years, hospital-based residencies with specific accreditation standards were implemented in health systems across the United States. By the 1980s calls began to grow for the creation of community pharmacy residency programs to improve clinical skills and prepare pharmacists for pharmacy ownership. In 1986, APhA created the pharmacy residency program initiative starting the process for developing community pharmacy post-graduate training programs [10]. By 1988, 200 ASHP residency programs had been accredited with 124 being in hospital pharmacy, 39 in clinical pharmacy, and 37 in specialty areas such as psychiatry and hospital administration. Furthermore, over 5800 residents had successfully graduated from an accredited ASHP residency program [9].

3.1. The Pharmaceutical Care Era

The term "pharmaceutical care" was first used in 1975, referring to the care a given patient requires and receives which assures safe and rational drug use [11,12]. The term manifested in response to renewed interest in shifting back to care for patients as opposed to the drug product, and coincided with the establishment of the clinical pharmacy era which recognized the value of pharmacists for their expert drug therapy knowledge [11]. The path of clinical pharmacy would be further developed in 1990 after a landmark article by Hepler and Strand was published outlining the patient care responsibilities of pharmacists that went beyond the traditional role of dispensing [13]. As a result, a new professional practice emerged that required a definition to aid in moving the idea from theory into application [11]. Thus, a pharmaceutical care practice is one in which the practitioner takes responsibility for all of a patient's drug-related needs and is also accountable for this commitment [11,13]. However, at the time, there was not an overall consensus for the best way to accomplish this expanded role of the pharmacist.

Therefore, initial demonstration projects and pilot programs were conducted to help add to the knowledge base of pharmacists as healthcare providers. For example, CPF awarded its very first grant in May of 2002 for a program that sought to evaluate the effectiveness of a community pharmacist-based home blood pressure monitoring program [14]. The study included 125 patients from 12 different community pharmacies. Patients were randomized to receive a high-intensity or low-intensity blood pressure intervention to determine differences in systolic and diastolic blood pressure from baseline to follow-up between the high-intensity and low-intensity patients. The results showed the high-intensity intervention achieved a lower diastolic blood pressure ($p = 0.03$) and could serve as a strategy for future patients with hypertension [14].

Another early study funded by CPF in 2002 examined pharmacy participation in the Wisconsin Medicaid Pharmaceutical Care Program (WMPCP) [15]. Pharmacies who participated in this program were provided an enhanced dispensing fee for pharmaceutical care actions. This study retrospectively reviewed administrative claims paid between 1997–2003 to investigate characteristics of claims submitted to WMPCP and claims paid for pharmaceutical care services. There were 359 pharmacies who participated in WMPCP for seven years. The claims per pharmacy ranged from 9.41–64.37, with an increasing volume trend observed at the end of the study period. The results showed that patient behavior, pharmacists resolving problems with patients, and patient response were the most common claims. Furthermore, some of the pharmacies had incorporated the program into their practice routinely. Also, pharmacists focused on drug therapy problems related to patient behavior, and worked directly with the patient to resolve these problems through education [15].

As more evidence became available about the value of pharmacists in helping improve patient outcomes expanded care delivery models began to be created. For example, CPF funded a study grant that was completed in 2006 and evaluated the effects of an extended diabetes care program compared to regular care on primary clinical outcomes such as hemoglobin A1c, low-density lipoprotein (LDL) cholesterol, and blood pressure [16]. The extended care diabetes program was provided by trained community pharmacists over 12-months with quarterly visits. The extended care program consisted of drug-therapy evaluation, patient education, and drug-therapy recommendations to the patient's physician as needed. Twelve pharmacists and eight community pharmacies participated in the program. A total of 67 subjects completed the study. The results showed pharmacist intervention helped to decrease LDL cholesterol levels significantly and resulted in a significant improvement in aggregate patient self-management of diabetes. There was no significant impact observed for blood glucose control or blood pressure levels. However, the overall program results were positive and helped to decrease the cardiovascular risks of the enrolled patients [16]. Additional CPF grants were awarded during the pharmaceutical care era that focused on pharmacy operations and furthering our understanding of the pharmacists' impact on disease state management [17–21].

At the same time, pharmacy education was also evolving to keep up with the changes in pharmacy practice. In 1997, APhA updated their post-graduate year-one (PGY1) community pharmacy residency program guidelines to reflect the new focus on pharmaceutical patient care [10]. These revised guidelines were then used to develop the first APhA-ASHP community pharmacy residency accreditation standards that were adopted in 1999. The adoption of the accreditation standards was an important step in the evolution of community pharmacy and for the development of community pharmacy residency programs. Further, accreditation standards increased program development, increased the perceived value of community pharmacy residencies, and allowed eligible student pharmacists to participate in the Residency Match Program [10].

3.2. Relationship of Medication Therapy Management to the Practice of Pharmaceutical Care

Medication therapy management (MTM) was the next development in the evolution of pharmacy practice. Origins of the term Medication Therapy Management can be traced to legislation proposed in the mid-1990s intended to reimburse pharmacists for pharmaceutical care services [22]. Then in 2002, the Medicare Payment Advisory Commission (MedPAC) prepared a report for Congress on Medicare payment for nonphysician providers describing medication management as an evolving approach in which drug therapy decisions are coordinated collaboratively by physicians, pharmacists, and other care providers together with the patient [23]. Shortly after this MedPAC Report was published, there were several noteworthy events that clarified MTM as a service provided within the practice of pharmaceutical care. A coalition of national pharmacy organizations collaborated with the American Medical Association's Current Procedural Terminology (CPT®) Editorial Panel in preparation of a proposal establishing reporting and billing codes for pharmacists' clinical services. In official health reporting nomenclature of CPT®, Medication Therapy Management Services (MTMS) is described as face-to-face assessment and intervention as appropriate, by a pharmacist, to optimize the response to medications or to manage treatment-related medication interactions or complications [24]. Furthermore, the comprehensiveness of MTMS in official health reporting nomenclature was further clarified as an assessment to identify, resolve and prevent drug therapy problems, formulating a medication treatment plan to achieve patients' goals of therapy, and follow-up monitoring and evaluation of patient outcomes [24,25]. CPF also supported a grant to develop educational tools to advance MTMS [26].

MTM service has also been characterized by the Centers for Disease Control and Prevention (CDC) as "a distinct service or group of services provided by healthcare providers, including pharmacists, to ensure the best therapeutic outcomes for patients. MTM includes five core elements: medication therapy review, a personal medication record, a medication-related action plan, intervention or referral, and documentation and follow-up" [27]. In addition, this service was also recognized in the Medicare Modernization Act of 2003 (MMA), which established the Medicare Part D drug benefit and requirements for controlling costs, quality improvement, and MTM programs [28]. As part of the MMA, broad goals were established to optimize therapeutic outcomes (e.g., reducing adverse events) for targeted beneficiaries. Afterward, several pilot programs were carried out across the US to increase knowledge of MTM (e.g., Asheville Project, Diabetes Ten City Challenge) [28]. These early pilot programs were essential in the process of creating a profession-wide-consensus about the process of MTM [29].

CPF's grant funding during this time also went through an evolution process by moving towards the funding of projects that were more outcomes based. A study by Isetts et al. compared the impact of CPF funding between the initial years and recent years of the foundation utilizing the AHRQ Impact Factor Framework (Table 1). Their study found a trend of more recently completed grants having a higher AHRQ impact level compared to those in the initial years. For example, 53% of projects completed in the initial years had an AHRQ impact of level 1 compared to 36% in recent years. Furthermore, grants completed more recently were more likely to have a higher impact at levels 2, 3, and 4 (36%, 26%, 3%, respectively) [2].

Table 1. The Four AHRQ Impact Factor Levels [2].

AHRQ Level	AHRQ Level Description
1	Studies that add to the knowledge base only and do not represent direct change in policy or practice
2	Studies that may lead to a policy or program change as a direct result of the research
3	Studies that may cause a potential change in what clinicians or patients do, or result in a change in a care pattern
4	Studies that may change actual health outcomes (clinical, economic quality of life, and/or patient satisfaction), or profoundly change practice

CPF grants during the early years of MTM also helped to contribute to a professional consensus about the viability of MTM. For example, CPF funded a grant that was completed in 2008 that evaluated the effect of implementing MTM services (pharmaceutical case management [PCM]) conducted by community pharmacists for a private health plan [30]. The PCM model had already demonstrated success with Iowa Medicaid beneficiaries and was an innovative model of care when initiated in 2000. Therefore, an 18-month pilot study was conducted with CPF support to assess the benefits of implementing the PCM model in a private sector health plan. The same PCM model used for Iowa Medicaid Beneficiaries was adopted; however, only pharmacists could be reimbursed in this program (including collaboration with some case managers and disease managers) [30].

The objectives of the PCM pilot program were to evaluate the effect of PCM on medication appropriateness, characterize drug-therapy problems identified by PCM pharmacists, compare healthcare utilization among patients eligible for PCM services, assess the impact of PCM on patient's self-reported health, and assess pharmacist barriers to providing PCM services [30]. The pilot program showed on average almost three drug-therapy problems were identified per patient over the study period, and 89.3% were resolved by the pharmacist. This early pilot program identified significant barriers such as the higher health status of private sector patients which may have led to a perception that they did not need the PCM service, and 50% of pharmacies had less than five eligible patients. Overall, PCM services were considered an opportunity to reduce overall healthcare costs and utilization; and served as a launching pad for future MTM studies conducted in the community pharmacy setting [30].

Another CPF grant awardee showed it was possible to set up a network of 135 pharmacists across seven states of the upper Midwest to provide MTM services to older adults [31]. As a result, the grantee was able to create a tool, called TIMER (Tool to Improve Medications in the Elderly via Review), which was shown to be helpful for pharmacists to provide MTM services to older adults [31]. There are multiple other examples of CPF funded grants in the early MTM era which also contributed to the knowledge base of pharmacists providing MTM services in the community pharmacy setting [32–36].

The funding of expanded MTM services with greater disease state complexity became commonplace after the viability of pharmacist-led MTM programs was established based upon

CPF grant funding. For example, a grant completed in 2009 implemented a pharmacist-led rapid strep test service in the community pharmacy setting [37]. Furthermore, the participating pharmacists also obtained prescriptive authority via collaborative practice agreements in order to provide antibiotic treatment after a positive rapid strep test. In total, 85 rapid strep tests were performed and showed pharmacists could conduct rapid strep tests, identify the presence or absence of group A Streptococcus, and whether or not antibacterial therapy should be initiated [37].

Similarly, a 2014 pilot project evaluated whether or not community pharmacists could identify patients at risk of worsening heart failure through the use of a clinical decision tool called the One Minute Clinic for Heart Failure (TOM-C HF) [38]. TOM-C HF was a simple six-item screening tool that would be used during routine patient encounters. Results showed application of the screening tool took about 1 to 5 min in over 80% of the patient interactions. Furthermore, of the 121 patients evaluated, 62% had one or more symptoms of worsening heart failure. The most common symptoms identified were edema (39%) and increased shortness of breath (17%). Also, self-reported weight gain (>5 lbs) was also found in 19% of patients. This study showed that pharmacists can help screen and identify patients for heart failure decompensation and may be an important link in disease state management of heart failure to help lower hospital readmission rates [38].

The establishment of community pharmacy residency programs also began to grow rapidly during this time, with the number of programs almost tripling between 1999 and 2001 [10]. This growth has been attributed to an increase in clinical services being offered in the community setting, increased buy-in from colleges of pharmacy, and significant funding for PGY1 residency programs by the Institute for the Advancement of Community Pharmacy (IACP). IACP provided over $900,000 (US dollars) and led to the establishment of 45 community pharmacy residency positions over six years [10]. CPF grant funding was also in line with the trend of increased focus on the value of community pharmacy residencies during the MTM era and in 2004, CPF partnered with the APhA Foundation to co-fund community pharmacy resident incentive grants to cultivate innovative research projects of pharmacy residents (https://www.aphafoundation.org/incentive-grants) [39].

In 2010, CPF funded a grant that surveyed the perceived value of providing community pharmacy residency training from the perspective of the colleges of pharmacy and pharmacy provider organizations [40]. Survey findings revealed the most common value responses were altruistic (e.g., pharmacy profession development and pharmacy education development). In addition, barriers to offering residency programs included operational issues and challenges related to accreditation [39]. In 2014, CPF also funded a project that created an implementation guide for PGY1 community pharmacy residency programs to support the growth and expansion of these programs and to contribute to the advancement of community pharmacy [41]. As a result of this grant, the "implementation guide provided critical resources and materials to assist organizational entities, community pharmacies, and colleges of pharmacy in their development, implementation, and accreditation of new community pharmacy residency programs" [41].

3.3. The Value-Based Care Era

Pharmacists are considered the most accessible healthcare provider, and are uniquely qualified to provide patient-centered care that engages patients in proper medication use and chronic disease state management [42]. The provision of MTM services within the practice of pharmaceutical care forever changed the way pharmacists would be involved in the care of patients with expanded roles such as patient assessment, identification of therapeutic interventions, medication synchronization, immunizations, point-of-care testing, chronic disease state management, and therapeutic monitoring and follow-up. As such, the trend in the healthcare industry has seen a movement from a fee-for-service care model to one that is value-based where patient outcomes result in pay-for-performance as opposed to the volume of services rendered [42]. Pharmacists have begun to take on even more responsibility in the care of patients concerning medication optimization, clinical status, patient satisfaction, and chronic disease state outcomes. As a result, there are expanded opportunities for pharmacists to partner with physicians, payers, and other healthcare stakeholders more than ever before to improve health outcomes, enhance the patient experience, and reduce the total cost of care.

Approximately 60% of the grants awarded by CPF are direct-patient care focused. For example, a CPF grant completed in 2017 evaluated the effects of individualized patient care services by pharmacists on total costs of care, an adherence measure, and the use of high-risk medications by older patients [43]. To accomplish this, the grantee setup a separate pharmacy-based medical clinic that was staffed by healthcare providers who were recognized by payers to bill for services. The pharmacists, in collaboration with the rendering providers, were able to increase the number of patients seen, the quality of patient clinical outcomes, and the number of clinical services the pharmacy offers. The clinic saw 309 patients between September 2014–December 2015. An A1c drop of −1.29 was observed (average 8.72 to 7.43), and the patient's body mass index dropped −3.28 (35.68–32.4) after six months of the intervention. As a result of the demonstrated value for services, the clinic pharmacy was able to establish a limited provider status with a large healthcare payer leading to direct pharmacist billing and payment (vs. incident-to-billing) [43].

Another CPF grant completed in 2017 utilized targeted medication reviews by pharmacists to deliver pre-conception care as a public health demonstration project [44]. Community pharmacists were provided an American College of Pharmacy Education (ACPE) accredited continuing education program on addressing pre-conception care needs of patients via the framework of MTM. The targeted medication reviews (TMRs) included women 15 to 45 years enrolled in an Ohio managed care plan and focused on medications that could cause fetal harm, folic acid use, and immunizations. TMRs were generated and assigned to pharmacies where the eligible patients filled prescriptions. Any pharmacy in Ohio that participated in the commercially available MTM platform received a TMR notification. Pharmacists then provided the service, documented, and billed for the service through the MTM platform. Results showed 1149 pharmacists from 818 pharmacies completed at least 1 TMR (n = 6602). The TMRs had a 33% completion rate with a 65% (n = 4266) success rate. This demonstration project showed new service programs could be rapidly implemented into existing MTM service processes over hundreds of pharmacies in Ohio. Furthermore, it also provides data demonstrating the value of pharmacists and can serve as justification for additional payers to reimburse for similar services. Finally, pharmacists may be able to assist with other similar preventative care services and utilize this model to improve patient health outcomes as well as obtain reimbursement for their service [44].

Value-based services will require the collaboration of multiple healthcare providers including pharmacists to help patients achieve the best health outcomes. To better understand this requirement, a CPF grant completed in 2017 was conducted to increase knowledge about collaborative working relationships between pharmacists and other healthcare providers throughout multiple practice settings [45]. The study sample included 16 community pharmacists, nine prescribers, and five care managers. There was an agreement between all participants for the need to have face-to-face meetings with other healthcare team members to determine shared goals. Prescribers and care managers identified that community pharmacists providing education on medications was very helpful and also helped them reinforce the education each time they saw a patient. Also, medication adherence packaging provided by community pharmacists was also stated as helpful in improving adherence to chronic medications per prescribers and case managers. Community pharmacists from the project felt personally responsible for a patient's medication regimen. Also, prescribers and care managers felt they had additional time to focus on other, non-medication related issues when they worked with a community pharmacist to manage the patient's medication regimen. As a result, this demonstration project showed that including community pharmacists into team-based care can potentially improve patient care and outcomes [45].

CPF grants supporting pharmacists in patient-centered medical homes (PCMH) are important for the understanding of community pharmacist roles and responsibilities in alternate payment models [46–49]. The collaboration of pharmacists with other interprofessional care teams has further expanded during the value-based care era with the creation of alternative payment models in both commercial and government health insurance programs, such as accountable care organizations (ACOs). An ACO according to the Centers for Medicare and Medicaid Services (CMS) is a "group of doctors, hospitals, and other healthcare providers who come together voluntarily to deliver coordinated high-quality care to Medicare patients" [50]. This coordinated care helps reduce healthcare costs and ensure patients are receiving proper care while preventing unnecessary duplication of services and preventing medical errors. Further, when ACOs are successful in providing coordinated care for chronic disease states while simultaneously lowering costs they share in the savings they achieve for the Medicare program [50].

CPF grant funding has also been awarded to projects that seek to evaluate and establish the role of community pharmacists in an ACO. For example, a grant completed in 2016 assessed the feasibility of integrating MTM services provided by community pharmacists into the clinical care teams and the health information technology (HIT) infrastructure for a Minnesota Medicaid ACO [51]. The study included 15 community pharmacies who were all integrated into the HIT infrastructure via Direct Secure Messaging. There were 32 recipients who received MTM services resulting from ACO referral at 5 out of the 15 community pharmacies over one year. The project was able to set up an electronic MTM referral system successfully, and there was consideration given to the community pharmacists providing MTM in future ACO shared savings agreements [51].

Pharmacy education has also continued to evolve as pharmacists take on more advanced patient care roles. Since June of 2013, 34,824 pharmacists have graduated from ASHP accredited residency programs [9]. Also, BPS now recognizes twelve distinct specialties and more than 41,000 pharmacists, national and internationally, are board certified [52]. CPF continues to fund grants that support pharmacy education and the expansion of community pharmacy practice. For example, a 2016 CPF grant supported the development of a vision and strategic action plan for the future of community-based residency training [53]. This funding is directly aligned with the further evolution of pharmacy practice and the goals of achieving provider status and expanding access to care. The strategic action plan will help ensure the future needs of community-based pharmacist practitioners are met [53].

4. Conclusions

In summary, the Community Pharmacy Foundation is a non-profit organization whose mission is to support the advancement of community pharmacy practice and patient care delivery through grant funding and resource sharing. The history of pharmacy within the United States dates back to the beginning of the colonies, when physicians, druggists, and apothecaries were essential to providing health care in the new world. As America became urbanized and continued to grow in population, the necessity for domestic sources of drugs and pre-manufactured medications drastically changed the business of pharmacy, placing the pharmacist in a dispensing role. However, the pharmacist's extensive drug therapy knowledge would create an environment to shift the focus back onto the patient and create new pharmacy care service models that have been the backbone of modern pharmacy practice in the United States. Since its founding, CPF has actively supported grants that are aligned with the evolution of pharmacy practice and CPFs mission. In the early years of the foundation, the majority of grants focused on building the pharmacy knowledge base, but have since shifted towards impacting the health outcomes of patients. In addition, the CPF grants awarded have also helped contribute to establishing reimbursement models for pharmacies and pharmacists who participate in advanced patient care and the advancement of the profession through education and training.

Author Contributions: Conceptualization (B.H.-E., A.M.K., B.J.I.); Data curation (B.H.-E., A.M.K.); Formal analysis (A.M.K., B.J.I.); Investigation (A.M.K., B.J.I.); Methodology (B.H.-E., A.M.K., B.J.I.); Project administration (B.H.-E., A.M.K., B.J.I.); Supervision (A.M.K., B.J.I.); Validation (B.H.-E., A.M.K., B.J.I.); Visualization (B.H.-E., A.M.K.); Writing—original draft preparation (B.H.-E., A.M.K., B.J.I.); and Writing—review and editing (B.H.-E., A.M.K., B.J.I.).

Funding: This opinion article received no external funding.

Acknowledgments: CPF Board of Directors—Phil Burgess, Chicago, Illinois; Linda Garrelts MacLean, Spokane, Washington; Matthew Osterhaus, Maquoketa, Iowa; Brian Jensen, Two Rivers, Wisconsin; Dorinda Martin, Austin, Texas; Randy Myers, Carey, Ohio; Carlos Ortiz, Amherst, Massachusetts; CPF Emeritus—Lonnie Hollingsworth,

Lubbock, Texas; Frank J. McGarr, US District Court, Downers Grove, Illinois; Robert J. Osterhaus, Maquoketa, Iowa; Louis M. Sesti, Williamston, Michigan.

Conflicts of Interest: The authors declare no conflict of interest.

References

1. Community Pharmacy Foundation. History & Origin. Community Pharmacy Foundation, 2019. Available online: https://communitypharmacyfoundation.org/about/default.asp (accessed on 24 April 2019).
2. Isetts, B.J.; Olson, A.W.; Kondic, A.M.; Schommer, J. An Evaluation of the Distribution, Scope, and Impact of Community Pharmacy Foundation Grants Completed by Academic Principal Investigators between 2002 and 2014. *Innov. Pharm.* **2017**, *8*, 1–10. [CrossRef]
3. Olson, W.A.; Isetts, B.J.; Kondic, A.M.; Schommer, J. Comparing the Research Contributions of Community Pharmacy Foundation Funding on Practice Innovation between Non-Academics and Academics. *Innov. Pharm.* **2017**, *8*, 1–8. [CrossRef]
4. Baker, D.M.; Colbert, J.; Miller, S.; Nagel-Edwards, K.; Wensel, T.M.; Samuel, E.; Jusczak, P. AACP History Special Interest Group Model PowerPoint Presentations. American Institute of the History of Pharmacy, 2019. Available online: https://aihp.org/historical-resources/teaching/aacp-sig-model-presentations/ (accessed on 21 April 2019).
5. Hogshire, J. *Pills-a-Go-Go: The Fiendish Investigation into Pill Marketing, Art, History, and Consumption*; Feral House: Los Angeles, CA, USA, 1999.
6. McCarthy, R. Lecture One: Early Pharmacy in America. American Institute of the History of Pharmacy, 2019. Available online: https://aihp.org/historical-resources/teaching/ (accessed on 23 April 2019).
7. Alpers, W.C. The history of the American Pharmaceutical Association. *J. Am. Pharm. Assoc.* **1912**, *1*, 972–992. [CrossRef]
8. Drug Topics. From Apothecary to PharmD: 160 Years of Caring for Patients. Drug Topics, 2016. Available online: https://www.drugtopics.com/chains-business/apothecary-pharmd-160-years-caring-patients (accessed on 25 April 2019).
9. Clark, T. Celebrating 50 years of advancement in pharmacy residency training. *Am. J. Health Syst. Pharm.* **2014**, *71*, 1190–1195. [CrossRef] [PubMed]
10. Stolpe, S.F.; Adams, A.J.; Bradley-Baker, L.R.; Burns, A.L.; Owen, J.A. Historical Development and Emerging Trends of Community Pharmacy Residencies. *Am. J. Pharm. Educ.* **2011**, *75*, 160. [CrossRef] [PubMed]
11. Isetts, B.J. Systems of pharmaceutical care. In *Managing Pharmacy Practice: Principles, Strategies, and Systems*; Peterson, A.M., Ed.; CRC Press: New York, NY, USA, 2004; pp. 233–260.
12. Mikeal, R.L.; Brown, T.P.; Lazarus, H.L.; Vinson, M.C. Quality of pharmaceutical care in hospitals. *Am. J. Health Syst. Pharm.* **1975**, *32*, 567–574. [CrossRef]
13. Hepler, C.D.; Strand, L.M. Opportunities and responsibilities in pharmaceutical care. *Am. J. Hosp. Pharm.* **1990**, *47*, 533–543. [CrossRef]
14. Zillich, A.J.; Sutherland, J.M.; Kumbera, P.A.; Carter, B.L. Hypertension Outcomes through Blood Pressure Monitoring and Evaluation by Pharmacists (HOME Study). *J. Gen. Intern. Med.* **2005**, *20*, 1091–1096. [CrossRef]
15. Mott, D. Pharmacy Participation in and Nature of Claims Submitted to the Wisconsin Medicaid Pharmaceutical Care Program. Community Pharmacy Foundation, 2005. Available online: https://communitypharmacyfoundation.org/resources/grant_docs/CPFGrantDoc_35597.pdf (accessed on 26 April 2019).
16. Doucette, W.R. Extended Diabetes Care through Diabetes Center-Community Pharmacy Collaboration. Community Pharmacy Foundation, 2006. Available online: https://communitypharmacyfoundation.org/resources/grant_docs/CPFGrantDoc_5689.pdf (accessed on 26 April 2019).
17. Chui, M. Evaluation of online prospective DUR programs in community pharmacy practice. *JMCP* **2000**, *6*, 27–32. [CrossRef]
18. Owen, J. Asthma Care Improvement Initiative Study. Community Pharmacy Foundation, 2005. Available online: https://communitypharmacyfoundation.org/resources/grant_docs/CPFGrantDoc_93056.pdf (accessed on 26 April 2019).

19. Wertheimer, A. Effect of Prior Authorization and Formulary Limitation on Community Pharmacy Practice and Profitability. Community Pharmacy Foundation, 2005. Available online: https://communitypharmacyfoundation. org/resources/grant_docs/CPFGrantDoc_86425.pdf (accessed on 26 April 2019).

20. Shepherd, M.D.; Richards, K.M.; Winegar, A.L. Time from Medicare Part D claim adjudication to community pharmacy payment. *J. Am. Pharm. Assoc.* **2007**, *47*, 695–701. [CrossRef]

21. Harrington, C. Pharmacy Based Activity to Reverse and Manage Disease (PHARMD): The Hypertension Project The Community Pharmacy Foundation. 2004. Available online: https://communitypharmacyfoundation.org/ resources/grant_docs/CPFGrantDoc_74116.pdf (accessed on 26 April 2019).

22. Isetts, B.J. The Global Perspective—United States. In *Pharmaceutical Care Practice*, 3rd ed.; Cipolle, R.J., Strand, L.M., Morley, P.C., Eds.; McGraw Hill: New York, NY, USA, 2012.

23. Medicare Payment Advisory Commission HGC. *Report to the Congress: Medicare Coverage of Nonphysician Practitioners*; Medicare Payment Advisory Commission: Washington, DC, USA, 2002.

24. Isetts, B.J.; Buffington, D.E. CPT code change proposal: National data on pharmacists medication therapy management services. *J. Am. Pharm. Assoc.* **2007**, *47*, 491–495. [CrossRef] [PubMed]

25. American Medical Association. *CPT Changes 2006: An Insider's View*; American Medical Association: Chicago, IL, USA, 2005; pp. 309–312.

26. Westberg, S.M.; Pittenger, A.; Dickson, K.; Brummel, A.; Odell, L.; Johnson, J.K. Advancing Medication Therapy Management Services: Creating increased awareness and utilization of MTMS CPT billing codes Community Pharmacy Foundation. 2010. Available online: https://communitypharmacyfoundation.org/ resources/grant_docs/CPFGrantDoc_68855.pdf (accessed on 29 April 2019).

27. Centers for Disease Control and Prevention. Community Pharmacists and Medication Therapy Management|CDC|DHDSP. Centers for Disease Control and Prevention, 2018. Available online: https: //www.cdc.gov/dhdsp/pubs/guides/best-practices/pharmacist-mtm.htm (accessed on 24 April 2019).

28. Isetts, B.J. Pharmaceutical care, MTM, & payment: The past, present, & future. *Ann. Pharmacother.* **2012**, *46*, S47–S56. [PubMed]

29. American Pharmacists Association; National Association of Chain Drug Stores Foundation. Medication therapy management in pharmacy practice: core elements of an MTM service model (version 2.0). *J. Am. Pharm. Assoc.* **2008**, *48*, 341–353. [CrossRef] [PubMed]

30. Temple, T.; Puentz, K.; Doucette, W.R. Implementation of the Pharmaceutical Case Management Model in a Private Sector Health Plan. Community Pharmacy Foundation, 2008. Available online: https: //communitypharmacyfoundation.org/grants/grants_list_details.asp?grants_id=70378 (accessed on 27 April 2019).

31. Doucette, W.R. An Initial Evaluation of Medication Therapy Management (MTM) Services in the Upper Midwest Region. Community Pharmacy Foundation, 2009. Available online: https://communitypharmacyfoundation.org/ resources/grant_docs/CPFGrantDoc_2886.pdf (accessed on 27 April 2019).

32. Osborne, M.A.; Snyder, M.E.; Hall, D.L.; Coley, K.C.; McGivney, M.S. Evaluating Pennsylvania Pharmacists' Provision of Community-based Patient Care Services. *Innov. Pharm.* **2011**, *2*, 1–9. [CrossRef]

33. Trapskin, K.; Johnson, C.; Cory, P.; Sorum, S.; Decker, C. Forging a novel provider and payer partnership in Wisconsin to compensate pharmacists for quality-driven pharmacy and medication therapy management services. *J. Am. Pharm. Assoc.* **2009**, *49*, 642–651. [CrossRef]

34. Rashed, S.M.; Goldstein, S.; Tolley, E.A.; Wilson-Relyea, B.J. Cost Outcomes of Diabetes Education in a specialized community pharmacy. *Am. J. Pharm. Benefits* **2010**, *2*, 421–428.

35. Pudlo, A.; Abernathy, M.; Peek, J. Financial analysis of MTM Services Implemented in a Non-MTM Participating Pharmacy. Community Pharmacy Foundation, 2011. Available online: https://communitypharmacyfoundation. org/resources/grant_docs/CPFGrantDoc_20787.pdf (accessed on 27 April 2019).

36. McDonough, R.P.; Doucette, W.R.; Urmie, J.M.; Patterson, B.J. A Comprehensive Longitudinal Assessment of an Innovative Community Pharmacy Practice Community Pharmacy Foundation. 2012. Available online: https://communitypharmacyfoundation.org/resources/grant_docs/CPFGrantDoc_54202.pdf (accessed on 29 April 2019).

37. Garrelts MacLean, L.; Schwartz, C.; Sclar, D.A.; Wu, A.; Whitcomb Henry, H. Community Pharmacy Based Rapid Strep Testing with Prescriptive Authority. Community Pharmacy Foundation, 2009. Available online: https://communitypharmacyfoundation.org/resources/grant_docs/CPFGrantDoc_12587.pdf (accessed on 29 April 2019).

38. Bleske, B.E.; Dillman, N.O.; Cornelius, D.; Ward, J.K.; Burson, S.C.; Diez, H.L.; Pickworth, K.K.; Bennett, M.S.; Nicklas, J.M.; Dorsch, M.P. Heart failure assessment at the community pharmacy level: A feasibility pilot study. *J. Am. Pharm. Assoc.* **2014**, *54*, 634–641. [CrossRef]

39. American Pharmacists Association Foundation. Incentive Grants. APhA Foundation. Available online: https://www.aphafoundation.org/incentive-grants (accessed on 2 June 2019).

40. Schommer, J.C.; Bonnarens, J.K.; Brown, L.M.; Venable, J.; Good, K.R. Value of community pharmacy residency programs: College of pharmacy and practice site perspectives. *J. Am. Pharm. Assoc.* **2010**, *50*, e72–e88. [CrossRef]

41. Owen, J.A. PGY1 Community Pharmacy Residency Implementation Guide. Community Pharmacy Foundation, 2014. Available online: https://communitypharmacyfoundation.org/resources/grant_docs/CPFGrantDoc_4805.pdf (accessed on 27 April 2019).

42. Pharmacy Quality Alliance. Strategies to Expand Value-Based Pharmacist-Provided Care. Action Guide: For Community Pharmacists, Healthcare Prayers, and Other Stakeholders. 2019. Available online: https://www.pqaalliance.org/pharmacist-provided-care (accessed on 27 April 2019).

43. Twigg, G.A.; Motsko, J.; Sherr, J.; El-Baff, S. Interprofessional Approach to Increase Billable Care-Events in a Rural Community. *Innov. Pharm.* **2017**, *8*, 1–8. [CrossRef]

44. Mager, N.A.; Bright, D.R.; Markus, D.; Weis, L.; Hartzell, D.M.; Gartner, J. Use of targeted medication reviews to deliver preconception care: A demonstration project. *J. Am. Pharm. Assoc.* **2017**, *57*, 90–94. [CrossRef]

45. Phillips, R.C.; Ferreri, S. Integrating Community Pharmacists into Team-Based Care Community Pharmacy Foundation. 2018. Available online: www.communitypharmacyfoundation.org/resources/grant_docs/CPFGrantDoc_52603.pdf (accessed on 27 April 2019).

46. Engstrom, K.A. Pharmacist Based Medication Therapy Management is an Essential Part of Patient Centered Medical Home Community Pharmacy Foundation. 2013. Available online: https://www.communitypharmacyfoundation.org/resources/grant_docs/CPFGrantDoc_59132.pdf.Published~2013 (accessed on 29 April 2019).

47. Heetderks, L.; Paluta, L. Demonstrating the Impact and Feasibility of a Business Model which includes a Community-Based Pharmacist in a Patient Centered Medical Home (PCMH) Practice. Community Pharmacy Foundation, 2014. Available online: https://www.communitypharmacyfoundation.org/resources/grant_docs/CPFGrantDoc_46853.pdf (accessed on 29 April 2019).

48. Luder, H.R.; Shannon, P.; Kirby, J.; Frede, S.M. Community pharmacist collaboration with a patient-centered medical home: Establishment of a patient-centered medical neighborhood and payment model. *J. Am. Pharm. Assoc.* **2018**, *58*, 44–50. [CrossRef]

49. Wilson, C.; Twigg, G.A. Pharmacist-led depression screening and intervention in an underserved, rural, and multi-ethnic diabetic population. *J. Am. Pharm. Assoc.* **2016**, *58*, 205–209. [CrossRef]

50. Centers for Medicare and Medicaid Services. Accountable Care Organizations (ACOs): General Information Center for Medicare & Medicaid Innovation. Centers for Medicare and Medicaid Services, 2019. Available online: https://innovation.cms.gov/initiatives/aco/ (accessed on 27 April 2019).

51. Isetts, B. Integrating Medication Therapy Management (MTM) Services Provided by Community Pharmacists into a Community-Based Accountable Care Organization (ACO). *Pharmacy* **2017**, *5*, 56. [CrossRef]

52. Board of Pharmacy Specialties. History. Board of Pharmacy Specialties, 2019. Available online: https://www.bpsweb.org/about-bps/history/ (accessed on 27 April 2019).

53. Skelton, J.B.; Owen, J.A. Developing a vision and strategic plan for future community-based residency training. *J. Am. Pharm. Assoc.* **2016**, *56*, 584–589. [CrossRef]

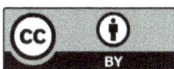

pharmacy

MDPI

Review

Community-Based Pharmacy Practice Innovation and the Role of the Community-Based Pharmacist Practitioner in the United States

Jean-Venable Goode [1,*], James Owen [2], Alexis Page [1] and Sharon Gatewood [1]

[1] Department of Pharmacotherapy and Outcomes Science, Virginia Commonwealth University, Richmond, VA 23298, USA
[2] Practice and Science Affairs, American Pharmacists Association, Washington, DC 20037, USA
* Correspondence: jrgoode@vcu.edu

Received: 1 June 2019; Accepted: 31 July 2019; Published: 4 August 2019

check for updates

Abstract: Community-based pharmacy practice is evolving from a focus on product preparation and dispensing to becoming a health care destination within the four walls of the traditional community-based pharmacy. Furthermore, community-based pharmacy practice is expanding beyond the four walls of the traditional community-based pharmacy to provide care to patients where they need it. Pharmacists involved in this transition are community-based pharmacist practitioners who are primarily involved in leading and advancing team-based patient care services in communities to improve the patient health. This paper will review community-based pharmacy practice innovations and the role of the community-based pharmacist practitioner in the United States.

Keywords: community-based pharmacy; community-based pharmacist practitioners

1. Introduction

1.1. An Overview of Health Care and the Role of Community-Based Pharmacists

There are substantial challenges related to public health including issues associated with health care inequalities, aging populations, increasing levels of chronic disease and urbanization [1]. There is a need to increase access to primary care services, control costs, and improve outcomes in health care for patients especially in the management of chronic conditions which puts a strain on health care systems worldwide [2]. Addressing these issues is critical for improving the health of patients in communities. To fully address these issues, all types of health care providers with the necessary knowledge, skills, abilities, and required competencies must be utilized whenever possible to provide needed care.

From a global perspective, community-based pharmacists represent the third largest health care professional group outnumbered only by physicians and nurses [2]. Community-based pharmacists are an underutilized health care provider who can improve access to care when and where patients want to receive it. Fortunately, a trend is emerging for community-based pharmacists to function as care extenders to counter primary care provider shortages and address the substantial problems and associated costs due to the inappropriate use of medication [2]. While the types of patient care services that community-based pharmacists are providing are extremely variable by country or even by provincial or state jurisdiction, more and more pharmacists are providing important emergency medication refills, renewals/extensions of prescriptions, changes to doses or formulations, therapeutic substitution, prescribing for minor ailments, initiation of prescription drug therapy, ordering and interpreting laboratory tests, and administering drugs by injection [2].

In the United States, the challenges to the health care system continue to mount. Despite changes to health care laws and coverage intended to insure more individuals and decrease costs, a substantial portion of the population remains without insurance coverage. Additionally, health care cost continues to be a significant portion of the gross domestic product in the United States (US) and is projected to grow by 5.5% from 2018–2027 [3]. Prescription drug costs are expected to increase an average of 6.1% per year during the same time due to the introduction of new drugs and a focused effort for patients with chronic disease to adhere to their medication regimen [3]. Pharmacists, who practice in community-based settings are key to improving adherence to prescribed medications. As the US health care system continues to evolve, a primary focus is on outcomes and quality as ways to manage costs effectively and efficiently [4].

Currently, there are shortages of health care providers with increasing shortages in primary care predicted for the future [4]. Specifically for physicians, it is predicted there will be a shortage of at least 43,000 primary care physicians and 140,000 total physicians in the US by 2030 [5]. Community-based pharmacists, however, can help to address this problem. The US Bureau of Labor Statistics estimates that there are more than 186,000 community-based pharmacists in the United States [6]. Increasingly, the pharmacists' role is being recognized as an important as the US health care environment changes and in initiatives to reform healthcare [7].

1.2. Defining Community-Based Pharmacist Practitioners

Community-based pharmacy settings positively impact patient care as a result of their convenience and as supported by the frequency of access by patients. One study revealed patients visited a community-based pharmacy 35 times per year compared with a primary care physician only four times per year [8]. Additionally, pharmacists are available in these settings with 58% of employed pharmacists in traditional community-based pharmacy settings (pharmacy, supermarket or general merchandise) [6]. Other community-based pharmacies include health-systems, Federally-Qualified Healthcare Centers, clinics, and specialty. Pharmacists are also in community-based settings beyond the traditional "four walls" of a pharmacy including physician offices, patient homes, churches, and work places [9,10].

Pharmacists practicing in community-based settings are health care providers who offer either generalist or specialist ambulatory care services to patients in the communities they serve [9]. The primary goal of a community-based pharmacist practitioner is to keep patients healthy [10]. Community-based pharmacist practitioners create, advance, and influence team-based care; strive to enhance management of community-based pharmacy practices to focus on the delivery of patient care services; serve as leaders within community-based pharmacy settings, local communities, and the profession of pharmacy; and provide direct patient care to meet the healthcare needs of the communities that they serve [9]. Regardless of the actual physical practice setting location, the focus of the community-based pharmacist practitioner is providing patients with the care they need, when and where they need it.

Community-based pharmacist practitioners provide a wide range of services including educational consultations, medication management and other medication optimization services, chronic condition management, patient empowerment, care coordination, health and wellness services, and other services that help to improve the lives of patients in the community [9]. Community-based pharmacist practitioners are essential health care professionals who provide direct patient care, advance team-based care, manage services that focus on the patient, and serve as leaders within their communities and the profession [9]. As a greater focus is placed on the importance of chronic disease management, wellness, and medication management the opportunities for community-based pharmacist practitioners are expected to continue to grow [11].

1.3. Challenges Facing Community-Based Pharmacist Practitioners in the United States

The underlying issues surrounding the expansion of community-based pharmacists' role in patient care no matter the country requires dedicated remuneration, primary care integration, and multidisciplinary education [2]. In traditional community-based pharmacies, there are multiple challenges for community-based pharmacist practitioners implementing innovative patient care services. The physical layout of the traditional community-based pharmacy does not facilitate patient care services. Many community-based pharmacist practitioners are adding semi-private counseling areas, private counseling rooms, exam rooms, and conference rooms for innovative patient care service delivery. The workflow process in community-based pharmacies can also be a challenge. The process for dispensing of prescription medications usually requires the pharmacist as the person responsible for drug utilization review and the verification of the prescription. The number of support staff can greatly impact the pharmacist's ability to be involved with other patient care services along with dispensing of product. Several methods have been used to overcome the issue of time for the pharmacist to provide patient care services including adding more support staff, pharmacist overlap (i.e., more than one pharmacist working at a time) and using a technician checking technician, if allowed by state law [12,13].

It is essential to change, update, and redesign the business model in community-based pharmacy practice. The focus of community-based pharmacist practitioner activities need to be on patient-centered care to maximize their impact in the communities they serve. Schommer and colleagues state that you must "create payment and business models for community-based pharmacy practice, advance pharmacy technician practice, expand community-based pharmacy residency programs, and begin seeing transformations through the patient's eyes" [14]. This fundamental paradigm shift to the business model of community-based pharmacy practices will establish the pharmacy practice location as a heath care access point where the practice is reimbursed for the public health services they are providing [14]. The redesign of community pharmacy practices as settings of care is essential including changing the business model, implementing strategies such as medication synchronization, integrating technology and maximizing technicians [15].

Another challenge for community-based pharmacist practitioners is integrating technology in community-based practices. Currently, the majority of community-based pharmacies use a dispensing system with or without the capability to document patient care services, limiting the ability to document services. Furthermore, the pharmacy systems usually do not integrate with the electronic health care record (EHR). Several recent articles have been published documenting the value of EHR integration [16,17]. There is also a movement for documentation and patient care services through the use of a pharmacist e-care plan [18]. New systems enabling standards and technology systems will hopefully help to address these issues primarily focusing on consistent electronic documentation methods and strategies for consistently coding and documenting care provided to patients [19].

Additionally, the location of community-based pharmacy practices can be a barrier to the provision of team-based care and integration [20]. However, as the community-based pharmacist practitioner expands beyond the four walls of the traditional based-community pharmacy it will become easier to engage in team-based care. Furthermore, the profession does not have a referral process that is similar to other health care providers. There needs to be process for referrals between pharmacists and other healthcare providers as well as other pharmacists. Integration of technology may help with team-based care and the referral process.

Expanding the role of pharmacists where they are practicing at the "top of their license" to improve care and drug therapy outcomes is essential to the activities of a community-based pharmacist practitioner and has been promoted by the World Health Organization [7,20]. In 2007, Canada enacted laws that enabled expanded scope in some provinces through the Additional Prescribing Authorization (APA) [20]. In the United States, the practice of pharmacy is regulated by individual state boards of pharmacy and scope of practice and authority varies greatly from state to state. States such as Oregon, California, Idaho, and Washington have begun to expand the scope of practice and authority for pharmacists to prescribe medications, perform point of care diagnostic tests, initiate hormonal contraception, and administer injectable medications [21]. However, continued expansion of changes remains a challenge in many states, but important to allow community-based pharmacist practitioners to provide the needed patient care services in the communities they serve.

A major obstacle for community-based pharmacists in the United States is that pharmacists lack formal designation as providers in the federal Medicare program. Specifically, pharmacists are not recognized as providers under Section 1861(s) (2) of the Social Security Act, as such pharmacists are not paid by the Federal government for health care services under the Medicare Part B program. To address this important barrier, professional associations, and other stakeholders have advocated for decades that action be taken through the US legislative process to include pharmacists and enable a payment mechanism for the services that pharmacists can provide to patients. It is important because other payers in the US typically follow Medicare payment policies, thus limiting the ability of pharmacists from receiving payment from these other public, private and commercial entities. The reason that recognition in the Federal Medicare program is viewed by many as the key to the establishment of successful payment models nationwide. However, it is important to note that many states have designated pharmacists as providers, however, this recognition may or may not guarantee payment for service. Pharmacist services need recognition as being valuable by patients and other payers [7].

While the overall number of potential community-based pharmacist practitioners is large; engaging and developing them as providers of care remains a challenge. There is a need for these individuals to undergo continuing professional development and training with a focus as on patient-centered, team-oriented, evidence-based care providers of care [22]. Additionally, there are needs for the credentialing and privileging of community-based pharmacist practitioners which facilitates provision of care and payment for service. Finally, there is an inherent difficulty in establishing value and attributing the outcomes to the pharmacist-provided patient care services [19]. What are the innovative community-based pharmacy services in the United States and the role of the community-based pharmacist practitioner?

2. Methods

This review was developed based on the author's knowledge of community-based pharmacy practice. The authors define the service delivery model and innovative services and provide support from the literature where available. The authors have developed a system for organizing the types of community-based pharmacy innovative patient care services characterizing all of the patient care services in six different categories. All of the types of innovative patient care services are incorporated in one of the six categories. Additionally, the authors describe the services with a focus on the role of the community-based pharmacist practitioner [9].

3. Findings

The findings include a description of community-based pharmacy practice innovations and the role of the community-based pharmacist practitioner in the United States. First, the service models are described to provide insight on the framework for the delivery of the patient care in community-based pharmacy practice. Then the types of the innovative patient care services are described with detail under the six categories. It is important to note that all of the types and categories of patient care services may be offered within the different service delivery models. Most of the innovative patient care services are supported by recent literature. Furthermore, a brief global context is offered about the impact of innovations in the US.

3.1. Models of Community-Based Patient Care Service Delivery

Traditionally, around the world, community pharmacists have been viewed as a distributor of medications [1]. This, however, is shifting as now with the public viewing pharmacists as health care providers. To support this, research has been published that indicates patient and pharmacist preferences for care provided in community-based pharmacies [23]. Published in this research, patients report that from their perspective, the optimal service model includes options for appointments with a health care provider in the pharmacy, having access to the full medical record, providing a point of care diagnostic testing, offering preventive health screening, limited physical examinations, and prescribing of medications [23]. As the profession of pharmacy continues to evolve to focus on patient care, a shift is occurring from product centered to a patient-centered model of care [14]. In the US, patient's medication experience includes both a social and personal experience [14]. Responding to these changes, the pharmacy profession has entered a new "patient-centered medication experience" era and pharmacy practices are employing principles of "collaboration theory" to implement new systems of care [14]. To address these changes, community-based pharmacist practitioners spend time and make connections to the community being visible, increasing health awareness and meeting the needs of the patients in the communities they serve [10].

The service model develops from the traditional community-based pharmacy or four walls and expands beyond to the community (Figure 1). Additionally, the four walls of the traditional community-based pharmacy are changing, becoming health care destinations which even include health care classes such as yoga. Community-based pharmacist practitioners are participating in outreach events in the communities, churches, workplaces, shopping malls, etc. Community-based pharmacist practitioners are conducting home visits form traditional community-based pharmacies. Community-based pharmacist practitioners are also being placed in physician offices to provide care. These patient care services are on a part-time basis where the community-based pharmacist practitioner spends some portion of their time in the physician office or the community-based pharmacist practitioner is embedded in the office on a full-time basis, but employed by the traditional community-based pharmacy. This article will focus on innovative community-based pharmacy services that are encompassed within this service delivery model.

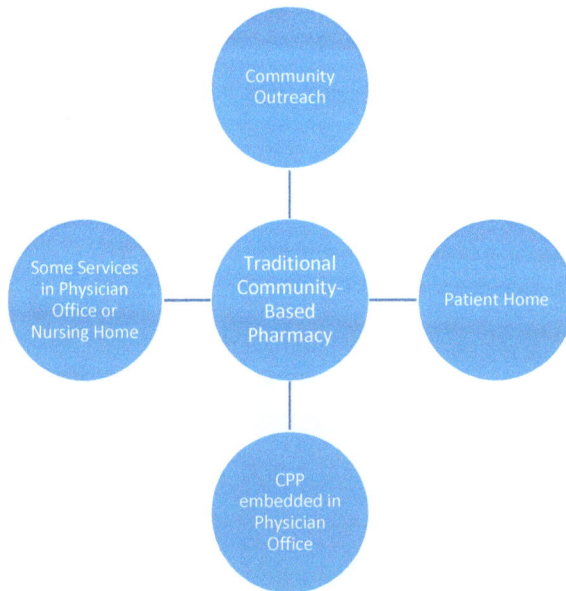

Figure 1. Community-based pharmacist practitioner service model.

3.2. Community-Based Pharmacy Services

Community-based pharmacist practitioners in community-based settings are providing innovative patient care services beyond preparing and dispensing prescription products. These services are categorized into the following areas: medication optimization, wellness and prevention, chronic care management, acute care management, patient education, and other services (Table 1). This manuscript will review those services and supporting literature, if available.

Table 1. Community-Based Patient Care Services.

Medication Optimization	Wellness and Prevention	Chronic Care Management	Acute Care Management	Patient Education	Other Patient Care Services
	Screenings				
	Blood pressure				
	Diabetes				
	Cholesterol				
	Osteoporosis				
	Body Fat				
	HIV				
	Hepatitis C				
	Allergy				
Medication Packing	Lead poisoning				
Home Delivery	**Risk Assessment**	Diabetes			
Medication Reconciliation	Falls	HTN		Store	
	Depression	Cholesterol			
	Asthma	Asthma		• Brochures	
Appointment-Based Medication Synchronization	Cardiovascular risk	Anticoagulation		• Videos	
	Weight management	Heart failure	Test and treat	• Shelf-talkers	Tuberculosis testing
Medication Adherence Programs	Tobacco cessation	Hepatitis C	(rapid diagnostics)	• Posters	
		Menopause	• Influenza	Individual	Telehealth
	Contraception	Monitoring through laboratory testing	• Strep	Group	Durable medical equipment
Comprehensive Medication Management Services	Bioidentical hormone replacement	• BHRT saliva testing	• *H. pylori*	Exercise classes	Care transitions
	Fluoride treatments		Urgent care (minor ailments)		Population health
	Naloxone	• Anticoagulation		Diabetes prevention program	Emergency preparedness
Targeted Medication Review	Needle exchange	• A1c	Triage and referral		
		• TSH		Diabetes education program	
Medication Administration	Drug take back	• Pharmacogenetics			
	Nutraceuticals	• Liver function			
Deprescribing	Annual wellness				
	• In physician office				
	Pharmacogenomics				
	Sleep assessment				
	Falls prevention				
	Immunizations				
	Pre-travel health services				

BHRT—biodentical hormone replacement therapy.

3.2.1. Medication Optimization

Medication optimization is defined as a patient-centered, collaborative approach to managing medication therapy that is applied consistently and holistically across care settings to improve patient care and reduce overall health care costs [24]. Medication optimization services are comprehensive and include services directly related to the medication including medication packaging and home delivery and other services such appointment-based medication synchronization, other adherence programs, comprehensive and targeted medication management, and deprescribing.

Community-based pharmacists are also making an impact on adherence through appointment-based medication synchronization. This process has been shown to increase adherence and improve chronic health conditions, as well as reduce overall cost [25,26]. Although synchronization can help remind patients, provide updates on their progress, simplify the process, and make refilling a prescription more convenient, nonadherence can be multifactorial. The monthly appointments with the pharmacist are critically important, because it allows the pharmacist to educate, engage, and solve problems [26]. However, some community-based pharmacist practitioners may provide only medication synchronization without the appointment with the pharmacist as a way to just align refills and avoid trips to the pharmacy. Other adherence programs include counseling and education by pharmacists and automatic refills [27]. Community-based pharmacist practitioners are helping through medication packing and home delivery. Medication packing helps patients to take their medications correctly and know if they have missed a dose. Community-based pharmacist practitioners package patient medications according to days of the week or time of day. Another mechanism for improving patient adherence is through community-based pharmacist practitioner administration of medications such as long-acting injectables (e.g., antipsychotics, contraceptives) and vitamin B-12 [28]. Home delivery of medications has increased patient access to their medications by taking away the barriers of transportation and proximity to a pharmacy.

Medication reconciliation is the process of creating the most accurate medication list to increase patient safety, decrease medication related problems, and improve health outcomes [29,30]. One of the barriers to maintaining an accurate medication list happens when the patient is discharged from a healthcare facility to another facility because there is loss to follow up. The Affordable Care Act in 2012 launched measurement of hospitals on performance with the Hospital Readmission Reduction Program. This program is administered by the Centers for Medicare and Medicaid Services (CMS) and penalizes hospitals with excess readmissions within 30 days of discharges for certain chronic diseases [31]. Community-based pharmacist practitioners are emerging in the transitions of care area to help decrease readmissions rates and emergency room visits and increase healthcare cost savings [32,33]. Physicians in multiple settings believe that community-based pharmacists should be a part of the transitions of care process because of their medication knowledge and access to patients [34,35].

Medication management services also contribute to medication optimization. Medication management services are a spectrum of patient-centered, pharmacist-provided, collaborative services that focus on medication appropriateness, effectiveness, safety, and adherence with the goal of improving health outcomes [36]. Typically, in practice there are two different distinct services; either comprehensive medication management or targeted medication review. Comprehensive medication management is defined as the standard of care that ensures each patient's medications (whether they are prescription, nonprescription, alternative, traditional, vitamins, or nutritional supplements) are individually assessed to determine that each medication is appropriate for the patient, effective for the medical condition, safe given the comorbidities and other medications being taken, and able to be taken by the patient as intended [37]. Several studies have documented the positive impact of community-based pharmacist practitioner engaged in comprehensive medication management [38–40]. Targeted medication review (TMR) assesses medication use, monitors whether any unresolved issues need attention, new drug therapy problems have arisen, or if there has been a transition in care. TMRs are also used when a potential medication therapy problem is identified and the community-based pharmacist practitioner verifies whether or not there is an actual problem and if a problem exists, an attempt is made to resolve it. Medication optimization also includes efforts by community-based pharmacist practitioners to be involved with deprescribing medications.

3.2.2. Wellness and Prevention

Community-based pharmacist practitioners have been involved in wellness and prevention services through point-of-care testing (POCT) for years, including blood glucose, cholesterol, and A1c. Many states allow pharmacists to perform these laboratory tests through the state's pharmacy practice act or by establishing a collaborative practice agreement with a provider. These services can be provided by a pharmacist once the pharmacy obtains and maintains Clinical Laboratory Improvement Amendments (CLIA) Certificate of Waiver through Centers for Medicare & Medicaid Services (CMS). The pharmacy must follow 'good laboratory practice' when performing tests, which address issues of proper physical environment and recording of test results with patient information in a retrievable file. The pharmacy also needs to follow Occupational Safety and Health Administration (OSHA) standards to provide a safe and healthy environment [41]. As of 2015, community pharmacies are the fourth highest-ranking entity of CLIA-waived laboratories, accounting for 5.4% of all CLIA-waived laboratory facilities [42,43]. More recently, community-based pharmacist practitioners have become involved in POCT for infectious diseases like Human Immunodeficiency Virus (HIV), Hepatitis C, streptococcus, and influenza [44,45]. As pharmacogenomics develops, POCT devices that measure drug metabolism are becoming available and community-based pharmacist practitioners with their drug expertise are a good choice to provide this service [46]. This would prevent someone from taking a medication that they cannot process and avoid having to try multiple medications to find the right one. For those states that do not allow pharmacists to provide these services, risk assessments can be provided to patients. These can determine the patient's risk of developing or assessing the severity of conditions like depression, asthma, and cardiovascular risks. These services have been performed by pharmacists as health screenings in patients who are undiagnosed and for monitoring a patient's chronic disease state [40].

One of the most successful services in wellness and prevention that community-based practitioners offer is immunizations [47]. Pharmacist-provided immunization services began with the administration of the influenza and pneumococcal vaccine. From there, services expanded to pharmacists administering routine adult immunizations. Pharmacist involvement with administering immunizations has increased vaccinations rates [47,48]. In 2000, pre-travel health services began to be offered to patients by community-based pharmacist practitioners [49,50]. These services not only include immunizations needed for international travel but also education, treatment, and prevention of non-vaccine preventable disease. Studies have shown that the pharmacist run pre-travel health clinics have an overall high patient satisfaction rate and recommendations are accepted by providers [51,52].

Community-based pharmacist practitioners provide tobacco cessation services and new scope of practice changes in individual state jurisdictions are facilitating the role by allowing pharmacists to prescribe medication [53,54]. Another service facilitated by practice change is the prescribing of contraceptive therapy for women [55]. Due to the increase in patient deaths from the opioid epidemic, a new role in most states is for community-based pharmacist practitioners to be involved with the dispensing and administering of naloxone. It has been shown that pharmacist involvement in the dispensing of naloxone had significant reductions in fatal opioid overdoses as opposed to just improving access [56]. Other wellness and prevention services include weight management, fluoride treatments, falls prevention, pharmacogenomics, sleep assessment, drug take back, nutraceuticals, and bioidentical hormone replacement [57–62]. Lastly, community-based pharmacist practitioners are involved in providing Medicare Annual Wellness Visits in physician offices [63].

3.2.3. Chronic Care Management

Chronic care management (CCM) is defined as services aim to deliver quality patient centered care, which can assist providers in improving patient outcomes and quality metrics [64,65]. CCM aims to increase non-face-to-face interactions with patient which helps to improve the coordination of care between provider office visits. Pharmacists are able to partner with qualified health professionals to provide CCM services under general supervision of providers, including those located in federally qualified health centers (FQHCs) or rural health centers (RHCs). Studies have shown community-based pharmacist practitioners are involved with CCM visits which make an impact on health indicators, like adherence and medication safety [66,67]. In another study, pharmacists proved that they could reduce the overall drug cost and increase the quality of care through medication management [68].

Community-based pharmacist practitioners also offer chronic care management sometimes known as disease management for chronic disease such as diabetes, hypertension, hyperlipidemia, heart failure, asthma, or hepatitis C [69]. Additionally, community-based pharmacists offer anticoagulation services. These chronic care management services may or may not be offered under collaborative practice agreements [21]. Some of these services may even be offered outside of the four walls of the community pharmacy in places such as barbershops [70]. Furthermore, the community-based pharmacist practitioner can use CLIA-waived tests for monitoring chronic disease states or these tests may be offered in the pharmacy without any association management services. These tests may include pharmacogenomics tests for ensuring patients are taking appropriate therapy. Community-based pharmacists are using saliva testing for biodentical hormone replacement therapy services.

3.2.4. Acute Care Management

Antibiotic resistance is one of the largest global health problems leading to extended inpatient hospitals stays, higher medical costs, and increased mortality [71]. Community-based pharmacist practitioners are well positioned to serve as gatekeepers for antibiotic prescribing due to their considerable training and knowledge of infectious disease pathophysiology, antibiotic indication, dosing, and appropriate length of treatment [72]. In addition to being competent antimicrobial stewards, community-based pharmacist practitioners' role in curbing antimicrobial resistance is expanding to increase patient access to care through physician-led collaborative practice agreements and CLIA waived POCT [73]. In community pharmacy-based CLIA-waived testing facilities, community-based pharmacist practitioners can screen for and treat acute infectious diseases, such as influenza A/B, Group A streptococcus (GAS) and *Helicobacter pylori*, decreasing time to therapy for patients [74].

It has been reported that patients who present with influenza-like symptoms and are not tested for influenza are twice as likely to be prescribed antiviral therapy [75]. The increasing prevalence of CLIA-waived POCT and rapid diagnostic testing (RDT) in community pharmacies can help mitigate unnecessary antimicrobial prescribing. A report on midwestern pharmacies offering influenza testing showed that of the 121 patients who presented to a community-pharmacy with influenza-like symptoms and screened for influenza, 75 patients were tested, with 8 tests yielding positive results. Seven of the eight patients who tested positive received a prescription for oseltamivir and six of these seven patients reported feeling better during 24–48-h follow-up call [76]. Initiation of appropriate antiviral therapy for patients infected with influenza is time sensitive. Community-based pharmacist practitioners offer extended hours and patients can access appropriate antiviral medications quicker by seeing a pharmacist for diagnosis and treatment than when a patient is referred to another provider [77].

Analogous to influenza POCT in community-based pharmacies is group A streptococcus (GAS) POCT, which has also grown as a community-based pharmacist provided service. Community-based pharmacist practitioners need to be conscientious antimicrobial stewards because adult pharyngitis is most commonly viral, yet it has been shown that up to 75% of patients are prescribed antibiotics [78]. *Streptococcus pyogenes* is the most common bacterial cause of adult pharyngitis, accounting for up to 15% of cases, indicating that antibiotics are only warranted for roughly 15% these adult pharyngitis cases [78]. GAS POCT can be implemented alongside influenza POCT within the same community-based pharmacies using a similar collaborative care model for managing patients that was used in several midwestern pharmacies [79]. Community pharmacy-based GAS POCT was found to be more cost effective for the diagnosis and treatment than physician-based diagnosis and treatment, in addition to being more convenient for patients. [80].

Community-based pharmacist practitioners are capable of managing and prescribing for other common acute diseases such as uncomplicated urinary tract infections (UTIs) [81]. Evidence is lacking in the US, but in a prospective trial in 39 community pharmacies in Canada, community pharmacists were able to achieve symptom resolution in 88.9% of patients who presented to the pharmacy with symptoms of a UTI, with high patient satisfaction [82]. In the United Kingdom, community pharmacists were able to screen patients for UTIs and provide trimethoprim to 73% patients, with the remaining patients receiving symptomatic management. Outcomes of this study suggest that community pharmacists can provide appropriate treatment for patients with uncomplicated UTIs and increase patient access to care [83].

3.2.5. Education

Community-based pharmacist practitioners are well prepared to educate patients about medications, wellness, and prevention and medical conditions. Community-based pharmacist practitioners are playing an even larger role within their community by promoting health and wellness programs. Pharmacists are coaching on healthy eating habits, assisting with smoking cessation, and combating sedentary lifestyles [84]. The Centers for Disease Control and Prevention (CDC) recognize community pharmacists' role in preventive health care and have even called upon them to facilitate the National Diabetes Prevention Program (DPP) throughout the country [85]. Community-based pharmacist practitioners are also providing accredited diabetes education programs through either the American Diabetes Association or American Association of Diabetes Educators [86].

3.2.6. Other Services

Community-based pharmacist practitioners are serving as transitions-of-care (TOC) champions when patients are discharged from inpatient settings to help minimize gaps in care, reduce hospital readmissions, and resolve medication-related problems. When community pharmacies provided medication management services within one week of hospital discharge to patients with congestive heart failure, chronic obstructive pulmonary disease, or pneumonia, the 30-day readmission rate was 13.1% less in patients compared to patients who did not receive the service [87]. Through community pharmacy-based TOC programs, patients' risk of readmission can be decreased by 28% and 31.9% at 30 and 180 days, respectively, when pharmacists are involved in discharge counseling, medication reconciliation, and telephone follow-up [88]. Through the utilization of pharmacists during health care setting transitions for patients, community-based pharmacist practitioners are capable of improving patient outcomes and reducing hospital readmission rates.

Teleheath is rapidly advancing, which provides increasing opportunities for community-based pharmacist practitioners to be involved in remote pharmacy operations and patient care. Virtual pharmacist services is a new innovative practice model that has been shown to improve patient outcomes and minimize costs [65,67,89]. When patients at risk for medication-related problems were referred to a telepharmacist for chronic care management at an outpatient family medicine clinic, pharmacists generated 200 interventions over a 6-month period. The physicians accepted 37.5% of the pharmacist's recommendations, over half of which were related to medication safety [65]. Pharmacists have also been able to show effective management of hypertension and diabetes through telepharmacy by providing medication management and lifestyle modification recommendations with medication adjustments [90,91].

Community-based pharmacist practitioners collaborate with local associations and public health agencies to provide education and serve as a resource during public health emergencies. In fact, community-based pharmacist practitioners are well positioned to respond to emergencies due to their wide distribution across urban, suburban, and rural settings, and their easy access for patients. Proposed disaster-readiness roles of pharmacists include "clinical" and "other", with the clinical category referring to ambulatory care, community-based or outpatient clinic pharmacists with strong pharmacotherapy backgrounds, working in a variety of settings during a disaster such as a shelter, hospital, clinic, or outreach site [92]. In an evaluation of community healthcare providers ability to respond to emergencies resulting from bioterrorist attacks, pharmacists scored higher (78.5%) than physicians (71.3%) and nurses (66.5%) in their ability to demonstrate creative problem solving and flexible thinking to unusual situations [93].

Some community-based pharmacist practitioners have started a new patient care service that is involves administering an intradermal injection; tuberculin skin testing. The first report of pharmacists conducting tuberculin skin testing was in 2008 in a national grocery chain pharmacy where 18 tuberculin skin tests were administered over 11 months by two pharmacists and 17 of the 18 patients returned within the allotted time for their reading. The pharmacists felt that this service was relatively simple to integrate into workflow, with each test taking less than 10 min per patient and that it was an important public service opportunity [94]. In 2011, New Mexico pharmacists became authorized to prescribe, administer, and read tuberculin skin tests. Trained pharmacists in rural and urban New Mexico administered 606 tuberculin skin tests with 578 patients having appropriate follow-up to read the test. The authors attributed the high follow-up rates at the community pharmacies to convenience and accessible locations [95].

4. Innovation in the US and Global Impact

It is beyond the scope of this paper to provide a comprehensive review of global innovative community-based pharmacy practice. However, it is important to note that there is a global shift in community-based pharmacy from a dispensing retail to a health care provider practice [2]. No country has been able to transform community-based pharmacy practice completely as a sustainable health care destination without the product driving the business model. However, some countries like the US have made substantial progress in certain innovations. This provides an opportunity for community-based pharmacists practitioners to learn from practice innovations in other countries. In 2016, the International Pharmaceutical Federation published a report on the global impact of pharmacy-based immunization [96]. Pharmacists in Australia, Canada, England, Netherlands, and Scotland have made substantial progress in expanding the role of the community-based pharmacist [2]. Examples of services related to medication optimization include providing emergency refills, renewing or extending prescriptions, changing drug dosage or formulation, and making therapeutic substitution [2]. Furthermore, in Canada and the United Kingdom, community-based pharmacists are offering comprehensive minor ailment services [97,98]. New Zealand has an opportunity to expand community-based pharmacy services through a new funding model [99]. Changes to qualifications of pharmacists in South Africa which will include prescriptive authority will facilitate expansion of community-based pharmacy services [100]. The United Arab Emirates is implementing initiatives to allow expansion of the role of the community pharmacist; however, other countries in the Middle East continue to struggle with practice expansion [101]. The expansion of the role of the community-based pharmacist has been inconsistent in Asia, but emerging with health assessment, health promotion and medication use reviews [102]. The Pharmaceutical Group of European Union (PGEU) issued a 2030 vision for community-based pharmacy in Europe including expanding pharmacy services to increase access and optimize medication use as part of collaborating primary care team, integrating digital health solutions in practice, showing leadership in personalized medicine, reducing the burden of chronic disease through wellness and prevention and education, identifying public health threats, and providing innovative and effective services to reduce the burden on other services [103]. These components of practice expansion are similar to innovations reported in this manuscript for the US community-based pharmacy practice.

5. Conclusions

Community-based pharmacist practitioners in the US are developing and delivering services that meet the needs of patients within the communities they serve. However, there are challenges to overcome but which may be accomplished through policy change, education and training, collaboration, and technology. Through the engagement of community-based pharmacist practitioners, patients will have additional access to more than 180,000 community-based pharmacists, substantially increasing provider capacity, improving care, and reducing overall health care costs to the US health care system.

Author Contributions: All authors contributed to the writing of the manuscript.

Funding: This research received no external funding.

Conflicts of Interest: The authors declare no conflict of interest.

References

1. Policarpo, V.; Romano, S.; António, J.H.; Correia, T.S.; Costa, S. A new model for pharmacies? Insights from a quantitative study regarding the public's perceptions. *BMC Health Serv. Res.* **2019**, *19*, 186. [CrossRef] [PubMed]
2. Mossialos, E.; Courtin, E.; Naci, H.; Benrimoj, S.; Bouvy, M.; Farris, K.; Noyce, P.; Sketris, I. From "retailers" to health care providers: Transforming the role of community pharmacists in chronic disease management. *Health Policy* **2015**, *119*, 628–639. [CrossRef] [PubMed]
3. Centers for Medicaid and Medicare Services. National Health Expenditure Projections 2018–2027. Available online: https://www.cms.gov/Research-Statistics-Data-and-Systems/Statistics-Trends-and-Reports/NationalHealthExpendData/Downloads/ForecastSummary.pdf (accessed on 13 April 2019).
4. Avalere Health. Exploring Pharmacists' Role in a Changing Health Care Environment. May 2014. Available online: https://avalere.com/insights/exploring-pharmacists-role-in-a-changing-healthcare-environment (accessed on 26 May 2019).
5. American Association of Medical Colleges. Workforce Projections. Available online: https://www.aamc.org/newsroom/newsreleases/458074/2016_workforce_projections_04052016.html (accessed on 25 May 2019).
6. United States Bureau of Labor Statistics. Available online: https://www.bls.gov/oes/current/oes291051.htm (accessed on 24 May 2019).
7. US Department of Health and Human Services. Reforming America's Healthcare System through Choice and Competition. Available online: https://www.hhs.gov/sites/default/files/Reforming-Americas-Healthcare-System-Through-Choice-and-Competition.pdf (accessed on 13 April 2019).
8. Moose, J.; Branham, A. Pharmacists as Influencers of Patient Adherence. *Pharmacy Times*. 21 August 2014. Available online: https://www.pharmacytimes.com/publications/directions-in-pharmacy/2014/august2014/pharmacists-as-influencers-of-patient-adherence- (accessed on 13 April 2019).
9. Bennett, M.; Goode, J.V. Recognition of community-based pharmacist practitioners: Essential health care providers. *J. Am. Pharm. Assoc.* **2016**, *56*, 580–583. [CrossRef] [PubMed]
10. Erickson, A. Community-Based Pharmacists Extend Care Far Beyond the Pharmacy Walls. Available online: https://www.pharmacytoday.org/article/S1042-0991(16)31227-0/fulltext (accessed on 25 May 2019).
11. Beatty, S.J.; Westberg, S.M.; Sharma, A. Professional responsibilities reported by pharmacists completing residencies in community-based settings. *J. Am. Pharm. Assoc.* **2019**, *59*, 217–221.e2. [CrossRef] [PubMed]
12. Andreski, M.; Myers, M.; Gainer, K.; Pudlo, A. The Iowa new practice model: Advancing technician roles to increase pharmacists' time to provide patient care services. *J. Am. Pharm. Assoc.* **2018**, *58*, 268–274.e1. [CrossRef] [PubMed]
13. Fleagle Miller, R.; Cesarz, J.; Rough, S. Evaluation of community pharmacy tech-check-tech as a strategy for practice advancement. *J. Am. Pharm. Assoc.* **2018**, *58*, 652–658. [CrossRef]
14. Schommer, J.C.; Olson, A.W.; Isetts, B.J. Transforming community-based pharmacy practice through financially sustainable centers for health and personal care. *J. Am. Pharm. Assoc.* **2019**, *59*, 306–309. [CrossRef]
15. McDonough, R. Embracing a New Business Model for Community-Based Pharmacy Practice. Pharmacy Today. Available online: https://www.pharmacytoday.org/article/S1042-0991(17)30604-7/fulltext (accessed on 25 May 2019).
16. Hughes, C.A.; Guirguis, L.M.; Wong, T.; Ng, K.; Ing, L.; Fisher, K. Influence of pharmacy practice on community pharmacists' integration of medication and lab value information from electronic health records. *J. Am. Pharm. Assoc.* **2011**, *51*, 591–598. [CrossRef]
17. Faiella, A.; Casper, K.A.; Bible, L.; Seifert, J. Implementation and use of an electronic health record in a charitable community pharmacy. *J. Am. Pharm. Assoc.* **2019**, *59*, S110–S117. [CrossRef]
18. Pharmacist ECare Plan Initiative. Available online: https://www.ecareplaninitiative.com/ (accessed on 26 May 2019).
19. Nguyen, E.; Holmes, J.T. Pharmacist-provided services: Barriers to demonstrating value. *J. Am. Pharm. Assoc.* **2019**, *59*, 117–120. [CrossRef]

20. Schindel, T.J.; Yuksel, N.; Breault, R.; Daniels, J.; Varnhagen, S.; Hughes, C.A. Perceptions of pharmacists' roles in the era of expanding scopes of practice. *Res. Soc. Adm. Pharm.* **2017**, *13*, 148–161. [CrossRef] [PubMed]

21. Adams, A.J.; Weaver, K.K. The continuum of pharmacist prescriptive authority. *Ann. Pharmacother.* **2016**, *50*, 778–784. [CrossRef] [PubMed]

22. Catizone, C.; Maine, L.; Menighan, T. Charting Accreditation's Future: Continuing our collaboration to create practice-ready, team oriented patient care pharmacists. *Am. J. Pharm. Educ.* **2013**, *77*, 43. [CrossRef] [PubMed]

23. Feehan, M.; Walsh, M.; Godin, J.; Sundwall, D.; Munger, M.A. Patient preferences for healthcare delivery through community pharmacy settings in the USA: A discrete choice study. *J. Clin. Pharm. Ther.* **2017**, *42*, 738–749. [CrossRef] [PubMed]

24. Easter, J.C.; DeWalt, D.A. The medication optimization value proposition aligning teams and education to improve care. *NCMJ* **2017**, *3*, 168–172. [CrossRef]

25. Nguyen, E.; Sobieraj, D. The impact of appointment based medication synchronization on medication taking behaviour and health outcomes: A systematic review. *J. Clin. Pharm. Ther.* **2017**, *42*, 404–413. [CrossRef]

26. Holdford, D.A.; Inocencio, T.J. Adherence and persistence associated with an appointment-based medication synchronization program. *J. Am. Pharm. Assoc.* **2013**, *53*, 576–583. [CrossRef]

27. Kadia, N.K.; Schroeder, M.N. Community pharmacy-based adherence programs and the role of the pharmacy technician: A review. *J. Pharm. Technol.* **2015**, *31*, 51–57. [CrossRef]

28. Mooney, E.V.; Hamper, J.G.; Willis, R.T.; Farinha, T.L.; Ricchetti, C.A. Evaluating patient satisfaction with pharmacist-administered long-acting injectable antipsychotics in a community pharmacy. *J. Am. Pharm. Assoc.* **2018**, *58*, S24–S29.e2. [CrossRef]

29. McNab, D.; Bowie, P.; Ross, A.; MacWalter, G.; Ryan, M.; Morrison, J. Systematic review and meta-analysis of the effectiveness of pharmacist-led medication reconciliation in the community after hospital discharge. *BMJ Qual. Saf.* **2018**, *27*, 308–320. [CrossRef]

30. Mueller, S.; Sponsler, K.; Kripalani, S.; Schnipper, J. Hospital-based medication reconciliation practices: A systematic review. *Arch. Int. Med.* **2012**, *172*, 1057–1069. [CrossRef]

31. Centers for Medicare and Medicaid Services. Hospital Readmissions Reduction Program. Available online: https://www.cms.gov/medicare/quality-initiatives-patient-assessment-instruments/value-based-programs/hrrp/hospital-readmission-reduction-program.html (accessed on 26 May 2019).

32. Kilcup, M.; Schultz, D.; Carlson, J.; Wilson, B. Postdischarge pharmacist medication reconciliation: Impact on readmission rates and financial savings. *J. Am. Pharm. Assoc.* **2013**, *53*, 78–84. [CrossRef]

33. Ravn-Nielsen, L.V.; Duckert, M.L.; Lund, M.L.; Henriksen, J.P.; Nielsen, M.L.; Eriksen, C.S.; Buck, T.C.; Pottegard, A.; Hansen, M.R.; Hallas, J. Effect of an in-hospital multifaceted clinical pharmacist intervention on the risk of readmission: A randomized clinical trial. *JAMA Int. Med.* **2018**, *178*, 375–382. [CrossRef]

34. Foster, A.; Gatewood, S.; Kaefer, T.; Goode, J. Decision-maker and staff perceptions of the pharmacist's role in transitions of care programs. *J. Am. Pharm. Assoc.* **2019**, *59*, S101–S105. [CrossRef]

35. Paul, S.; DiDonato, K.L.; Liu, Y. Rural health systems' perceptions of referral to community pharmacists during transitions of care. *J. Am. Pharm. Assoc.* **2016**, *56*, 562–567. [CrossRef]

36. Joint Commission of Pharmacy Practitioners. Medication Management Services (MMS) Definition and Key Points. 14 March 2018. Available online: https://jcpp.net/wp-content/uploads/2018/05/Medication-Management-Services-Definition-and-Key-Points-Version-1.pdf (accessed on 31 May 2019).

37. Patient-Centered Primary Collaborative. The Patient-Centered Medical Home: Integrating Comprehensive Medication Management to Optimize Patient Outcomes. June 2012. Available online: https://www.pcpcc.org/sites/default/files/media/medmanagement.pdf (accessed on 26 May 2019).

38. Viswanathan, M.; Kahwati, L.C.; Golin, C.E.; Blalock, S.; Coker-Schwimmer, E.; Posey, R.; Lohr, K.N. Medication therapy management interventions in outpatient settings. *JAMA Int. Med.* **2015**, *175*, 76–87. [CrossRef]

39. Isetts, B.J.; Schondelmeyer, S.W.; Artz, M.B.; Lenarz, L.A.; Heaton, A.H.; Wadd, W.B.; Brown, L.M.; Cipolle, R.J. Clinical and economic outcomes of medication therapy management services: The Minnesota experience. *J. Am. Pharm. Assoc.* **2008**, *48*, 203–211. [CrossRef]

40. Doucette, W.R.; McDonough, R.P.; Klepser, D.; McCarthy, R. Comprehensive medication therapy management: Identifying and resolving drug-related issues in a community pharmacy. *Clin. Ther.* **2005**, *27*, 1104–1111. [CrossRef]

41. Kehrer, J.; James, D. The Role of Pharmacists and Pharmacy Education in Point-of-Care Testing. *Am. J. Pharm. Educ.* **2016**, *80*, 129.

42. Buss, V.H.; Naunton, M. Analytical quality and effectiveness of point of care testing in community pharmacies: A systematic literature review. *Res. Soc. Adm. Pharm.* **2019**, *15*, 483–495. [CrossRef]

43. Klepser, M.E.; Adams, A.J.; Srnis, P.; Mazzucco, M.; Klepser, D. U.S. community pharmacies as CLIA-waived facilities: Prevalence, dispersion, and impact on patient access to testing. *Res. Soc. Adm. Pharm.* **2016**, *12*, 614–621. [CrossRef]

44. Gubbins, P.O.; Klepser, M.E.; Dering-Anderson, A.M.; Bauer, K.A.; Darin, K.M.; Klepser, S.; Matthias, K.R.; Scarsi, K. Point-of-care testing for infectious disease: Opportunities, barriers, and considerations in community pharmacy. *J. Am. Pharm. Assoc.* **2014**, *54*, 163–171. [CrossRef]

45. Weidle, P.J.; Lecher, S.; Botts, L.W.; Jones, L.; Spach, D.H.; Alvarez, J.; Jones, R.; Thomas, V. HIV testing in community pharmacies and retail clinics: A model to expand access to screening for HIV infection. *J. Am. Pharm. Assoc.* **2014**, *54*, 486–492. [CrossRef]

46. Haga, S.B.; Moaddeb, J.; Mills, R.; Voora, D. Assessing feasibility of delivering pharmacogenetic testing in a community pharmacy setting. *Pharmacogenomics* **2017**, *18*, 327–335. [CrossRef]

47. Hogue, M.D.; Grabenstein, J.D.; Foster, S.L.; Rothholz, M.C. Pharmacist involvement with immunizations: A decade of professional advancement. *J. Am. Pharm. Assoc.* **2006**, *46*, 168–179. [CrossRef]

48. Isenor, J.E.; Edwards, N.T.; Alia, T.A.; Slaytor, K.L.; MacDougall, D.M.; McNeil, S.A.; Bowles, S.K. Impact of pharmacists as immunizers on vaccination rates: A systematic review and meta-analysis. *Vaccine* **2016**, *34*, 5708–5723. [CrossRef]

49. Baroy, J.; Chung, D.; Frisch, R.; Apgar, D.; Slack, M.K. The impact of pharmacist immunization programs on adult immunization rates: A systematic review and meta-analysis. *J. Am. Pharm. Assoc.* **2016**, *56*, 418–426. [CrossRef]

50. Gatewood, S.B.S.; Stanley, D.D.; Goode, J.R. Implementation of a Pre-Travel Health Clinic in a Supermarket Pharmacy. *J. Am. Pharm. Assoc.* **2009**, *49*, 110–119. [CrossRef]

51. Hurley-Kim, K.; Goad, J.; Seed, S.; Hess, K.M. Pharmacy-Based Travel Health Services in the United States. *Pharmacy* **2018**, *7*, 5. [CrossRef]

52. Hess, K.M.; Dai, C.W.; Garner, B.; Law, A.V. Measuring outcomes of a pharmacist-run travel health clinic located in an independent community pharmacy. *J. Am. Pharm. Assoc.* **2010**, *50*, 174–180. [CrossRef]

53. Tran, D.; Gatewood, S.; Moczygemba, L.R.; Stanley, D.D.; Goode, J.V. Evaluating health outcomes following a pharmacist-provided comprehensive pretravel health clinic in a supermarket pharmacy. *J. Am. Pharm. Assoc.* **2015**, *55*, 143–152. [CrossRef]

54. Patwardhan, P.D.; Chewning, B.A. Tobacco users' perceptions of a brief tobacco cessation intervention in community pharmacies. *J. Am. Pharm. Assoc.* **2010**, *50*, 568–574. [CrossRef]

55. National Alliance of State Pharmacy Associations. Pharmacists Prescribing for Tobacco Cessation Medications. Available online: https://naspa.us/resource/tobacco-cessation/ (accessed on 26 May 2019).

56. National Alliance of State Pharmacy Associations. Pharmacists Authorized to Prescribe Birth Control in More States. Available online: https://naspa.us/2017/05/pharmacists-authorized-prescribe-birth-control-states/ (accessed on 26 May 2019).

57. Abouk, R.; Pacula, R.L.; Powell, D. Association between state laws facilitating pharmacy distribution of naloxone and risk of fatal overdose. *JAMA Int. Med.* **2019**, *179*, 805–811. [CrossRef]

58. Rosenthal, M.; Ward, L.M.; Teng, J.; Haines, S. Weight management counseling among community pharmacists: A scoping review. *Int. J. Pharm. Pract.* **2018**, *26*, 475–484. [CrossRef]

59. Mott, D.A.; Martin, B.; Breslow, R.; Michaels, B.; Kirchner, J.; Mahoney, J.; Margolis, A. The Development of a Community-Based, Pharmacist-Provided Falls Prevention MTM Intervention for Older Adults: Relationship Building, Methods, and Rationale. *Innov. Pharm.* **2014**, *5*, 140. [CrossRef]

60. Ferreri, S.P.; Greco, A.J.; Michaels, N.M.; O'Connor, S.K.; Chater, R.W.; Viera, A.J.; Faruki, H.; McLeod, H.L.; Roederer, M.W. Implementation of a pharmacogenomics service in a community pharmacy. *J. Am. Pharm. Assoc.* **2014**, *54*, 172–180. [CrossRef]

61. Nacopoulos, A.G.; Lewtas, A.J.; Ousterhout, N.M. Syringe exchange programs: Impact on injection drug users and the role of the pharmacist from a U.S. perspective. *J. Am. Pharm. Assoc.* **2010**, *50*, 148–157. [CrossRef]

62. Lystlund, S.; Stevens, E.; Planas, L.G.; Marcy, T.R. Patient participation in a clinic-based community pharmacy medication take-back program. *J. Am. Pharm. Assoc.* **2014**, *54*, 280–284. [CrossRef]

63. Shepard, J.E.; Bopp, J. Pharmacy-based care for perimenopausal and postmenopausal women. *J. Am. Pharm. Assoc.* **2002**, *42*, 700–711.

64. Evans, T.A.; Fable, P.H.; Ziegler, B. Community-pharmacist delivered Medicare Annual Wellness Visits within a family medicine practice. *J. Am. Pharm. Assoc.* **2017**, *57*, S247–S251. [CrossRef]

65. Department of Health and Human Services. Centers for Medicare & Medicaid Services. Chronic Care Management Service. Available online: www.cms.gov/outreach-and-education/medicare-learning-networkmln/mlnproducts/downloads/chroniccaremanagement.pdf (accessed on 24 May 2019).

66. American Pharmacists Association. Chronic Care Management (CCM): An Overview for Pharmacists. Available online: www.pharmacist.com/sites/default/files/CCM-An-Overview-forPharmacists-FINAL.pdf (accessed on 23 May 2019).

67. Taylor, A.M.; Bingham, J.; Schussel, K.; Axon, D.R.; Dickman, D.J.; Boesen, K.; Martin, R.; Warholak, T.L. Integrating innovative telehealth solutions into an interprofessional team-delivered chronic care management pilot program. *J. Manag. Care Spec. Pharm.* **2018**, *24*, 813–818. [CrossRef]

68. Johnson, M.; Jastrzab, R.; Tate, J.; Johnson, K.; Hall-Lipsy, E.; Martin, R.; Taylor, A.M.; Warholak, T. Evaluation of an academic-community partnership to implement MTM services in rural communities to improve pharmaceutical care for patients with diabetes and/or hypertension. *J. Manag. Care Spec. Pharm.* **2018**, *24*, 132–141. [CrossRef]

69. Armour, C.L.; Smith, L.; Krass, I. Community pharmacy, disease state management, and adherence to medication. *Dis. Manag. Health Outcomes* **2008**, *16*, 245–254. [CrossRef]

70. Victor, R.G.; Lynch, K.; Blyler, C.; Muhammed, E.; Handler, J.; Brettler, J.; Rashid, M.; Hsu, B.; Fox-Drew, D.; Moy, N.; et al. A cluster-randomized trial of blood-pressure reduction in black barbershops. *N. Engl. J. Med.* **2018**, *378*, 1291–1301. [CrossRef]

71. World Health Organization. Antibiotic Resistance Fact Sheet. 2018. Available online: https://www.who.int/news-room/fact-sheets/detail/antibiotic-resistance (accessed on 7 May 2019).

72. Essack, S.; Bell, J.; Shepard, A. Community pharmacists—leaders for antibiotic stewardship in respiratory tract infection. *J. Clin. Pharm. Ther.* **2018**, *43*, 302–307. [CrossRef]

73. Gubbins, P.O.; Klepser, M.E.; Adam, A.J.; Jacobs, D.M.; Percival, K.M.; Tallman, G.B. Potential for pharmacy-public health collaborations using pharmacy-based point-of-care testing services for infectious disease. *J. Public Health Manag. Pract.* **2017**, *23*, 593–600. [CrossRef]

74. Weber, N.C.; Klepser, M.E.; Akers, J.M.; Klepser, D.G.; Adams, A.J. Use of CLIA-waived point-of-care tests for infectious diseases in community pharmacies in the United States. *Expert Rev. Mol. Diagn.* **2016**, *16*, 253–264. [CrossRef]

75. Klepser, D.G.; Corn, C.E.; Schmidt, M.; Dering-Anderson, A.M.; Klepser, M.E. Health care resource utilization and costs for influenza-like illness among Midwestern health plan members. *J. Manag. Care Spec. Pharm.* **2015**, *21*, 568–573. [CrossRef]

76. Klepser, M.E.; Klepser, D.G.; Dering-Anderson, A.M.; Morse, J.A.; Smith, J.K.; Klepser, S.A. Effectiveness of a pharmacist-physician collaborative program to manage influenza-like illness. *J. Am. Pharm. Assoc.* **2016**, *56*, 14–21. [CrossRef]

77. Klepser, M.E.; Hagerman, J.K.; Klepser, S.A.; Bergman, S.J.; Klepser, D.G. A community pharmacy-based influenza screening and management program shortens time to treatment versus pharmacy screening with referral to standard of care. *Ill. Pharm.* **2014**, *76*, 12–18.

78. Klepser, D.G.; Klepser, M.E.; Dering-Anderson, A.M.; Morse, J.A.; Smith, J.K.; Klepser, S.A. Community pharmacist-physician collaborative streptococcal pharyngitis management program. *J. Am. Pharm. Assoc.* **2016**, *56*, 323–329. [CrossRef]

79. Klepser, D.G.; Klepser, M.E.; Smith, J.K.; Dering-Anderson, A.M.; Nelson, M.; Pohren, L.E. Utilization of influenza and streptococcal pharyngitis point-of-care testing in the community pharmacy practice setting. *Res. Soc. Adm. Pharm.* **2018**, *14*, 356–359. [CrossRef]

80. Klepser, D.G.; Bisanz, S.E.; Klepser, M.E. Cost-Effectiveness of pharmacist-provided treatment of adult pharyngitis. *Am. J. Manag. Care* **2012**, *4*, e145–e154.

81. Idaho Pharmacists can Prescribe more than 20 Categories of Medications. Pharmacy Today 2018. Available online: https://www.pharmacytoday.org/article/S1042-0991(18)31417-8/pdf (accessed on 26 May 2019).

82. Beahm, N.P.; Smyth, D.J.; Tsuyuki, R.T. Outcomes of urinary tract infection management by pharmacists (RxOUTMAP): A study of pharmacist prescribing and care in patients with uncomplicated urinary tract infections in the community. *Can. Pharm. J.* **2018**, *15*, 305–314. [CrossRef]

83. Booth, J.L.; Mullen, A.B.; Thomson, D.A.; Johnstone, C.; Galbraith, S.J.; Bryson, S.M.; McGovern, E.M. Antibiotic treatment of urinary tract infection by community pharmacists: A cross-sectional study. *Br. J. Gen. Pract.* **2013**, *63*, e244–e249. [CrossRef]

84. DiDonato, K.L.; May, J.R.; Lindsey, C.C. Impact of wellness coaching and monitoring services provided in a community pharmacy. *J. Am. Pharm. Assoc.* **2013**, *53*, 14–21. [CrossRef]

85. Centers for Disease Control and Prevention. Rx for the National Diabetes Prevention Program: Action Guide for Community Pharmacists. Centers for Disease Control and Prevention, US Dept of Health and Human Services: Atlanta, GA, USA, 2018. Available online: https://www.cdc.gov/diabetes/prevention/pdf/pharmacists-guide.pdf (accessed on 14 May 2019).

86. Ragucci, K.R.; Fermo, J.D.; Wessell, A.M.; Chumney, E.C. Effectiveness of pharmacist-administered diabetes mellitus education and management services. *Pharmacotherapy* **2005**, *25*, 1809–1816. [CrossRef]

87. Luder, H.R.; Frede, S.M.; Kirby, J.A.; Epplen, K.; Cavanaugh, T.; Martin-Boone, J.E.; Conrad, W.F.; Kuhlmann, D.; Heaton, P.C. TransitionRx: Impact of community pharmacy postdischarge medication therapy management on hospital readmission rate. *J. Am. Pharm. Assoc.* **2015**, *55*, 246–254. [CrossRef]

88. Ni, W.; Colayco, D.; Hasimoto, J.; Komoto, K.; Gowda, C.; Wearda, B.; McCombs, J. Impact of a pharmacy-based transitional care program on hospital readmissions. *Am. J. Manag. Care* **2017**, *23*, 170–176.

89. Garrelts, J.C.; Gagnon, M.; Eisenberg, C.; Moerer, J.; Carrithers, J. Impact of telepharmacy in a multihospital health system. *Am. J. Health Syst. Pharm.* **2010**, *67*, 1456–1462. [CrossRef]

90. Omboni, S.; Tenti, M. Telepharmacy for the management of cardiovascular patients in the community. *Trends Cardiovasc. Med.* **2019**, *29*, 109–117. [CrossRef]

91. Baker, J.W.; Forkum, W.; McNeal, J. Utilizing clinical video to improve access and optimize pharmacists' role in diabetes management. *J. Am. Pharm. Assocc.* **2019**, *59*, S63–S66. [CrossRef]

92. Pincock, L.L.; Montello, M.J.; Tarosky, M.J.; Pierce, W.F.; Edwards, C.W. Pharmacist readiness roles for emergency preparedness. *Am. J. Health Syst. Pharm.* **2011**, *68*, 620–623. [CrossRef]

93. Crane, J.S.; McCluskey, J.D.; Johnson, G.T.; Harbison, R.D. Assessment of community healthcare providers ability and willingness to respond to emergencies resulting from bioterrorist attacks. *J. Emerg. Trauma Shock* **2010**, *3*, 13–20. [CrossRef]

94. Hecox, N. Tuberculin skin testing by pharmacists in a grocery store setting. *J. Am. Pharm. Assoc.* **2008**, *48*, 86–91. [CrossRef]

95. Jakeman, B.; Gross, B.; Fortune, D.; Babb, S.; Tinker, D.; Bachyrycz, A. Evaluation of a pharmacist-performed tuberculosis testing initiative in New Mexico. *J. Am. Pham. Assoc.* **2015**, *55*, 307–312. [CrossRef]

96. International Pharmaceutical Federation (FIP). An overview of Current Pharmacy Impact on Immunization: A Global Report 2016. International Pharmaceutical Federation: The Hague, The Netherlands, 2016. Available online: https://www.fip.org/files/fip/publications/FIP_report_on_Immunisation.pdf (accessed on 29 July 2019).

97. Taylor, J.G.; Joubert, R. Pharmacist-led minor ailment programs: A Canadian perspective. *Int. J. Gen. Med.* **2016**, *9*, 291–302. [CrossRef]

98. Paudyal, V.; Watson, M.C.; Sach, T.; Porteous, T.; Bond, C.M.; Wright, D.J.; Cleland, J.; Barton, G.; Holland, R. Are pharmacy-based minor ailment schemes a substitute for other service providers? A systematic review. *Br. J. Gen. Pract.* **2013**, *63*, e472–e481. [CrossRef]

99. Smith, A.J.; Scahill, S.L.; Harrison, J.; Carroll, T.; Medlicott, N.J. Service provision in the wake of a new funding model for community pharmacy. *BMC Health Serv. Res.* **2018**, *18*, 307. [CrossRef]

100. Malangu, N. The future of community pharmacy practice in South Africa in the light of the proposed new qualification for pharmacists: Implications and challenges. *Glob. J. Health Sci.* **2014**, *6*, 226–233. [CrossRef]

101. Sadek, M.M.; Elnour, A.A.; Al Kabini, N.M.; Bhagavathula, A.S.; Baraka, M.A.; Aziz, A.M.; Shehab, A. Community pharmacy and the extended community pharmacist practice roles: The UAE experiences. *Saudi Pharm. J.* **2016**, *24*, 563–570. [CrossRef]
102. Lee, S.; Bell, J.S. Pharmaceutical Care in Asia. In *The Pharmacist Guide to Implementing Pharmaceutical Care*; Da Costa, F.A., van Mil, J.W.F., Alvarez-Risco, A., Eds.; Springer International: Cham, Switzerland, 2019.
103. Pharmaceutical Group of the European Union (PGEU). Pharmacy 2030: A Vision for Community Pharmacy in Europe. Belgium. Available online: https://www.pgeu.eu/wp-content/uploads/2019/03/Pharmacy-2030_-A-Vision-for-Community-Pharmacy-in-Europe.pdf (accessed on 29 July 2019).

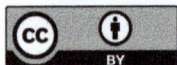

pharmacy

Review

Using Service Blueprints to Visualize Pharmacy Innovations

David A. Holdford

Center for Pharmacy Practice Innovation, School of Pharmacy, Virginia Commonwealth University, Richmond, VA 23298, USA; david.holdford@vcu.edu

Received: 10 April 2019; Accepted: 1 May 2019; Published: 8 May 2019

Abstract: Background: Applying the principles of service design can help pharmacists manage both the quality and patient perceptions of the services they provide. Service blueprints are a widely used service design tool that are rare in the healthcare literature. They can be used to design new services or revisit the design of established services. This paper describes service blueprints and their uses, and illustrates how to build one using an example. **Methods**: A blueprint is built for appointment-based medication synchronization services to illustrate the tool. **Conclusions**: Service blueprints permit pharmacists to better see and understand service processes. They clarify the process of service delivery and the roles of customers, service providers, and supporting services. They provide a way of depicting complex services in a concise visual way that communicates details at a glance. Pharmacists who utilize service blueprints can improve the consistency and quality of services provided, and they can increase the chance that every interaction with patients sends a positive message about the value of pharmacist services.

Keywords: serviced marketing; design thinking; medication synchronization; community pharmacists; innovation science; adherence; competitive advantage

1. Introduction

Pharmacy is a service profession. Although pharmacy practice revolves around the provision of a tangible product, the value of pharmacists lies in the intangible acts delivered along multiple touchpoints of the service experience. Yet, the public stills sees pharmacists as a dispenser of drugs due to the distinct nature of services [1–4].

When compared to tangible products, services are much harder to promote due to four distinct attributes they have known as the 4I's [5]. The first "I" is intangibility, which characterizes services as intangible actions or events. Services are intangible because they cannot be seen, held, or touched. Thus, their quality cannot be measured, tested, or verified in advance of the sale to ensure excellence. The second "I" is inconsistency in that no two service performances are identical—meaning that they vary from person to person, transaction to transaction, and even time to time. Service quality cannot be easily standardized because of the variations among interactions between buyer and seller. The third characteristic is inseparability—referring to the fact that the service provider, customers, and service itself are inseparable because the service is co-created by both the provider and the customer. Each participates in and determines the quality of the service experience. In pharmacy practice, the more engaged the patient, the more likely that better outcomes will occur. The fourth and final characteristic is inventory, which describes how face-to-face services cannot be put into inventory or on a shelf for later use. With online and mobile services, this characteristic is less applicable because technology now allows us to store many services electronically. The fourth "I" only applies to person-to-person services that are provided in a real-time, synchronous manner. When added up, the "4I's" of services present special challenges in marketing the value of pharmacists [5].

2. Challenges in Marketing Pharmacy Services

It is a challenge for pharmacists to get customers to appreciate and desire an intangible product they cannot see or touch. The intangible nature of pharmacist services makes it hard for consumers to mentally appreciate what pharmacists do. It is much easier for people to grasp the purpose of a drug than to comprehend the pharmacist services associated with that drug.

Intangible services are hard for consumers to assess. Although some aspects of pharmacy services are easy to evaluate (e.g., fast, friendly, inexpensive), the clinical and technical aspects of the service experience are difficult to evaluate even with extensive experience. For instance, consumers cannot typically tell if a pharmacist omits critical drug-related information during patient counseling, fails to screen for drug interactions, or misses a chance to intervene in avoiding a drug-related problem. Instead, patients tend to rely on variables that they can assess, such as how a pharmacist looks and acts [6].

The variability of pharmacist services also makes them a challenge to provide and assess. Pharmacists and pharmacy technicians are imperfect human beings whose service performances can vary from minute-to-minute with changing service conditions. Each service experience can be affected by a host of factors including the atmospherics of the work environment, the engagement of patients, the characteristics of individual pharmacists and technicians, and the workload. Demand for service varies throughout the day and week; there are times when business is relatively slow and other times when it gets quite hectic. It is a problem to synchronize customers' demand for services with the availability of pharmacy personnel to serve them. When combined with the fact that most pharmacist services are performed behind the scenes out of view of the customer, patients have an uneven and unclear understanding of the value of what a pharmacist does.

Applying the principles of service design can help pharmacists manage both the quality and patient perceptions of the service provided [7,8]. Service design is the process of planning and organizing the customer service experience using a number of methods and tools derived from disciplines as diverse as ethnography, systems engineering, management science, and informatics. Service design tools and methods typically attempt to portray services visually, using flow diagrams of the customers, front-facing service providers, and supporting individuals and processes. An established service design tool that would benefit pharmacists is the service blueprint [9].

3. Service Blueprints

Service blueprints are pictures or maps of service processes intended to help providers and service marketers to design, deliver, and manage new and established service offerings [10]. They depict the service process and the roles of consumers, service providers, and supporting services involved. These visual depictions help improve the delivery of pharmacy services by identifying gaps and potential points of failure in processes. They are able to improve communications between consumers, pharmacists, support staff, and backstage services by mapping out the various points of contact throughout the service process. Service blueprints can visually communicate complex service processes to stakeholders more clearly and efficiently than verbal descriptions of the services.

Although widely used and accepted by service designers in many industries, evidence of the use of service blueprints is lacking in pharmacy. Holdford and Kennedy [9] used service blueprints in describing the dispensing process for a new prescription and for a smoking cessation program. Other than that single instance, no other mention of service blueprints can be found in the pharmacy literature. This paper will describe how to build service blueprints and discuss how they can be used by pharmacists and when.

4. Uses of Service Blueprints

Service blueprints can be used whenever there is interest in improving a service experience. It can be used to design new services or revisit the design of established services. A major benefit of developing a service blueprint is that it forces pharmacists to conduct a detailed analysis of each step in the service process. It challenges pharmacists to question the value of each step and clarify the roles of everyone involved. Pharmacists who utilize service blueprints can improve the consistency and quality of services provided, and they can increase the chance that every interaction with patients sends a positive message about the value of pharmacist services.

Blueprints can be used in research to provide explicit details of interventions. A clearly written blueprint can be used in implementation science to allow comparisons at a glance of the exact nature of service innovations in comparison to the status quo. They are also helpful in describing the competitive advantage of one innovation over another, allowing pharmacists to develop service offerings that are sustainable over time [11].

Service blueprints are especially useful in designing complex services that might include multiple people, processes, and channels of communication. The greater the complexity, the increased likelihood of miscommunication, fumbled handoffs between individuals, and lack of accountability between people. A blueprint can clarify problems and coordinate complicated processes.

Finally, blueprints can be used to promote a positive image of pharmacists [7,9]. Because customers often have difficulty evaluating pharmacist services due to the intangible nature of services, they look for tangible clues to quality. Tangible clues are things such as signs, parking, landscaping, cleanliness, advertising, pharmacy layout, and how service personnel are dressed. Service blueprints can be used to identify these visual and physical aspects of services that customers often use as tangible cues of quality. By seeing services from the customer's perspective, pharmacists can ensure that these tangible cues send the same positive message of professionalism delivered by other touchpoints of the service experience.

5. Components of a Service Blueprint

There are no concrete rules for designing service blueprints allowing for a lot of flexibility in their purpose and use. However, most service blueprints have the following key components [12]: customer actions, "frontstage" contact employee actions, "backstage" contact employee actions, and support processes—as explained below and illustrated in Figure 1.

Customer actions. These are actions performed by the customer when interacting with a service provider. "Customers" can be any recipient of the service including patients, family caregivers, physicians, and nurses, depending on the process. Customer actions associated with a pharmacy visit can be contacting the pharmacy website prior to the visit, driving to the pharmacy, dropping off a prescription, providing information to the pharmacist, waiting, receiving the prescription along with counseling, and leaving the pharmacy. Each customer action is a touchpoint or moment-of-truth where customers judge the quality of pharmacy services and make decisions about whether to continue visiting the pharmacy in the future. The number of customer actions and the level of detail about each depends on the depth of the analysis desired.

Frontstage actions. These are the service actions that are directly visible to the customer. They can be actions between the customer and service personnel or with technology, such as a website or mobile app. Frontstage actions associated with a pharmacy visit could include interfacing with the pharmacy website prior to the visit, talking to pharmacy personnel throughout the steps of the dispensing process, and a follow-up phone call to help resolve any concerns the patient has about their medications. Frontstage actions do not always match every customer action. Some customer actions, like waiting for a prescription to be filled, are things that the customer does alone.

Backstage actions. These are any actions done for the customer that are not visible. Backstage actions in a pharmacy might include professional decisions made by pharmacists (e.g., checking the patient profile for drug allergies, interactions, and duplicate medications), consultations with physicians about therapy, resolving insurance claims, and remote filling of prescriptions.

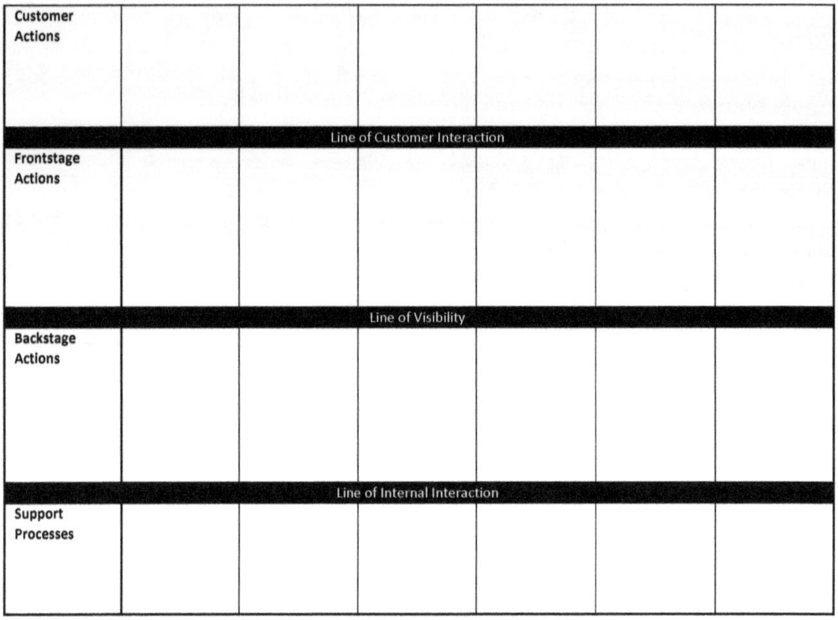

Figure 1. Basic components of a service blueprint.

Support processes. Support processes are any actions that support frontstage and backstage actions in service delivery. For pharmacists, these might include computer support services, billing, prescription claims adjudication, web design, and inventory control.

In service blueprints, key components of the blueprint are separated by three horizontal lines: the line of interaction, the line of visibility, and the line of internal interaction (Figure 1). The line of interaction is where customers and providers interact. Service encounters occur wherever a vertical line crosses the line of interaction. The line of visibility separates frontstage contact employee actions and backstage employee actions. Actions below this line are invisible to the customer. This line is critical because patients' image of a pharmacist is determined to a great extent by what they see the pharmacist do. If the patient's primary view is of the pharmacist counting and pouring, then the image of pharmacists will be consistent with that view. The line of internal interaction separates frontline employees from supporting individuals. Any action that crosses this line indicates a process that supports the frontline employee.

Optional Components of Service Blueprints

Additional components can be added to service blueprints depending on the purpose and goals of completing one. These components include physical evidence, arrows, and time.

Physical evidence. This describes the tangible features of each step in the service process that might influence a customer's perception of the service experience and service firm. Physical evidence includes the dress of service employees, the signage in the pharmacy, location, advertising, website design, delivery vehicles, and pharmacy layout. These and other forms of tangible evidence set expectations of service and influence evaluation of service quality. Clarifying the physical evidence of services can help ensure a consistent message across all elements of the service experience.

Arrows. Arrows are used to visualize relationships between key components of the blueprints. Arrows are used to indicate dependent relationships between customer and service provider actions. Single arrows indicate linear one-way relationships and double arrows signify collaborative two-way relationships.

Time. Time can be added to service blueprints to map out the amount of time needed for the total service experience or elements of it. This can be useful in estimating personnel costs in providing services and estimating the cost effectiveness of each step in the process.

6. Building a Blueprint

Building a service blueprint starts by developing an intimate understanding of the customers' service experience as well as a clear delineation of all of the people, processes, and systems involved. Whether the pharmacy service experience is face-to-face, online, via an app, over the phone, or via multiple service channels, a service blueprint can be used to map out the process.

Service blueprints can be developed using a provider-centered or a customer-centered perspective. Provider-centered perspectives start by mapping out the details of the service delivery process and then seeing where customers interact with this process. Provider-centered perspectives might be taken when analyzing an established service for gaps, redundancies, and other inefficiencies in delivery. A customer-centered approach starts by mapping out the service experience from the customer's perspective. It begins by outlining the points of contact between customers and the service—customer experiences with the pharmacy parking lot, the pharmacy building itself, signage, website, phone calls, printed bag, self-service machines, and contact with frontline employees like clerks, technicians, and pharmacists. Each time a customer interacts with a touchpoint, they have a service encounter that is mapped on the blueprint. The following description of building a service blueprint will use a customer-centered perspective.

The process of building a customer-centered service blueprint commences by asking what the customer hopes to achieve by interacting with a pharmacy service. The blueprint will vary depending on whether the visit is to fill a prescription, ask advice, enroll in a smoking cessation program, seek a nonprescription medication, or some other reason. Another question to be asked is the breadth and level of detail desired in mapping the service. An entire service process (e.g., dispensing) can be mapped, or the focus can be on a specific component of the process (e.g., patient counseling). Once these decisions are made, the blueprint is built through the following steps [12], which will be illustrated using the service blueprint illustrating an appointment-based medication synchronization program shown in Figure 2 [13].

1. Draw a template similar to the one in Figure 1 delineating the components of the service blueprint including lines of interaction and any optional components like physical evidence and time. Note that arrows can only be added as the actions are added.
2. Map the customer's journey through the service experience. From the customer's perspective, chart each action and choice made by the customer and place them sequentially in the customer actions of the blueprint template. For the appointment-based medication synchronization program in Figure 2, customer actions are patient learns details of the program, signs a contract, brings in prescriptions to the pharmacy to choose synch date, participates in establishing an appointment and adherence plan, receives a monthly call prior to picking up the medications, and receives the medications and discusses any issues with adherence or therapy.
3. Map frontstage actions. List all of the visible points of contact between the customer and specific service personnel, technologies (e.g., website), or processes. They should generally match the temporal sequence of the customer's journey throughout the service process although there may not always be a matching frontstage action with each customer action. For the program in Figure 2, frontstage actions are a discussion of the program with patients, having the patient sign the contract, the pharmacist conducting a comprehensive medication review, the cocreation of a treatment plan, a reminder call, and the interaction with the patient when they visit the pharmacy.
4. Map backstage actions. List all of the service actions which are invisible to customers. In many cases, these are actions in support of frontstage actions but sometimes they involve interactions with other healthcare professionals, healthcare insurers, and other stakeholders.

5. Map internal support activities. Support activities may serve either frontstage or backstage actions. In Figure 2, internal support activities serve both frontstage and backstage actions and consist of support from information technology, marketing, website design, and the business office.

6. Add additional details as needed including physical evidence, arrows, and time. The blueprint in Figure 2 has single arrows to illustrate one-way relationships (e.g., patient signs the ABMS contract and gives it to a technician or pharmacist). Double arrows illustrate two-way relationships where both customer and provider collaborate in the task (e.g., establishing a patient appointment and adherence plan). Note that some arrows may cross more than one line of interaction.

Customer Actions	Patient learns details of ABMS program	Patient signs ABMS contract	Patient brings new and/or refill prescriptions to pharmacy to choose synch date	Patient appointment and adherence plan is established	Patient receives monthly call prior to picking up the meds	Patient receives meds and discusses any issues with adherence or therapy
Line of Customer Interaction						
Frontstage Actions	Technician or pharmacist discusses program with patients or patient learns from website	Technician or pharmacist takes signed contract and forwards it to business office	Pharmacist conducts comprehensive medication review	Pharmacist and patient co-create a treatment plan	Reminder call by technician to resolve issues and set time when prescription will be ready	Pharmacist gives medication and probes for patient concerns or issue
Line of Visibility						
Backstage Actions		Contract filed and entered by business office	Documentation of comprehensive medication review		Remote filling of prescription and delivery to pharmacy on synched date	
Line of Internal Interaction						
Support Processes	Information technologies and marketing personnel develop website and promotional messaging	Physician, insurance company, and business office coordinate enrollment		Physician, insurance company, and business office coordinate treatment plan and financing	Physician, insurance company, and pharmacy coordinate on changes	Payment and billing by business office

Figure 2. Service blueprint of an appointment-based medication synchronization (ABMS) program.

7. Managerial Uses of Service Blueprints

The process of completing service blueprints requires pharmacists to clarify each step of the service experience. This process often leads to obvious opportunities for improving service delivery. Blueprints might suggest a need for minor improvements or a complete overhaul of the service system. The following is a list of actions that might be taken in response to an analysis of a service blueprint:

- Standardize service delivery by ensuring every frontstage, backstage, and support action is consistently provided. Time-and-motion studies and quality improvement cycles can assist in this standardization.
- Identify added service steps that might appeal to other customer segments. For instance, some segments might benefit from comprehensive medication reviews in appointment-based medication synchronization while others may not need or want it.
- Incorporate physical evidence into marketing communications plans. Although some pharmacists only see marketing communications in terms of paid advertising, every touchpoint in the service delivery process is a way of communicating a message of quality to patients. Therefore, cues to quality should be identified within the service experience and changed if needed to provide the messaging desired.

- Simplify service delivery. Look at every step of the process and remove any that do not add value.
- Identify those moments of truth that drive customer perceptions of the service process. There may only be a few touchpoints that drive loyalty to a pharmacy. Make certain that delivery at those touchpoints exceeds customer expectations.

8. Conclusions

Service blueprints permit pharmacists to better see and understand service processes. It clarifies the process of service delivery and the roles of customers, service providers, and supporting services. It breaks down the service into components and arranges them according to their purpose.

Service blueprints are rare in healthcare although they can be used in implementation research, interprofessional service delivery, business modeling, quality improvement interventions, and outcomes studies. They provide a way of depicting complex services in a concise visual way that communicates details at a glance. Services blueprints also use a customer-centered approach to design in which each customer action is matched to service providers and processes. When combined with physical cues to quality, pharmacists can send a consistent positive message to customers.

Service blueprints force a careful analysis of each step in the service process and help communicate that information to people such as the frontline employees who help determine its success. When everyone in the service process engages in the development of blueprints, they can understand each step in the process, probe for difficulties, and identify problem areas.

Finally, blueprints can facilitate the analysis of cost–benefit tradeoffs in providing services. They provide a template for quantifying the value of each patient contact, customer touchpoint, and support process. In some cases, some frontstage and backstage actions may be added if they add value to the service experience. In other cases, low value activities may be deleted without any impact on perceived value. Service blueprints allow pharmacists to be more strategic in the design and delivery of their services.

Funding: This research received no external funding.

Conflicts of Interest: The author declares no conflicts of interest.

References

1. Chewning, B.; Schommer, J.C. Increasing Clients' Knowledge of Community Pharmacists' Roles. *Pharm. Res.* **1996**, *13*, 1299–1304. [CrossRef] [PubMed]
2. Schommer, J.C.; Gaither, C.A. A segmentation analysis for pharmacists' and patients' views of pharmacists' roles. *Res. Soc. Adm. Pharm.* **2014**, *10*, 508–528. [CrossRef] [PubMed]
3. Gammie, S.M.; Rodgers, R.M.; Loo, R.L.; Corlett, S.A.; Krska, J. Medicine-related services in community pharmacy: Public preferences for pharmacy attributes and promotional methods and comparison with pharmacists' perceptions. *Patient Prefer. Adherence* **2016**, *10*, 2297–2307. [CrossRef] [PubMed]
4. Worley, M.M.; Schommer, J.C.; Brown, L.M.; Hadsall, R.S.; Ranelli, P.L.; Stratton, T.P.; Uden, D.L. Pharmacists' and patients' roles in the pharmacist-patient relationship: Are pharmacists and patients reading from the same relationship script? *Res. Soc. Adm. Pharm.* **2007**, *3*, 47–69. [CrossRef] [PubMed]
5. Holdford, D.A. Characteristics of Services. In *Marketing for Pharmacist: Providing and Promoting Pharmacy Services*, 3rd ed.; PharmacoEnterprise Publishing: Richmond, VA, USA, 2015; Chapter 7, pp. 125–146.
6. Holdford, D.; Schulz, R. Effect of technical and functional quality on patient perceptions of pharmaceutical service quality. *Pharm. Res.* **1999**, *16*, 1344–1351. [CrossRef] [PubMed]
7. Holdford, D.A. Designing Pharmacy Services. In *Marketing for Pharmacist: Providing and Promoting Pharmacy Services*, 3rd ed.; PharmacoEnterprise Publishing: Richmond, VA, USA, 2015; Chapter 9; pp. 164–189.
8. Isetts, B.J.; Schommer, J.C.; Westberg, S.M.; Johnson, J.K.; Froiland, N.; Hedlund, J.M. Evaluation of a Consumer-Generated Marketing Plan for Medication Therapy Management Services. 2012. Available online: https://conservancy.umn.edu/handle/11299/122757 (accessed on 6 May 2019).
9. Holdford, D.A.; Kennedy, D.T. The service blueprint as a tool for designing innovative pharmaceutical services. *J. Am. Pharm. Assoc.* **1999**, *39*, 545–552. [CrossRef]

10. Shostack, G.L. Designing Services that Deliver. *Harv. Bus. Rev.* **1984**, *62*, 133–139.
11. Holdford, D.A. Resource-based theory of competitive advantage—A framework for pharmacy practice innovation research. *Pharm. Pract. (Granada)* **2018**, *16*, 1351. [CrossRef] [PubMed]
12. Bitner, M.J.; Ostrom, A.L.; Morgan, F.N. Service Blueprinting: A Practical Technique for Service Innovation. *Calif. Manag. Rev.* **2008**, *20*. [CrossRef]
13. Holdford, D.A.; Inocencio, T.J. Adherence and persistence associated with an appointment-based medication synchronization program. *J. Am. Pharm. Assoc.* **2013**, *53*, 576–583. [CrossRef] [PubMed]

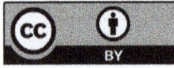

pharmacy

MDPI

Commentary

Applying Contemporary Management Principles to Implementing and Evaluating Value-Added Pharmacist Services

Shane P. Desselle [1],*, Leticia R. Moczygemba [2], Antoinette B. Coe [3], Karl Hess [4] and David P. Zgarrick [5]

[1]   California College of Pharmacy, Touro University, Vallejo, CA 94952, USA
[2]   College of Pharmacy, University of Texas at Austin, Austin, TX 78712, USA
[3]   College of Pharmacy, University of Michigan, Ann Arbor, MI 48109, USA
[4]   Keck Graduate Institute, School of Pharmacy and Health Sciences, Claremont, CA 91711, USA
[5]   Bouve College of Health Sciences, School of Pharmacy, Northeastern University, Boston, MA 02115, USA
*   Correspondence: shane.desselle@tu.edu

Received: 8 June 2019; Accepted: 18 July 2019; Published: 20 July 2019

check for updates

Abstract: Value-added pharmacy services encompass traditional and emerging services provided by pharmacists to individual and entire populations of persons increasingly under the auspices of a public health mandate. The success of value-added pharmacy services is enhanced when they are carried out and assessed using appropriate theory-based paradigms. Many of the more important management theories for pharmacy services consider the "servicescape" of these services recognizing the uniqueness of each patient and service encounter that vary based upon health needs and myriad other factors. In addition, implementation science principles help ensure the financial viability and sustainability of these services. This commentary reviews some of the foundational management theories and provides a number of examples of these theories that have been applied successfully resulting in a greater prevalence and scope of value-added services being offered.

Keywords: pharmacist; services marketing; management; value-added services

1. Introduction

Pharmacists have always been in a service industry, including those in the community sector selling medicines and other health products, specifically for the delivery of health and medication-related services. The role of the pharmacist has evolved over the years, from compounding remedies from raw materials; to dispensing pre-manufactured dosage forms; to educating, advising, managing, and monitoring the outcomes of drug therapy for both patients and populations. All of these services add value to medication and patient care outcomes. Additionally, pharmacists have continued to develop services that add value to the medication use process and encompass a variety of individual and public health services. The more "traditional" and newly emerging services can be regarded as "value-added" services, or those that are likely to positively impact medication outcomes [1]. These services are especially salient for certain populations of vulnerable or high-risk persons, such as those with multiple comorbidities, younger and older patients, those with diminished access to care, those with marginal or low health literacy, and the medically underserved, to name a few. As such, value-added services aim to contribute toward and improve public health and health outcomes across diverse settings. Among the more common value-added services of pharmacists and pharmacy personnel under the aegis of public health is the provision of immunizations for various infectious diseases, such as for influenza, herpes zoster and pneumococcal [2] as well as provision of education and advocacy related to vaccinations [3,4]. Pharmacists are also increasing their roles in public health issues such as health literacy [5,6] opioid misuse and naloxone training and education [7–10], emergency preparedness planning [11] and safe medication disposal [12,13]. Pharmacists are also members of health care teams in ambulatory care settings and provide medication and disease management for chronic conditions such as diabetes, hypertension, and congestive heart failure [14–17]. In the hospital setting, pharmacists have roles in antibiotic stewardship [18,19], medication reconciliation [20,21] and therapeutic drug monitoring [22,23].

2. Business Planning for Successful Implementation of Pharmacist Services

Careful planning and management is needed to evaluate whether a value-added pharmacist service should be pursued or not. Thus, the creation of a business plan is a foundational step in beginning a new service. A business plan helps stakeholders (e.g., administrators, investors, payers, other health care professionals) decide whether to devote resources and energy to a new service. The first step of a business plan is to identify how a value-added service aligns with an organization's strategic plan, mission statement, and current priority areas. For example, an organization that is focused on improving diabetes outcomes will likely not be interested in a service that focuses on asthma [24]. Next, input from stakeholders such as pharmacists, technicians, physicians and other health professionals, and patients should be sought to refine ideas and tailor a new service to stakeholders' needs. Given that pharmacists have an established track record of implementing services ranging from medication therapy management to chronic disease management to immunization programs, it is likely that a review of the primary literature and pharmacy organization websites would provide guidance and examples of successful models that could be replicated [24].

It is also worthwhile to consider the flexibility level of the pharmacy organization when deciding what type of value-added service to pursue. Feletto has described four states of flexibility that a pharmacy organization may be in when transitioning to provision of value-based services. These include steady-state, operational, structural, and strategic flexibility [25]. A pharmacy in steady-state does not offer services beyond traditional dispensing activities. Operational flexibility occurs when a pharmacy is beginning to expand offerings to increase the number of customers but not providing a value-based service. A pharmacy that has developed at least one value-based service and begun to implement internal infrastructure to support the service is exhibiting structural flexibility, although at this point there is not a plan for long-term success. Strategic flexibility occurs when a pharmacy has successfully implemented value-based services and has infrastructure and processes in place for sustainability [25]. A pharmacy in a steady-state may venture into value-based services by offering immunization services whereas a pharmacy in strategic flexibility may be in a position to partner with providers for a diabetes management service.

3. The Market for Pharmacist Services

No matter how valuable the service might be in the mind of the pharmacist and no matter how well executed, if that service does not fulfill a perceived or actual need by its target market, it will likely fail. Thus, it is essential to consider the target market for the service. Collaboration with other health care professionals is usually needed for a successful pharmacist service [24,26]. Building relationships with health care professionals who could benefit from a pharmacist service is important to facilitate patient referrals, medical information exchange, and billing for pharmacist services. Pharmacists and health care providers are likely aware of each other in a community but that does not automatically translate to meaningful collaboration. Thus, pharmacists will need to spend some effort increasing interactions with local providers to develop successful services. Once a provider recognizes that a pharmacist can provide nondispensing services, a pharmacist can begin to build trust and rapport to lead to sharing of patient information, referrals, etc. To build rapport it is important to be able to clearly articulate the purpose of the service and how it benefits a health care professional, such as a physician. For example, a pharmacist seeking referrals for medication therapy management in a community setting may highlight benefits such as improved medication adherence which can in turn lead to a decrease in use of acute services such as hospitalization. Physicians are under increasing pressure to meet quality metrics such as controlling high blood pressure in their patients, and this creates opportunities to align value-based pharmacist services with blood pressure monitoring and medication therapy management [24].

Payment for services should always be considered when thinking about a new pharmacist service. Thus, health care payers are another stakeholder to consider when marketing a new service. Pharmacists have had some success with payers reimbursing for nondispensing services such as medication therapy management (MTM) and diabetes management [27,28]. However, the fact that pharmacists are not recognized as providers by most payers can present challenges to pharmacists negotiating service payment. It is important that pharmacist services align with priorities of payers, which often means reducing high-cost expenditures such as emergency department visits or hospitalizations for chronic conditions. The "value-add" of a service for a payer often means decreasing costs while improving patient outcomes [29,30]. Effective management would entail understanding of various reimbursement mechanisms and leveraging them not only for the success of the pharmacy, but perhaps even a larger organization. For example, Wu et al. used monies acquired for participating in the 340B drug discount program to create a financially viable and more clinically relevant hospital discharge service associated with improved patient outcomes, such as a reduction in 30-day readmissions [31].

A market evaluation should also consider the competition for services. Depending upon the type of service being provided, competitors could include physicians, nurse practitioners, and even other pharmacists/pharmacies [24,32]. In addition to pharmacists, diabetes education can be provided by physicians, nurse practitioners, and other health professionals. A payer would want to know why a pharmacist versus other qualified health professional should provide diabetes education to its beneficiaries. In a community pharmacy, perhaps the value-add is the convenience of providing the service on a walk-in basis with little to no waiting whereas in a patient-centered medical home, the value-add could be increasing physician time to focus on other patients or services. To effectively mitigate the impact of competitors, a pharmacist should be able to describe how a service is unique from similar services [24,33].

The viability of a pharmacist service is also impacted by the volume of potential consumers (i.e., patients) in its service area. Internal and external data can be used to help assess market size for a pharmacist service. Internal data, such as patient profiles, purchasing, and financial records can help examine the number of potentially eligible patients within the organization. Often, a new service has a goal of attracting new patients. In this case, local information about desired health outcomes can be obtained from interviews of other health care professionals in the pharmacy's market area or a review of the local health department website to identify indications and prevalence of the area's major health burdens. A market research study could also be undertaken to collect feedback and perceptions about a service from potential patients [24,34,35].

Although market research may indicate patient interest in a particular service, ultimately patients may not be willing to pay for a service if they cannot afford it or if they do not perceive value in the service [24,29]. This may be especially true if a service is not covered by insurance and a patient would have to pay out-of-pocket. Although Medicare recognizes pharmacists as a provider for MTM provided to Medicare Part D beneficiaries and some state Medicaid programs and commercial payers will pay for pharmacist services, most payers do not pay for pharmacist services in the United States [29]. Government sponsorship helps cover costs for other services in other countries such as U.K.'s minor ailment service [36] and Australia's Home Medicines Review program [37].

4. Patient Engagement and Participation in Services Delivery

Consumers' willingness to pay and even their impressions and experiences with a service will likely be enhanced if they are engaged and participatory in the service encounter [38]. For example, if a pharmacist has effectively engaged a patient in a lipid management service, the patient will likely be more successful in the endeavor to maintain control, or keep their lipid levels below target goal.

Further, if the pharmacist is able to get that same patient to relay successes and strategies for how they are succeeding and engage them in provocative discussion, then the patient will enjoy the entirety of the service to a greater degree. This behooves the pharmacist to ascertain the degree that patients might want to engage, thus tailoring strategies of service delivery to reflect patient desires. As such, any service designed must be flexible, and pharmacists and support personnel providing the service must be adaptive to the situation. With this in mind, research has demonstrated that the transtheoretical model (TTM), health belief model, and theory of planned behavior can be useful guides for pharmacists in designing and implementing value-added services [39]. This extends toward contemporary patient needs and public issues, such as that with the opioid crisis. Fleming et al. effectively employed the theory of planned behavior to identify challenges to overcome in pharmacists' engagement of patients in an attempt to curb their misuse of drug substances [40].

5. Meeting Patient Needs

Assuming that there is a consumer need and a market for a particular value-added pharmacist service, business planners must ascertain whether the service is meeting a need. One way to discern this is through a SWOT (i.e., strengths, weaknesses, opportunities, and threats) analysis [24]. In a SWOT analysis, internal opportunities and weaknesses and external opportunities and threats are examined. Generally, internal opportunities and weaknesses are easier to control than external opportunities and threats. Internally, resources such as personnel, training requirements for pharmacists and staff, space, equipment (e.g., computers and software) and supplies (e.g., medical and office supplies) needed to deliver a service should be determined. This can help decide the amount of working capital necessary to support development of a new service. Initially, an organization may leverage existing resources, such as reallocation of pharmacist time to include a percentage of time to deliver MTM, before investing large amounts of capital into a service. At a minimum, resources for equipment, supplies, and market are often needed [24]. Administrative support and buy-in for a new service is critical to getting support for resources needed for the service. Evaluating the culture is also part of the homework that needs to be done. Organizational culture has shown to be the primary driver in the success of many value-added pharmacy services. The organization's culture might or might not be receptive to new ideas, might infer a preference as to who or what types of persons approach upper administration with ideas, and also how to couch, or frame the discussion when pitching the idea [41].

Externally, a number of factors, such as demographic trends of patients and providers, state scope of practice laws and regulations, and the number and type of competitors in a market, can represent opportunities or threats for a value-added pharmacist service. For example, an aging population might represent an opportunity for disease management, but a threat in lack of time to devote to non-dispensing activities. If a pharmacist has identified the potential opportunities or threats to a service, they can apply some of the management principles described above to manage the impact.

Patients often understand their own needs, but in some cases, might not perceive a need for a particular service or even see its relevance unless they have been properly engaged. While some patients are undertreated, many patients with comorbid disease states are on too many medications that may result in untoward outcomes, even idiosyncratic conditions. Historically referred to as "polypharmacy", the term "deprescribing" refers to systematic and evidence-based practices to deprescribe, or streamline a patient's therapeutic regiment to maximize outcomes. Trenament et al. described a service in which they engaged patients in a deprescribing program to promote those patients' buy-in, have greater confidence in and thus better adherence to their new medication regimen [42].

6. Managing the Servicescape

The ability of pharmacists to manage internal and even some external factors in service deliveries provides them great opportunities in what has been referred to as the "servicescape" [43]. It refers to physical and other constructs wherein a service is performed, delivered, and consumed [44]. There are objective stimuli generated during the performance and consumption/use of a service that are measurable and controllable to enhance employee/patient interactions. The servicescape influences the patient's experience and thus their satisfaction with service experience. For example, the layout and structural design of the pharmacy, along with job descriptions and workflow, will determine where a patient drops off their prescription, how long it is they might have to wait before being greeted, who takes responsibility for greeting them and for initial medication history-taking and other services, and the extent to which privacy can be offered and even the types or array of services that could potentially be offered for each patient. In the background, various "physical" attributes ranging from such phenomena even as the type [or lack] of music playing in the background of the pharmacy has an impact on the overall sensory experience of the patient. Design of the servicescape can be informed by any number of questions such as:

How can the servicescape be designed to attract the most profitable customer/patient segments to the service?

How can the servicescape be designed to maximize customer satisfaction and retention?

How much money and resources should be invested into the servicescape? These questions get to the core business mission, vision, and values of the organization and thus translate into consideration of which service, or services might be offered from an array of possibilities.

7. Array of Value-Added Pharmacist Services

Value-added pharmacist services range from focused, one-time interventions to resolve medication issues identified during the dispensing process to nondispensing direct patient care services that focus on comprehensive and longitudinal management of medications for chronic conditions. Prevention and wellness services are another type of pharmacist service [24].

Recently, there has been a focus on creating opportunities in the community pharmacy setting for increased engagement between pharmacists and patients and to enhance clinical services [44]. Continuous medication monitoring (CoMM) is one approach to that has been gaining momentum [45]. In CoMM, "pharmacists systematically review the patients' medication record and monitor every medication being dispensed to prevent, identify, and resolve drug therapy problems or obstacles to optimal therapy during the dispensing process" [45]. Traditional MTM, especially for Medicare Part D beneficiaries whereby pharmacists can be reimbursed, remains a clinical service offered in many pharmacies. MTM generally includes five key steps, including comprehensive medication review, medication action plan, personalized medication record, intervention and referral, and documentation and follow-up [46].

Value-added services, such as appointment-based models (ABM), may be integrated with existing services such as CoMM or MTM. The goal of ABM is to increase medication adherence and efficiency for pharmacies and patients [47]. ABM is comprised of three components: medication synchronization which includes refilling all medications on the same day each month, monthly phone call to patient to confirm refill order and identify any medication-related issues, and scheduled monthly appointment to pick up the medications [48]. At the monthly appointment, additional services such as MTM may be provided to address medication-related problems.

Whereas MTM is a holistic approach to managing all medications, disease state management is a more focused type of service that pharmacists provide. In disease management, pharmacists educate and monitor medication therapy to achieve therapy goals over a period of time, make recommendations about drug therapy to providers, and may be able to directly initiate or change therapy under a collaborative practice agreement (depending upon each state's scope of practice). Examples of conditions that pharmacists commonly manage include hypertension [49], heart failure [50], diabetes [51,52], and asthma [53,54].

Finally, pharmacists have an established history of delivering monitoring/screening services and wellness/health-promotion programs. Examples include anticoagulation services [54–57], travel health [55,58], hormonal contraception prescribing [59], naloxone dispensing and education [60], smoking cessation counseling [61], osteoporosis screenings [62], and lipid screenings [63]. Point-of-care testing for conditions such as influenza, strep throat, and hepatitis C is also increasing [64,65].

8. The Aesthetics of Services Delivery and Consumption

There are various idioms referring to the importance of making a good first impression, or a good impression, overall. Service companies depend on front-line service workers to control and communicate a certain image that consumers/patients will associate with the business and with the service [66]. In community practice, technicians have been referred to by pharmacists as the "face" of the pharmacy [67]. Image control demands that service workers act according to scripts that diverge from their actual preferences and capacities. Additionally, service recipients are also acting on social norms, as well as to gauge the intent of the service provider and to potentially acquire a higher level of service or enhance their own experiences. Given the acting of both parties, a number of conflicts arise regarding the truthfulness of sincerity regarding service performance. The expected set of behaviors each actor in the process plays out are often referred to as roles; and thus role theory might be helpful in determining proper training for pharmacy staff and for the expectations one might have of patients. The aesthetic appeal of services is thus under significant control and can be managed effectively by the pharmacy. This includes ascribing proper roles to workers, training patients on the roles they might assume in receiving services, and strategizing to optimize the impression by patients of the service. The impression of those using or experiencing the service will go a long way toward successful marketing of the service, particularly in an age where reviews of experiences are proliferated so quickly on web-based ratings platforms. It is important, then, to manage not only the entirety or "gestalt" of the service but also its individual components. A recent study of both "traditional" and emerging pharmacist services found that visual appeal of the pharmacy and its aesthetics, including the image projected by service personnel (pharmacists and technicians) impacts the relationship between perceived quality of the service and thus customer loyalty [68].

9. Components of A Value-Added Pharmacist Service

Once the decision is made to implement a new service, patient eligibility criteria for the service needs to be established and roles and responsibilities of the pharmacist and other supporting staff need to be defined and agreed upon by all stakeholders [69,70]. Patient eligibility will vary depending upon the service but may include patients who are not meeting goals for a particular chronic disease, patients with multiple chronic conditions, or patients taking multiple chronic medications [66]. Also, workflow for delivery of the intervention and processes such as identification of eligible patients, data collection, and documentation, needs to be developed. A detailed workflow can help guide next steps needed for implementation such as reallocation of existing pharmacist resources to deliver the service or engaging information technology personnel to create a flag in an electronic health record to identify eligible patients [71].

9.1. Patient Data Collection

A well-developed data collection plan is important to ensure that relevant baseline and monitoring variables are systematically recorded when the service is provided. A pharmacy management system or electronic health record may need to be modified in order to collect the desired data [24]. This process should begin early because it can be time-intensive as it often involves additional organizational approvals and may depend upon availability of personnel from nonpharmacy departments such as information technology [72]. A data collection plan should also include details about security of data and compliance with rules and regulations such as the Health Insurance Portability and Accountability Act of 1996 HIPAA [24].

9.2. Pharmacy-Based Laboratory

While laboratory data are often obtained from external sources, it may be advantageous or even necessary to conduct laboratory monitoring/screening as part of a broader service. Thus, some pharmacists have equipment and supplies available to measure blood glucose, A1C, international normalization ratio, lipids, or bone mineral density at the point-of-care. Any pharmacy performing tests that involve collecting blood or saliva must follow guidelines according to the Clinical Laboratory Improvement Amendments of 1988. Other considerations include being familiar with the Occupational Safety and Health Act (OSHA) and having a plan in place for blood-borne pathogen exposure [24]. In some U.S. states, pharmacists are permitted to order laboratory tests when needed to assess and monitor medication-related problems [73].

9.3. Medication Management Protocols/Collaborative Practice Agreements

A protocol or collaborative practice agreement (CPA) is useful to provide a framework for consistent delivery and guide treatment decisions for a medication or disease management service, which typically includes a comprehensive assessment of medications for appropriateness and whether or not treatment goals are being reached, identification and resolution of medication-related problems, development of a medication care plan and follow-up and monitoring [74,75]. Protocols or CPAs formalize collaborations between pharmacists and providers and "define certain patient care functions that a pharmacist can autonomously provide under specified situations and conditions" [76].Treatment pathways in protocols or CPAs should adhere to national guidelines and evidence-based recommendations and reflect input and feedback from collaborating providers, such as physicians and nurse practitioners. The roles and responsibilities of each team member should also be clearly defined. While a protocol or CPA is typically not required for pharmacist services, it is advantageous to outline a process to support decision-making. Further, a protocol or CPA improves efficiency of a pharmacist being able to directly implement therapy recommendations rather than wait for provider approval [24].

CPAs, or as they are otherwise known as collaborative practice agreements (CPAs), can become so commonplace and so successful as to eventually actuate or serve as a foundation for changes in scope of practice. For example, Farris et al. utilized a CPA to extend pharmacists' roles in providing oral contraceptive medications and other related services [77]. This and other programs like it, along with regulatory and societal attitude evolutions about oral contraception, have resulted in more commonplace pharmacist involvement in such services [78].

9.4. Patient Education

Patient education is commonly included as part of a value-added pharmacist service although the extent of education varies by the type of service being delivered. Patient education may be brief such as discussing benefits/risks of immunizations for an immunization service or providing one-time education about how a medication works and expected outcomes from taking a medication [24]. Pharmacists are increasingly expanding their roles in managing patient education services, such as is the case with nutrition education [79] and in engaging patients in successful weight loss programs using individualized and group education, as well as other tailored interventions [80]. More comprehensive education may be provided over time for disease management services. For example, in diabetes management pharmacists may spend time training a patient on how to use a blood glucose monitor and/or insulin injections and providing education about healthy eating, signs and symptoms of hypoglycemia, and assessing patient goals for treatment over multiple visits. For education services, it is important for a pharmacist to consider literacy levels and needs of local populations, such as availability of educational materials in English and Spanish, when applicable [24].

10. Outcome Measurements

Pharmacists need to think about which outcomes should be assessed to determine the effectiveness and value of services. It is a good practice to obtain feedback from key stakeholders about outcomes as well. For example, pharmacists often focus on clinical outcomes whereas an administrator may be primarily focused on economic outcomes. A combination of process, clinical, and economic outcomes are useful to be able to have a full picture of the impact of a service. Process measures may include the number and type of medication-related problems identified and resolved. Examples of clinic measures include systolic and diastolic blood pressure, A1C, and lipid levels. Economic outcomes can range from total health care costs to costs of medications, hospitalizations or emergency department visits. Some stakeholders may also be interested in the return-on-investment for a particular service [24]. Pharmacists should determine if desired outcome data is easily available in a pharmacy management system or electronic health record. Often, a pharmacist has to work with information technology personnel to develop templates to systematically collect and document outcomes for reporting purposes [72,81]. Humanistic outcomes, such as patient satisfaction, often require collecting data from patients with a tool such as a survey. For some outcomes, such as cost data, partnering with payers for claims data may be necessary. Thus, it is important to create an evaluation plan early to have the necessary infrastructure in place for successful outcome reporting.

Outcomes are not necessarily mutually exclusive to one another. More often than not, when exemplary clinical and humanistic outcomes are being achieved, financial outcomes are in lock-step with them. As mentioned previously, pharmacies develop services in agreement with their mission and to advance the profession and to diversify their revenue streams. Relying solely on product distribution or even hanging one's hat on one particular service can be especially problematic in an environment of shrinking profit margins. It is healthy and wise to consider concomitant services that leverage one another in use of resources and in marketing, while also focusing on a comprehensive set of operations management strategies that seek to optimize concurrent and various types of outcomes. It has been suggested that pharmacies develop and succeed in distinctive competencies, ranging from unique services delivery, to distribution efficiency, and marketing efforts to maximize the likelihood of clinical and economic success [82].

11. Pharmacist and Staff Training

For a service to be successful and attractive to payers, the service needs to be consistently and systematically delivered to all patients [83]. To ensure this, pharmacists and staff should be trained and proficient in delivering the service. The type and extent of training varies according to the type of service being provided. For services such as MTM, pharmacists may adopt national programs such as the American Pharmacists Association MTM Certificate program [84]. A component of training should also focus on documentation and outcome reporting procedures. It also useful to provide scripts or workflow diagrams (may be electronic or on paper) as part of the training to guide pharmacists in consistent delivery of an intervention. Adequate training of support personnel is demonstrated repeatedly for successful expansion of pharmacist services, such as when technicians accept medication histories of patients being admitted into the hospital, thus affording pharmacists the ability to effectively work with prescribers on medication care planning [85]. Annual booster trainings should also be considered to maintain quality [83]. Technicians and support personnel involved in record-keeping, coordination, and assistance with data retrieval as a component of the service process should receive training as well as the overall goals of the service, how the service fits with the organization's mission, and what value they (as support staff) bring to the table in executing the service [24].

12. Management and Marketing Services—The Services as Theatre Paradigm

There are many ways one can conceptualize services so as to proffer management and marketing best practices for their development and implementation. Grove et al. envisage service as a human drama depicting the service experience [77]. Those performing the service are actors aiming to create a desired impression before the audience on the "front stage" [86]. The "rehearsal" for the performance takes place "backstage" away from the audience and where strategies for design and implementation are laid out. In drama, the service is carried out not in the absence, but rather, with the audience's input. Similarly, a performance of a service often requires stakeholder (i.e., patients, physicians and other health professionals, and payers) participation in the process. Like theatrical performances, services delivery can be tenuous and fragile as processes can be disrupted by minor mishaps. As such, both service provision and drama performance employ strategies to create a desirable impression. This includes avoidance of service mistakes, of which things like poor service design are obvious (e.g., not aligning a service with organizational needs), but also avoidance of "simple" errors like misspelling a patient's name on a communication that might connote laziness or apathy. Organizations that are skillful in their management of stakeholder expectations and interactions with them can improve the value of the service from the view of those stakeholders.

Much of this metaphor would suggest the performance of the actors in delivery. However, the scenery cannot be ignored. Just like an audience might be favorably impressed with superior stage setting, design, and props, the health care service delivery must be provided in a place that is clean, professional, and connotes the appropriate atmosphere. To that end, to be successful, service performance is about managing the expectations and meeting the needs of stakeholders. In one particular interdisciplinary collaborative, pharmacists worked with other healthcare professionals to manage the expectations of kidney transplants patients during medical and education services, as well as with self-monitoring activities, to better regulate their expectations and elevate their experiences throughout the process [87].

13. Monitoring and Sustaining Value-Added Pharmacist Services Through Implementation Science

Although there are many steps involved in getting a new service started, part of implementation activities also includes thinking about what needs to be achieved for sustainability (or not) [88]. Additionally, in the spirit of public health discussed previously, pharmacy organizations will advance the profession and best serve the community and its vulnerable populations when it develops sustainable services that treat and monitor patient progress for positive outcomes over the long haul. When approaching the value-added services concept, a useful paradigm to consider is implementation science, which is defined as the "scientific study of methods to promote the systematic uptake of research findings and other evidence-based practices into routine practice, and, hence, to improve the quality and effectiveness of health services" [89]. As pharmacy, continues to work towards advancing practice, implementation science offers a key to promote the systematic uptake of newer evidence-based practices and a frame on how to improve the quality and effectiveness of existing services, such as MTM [90].

Within implementation science, a useful approach for the implementation of value-added pharmacy services is the Consolidated Framework for Implementation Research (CFIR) model [91]. The model has designers of services consider the following to help ensure service longevity: evidence strength and quality advantage; adaptability; trialability; complexity; design quality and packaging; and cost. The CFIR and similar implementation science frameworks have demonstrated success in service design and monitoring. The aforementioned appointment-based model (ABM) can have an even more positive impact on the pharmacy and its patients when designed using a CFIR approach [44]. Use of an implementation model approach was associated with greater longevity for an pharmacist-driven asthma service in the community setting [92]. This type of framework might be especially valuable for other "non-routine" or "outside the box" types of pharmacy services, such as those associated with assisting breastfeeding mothers with their particular medication-taking needs [93] and mental health services [94]. In one study, success rates of MTM services (defined as completed and reimbursable claims) rose from 42.9% to 64% of attempts following the adoption of a

CFIR framework [95]. Again, the adoption of CFIR and other implementation science frameworks approaches service design and implementation from many aspects, but principle among them is the mindset of ongoing evaluation and the need to ensure program quality.

The CFIR provides an excellent framework for executing services that promote positive outcomes for all stakeholders, thus potentiating its success well after its initial design. However, there are still additional considerations for ensuring long-term sustainability of a service even well after its implementation. Lennox et al. reviewed the implementation literature for successful program sustainability and produced a comprehensive model that involves patients/clients, infrastructure, staff training and support, maintaining organizational readiness, continuously raising the organization's profile, and keep attuned to socioeconomic and political changes in force [96]. Shelton and Cooper concurred, emphasizing the dynamic nature of sustainability and thus the organization's ability to adapt to change [97].

14. Receiving Payment for Value-Added Services

Ultimately, for a value-added service to be successful, payment must be received for it. This can be complex for value-added pharmacist services because traditionally payment for pharmacist dispensing services has been tied to a medication and pharmacists are not recognized as providers by most payers. A first step is to set a price for the service. In order to do this, one must determine all of the costs (e.g., personnel, equipment and supplies, space) related to delivery of the service. One paradigm that has been used is that a service should result in revenue that is two to three times a pharmacist's salary [24]. Assuming that a pharmacist earns $60/hour, this may mean charging $2.00 to $3.00 per minute for a value-added pharmacy service [98]. It also important to remember that setting a price for a service does not mean that a payer (or patient) is willing to pay that price [24].

Next, various pricing methodologies should be reviewed to determine which one aligns best with the service. Fee-for-service pricing, which charges a set rate based on time or a specific intervention, is a common approach. However, it might not maximize revenue for the provider or might create disadvantages for promoting the service to patients. This strategy does not consider external factors, such as competitors' prices and could also overestimate or underestimate its value to clients. Another pricing method is based on the resources used, or resource-based relative-value scale (RBRVS) used commonly in the U.S.[24] There are available pharmacy-specific Current Procedural Technology (CPT) codes that might be accepted by Medicare carriers and other payers, including [99]:

99605: An initial encounter service performed face-to-face with a patient in a time increment of up to 15 min.

99606: For use for a subsequent or follow-up encounter with the same patient in a time increment of up to 15 min.

99607: An add-on code that may be used to bill for additional increments of 15 min of time to either of the above codes.

CPT code 99211 is another code which has been used by pharmacists providing patient care incident to a physician [99]. There are various codes for specific procedures such as for fasting lipid panel, finger stick, and others. In partnership with providers, pharmacists may also be able to use codes such as CPT code 99490 for chronic care management [99].

As mentioned previously, the use of implementation science and CFIR frameworks can assist not only in sustainability, but also with quality assurance and reimbursement for services. Increasingly, payers are looking for value; that is, payment for services that will save money for the insurer and its patients in the long term, when considering all medical costs. Alternative payment models reward performance, sustainment, and quality metrics. Therefore, it makes sense to identify and resolve medication-related problems "upstream" at the point-of-care to avoid clinical inertia, medication errors, and prevent more costly "downstream" care such as hospitalizations, readmissions, or emergency room visits [100]. This inertia, or momentum, often tempts pharmacy managers to focus on quantity (volume) and efficiency, which is important; however, reimbursement is often attained at higher levels and at higher rates when the goals of design and implementation focus on quality.

15. Conclusions

There are numerous opportunities for pharmacists to engage in the provision of valued-added services. Successful implementation of value-added services requires careful planning, evaluation and monitoring. The use of business and management principles as well as theory-based frameworks can facilitate a path to financial viability and sustainability of value-based pharmacist services.

Author Contributions: S.P.D., D.P.Z., and L.R.M. conceptualized this commentary. A.B.C. and K.H. provided valuable updates and recent literature, along with additional editing.

Funding: This research received no external funding.

Conflicts of Interest: The authors declare no conflicts of interest.

References

1. Marcrom, R.E.; Horton, R.M.; Shepherd, M.D. Creating value-added services to meet patient needs: Use these practical suggestions to help tailor your services to various market segments and expand your practice. *J. Am. Pharm. Assoc.* **1992**, *32*, 48–57.
2. Westrick, S.C. College/school of pharmacy affiliation and community pharmacies' involvement in public health activities. *Am. Assoc. Coll. Pharm. Annu. Meet.* **2009**, *73*, 123. [CrossRef]
3. Queeno, B.V. Evaluation of inpatient influenza and pneumococcal vaccination acceptance rates with pharmacist education. *J. Pharm. Pract.* **2017**, *30*, 202–208. [CrossRef]
4. Gonzalvo, J.D.; Lantaff, W.M. CDE pharmacists in the United States. *Diabetes Educ.* **2018**, *44*, 278–292. [CrossRef]
5. Vargas, J.; Dang, C.; Subramaniam, V. Public health approaches in ethnically diverse populations. *Drug Top.* **2011**, *155*, 4.
6. Gerber, B.S.; Cano, A.I.; Caceres, M.L.; Smith, D.E.; Wilken, L.A.; Michaud, J.B.; Ruggiero, L.A.; Sharp, L.K. A pharmacist and health promoter team to improve medication adherence among Latinos with diabetes. *Ann. Pharmacother.* **2010**, *44*, 70–79. [CrossRef]
7. Cochran, G.; Hruschak, V.; De Fosse, B.; Hohmeier, K.C. Prescription opioid abuse: pharmacists' perspective and response. *Integr. Pharm. Res. Pract.* **2016**, *5*, 65–73. [CrossRef]
8. Strand, M.A.; Eukel, H.; Burck, S. Moving opioid misuse prevention upstream: A pilot study of community pharmacists screening for opioid risk. *Res. Soc. Adm. Pharm.* **2019**, *15*, 1032–1036. [CrossRef]
9. Hill, L.G.; Sanchez, J.P.; Laguado, S.A.; Lawson, K.A. Operation naloxone: Overdose prevention service learning for student pharmacists. *Curr. Pharm. Teach. Learn.* **2018**, *10*, 1348–1353. [CrossRef]
10. Substance Abuse and Mental Health Services Administration (SAMHSA), Center for the Application of Prevention Technologies. Preventing the Consequences of Opioid Overdose: Understanding Naloxone Access Laws. 2018. Available online: https://www.samhsa.gov/capt/sites/default/files/resources/naloxone-access-laws-tool.pdf (accessed on 12 January 2019).
11. Fitzgerald, T.J.; Kang, Y.; Bridges, C.B.; Talbert, T.; Vagi, S.J.; Lamont, B.; Graitcer, S.B. Integrating pharmacies into public health program planning for pandemic influenza vaccine response. *Vaccine* **2016**, *34*, 5643–5648. [CrossRef]
12. Athern, K.M.; Linnebur, S.A.; Fabisiak, G. Proper disposal of unused household medications: The role of the pharmacist. *Consult. Pharm.* **2016**, *31*, 261–266. [CrossRef]
13. Eerry, L.A.; Shinn, B.W.; Stanovich, J. Quantification of an ongoing community-based medication take-back program. *J. Am. Pharm. Assoc.* **2014**, *54*, 275–279.
14. Benedict, A.W.; Spence, M.M.; Sie, J.L.; Chin, H.A.; Ngo, C.D.; Salmingo, J.F.; Vidaurreta, A.T.; Rashid, N. Evaluation of a Pharmacist-Managed Diabetes Program in a Primary Care Setting Within an Integrated Health Care System. *J. Manag. Care Spec. Pharm.* **2018**, *24*, 114–122. [CrossRef]
15. Choe, H.M.; Farris, K.B.; Stevenson, J.G.; Townsend, K.; Diez, H.L.; Remington, T.L.; Rockafellow, S.; Shimp, L.A.; Sy, A.; Wells, T.; et al. Patient-centered medical home: Developing, expanding, and sustaining a role for pharmacists. *Am. J. Health Syst. Pharm.* **2012**, *69*, 1063–1071. [CrossRef]

16. Moczygemba, L.R.; Goode, J.V.; Gatewood, S.B.; Osborn, R.D.; Alexander, A.J.; Kennedy, A.K.; Stevens, L.P.; Matzke, G.R. Integration of collaborative medication therapy management in a safety net patient-centered medical home. *J. Am. Pharm. Assoc.* **2011**, *51*, 167–172. [CrossRef]

17. Hirsch, J.D.; Steers, N.; Adler, D.S.; Kuo, G.M.; Morello, C.M.; Lang, M.; Singh, R.F.; Wood, Y.; Kaplan, R.M.; Mangione, C.M. Primary-care based, pharmacist-physician collaborative medication-therapy management of hypertension: A randomized, pragmatic trial. *Clin. Ther.* **2014**, *36*, 1244–1254. [CrossRef]

18. Parente, D.M.; Morton, J. Role of the pharmacist in antimicrobial stewardship. *Med. Clin. N. Am.* **2018**, *102*, 929–936. [CrossRef]

19. Baker, S.N.; Acquisto, N.M.; Ashley, E.D.; Fairbanks, R.J.; Beamish, S.E.; Haas, C.E. Pharmacist-managed antimicrobial stewardship program for patients discharged from the emergency department. *J. Pharm. Pract.* **2011**, *25*, 190–194. [CrossRef]

20. Patel, E.; Pevnick, J.M.; Kennelty, K.A. Pharmacists and medication reconciliation: A review of recent literature. *Integr. Pharm. Res. Pract.* **2019**, *8*, 39–45. [CrossRef]

21. Splawski, J.; Minger, H. Value of the pharmacist in the medication reconciliation process. *Pharm. Ther.* **2016**, *41*, 176–178.

22. Balch, A.H.; Constance, J.E.; Thorell, E.A.; Stockmann, C.; Korgenski, E.K.; Campbell, S.C.; Spigarelli, M.G.; Sherwin, C.M. Pediatric vancomycin dosing: Trends over time and the impact of therapeutic drug monitoring. *J. Clin. Pharmacol.* **2015**, *55*, 212–220. [CrossRef]

23. Wong, K.R.; Nelson, L.A.; Elliott, E.S.; Liu, Y.; Sommi, R.W.; Winans, E.A. Utilization of antipsychotic therapeutic drug monitoring at a state psychiatric hospital. *Ment. Health Clin.* **2016**, *6*, 1–7. [CrossRef]

24. Zgarrick, D.; Moczygemba, L.R.; Alston, G.L.; Desselle, S.P. *Pharmacy Management: Essentials for All Practice Settings*, 5th ed.; McGraw-Hill: New York, NY, USA, 2016.

25. Feletto, E.; Wilson, L.K.; Roberts, A.S.; Benrimoj, S.I. Building capacity to implement cognitive pharmaceutical services: Quantifying the needs of community pharmacies. *Res. Soc. Adm. Pharm.* **2010**, *6*, 163–173. [CrossRef]

26. Kennedy, A.G.; Biddle, M.A. Practical Strategies for Pharmacist Integration with Primary Care: A Workbook. Available online: http://contentmanager.med.uvm.edu/docs/default-source/ahec-documents/practicalstrategiesforpharmacistintegrationwithprimarycare-workbook_000.pdf?sfvrsn=2 (accessed on 13 January 2019).

27. Cowart, K.; Olson, K. Impact of pharmacist care provision in value-based care settings: How are we measuring value-added services? *J. Am. Pharm. Assoc.* **2019**, *59*, 125–128. [CrossRef]

28. McAdam-Marx, C.; Dahal, A.; Jennings, B.; Singhal, M.; Gunning, K. The effect of a diabetes collaborative care management program on clinical and economic outcomes in patients with type 2 diabetes. *J. Manag. Care Spec. Pharm.* **2015**, *21*, 452–468. [CrossRef]

29. American Pharmacists Association (APhA). Pharmacists' Patient Care Services Digest. Building Momentum. Increasing Access. 2016. Available online: http://media.pharmacist.com/documents/APhA_Digest.pdf (accessed on 13 January 2019).

30. Smith, M.; Cannon-Breland, M.L.; Spiggle, S. Consumer, physician and payer perspectives on primary care medication management services with a shared resource pharmacists network. *Res. Soc. Adm. Pharm.* **2014**, *10*, 539–553. [CrossRef]

31. Wu, T.; Williams, C.; Vranek, K.; Mattingly, T.J. Using 340B discounts to provide a financially stable medication discharge service. *Res. Soc. Adm. Pharm.* **2019**, *15*, 114–116. [CrossRef]

32. Zrebiec, J. A national study of the certified diabetes educator: Implications for future certification examinations. *Diabetes Educ.* **2014**, *40*, 470–475. [CrossRef]

33. Doucette, W.R.; McDonough, R.P. Beyond the 4 P's: Using relationship marketing to build value and demand for pharmacy services. *J. Am. Pharm. Assoc.* **2002**, *42*, 183–194.

34. Feehan, M.; Walsh, M.; Godin, J.; Sundwall, D.; Munger, M.A. Patient preferences for healthcare delivery through community pharmacy settings in the USA: A discrete choice study. *J. Clin. Pharm. Ther.* **2017**, *42*, 738–749. [CrossRef]

35. Painter, J.T.; Gressler, L.; Kathe, N.; Slabaugh, L.; Blumenschein, K. Consumer willingness to pay for pharmacy services: An updated review of the literature. *Res. Soc. Adm. Pharm.* **2018**, *14*, 1091–1105. [CrossRef]

36. Nazar, H.; Nazar, Z. Community pharmacy minor ailment services: Pharmacy stakeholder perspectives on the factors affecting sustainability. *Res. Soc. Adm. Pharm.* **2019**, *15*, 292–302. [CrossRef]

37. White, L.; Klinner, C.; Carter, S. Consumer perspectives of the Australia Home Medicines Review Program: Benefits and barriers. *Res. Soc. Adm. Pharm.* **2012**, *8*, 4–16. [CrossRef]

38. Dabholkar, P.A. How to improve perceived service quality by increasing customer participation. In *Proceedings of the 1990 Academy of Marketing Science (AMS) Annual Conference. Developments in Marketing Science: Proceedings of the Academy of Marketing Science*; Dunlap, B., Ed.; Springer: Cham, Switzerland, 2015.

39. Patwardhan, P.D.; Amin, M.E.; Chewning, B.A. Intervention research to enhance community pharmacists' cognitive services: A systematic review. *Res. Soc. Adm. Pharm.* **2014**, *10*, 475–493. [CrossRef]

40. Fleming, M.L.; Bapat, S.S.; Varisco, T.J. Using the theory of planned behavior to investigate community pharmacists' beliefs regarding engaging patients about prescription drug misuse. *Res. Soc. Adm. Pharm.* **2019**, *15*, 992–999. [CrossRef]

41. Holiday-Goodman, M. Entrepreneurship, resource management, organizational culture and other "business" factors influencing pharmacy practice change. *Res. Soc. Adm. Pharm.* **2012**, *8*, 269–271. [CrossRef]

42. Treneman, S.; Willison, M.; Robinson, B.; Andrew, M. A collaborative intervention for deprescribing: The role of stakeholder and patient engagement. *Res. Soc. Adm. Pharm.* **2019**, *15*. [CrossRef]

43. Bitner, M.J. The servicescape. In *Handbook of Services Marketing*; Swartz, T.A., Iacobucii, D., Eds.; Sage: Thousand Oaks, CA, USA, 2000; pp. 37–50.

44. Zeithaml, V.; Bitner, M.J. *Services Marketing*; McGraw-Hill: New York, NY, USA, 1996.

45. Goedken, A.M.; Butler, C.M.; McDonough, R.P.; Deninger, M.J.; Doucette, W.R. Continuous medication monitoring (CoMM): A foundational model to support the clinical work of community pharmacists. *Res. Soc. Adm. Pharm.* **2018**, *14*, 106–111. [CrossRef]

46. Medication Therapy Management in Pharmacy Practice: Core Elements of an MTM Service Model, Version 2.0. American Pharmacists Association and National Association of Chain Drug Stores Foundation. 2008. Available online: https://www.pharmacist.com/sites/default/files/files/core_elements_of_an_mtm_practice.pdf (accessed on 6 June 2019).

47. Patterson, J.; Holdford, D. Understanding the dissemination of appointment-based synchronization models using the CFIR framework. *Res. Soc. Adm. Pharm.* **2017**, *13*, 914–921. [CrossRef]

48. Watson, L.L.; Bluml, B.M. Pharmacy's Appointment Based Model: Implementation Guide for Pharmacy Practices. APhA Foundation. 2013. Available online: https://www.aphafoundation.org/sites/default/files/ckeditor/files/ABMImplementationGuide-FINAL-20130923.pdf (accessed on 3 June 2019).

49. Khazan, E.; Anastasia, E.; Hough, A.; Parra, D. Pharmacist-managed ambulatory blood pressure monitoring service. *Am. J. Health Syst. Pharm.* **2017**, *74*, 190–195. [CrossRef]

50. Milfred-LaForest, S.K.; Gee, J.A.; Pugacz, A.M.; Pina, I.L.; Hoover, D.M.; Wenzell, R.C.; Felton, A.; Guttenberg, E.; Ortiz, J. Heart failure transitions of care: A pharmacist-led post-discharge pilot experience. *Prog. Cardiovasc. Dis.* **2017**, *60*, 249–258. [CrossRef]

51. Halalau, A.; Shelden, D.; Keeney, S.; Hehar, J. Pharm-MD; an open-label, randomized controlled, phase II study to evaluate the efficacy of a pharmacist-managed diabetes clinic in high-risk diabetes patients study protocol for a randomized controlled trial. *Trials* **2018**, *19*, 458. [CrossRef]

52. Schultz, J.L.; Horner, K.E.; McDanel, D.L.; Miller, M.L.; Beranek, R.L.; Jacobsen, R.B.; Sly, N.J.; Miller, A.C.; Mascardo, L.A. Comparing clinical outcomes of a pharmacist-managed diabetes clinic to usual physician-based care. *J. Pharm. Pract.* **2018**, *31*, 268–271. [CrossRef]

53. Pett, R.G.; Nye, S. Evaluation of a pharmacist-managed asthma clinic in an Indian Health Service clinic. *J. Am. Pharm. Assoc.* **2016**, *56*, 237–241. [CrossRef]

54. Hale, A.; Merlo, G.; Nissen, L.; Coombes, I.; Graves, N. Cost-effectiveness analysis of doctor-pharmacist collaborative prescribing for venous thromboembolism in high risk surgical patients. *BMC Health Serv. Res.* **2018**, *18*, 749. [CrossRef]

55. Lee, J.C.; Horner, K.E.; Krummel, M.L.; McDanel, D.L. Clinical and financial outcomes evaluation of multimodal pharmacist warfarin management of a statewide urban and rural population. *J. Pharm. Pract.* **2018**, *31*, 150–156. [CrossRef]

56. Manzoor, B.S.; Cheng, W.H.; Lee, J.C.; Uppuluri, E.M.; Nutescu, E.A. Quality of pharmacist-managed anticoagulation therapy in long-term ambulatory settings: A systematic review. *Ann. Pharmacother.* **2017**, *51*, 1122–1137. [CrossRef]

57. Durham, M.J.; Goad, J.A.; Neinstien, L.S.; Lou, M.A. A comparison of pharmacist travel-health specialists' versus primary care providers' recommendations for travel-related medications, vaccination, and patient compliance in a college health setting. *J. Travel Med.* **2011**, *18*, 20–25. [CrossRef]

58. Hess, K.M.; Dai, C.W.; Garner, B.; Law, A.V. Measuring outcomes of a pharmacist-run travel health clinic located within an independent community pharmacy. *J. Am. Pharm. Assoc.* **2010**, *50*, 174–180. [CrossRef]

59. Manchikanti Gomez, A. Availability of pharmacist-prescribed contraception in California. *J. Am. Med. Assoc.* **2017**, *318*, 2253–2254. [CrossRef]

60. Puzantian, T.; Gasper, J.J. Provision of naloxone without a prescription by California pharmacists 2 years after legislation implementation. *J. Am. Med. Assoc.* **2018**, *320*, 1933–1934. [CrossRef]

61. Smalls, T.D.; Broughton, A.D.; Hylick, E.V.; Woodard, T.J. Providing medication therapy management for smoking cessation patients. *J. Pharm. Pract.* **2015**, *28*, 21–25. [CrossRef]

62. Salvig, B.E.; Gulum, A.H.; Walters, S.A.; Edwards, L.B.; Fourakre, T.N.; Marvin, S.C.; McKenzie, M.S.; Moseley, M.V.; Ansari, I.J. Pharmacist screening for risk of osteoporosis in elderly veterans. *Consult. Pharm.* **2016**, *31*, 440–449. [CrossRef]

63. Smith, M.C.; Boldt, A.S.; Waston, C.M.; Zillich, A.J. Effectiveness of a pharmacy care management program for veterans with dyslipidemia. *Pharmacotherapy* **2013**, *33*, 736–743. [CrossRef]

64. Isho, N.Y.; Kachlic, M.D.; Marcelo, J.C.; Martin, M.T. Pharmacist-initiated hepatitis C virus screening in a community pharmacy to increase awareness and link to care at the medical center. *J. Am. Pharm. Assoc.* **2017**, *57*, S259–S264. [CrossRef]

65. Klepser, D.G.; Klepser, M.E.; Smith, J.K.; Dering-Anderson, A.M.; Nelson, M.; Pohren, L.E. Utilization of influenza and streptococcal pharyngitis point-of-care testing in the community pharmacy practice setting. *Res. Soc. Adm. Pharm.* **2017**, *14*, 356–359. [CrossRef]

66. Grayson, G.; Shulman, D. Impression management in services marketing. In *Handbook of Services Marketing*; SwartZ, T.A., Iacobucci, D., Eds.; Sage: Thousand Oaks, CA, USA, 2000; pp. 51–68.

67. Guhl, D.; Blankart, K.E.; Stargardt, T. Service quality and perceived customer value in community pharmacies. *Health Serv. Manag. Res.* **2018**, *32*, 36–48. [CrossRef]

68. Desselle, S.P. An in-depth examination of pharmacy technician worklife through an organizational behaviour framework. *Res. Soc. Adm. Pharm.* **2016**, *12*, 722–732. [CrossRef]

69. Ghorob, A.; Bodenheimer, T. Building teams in primary care: A practical guide. *Fam. Syst. Health* **2015**, *33*, 182–192. [CrossRef]

70. Brummel, A.; Lustig, A.; Westrich, K.; Evans, M.A.; Plank, G.S.; Penso, J.; Dubois, R.W. Best practices: Improving patient outcomes and costs in an ACO through comprehensive medication therapy management. *J. Manag. Care Pharm.* **2014**, *20*, 1152–1158. [CrossRef]

71. MacKeigan, L.D.; Ljaz, N.; Bojarski, E.A.; Dolovich, L. Implementation of a reimbursed medication review program: Corporate and pharmacy level strategies. *Res. Soc. Adm. Pharm.* **2017**, *13*, 947–958. [CrossRef]

72. Musselman, K.T.; Moczygemba, L.R.; Pierce, A.L.; Plum, M.B.; Brokaw, D.K.; Kelly, D.L. Development and implementation of clinical pharmacist services within an integrated medical group. *J. Pharm. Pract.* **2017**, *30*, 75–81. [CrossRef]

73. American Pharmacists Association. Pharmacist Scope of Services. Available online: https://www.pharmacist.com/sites/default/files/files/APhA%20-%20PAPCC%20Scope%20of%20Services.pdf (accessed on 1 January 2019).

74. Collaborative Practice Agreements and Pharmacists' Patient Care Services: A Resource for Pharmacists. National Center for Chronic Disease Prevention and Health Promotion. Available online: https://www.cdc.gov/dhdsp/pubs/docs/Translational_Tools_Pharmacists.pdf (accessed on 6 June 2019).

75. Collaborative Practice Agreements: Resources and More. NASPA. Available online: https://naspa.us/resource/cpa/ (accessed on 6 June 2019).

76. Collaborative Practice Agreements (CPA) and Pharmacists' Patient Care Services. APhA Foundation. Available online: https://www.aphafoundation.org/collaborative-practice-agreements (accessed on 6 June 2019).

77. Farris, K.B.; Ashwood, D.; McIntosh, J.; DiPietro, N.A.; Maderas, N.M.; Landau, S.C.; Swegle, J.; Solemani, O. Preventing unintended pregnancy. Pharmacists' roles in practice and policy via partnerships. *J. Am. Pharm. Assoc.* **2010**, *50*, 604–612. [CrossRef]

78. Beal, J.L.; Plake, K.S.I. Social and legislative shaping of access to to contraceptives and the pharmacist's role: A literature review. *Res. Soc. Adm. Pharm.* **2019**. [CrossRef]

79. Parsai, S. Nutrition education improves patient care. *J. Am. Pharm. Assoc.* **2016**, *56*, 225–226. [CrossRef]

80. Harmon, M.; Pogge, B.; Boomershine, V. Evaluation of a pharmacist-led, 6-month weight loss program for obese patients. *J. Am. Pharm. Assoc.* **2014**, *54*, 302–307. [CrossRef]

81. Matzke, G.R.; Czar, M.J.; Lee, W.T.; Moczygemba, L.R.; Harlow, L.D. Improving health of at risk rural patients: A collaborative care model. *Am. J. Health Syst. Pharm.* **2016**, *73*, e583–e591. [CrossRef]

82. McGee, J.E.; Love, J.G.; Festervand, T.A. Competitive advantage and the independent retail pharmacy: The role of distinctive competencies. *J. Pharm. Mark. Manag.* **2000**, *13*, 31–46. [CrossRef]

83. Planas, L.G. Intervention design, implementation, and evaluation. *Am. J. Health Syst. Pharm.* **2008**, *65*, 1854–1863. [CrossRef]

84. Delivering Medication Therapy Management Services. American Pharmacists Association. Available online: https://www.pharmacist.com/education/advanced-training-programs/delivering-medication-therapy-management-services?is_sso_called=1 (accessed on 6 June 2019).

85. Jobin, J.; Irwin, A.N.; Pimentel, J.; Turner, M.C. Accuracy of medication histories collected by pharmacy technicians during hospital admission. *Res. Soc. Adm. Pharm.* **2018**, *14*, 695–699. [CrossRef]

86. Grove, S.J.; Fisk, R.P.; John, J. Services as theatre: Guidelines and implications. In *Handbook of Services Marketing and Management*; Swartz, T.A., Iacobucci, D., Eds.; Sage: Thousand Oaks, CA, USA, 2000; pp. 2–36.

87. Crawford, C.; Low, J.K.; Manias, E.; Williams, A. Healthcare professionals can assist patients with managing post kidney transplant expectations. *Res. Soc. Adm. Pharm.* **2017**, *13*, 1204–1207. [CrossRef]

88. Crespo-Gonzalez, C.; Garcia-Cardenas, V.; Benrimoj, S.I. The next phase in professional services research: From implementation to sustainability. *Res. Soc. Adm. Pharm.* **2017**, *13*, 896–901. [CrossRef]

89. Eccles, M.P.; Mittman, B.S. Welcome to implementation science. *Implement. Sci.* **2006**, *1*, 1. [CrossRef]

90. Curran, G.M.; Shoemaker, S.J. Advancing pharmacy practice through implementation science. *Res. Soc. Adm. Pharm.* **2017**, *13*, 889–891. [CrossRef]

91. Shoemaker, S.J.; Curran, G.M.; Swan, H.; Teeter, B.S.; Thomas, J. Application of the Consolidated Framework for implementation research to community pharmacy: A framework for implementation research on pharmacy services. *Res. Soc. Adm. Pharm.* **2017**, *13*, 905–913. [CrossRef]

92. Fuller, J.M.; Saini, B.; Bosnic-Anticevich, S.; Cardenas, V.G.; Benrimoj, S.I.; Armour, C. Testing evidence routine practice: Using an implementation framework to embed a clinically proven asthma service in Australian community pharmacy. *Res. Soc. Adm. Pharm.* **2017**, *13*, 989–996. [CrossRef]

93. Sim, T.F.; Hattingh, H.L.; Sherriff, J.; Tee, L.B.G. Towards the implementation of breastfeeding-related health services in community pharmacies: Pharmacists' perspectives. *Res. Soc. Adm. Pharm.* **2017**, *13*, 980–988. [CrossRef]

94. Hattingh, H.L.; Kelly, F.; Fowler, J.; Wheeler, A.J. Implementation of a mental health medication management intervention in Australian community pharmacies: Facilitators and challenges. *Res. Soc. Adm. Pharm.* **2017**, *13*, 969–979. [CrossRef]

95. Stafford, R.; Thomas, J.; Payakachat, N.; Diemer, T.; Lang, M.; Kordsmeier, B.; Curran, G. Using an array of implementation strategies to improve success rates of pharmacist-initiated medication therapy management services in community pharmacies. *Res. Soc. Adm. Pharm.* **2017**, *13*, 98–946. [CrossRef]

96. Lennox, L.; Maher, L.; Reed, J. Navigating the sustainability landscape: A systematic review of sustainability approaches in healthcare. *Implement. Sci.* **2018**, *13*, 27. [CrossRef]

97. Shelton, R.C.; Cooper, B.R.; Stirman, S.W. The Sustainability of Evidence-Based Interventions and Practices in Public Health and Health Care. *Annu. Rev. Public Health* **2018**, *39*, 55–76. [CrossRef]

98. DaVanzo, J.; Dobson, A.; Koenig, L.; Book, R. Medication Therapy Management Services: A Critical Review. 2005. Available online: https://www.acccp.com/docs/positions/commentarties/memts/pdf (accessed on 6 June 2019).

99. Payment Methods in Outpatient Team-Based Clinical Pharmacy Practice, Part 1. ACCP Practice Advancement Issue Brief. 2018. Available online: https://www.accp.com/docs/positions/misc/IB1PaymentPart1-ACCPPracticeAdvancement.pdf (accessed on 6 June 2019).

100. Smith, M.A. Implementing primary care pharmacist services: Go upstream in the world of value-based payment models. *Res. Soc. Adm. Pharm.* **2017**, *13*, 892–895. [CrossRef]

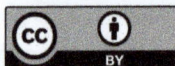

pharmacy

MDPI

Commentary

Co-located Retail Clinics and Pharmacies: An Opportunity to Provide More Primary Care

Katherine Knapp [1,*], **Keith Yoshizuka** [1], **Debra Sasaki-Hill** [1] **and Rory Caygill-Walsh** [2]

[1]   College of Pharmacy, Touro University California, 1310 Club Drive, Vallejo, CA 94592, USA
[2]   Zuckerberg San Francisco General Hospital, 1001 Potrero Ave, San Francisco, CA 94702, USA
*   Correspondence: Katherine.knapp@tu.edu

Received: 10 April 2019; Accepted: 18 June 2019; Published: 26 June 2019

check for updates

Abstract: This paper proposes that co-located retail clinics (RCs) and community pharmacies can increase opportunities to provide more accessible, affordable, and patient-friendly primary care services in the United States. RCs are small businesses of about 150–250 square feet with a clientele of about 10–30 patients each day and most frequently staffed by nurse practitioners (NPs). Community pharmacies in the U.S. at ~67,000 far outnumber RCs at ~2800, thereby opening substantial opportunity for growth. Community pharmacies and pharmacists have been working to increase on-site clinical services, but progress has been slowed by the relative isolation from other practitioners. An ideal merged facility based on an integrated platform is proposed. NPs and pharmacists could share functions that fulfill documented consumer preferences and still maintain separate practice domains. Potential benefits include a broader inventory of clinical services including laboratory tests, immunizations, patient education, and physical assessment, as well as better patient access, interprofessional training opportunities, and economies related to the use of resources, day-to-day operations, and performance metrics. Challenges include the availability of sufficient, appropriately trained staff; limitations imposed by scope of practice and other laws; forging of collaborative relationships between NPs and pharmacists; and evidence that the merged operations provide economic benefits beyond those of separate enterprises.

Keywords: community pharmacy; retail clinics; pharmacists; nurse practitioners; interprofessional training; primary care; healthcare access

1. Purpose

We propose that the growing presence of co-located retail clinics (RCs) and pharmacies in the United States provides an opportunity to improve the delivery of accessible, affordable, and patient-friendly primary care services in the United States. In this paper, we present the case for the gains that could be made and the challenges that could reduce benefits and/or stand in the way of continued, successful implementation.

2. Methods

A three-person team with practice and research experience searched PubMed, Google Scholar, and Google for articles and papers about retail clinics, community pharmacy practice trends, training and clinical activities of nurse practitioners and pharmacists, primary care delivery trends, and approaches to merging business operations. Search terms included community pharmacy, retail clinics, pharmacist, nurse, and primary care. Previously collected resources were added to relevant articles. Based on the importance of legal issues, we only considered papers from the United States. The resource articles and follow-up discussions were used to identify benefits and challenges in establishing a successful, merged operation in co-located RCs and community pharmacies.

3. Background

3.1. Retail Clinics

The retail clinic (RC) is a relatively new site for providing primary healthcare services. These ambulatory sites render preventive and therapeutic services and are generally staffed by nurse practitioners (NPs) or physician assistants (PAs) [1–3]. In 2018, RC numbers in the U.S. were estimated at 2800, and the numbers continue to grow [4]. The potential value of RCs was explored in a landmark 2009 study that provided evidence that the cost of a typical RC visit ($110) was significantly less than similar visits to physician offices ($166), urgent care centers ($156), or emergency departments ($570), while the quality of care was equivalent or better [5]. The RCs are generally co-located with pharmacies. To date, CVS and Walgreens have sponsored the greatest numbers of RCs. Also sponsoring RCs, either directly or by contract, are mass merchandise corporations such as Target and Walmart and some grocery operations [2]. Here also, co-location with pharmacies is generally the rule. To give an idea of the potential for expansion, in 2015, <3% of the approximate 67,000 pharmacies in the U.S. had co-located RCs [6].

A 2015 report described RCs as small businesses of about 150–250 square feet with a clientele of about 10–30 patients each day [7]. It is hard to imagine RCs flourishing as independent, stand-alone entities; indeed, the business model pairing them with pharmacies has many potential advantages, a number of which we explore in this paper. With cost a critical issue for sustainability and expansion, it seems that co-located RCs and pharmacies should explore all reasonable economies by virtue of co-location.

3.2. Nurse Practitioners

NPs are generally preferred over PAs to lead RC operations. This is because scope of practice laws, which are generated at the state level, have allowed NPs in most states to have more autonomy from physician oversight. Given the small percentage of pharmacies co-located with RCs, a basic question for potential RC growth is the availability of sufficient numbers of appropriately prepared NPs.

Advanced Practice Registered Nurses (APRNs) provide diagnostic and therapeutic services for acute, episodic, or chronic illnesses [8,9]. APRNs include three cohorts, with NPs representing about 76% by number and nurse midwives and nurse anesthetists representing the rest. (Clinical nurse specialists are a fourth cohort of APRNs. This group is not currently represented in Bureau of Labor Statistics (BLS) data.) Bureau of Labor Statistics (BLS) data for 2017 report 166,280 employed NPs in the U.S. with mean annual wages of $107,480 [9]. There are several specialty areas for NPs based on the patient populations they are trained to care for. Some examples are pediatrics, acute care, psychiatry, and family care [10]. Family NPs (FNPs) are the only group licensed to treat both adults and children. This is an important consideration given that RCs treat both adult and pediatric patients, and it makes the FNP the best candidate for RC positions.

Requirements for licensure as an NP vary by state. Most states require RN status, completion of a Master's degree or higher with emphasis on nursing skills from an accredited institution, and national certification from either the American Association of Nurse Practitioners or the American Nurses Credentialing Center [11]. Achieving NP status takes about two years beyond RN status. Nationally, there is a trend toward common licensure requirements for NPs. While every state would still require NP licensure to practice in that state, common licensure requirements could benefit RCs expanding across state lines by allowing NPs to gain licensure in another state more easily.

Health-related services that NPs can offer are determined by state-based scope of practice laws, a circumstance which has implications for RCs. Practice activities of NPs in California, for example, must meet the requirements for "standardized procedures" (SPs), meaning that only procedures that have been developed, reviewed, and approved by an interdisciplinary team can be legally performed [12]. Standardized procedures apply to diagnostic and treatment activities. One such procedure is the ability to prescribe medications under protocol. (In California, the term "furnish" is used in legal language regarding prescribing activities for both NPs and pharmacists.) For RCs, a particular advantage of co-location with pharmacies is this authority—an approved practice activity which is generally broader than allowed for pharmacists. The ability to obtain prescriptions which can potentially be filled under the same roof has been cited as a preference by patients [13]. There are, however, limitations on prescribing activities which are discussed below. A new direction related to services that can be offered is reflected in a bill that has been introduced in the California legislature that would allow NPs and physician assistants to practice independent of a supervising physician [14,15].

3.3. Pharmacists

By way of comparison with NPs, pharmacists are greater in number. According to the BLS [16], 309,330 pharmacists were employed in the United States in 2017. Their mean annual wage was $121,710. To become a pharmacist, one must earn a Doctor of Pharmacy (PharmD) through a program accredited by the Accreditation Council of Pharmacy Education (ACPE). The PharmD program requires four years, sometimes three years, depending on the curriculum of the institution. Once graduated, two sets of exams must be passed to obtain licensure: the North American National Pharmacist Licensure Examination (NAPLEX) and the Multistate Pharmacy Jurisprudence Examination (MJPE) or a state-specific law exam. Some pharmacists will continue training by completing a residency or fellowship. Some will pursue board certification in a specialty area by passing an examination. Currently, there are 41,000 [17] pharmacists worldwide that are Board of Pharmacy Specialties (BPS)-certified in 11 specialty areas such as pharmacotherapy, geriatrics, ambulatory care, and cardiology.

Pharmacists have been working professionally and politically to increase clinical involvement in patient care, especially in areas that relate to primary care. Through education and training, as well as expansion of scope of practice laws, progress has occurred. Indeed, pharmacists have been identified as part of the solution to reducing the shortage of primary care providers in this country [18,19]. Some states have passed laws allowing qualified pharmacists to expand their scope of practice and a pathway has been created to support another level of licensure: Advanced Practice Pharmacist (APP). California, North Carolina, Minnesota, New Mexico, Oregon, and Washington now support APP licensure. However, despite these advances, community pharmacies' physical locations, somewhat isolated from other healthcare providers, have slowed this progress. The prospect of pharmacists partnering with NPs whose practice privileges overlap—but usually extend beyond those of pharmacists—opens the door to expanding services as a merged, joint operation.

3.4. Pharmacies

Health services offered in pharmacies have been expanding since the early 2000s when immunizations started being offered widely at pharmacies. More recently, but only in some states, pharmacies became able to prescribe naloxone for opioid overdose, hormonal contraceptives, and medications recommended for international travel. Pharmacies are providing smoking cessation programs, and there has recently been a proposal for pharmacists to prescribe medications to prevent the transmission of HIV [20–22]. Ohio recently passed SB 265 to provide reimbursement to pharmacists for clinical services by the state Medicaid program [23]. This trend toward expanding health services in community pharmacies has continued with both CVS and Walgreens recently launching initiatives. For example, CVS has opened three concept stores in the Houston area featuring "HealthHUBs" that offer assistance with durable medical equipment, yoga classes, blood tests, and nutritional advice in addition to their RCs (MinuteClinics) and pharmacies. CVS also announced the availability of telehealth services through its MinuteClinics [24]. Additionally, Walgreens renovated a store in Deerfield, Illinois to house a "Health Corner" offering such services as vision care, lab tests, and hearing services [25]. These initiatives by pharmacy industry giants may be an indication of the future direction of community pharmacies. Most recently, health insurer Aliera signed an agreement with CVS's MinuteClinics to provide their members "with access to MinuteClinic services at no cost and with no applicable co-pays or deductibles" [26].

Besides these new ventures by pharmacy corporations, there is evidence that customers/patients are looking for an expanded service package when they go to a pharmacy. Table 1 combines results from three studies about consumer preferences for pharmacy-based health services. The first of these is a 2017 study of over 9000 people ≥18 years of age [27]. The second is a 2018 study of >1000 U.S. adults ≥40 years of age [13]. The third is a 2018 study that showed agreement among pharmacists, physicians, and patients that "minor ailments" could be well treated in rural community pharmacy settings by pharmacists, NPs, and/or PAs [28]. In these studies, participants identified preferred services they would like to see in community pharmacies. Table 1 suggests that, under the right circumstances, NPs and pharmacists could share several of these functions and still maintain separate practice domains. The shared services could allow for flexibility depending on the demand for services in either the RC or the pharmacy. This topic is explored further in a later section.

Table 1. Customer/Patient preferences from three studies.

Clinical Service	More Specific Details	Deliverable by Pharmacist or Pharmacy	Deliverable by NP or RC
Access by appointment or walk-in	Ability to make an appointment for service(s)	Some	Some
Preventive health services	Cholesterol, blood pressure, diabetes, osteoporosis screening, immunizations, life style evaluation, vitamins and supplements, lung function	Sometimes *	Yes, in California (CA) with standardized procedures (SPs)
Diagnostic testing	Diabetes mellitus, lipid/cholesterol measurements, testing for common infections including flu, strep, hepatitis, tuberculosis, HIV and chemistry tests (urine, saliva, and blood)	Yes	Yes, in CA with SPs
(Quick) OTC treatments and/or recommendations	Allergies, skin rashes, cough and cold, gastro-intestinal issues, feminine issues, sleeping aids, first aid, eye and ear problems, analgesics	Yes	Yes, in CA with SPs
Patient education	Advice on prescriptions, Medicare plans, medication interactions, side effects, over-the-counter medications, Medication Therapy Management, patient safety, behavioral counseling	Yes	Yes
Prescription ordering, availability, information	Managing prescriptions, procurement, inventory, recalls, counseling	Yes	No
Medical records	Keep records on medications, patient profiles, e.g., allergies	Sometimes ** Depends	Yes
Physical examinations	Blood pressure, heart rate, breathing rate, extremities	Yes	Yes
Medication services	New prescriptions, refill reminders, delivery, counseling	Yes	Yes, in CA with SPs
Immunizations	Vaccinations: flu, pneumonia, zoster, travel medications	Yes	Yes, in CA with SPs

Table 1. *Cont.*

Clinical Service	More Specific Details	Deliverable by Pharmacist or Pharmacy	Deliverable by NP or RC
Drug prescribing	Oral contraceptives, smoking cessation, adjustment of dose	Yes ***	Yes, in CA with SPs
Advice and monitoring	Weight loss, diabetes, cholesterol, blood pressure	Yes	Yes

* Some screenings may be performed by the pharmacist, while others require specialized equipment not available in the pharmacy. ** In most cases, a patient's electronic health record is not readily available to the pharmacist, and a patient's electronic health record is not readily available to the NP. However, in some pharmacies affiliated with a medical care system, this information can be available to both parties. *** Pharmacist prescribing is dependent upon the setting (a provider who contracts with a licensed health care service plan with regard to the care or services provided to the enrollees of that health care service plan [29]) or the level of license of the pharmacist (Advanced Practice Pharmacist (APP)).

4. An Ideal Co-located Facility

4.1. Advantages of an Integrated Platform

Imagine for a moment that RCs and pharmacies could develop an integrated platform for delivering health services that are both preventive and therapeutic and that could also address customer preferences. What might it look like? The preferences in Table 1 indicate that customers and patients want their access to health care to be uncomplicated, quick, and convenient. In our ideal facility, for example, a patient could use a single access point—electronic, telephonic, or otherwise—to make an appointment for an immunization or blood pressure check, to get answers to questions about medication interactions, and/or to schedule a diabetic foot examination. Both NPs and pharmacists are trained to offer these services, although NPs perform diagnostic procedures more frequently. So, depending on the issue and overall workload, the patient's appointment could be with either an NP or a pharmacist or both. In an ideal situation, staff could be cross-trained in areas that do not require specialized licenses or certificates to fill in for the other service area to prevent delaying or denying services to the patient. For situations requiring prescription medications, patients would have the option of filling their prescription and receiving counseling a few steps away, although there are caveats about getting prescriptions filled that are discussed below. In short, an integrated RC/pharmacy platform could mimic, on a smaller scale, a well-established and reputable health maintenance organization where a patient could receive several different healthcare services under one roof.

4.2. Clinical Laboratory Tests

Regarding customer preferences around clinical tests, the Clinical Laboratory Improvement Amendments 1988 (CLIA) describe quality standards for testing in clinical laboratories. For >1400 test systems that are non-technical and unlikely to provide erroneous results, CLIA requirements have been waived. These include, for example, blood glucose testing, cholesterol and hemoglobin A1c measurement, and testing for the presence of HIV-1 and HIV-2. Both pharmacies and RCs can offer diagnostic tests that are CLIA-waived after obtaining a CLIA Certificate of Waiver (COW). An integrated operation under the same roof and address could allow a single COW for the facility—a valuable efficiency saving time and money. In like fashion, inventories of vaccines could serve both the pharmacy and the RC.

4.3. Interprofessional Training Opportunities

Both pharmacist and NP training programs struggle with meeting mandates for interprofessional training as part of their programs. Such training is now mandated by accreditation agencies for most health professions [30,31]. An integrated, co-located RC and pharmacy could provide an ideal site for NP and pharmacy students to work with other health professionals—and one another—as part of providing care and being part of a care team. From a training perspective, these sites could help schools achieve accreditation requirements. From an economic perspective, students could augment the amount of service that can be offered to patients. From a student perspective, there is the opportunity for concrete experience working as a team in a primary care arena. One caveat would be that it is probably optimal that a site used for training be "mature" in the sense that integration is operational and the staff are experienced in working as a team.

4.4. Other Advantages

Some other advantages that could be realized with an integrated platform include providing more flexibility with hours of operation, providing more and richer patient education, creating in-house consultation on clinical issues, and expanding the service list that a single facility can offer.

5. Challenges

5.1. NP Supply

Despite the several clinical, financial, and convenience advantages cited above, there are barriers to consider and overcome. First, adequate numbers of appropriately trained NPs are needed to staff RCs. As noted earlier, only Family NPs (FNPs) are licensed to provide care for children and adults and would therefore be preferred to staff RCs. Approximately 67% of the NP cohort are FNPs [32], which, using BLS data, would be about 110,000 persons, an attractive pool for RC recruitment. Moreover, the BLS projects the number of NPs to grow by 31% between 2016 and 2026, a growth rate which is "much faster than average" [9]. However, given that NPs must provide evidence of registered nurse (RN) status to qualify for NP licensure, a shortage of RNs in the U.S., reported as recently as 2019, is relevant to the issue of sustained supply [33]. The same report lists reasons for the RN shortage to include a shortage of faculty that limits enrollment, an aging population of RNs, workplace stress, and difficulties finding appropriate training sites [34]. Based on the relationship between RN and NP supply, sustained RN growth will be an important factor in having sufficient FNPs to staff RCs.

5.2. Collaborative Practice Agreements

This paper discusses the topic of RCs located within a pharmacy on a national basis. There are still a handful of states where collaborative practice for pharmacists is severely restricted (such as the state of New York, where pharmacist collaborative practice agreements are restricted to teaching hospitals). Even in those states that allow collaborative practice agreements, some are so restrictive that a separate agreement must be established for each patient. The strategy of inserting the NP as the provider in RCs definitely has advantages, but state legal restrictions could limit the applicability of this strategy.

5.3. Antitrust and Stark Laws

The management of prescription medications is another issue that is potentially challenging. While it may seem logical that a prescription generated by a RC co-located with a pharmacy be filled at that pharmacy, the patient always has the choice of where to get that prescription filled. Limiting that choice may possibly violate antitrust laws [35] and the Stark laws [34] regarding illegal referrals. The prescriber may not direct the patient to use a particular pharmacy, nor can a lease agreement contain any requirements or incentives regarding the number of prescriptions generated. The Stark law specifically states in 42 USC §1395nn(a)(1)(A) " ... the physician may not make a referral to the entity (where there is a financial arrangement) for the furnishing of designated health services for which payment otherwise may be made under this subchapter", and the definition of health services specifically lists outpatient prescription drugs [36].

5.4. Pharmacist Reimbursement

Reimbursement for clinical services provided by pharmacists could be an impediment to the business success of co-located RCs and pharmacies. While pharmacists may bill Medicare for certain services as "incident-to" a visit [37], efforts to pass legislation for direct reimbursement to pharmacists under Medicare Part B have failed to make it out of committee in Congress [36,38]. There are some signs of progress; however, these are not without complications. For example, in California, a bill passed both houses and was signed by the governor in 2016 authorizing payment to pharmacists by MediCal (Medicaid) for clinical services allowed by SB 493 [39]. However, it has taken MediCal three years to issue billing codes to allow pharmacists to bill for such services. On the positive side, Washington State was successful in passing a bill in 2015 requiring commercial health plans to enroll pharmacists as providers and pay for services permitted within their scope of practice [40], and, as noted earlier, the Ohio legislature recently passed a bill to provide reimbursement to pharmacists for clinical services by the state Medicaid program [23]. Some commercial health plans have taken the initiative to recognize and reimburse pharmacists for clinical services, but this is more the exception than the rule.

One area where pharmacists have found success is by contracting with Accountable Care Organizations (ACOs) created by the Patient Protection and Affordable Care Act [41] to work within their scope of practice to improve the quality of care, improve accessibility, and reduce costs. The ACO is based upon population management as opposed to fee-for-service, so there is incentive to provide improved-quality care while reducing costs. Overall, these fragmented and state-based approaches to pharmacy/pharmacist reimbursement for clinical services have not made a major breakthrough and can still obstruct efforts to expand services in pharmacies whether or not they are co-located with RCs.

5.5. Business Relationship between the RC and Pharmacy

The last challenge we present is based on the financial and operational arrangements between the RC and pharmacy. Current models may not allow crossover in financial areas including payroll, reimbursements, and cost of supplies. This practice effectively places the pharmacy in competition with the RC. We would propose that the best chance for the success of co-located facilities to be greater than the individual successes of each entity is to establish an integrated platform that merges the use of resources, the inventory of clinical services, rules for day-to-day operations, and performance metrics while paying attention to customer preferences. This merging will be no easy task and will rely heavily on the development and use of skills and methods involving collaboration. To the best of our knowledge, there is currently no model that achieves a sustainable, merged organization, but a recent study outlines the characteristics of such a model and actions that can build the needed collaborative relationships [42]. With the continued deficit in primary care access and affordability in the United States and the potential to use existing facilities to a broader extent, it seems reasonable to explore, experimentally implement, and assess a merged operation. We hope that the information and ideas presented here can promote efforts toward a model that capitalizes on the advantages of co-locating RCs and community pharmacies.

6. Summary

Retail clinics (RC) co-located with pharmacies have the potential to increase the delivery of primary care in the United States. The advantages in merging the two operations include the ability to address customer preferences, to expand clinical services, to achieve efficiencies in managing supplies and materials, and to create more interprofessional training sites. Challenges to achieving a successful merged operation include the limitations imposed by scope of practice and other laws, difficulties with pharmacist reimbursement for clinical services, a possible shortage of family nurse practitioners, and the development of a practice model that achieves these goals while being financially successful.

At this point, while the concept of co-located RCs and pharmacies is young, it is recommended to develop, implement, and assess a model or models based on merged, integrated operations.

Author Contributions: Conceptualization: K.K., D.S.-H. and K.Y.; data curation: all authors; formal analysis: K.K., D.S.-H. and K.Y.

Funding: This research received no external funding.

Conflicts of Interest: The authors declare no conflict of interest.

References

1. Rand Corporation. The Evolution of Retail Clinics. Available online: https://www.rand.org/pubs/research_briefs/RB9491-2.html (accessed on 24 September 2018).
2. Iglehart, J.K. The expansion of retail clinics—Corporate titans vs. organized Medicine. *N. Engl. J. Med.* **2015**, *373*, 301–303. [CrossRef] [PubMed]
3. Convenient Care Association. Retail Health Workforce: Creating Effective Experiences for Future Retail Health Clinics. Available online: https://www.scribd.com/document/367742288/Think-Tank-2017-Report (accessed on 15 January 2019).
4. Statista. Number of Retail Clinics in the United States from 2008–2018. 2019. Available online: https://www.statista.com/statistics/307264/number-of-us-retail-clinics/ (accessed on 15 January 2019).
5. Mehrotra, A.; Liu, H.; Adams, J.L.; Wang, M.C.; Lave, J.R.; Thygeson, N.M.; Solberg, L.I.; McGlynn, E.A. Comparing costs and quality of care at retail clinics with that of other medical settings for 3 common illnesses. *Ann. Intern. Med.* **2009**, *151*, 321–328. [CrossRef] [PubMed]
6. Qato, D.M.; Zenk, S.K.; Wilder, J.; Harrington, R.; Gaskin, D.; Alexander, G.C. The availability of pharmacies in the United States: 2007–2015. *PLoS ONE* **2017**, *12*, e0183172. [CrossRef] [PubMed]
7. Bachrach, D.; Frohlich, J.; Garcimonde, A.; Nevitt, K. Building a Culture of Health: The Value Proposition of Retail Clinics. 2015. Available online: http://www.manatt.com/uploadedFiles/Content/5_Insights/White_Papers/Retail_Clinic_RWJF.pdf (accessed on 24 January 2019).
8. Bureau of Labor Statistics. Occupational Employment Statistics. 2019. Available online: https://www.bls.gov/oes/2017/may/oes291171.htm (accessed on 10 January 2019).
9. Bureau of Labor Statistics. Occupational Outlook Handbook: Nurse Anesthetists, Nurse Midwives and Nurse Practitioners. 2019. Available online: https://www.bls.gov/ooh/healthcare/nurse-anesthetists-nurse-midwives-and-nurse-practitioners.htm (accessed on 10 January 2019).
10. Nurse Practioner Schools. Nurse Practitioners Programs by Specialty. Available online: https://www.nursepractitionerschools.com/programs/ (accessed on 31 May 2019).
11. Nurse Practitioner License Requirements: Change is in the Air. Available online: https://www.nursinglicensure.org/articles/nurse-practitioner-license.html (accessed on 16 January 2019).
12. State of California. An Explanation of Standardized Procedure Requirement for Nurse Practitioner Practice. Available online: https://www.rn.ca.gov/pdfs/regulations/npr-b-20.pdf (accessed on 14 January 2019).
13. Redman, R. Patients Want Pharmacies to Go 'Beyond the Fill'. Available online: www.chaindrugreview.com/patients-want-pharmacies-to-go-beyond-the-fill/ (accessed on 11 January 2019).
14. California State Assembly Bill 890. Available online: http://leginfo.legislature.ca.gov/faces/billNavClient.xhtml?bill_id=201920200AB890 (accessed on 8 March 2019).
15. California State Assembly Bill 697. Available online: http://leginfo.legislature.ca.gov/faces/billNavClient.xhtml?bill_id=201920200AB697 (accessed on 8 March 2019).
16. Bureau of Labor Statistics. Occupational Employment Statistics. Available online: https://www.bls.gov/oes/2017/may/oes291051.htm (accessed on 11 January 2019).
17. Board of Pharmacy Specialties. Available online: https://board-of-pharmacy-specialties.dcatalog.com/v/2017-Annual-Report/?page=3 (accessed on 9 April 2019).
18. Jain, S.H. Can Pharmacists Help Reinvent Primary Care in the United States? Available online: https://www.forbes.com/sites/sachinjain/2018/10/10/can-pharmacists-help-reinvent-primary-care-in-the-united-states/#185a7c1b590b (accessed on 27 December 2018).
19. Gums, J. Can Pharmacists Help Fill the Growing Primary Care Gap? Available online: https://theconversation.com/can-pharmacists-help-fill-the-growing-primary-care-gap-51015 (accessed on 27 December 2018).

20. California State Senate Bill 493. Available online: http://leginfo.legislature.ca.gov/faces/billTextClient.xhtml?bill_id=201320140SB493 (accessed on 8 March 2019).
21. California State Assembly Bill 1535. Available online: http://leginfo.legislature.ca.gov/faces/billNavClient.xhtml?bill_id=201320140AB1535 (accessed on 8 March 2019).
22. California State Senate Bill 159. Available online: http://leginfo.legislature.ca.gov/faces/billNavClient.xhtml?bill_id=201920200SB159 (accessed on 8 March 2019).
23. Ohio State Senate Bill 265. Available online: https://www.legislature.ohio.gov/legislation/legislation-summary?id=GA132-SB-265 (accessed on 8 March 2019).
24. CVS Health. CVS Health's MinuteClinic Introduces New Virtual Care Offering. Available online: https://cvshealth.com/newsroom/press-releases/cvs-healths-minuteclinic-introduces-new-virtual-care-offering (accessed on 30 May 2019).
25. Walgreens and CVS Are Redesigning Their Drugstores to Focus More on Health. Available online: https://www.cnbc.com/2019/02/18/look-at-walgreens-and-cvs-remodeled-stores-that-focus-more-on-health.html (accessed on 8 March 2019).
26. Aliera Healthcare Enters Agreement with MinuteClinic. Available online: https://apnews.com/Business%20Wire/c523982f4eff488a8a3ce5c18ec5421f (accessed on 29 March 2019).
27. Feehan, M.; Walsh, M.; Sundwall, D.; Munger, M.A. Patient Preferences for Healthcare Delivery Through Community Pharmacy Settings in the USA: A Discrete Choice Study. *J. Clin. Pharm. Ther.* **2017**, *42*, 737–749. [CrossRef] [PubMed]
28. McKeirnan, K.C.; MacLean, L.G. Pharmacist, physician, and patient opinions of pharmacist-treated minor ailments and conditions. *J. Am. Pharm. Assoc.* **2018**, *58*, 599–607. [CrossRef] [PubMed]
29. California Business & Professions Code §4052.2. Available online: https://codes.findlaw.com/ca/business-and-professions-code/bpc-sect-4052-2.html (accessed on 20 June 2019).
30. Accreditation Council of Pharmacy Education. Accreditation Standards and Key Elements for the Professional Program in Pharmacy Leading to the Doctor of Pharmacy Degree. Available online: https://www.acpe-accredit.org/pdf/Standards2016FINAL.pdf (accessed on 5 April 2019).
31. American Association of Colleges of Nursing. *Criteria for Evaluation of Nurse Practitioners Programs*, 5th ed.; American Association of Colleges of Nursing: Washington, DC, USA, 2016; Available online: https://www.aacnnursing.org/Portals/42/AcademicNursing/CurriculumGuidelines/Criteria-Evaluation-NP-2016.pdf (accessed on 5 April 2019).
32. American Association of Nurse Practitioners. NP Fact Sheet. Available online: https://www.aanp.org/about/all-about-nps/np-fact-sheet (accessed on 17 February 2019).
33. Haddad, L.M.; Toney-Butler, T.J. Nursing Shortage. Available online: https://www.ncbi.nlm.nih.gov/books/NBK493175/ (accessed on 10 March 2019).
34. Office of the Inspector General. OIG Advisory Opinion No. 18-03. Available online: https://oig.hhs.gov/fraud/docs/advisoryopinions/2018/AdvOpn18-03.pdf (accessed on 9 January 2019).
35. Government Publishing Office. Title 42—The Public Health and Welfare (42 USC §1395nn) Limitation on Certain Physician Referrals. Available online: https://www.govinfo.gov/content/pkg/USCODE-2010-title42/pdf/USCODE-2010-title42-chap7-subchapXVIII-partE-sec1395nn.pdf (accessed on 9 January 2019).
36. American Society of Health-System Pharmacy. Pharmacist Billing for Ambulatory Pharmacy Patient Care Services in a Physician-Based Clinic and Other Non-Hospital-Based Environments—FAQ. Available online: https://www.ashp.org/-/media/assets/ambulatory-care-practitioner/docs/sacp-pharmacist-billing-for-ambulatory-pharmacy-patient-care-services.pdf (accessed on 8 February 2019).
37. U.S. House of Representatives Bill 592. Available online: https://www.congress.gov/bill/115th-congress/house-bill/592 (accessed on 8 February 2019).
38. U.S. Senate Bill 109. Available online: https://www.congress.gov/115/bills/s109/BILLS-115s109is.pdf (accessed on 8 February 2019).
39. California State Assembly Bill 1114. Available online: http://www.leginfo.ca.gov/pub/15-16/bill/asm/ab_1101-150/ab_1114_bill_20160925_chaptered.pdf (accessed on 8 February 2019).
40. Washington State Senate Bill 5557. Available online: http://lawfilesext.leg.wa.gov/biennium/2015-16/Pdf/Amendments/House/5557-S.E%20AMH%20SHOR%20H2682.1.pdf (accessed on 8 February 2019).

41. Patient Protection and Affordable Care Act. Available online: https://www.govtrack.us/congress/bills/111/hr3590/text (accessed on 8 February 2019).
42. Knapp, K.K.; Olson, A.W.; Schommer, J.; Gaither, C.A.; Mott, D.A.; Doucette, W.R. Retail clinics co-located with pharmacies: A Delphi study of pharmacist impacts and recommendations for optimization. *J. Am. Pharm. Assoc.* **2019**, in press. [CrossRef] [PubMed]

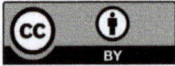

pharmacy

MDPI

Perspective

Establishing a New Ambulatory Care Practice Site as a Pharmacy Practice Faculty

Vasudha Gupta * and Evan Williams

College of Pharmacy, Roseman University of Health Sciences, 11 Sunset Way,
Henderson, NV 89014, USA; ewilliams1@roseman.edu
* Correspondence: vgupta@roseman.edu; Tel.: +1-702-968-1681

Received: 29 August 2018; Accepted: 9 October 2018; Published: 11 October 2018

check for updates

Abstract: There is an imminent need to identify and develop new ambulatory care practice sites with the increase in the number of colleges of pharmacy across the nation. This manuscript provides recommendations to help clinical faculty determine whether a potential pharmacy practice site will be able to provide adequate resources and support to establish a successful practice. This may be challenging to pharmacy practice faculty in settings where clinical pharmacy services have never been utilized. Topics include the pre-work needed prior to approaching a new practice site, assessing the need for physical requirements, meeting key personnel, marketing clinical skills and services, implementing, and evaluating practice site. Preparation includes having a clear vision of the pharmacist services, ensuring that stakeholders have an understanding of the pharmacy services inquiring the site support and resources for the pharmacist, and regularly communicating.

Keywords: ambulatory care; pharmacy practice faculty; pharmacy learners; clinical practice; pharmacist services

1. Purpose

The Accreditation Council for Pharmacy Education (ACPE) Standards 2016 requires all colleges of pharmacy across the United States to provide ambulatory care practice experiences to pharmacy students as a requirement for graduation [1]. With the increase in the number of colleges of pharmacy across the nation, there is an imminent need to identify and develop new ambulatory care practice sites [2,3]. This provides unique challenges for pharmacy practice faculty, as well as colleges of pharmacy, to establish a rewarding clinical practice while also providing opportunities for learners, including pharmacy students and residents. Additionally, faculty may be working with providers who may be unfamiliar with the clinical services ambulatory care pharmacists can provide [4]. Since many of these new programs are being established in areas where ambulatory care clinical pharmacy services are relatively novel, pharmacy practice faculty often find themselves describing the utility of an ambulatory care pharmacist.

Previous publications have focused on the establishment of a practice site that will exhibit clear evidence of outcome improvement and create financial incentives for clinics to thrive and justify salary requirements [5–10]. Pharmacy practice faculty have a different priority when establishing new ambulatory care clinic sites. Thus, it is imperative that the pharmacy practice faculty and academic unit closely evaluate the practice site for suitability towards their purpose. This purpose includes a collaborative learning environment to foster development of learners and building a practice site in his or her area of expertise. Literature is lacking for faculty hopeful in establishing a new practice site that will fulfill their goals and objectives. Based on experience establishing new ambulatory care practice at sites which have not previously had a pharmacy practice faculty, the authors have identified various factors to consider in order to create a successful practice model. These experiences include creating disease-state specific clinics, initiating interprofessional patient health programs, improving meaningful use and quality metrics as part of accountable care organizations, and coordinating activities at multiple clinics within an organization. The authors have also had experience with establishing practice initiatives that did not thrive to their full potential, allowing for reflection on the key issues that lead to unsuccessful implementation and identification of strategies to improve future forays.

Evaluation of the practice site is a multifaceted process and the importance of each section below needs to be weighed determine if the site will fit the needs of the pharmacist and the college of pharmacy. As a result, a formulaic approach is unlikely to be successful as each situation will require a nuanced understanding of various factors. The recommendations below are not in a sequential order and may need to be adapted to circumstances and preliminary conversations with the practice site.

2. Summary

2.1. Preparation

Prior to a meeting with individuals at the practice site, the first discussion that will occur will be between the pharmacy practice faculty and the college leadership, such as the dean of the college of pharmacy, clinical department chair or experiential director. This conversation will be focused on various responsibilities of the pharmacy practice faculty, related to expectations for both didactic and experiential teaching, service to the college and the profession, as well as scholarly activities. It's critical for the faculty and the college leadership to establish expectations related to how much time will be devoted to each of the faculty's roles, and specifically the time devoted to the practice site. Additional consideration should be given if the faculty position is split funded, with the clinic or health system providing some salary offset, either directly to the pharmacist or though remuneration to the school. In these situations, the clinic may have higher expectations regarding how much time the faculty member should be providing services at the site. Thus, clear delineation of roles and responsibilities is crucial during initial conversations between the college and the practice site leadership. As successful implementation of a new practice site may take up to 6–12 months, additional time may be devoted to the practice site during that period, with limited focus on other faculty responsibilities. The time commitment of the pharmacy practice faculty to the practice site will need to be discussed again in collaboration with the clinic leadership to establish clear expectations.

A practice protocol may help pharmacy practice faculty interested in pursuing a new practice site. The protocol can describe proposed clinical services and how the service may fit patients' needs, outlines key components of the practice flow, and includes the goals and the vision for the pharmacy services. The goals and vision may include conducting comprehensive medication reviews, identifying and solving complex drug-related problems, ensuring evidence-based and cost-effective therapies, and educating patients about appropriate medication use. Faculty also need to identify which disease states they would like to address, the types of collaborative drug therapy management that would be offered, and the scope of practice desired. Although it's essential to have a vision for services based upon the faculty's practice interest, it's important to keep in mind that the actual services provided at the site may be modified based upon a needs assessment of the patients seen at the practice site. However, the services may be extended after a period of time to also include some of the faculty's practice interest.

The description should include information such as hours of operation of the clinical services, how patients will be referred, what will be accomplished during the appointment with the patient, how interactions with patients will be documented, changes to therapy communicated to providers, what follow-up will look like, and how providers will be able to contact the pharmacist. Beyond the clinical components of practice, faculty also need to consider how the environment will foster teaching and learning, including opportunities for interprofessional education. Writing these components into a practice protocol will help define the pharmacist's role in patient care, but may need to be revised after discussions with key clinic personnel.

Faculty should consider gathering some evidence demonstrating that pharmacy services can help improve patient care in various practice settings as part of the preparation [11–14]. The pharmacist should also have an updated curriculum vitae (CV) that includes his or her training and experiences in implementing pharmacy services to help key clinic personnel to gain an understanding of role of the pharmacist.

Laws regarding the scope of practice and collaborative drug therapy management (CDTM) play a large role in delineating what is achievable in a new practice. This may be especially important in areas where ambulatory care clinical pharmacy services have not been fully established and widely adopted. Enhancing the scope of pharmacy practice may be difficult as it requires buy-in from several different stakeholders. While there are collaborative practice laws in nearly every American jurisdiction, the level of practicality written into these regulations varies widely across the nation and dictates limitations to the practice culture [15]. These laws must be considered in order to develop the clinical practice site. Consider preparing a collaborative practice agreement (CPA) or modify one that has been previously created taking state laws into consideration [16]. This may serve useful during conversations with the medical director to help develop a mutual understanding of the pharmacist's scope of practice.

One barrier encountered involves unfamiliarity with the role of the pharmacy practice faculty in an ambulatory care practice. Resolution of this issue may require education about the pharmacist's role in direct patient care prior to discussions regarding the model of practice at the clinic. It's important to emphasize that the pharmacist's role is to augment the productivity of the clinic and optimize patient outcomes in collaboration with other healthcare providers (HCPs) and does not replace the other providers' patient encounters [3,4]. The Pharmacist Patient Care Process model (PPCP) has been created to assist with succinctly explaining the role of a pharmacist in patient care, and may prove useful for discussions with providers and other clinic staff [17].

Other issues that may arise and limit the full implementation of the original practice vision may be the patient population, reimbursement constraints, or access to health resources. Careful consideration of potential barriers must be taken and the original practice protocol revised as necessary to create a plan that can be implemented within the required boundaries.

2.2. Physical Requirements

Consideration of physical requirements including space, access, and equipment are important to successfully establish pharmacy services. The discussion regarding these essentials will likely need to occur in collaboration with college and clinic leadership as the finances related to any physical space modifications, electronic health record (EHR) access, supplies and equipment for the faculty as well as the students will need to be delineated.

2.2.1. Space

Many clinic managers may be unfamiliar with the role of an ambulatory care pharmacist or have little insight as to the physical space and access requirements that a pharmacy practice faculty might need. Request adequate space for the number of patients that will be seen and the number of learners who will be on rotation at one time. There will be a need for an exam room or private space if direct patient care is offered. In the authors' experiences, two exam rooms are optimal if patients are scheduled back-to-back (every 30 or 45 min), as this allows for the rooming of one patient while the pharmacist is seeing another patient, improving efficiency.

Another key consideration for a successful practice is office space. Consideration regarding where documentation of encounters will be completed and where learners will look up information and prepare to interview patients is important. Determine the need for desks, chairs, work terminals, and storage space for educational materials. Having a dedicated workstation for the pharmacist and one workstation per learner is optimal. The pharmacist should also consider the space needed to have discussions with learners about work related to patient care or other assignments required for the rotation. Having access to a conference room, if available, provides adequate space to better facilitate topic discussions, and journal article presentations.

2.2.2. Access and Equipment

Electronic health record (EHR) access is key to any successful ambulatory care practice, and is becoming more prevalent even in community [18,19]. The clinic site must ensure that, as a HCP, the pharmacist will have access to the full medical record, as well as the ability to document in the EHR. The ability to modify medication orders will vary between locations based on local collaborative practice laws and practice culture. The pharmacist should advocate to practice at the top of his or her license and promote themselves as an integral part of the healthcare team. It may be appropriate for the pharmacist to initially attain limited authority to establish rapport with the providers until providers are comfortable with the pharmacist's clinical decision making.

The pharmacist should consider the resources that are available for scheduling and seeing patients in addition to EHR access and permissions. Considerations may include equipment needed for practice. These resources can include a blood pressure machine or point of care testing devices, availability of a medical assistant to help with scheduling and taking vitals for patients, and a phone for contacting and following-up with patients.

2.3. Meeting Key Personnel

2.3.1. Finding a Niche

One of the first meetings that will likely occur is with the medical director and the manager of the clinic to assess their interest in clinical pharmacy services. The medical director will be an essential partner to advocate for the clinical pharmacy services to other providers as they oversee all the HCPs at the site. The clinic manager will be a key asset during day-to-day operations as the pharmacist is learning to practice in a new environment. Other key personnel, such as a compliance officer, other medical leaders, human resources, or chief financial officer, may also be present during one of the first meetings to provide additional perspectives.

Pharmacy practice faculty must inquire about the patient population seen at the clinic and the needs of the patients from the medical director and clinic manager. Knowing basic information such as patient age, literacy, ethnicity, and socioeconomic status will help to tailor services to meet patients' needs. Ask the medical director about any current needs of the clinic or any gaps in care that the providers are hoping to improve. Identifying these will aid in matching the skill-set of the pharmacist with the needs of the site, creating a symbiotic relationship.

Faculty should provide a draft of the practice protocol for overview, which details a description of proposed clinical services and outlines key components of the flow of the practice. This will allow the medical director and the clinic manager to have a sound understanding of the day-to-day operations and how the patients will benefit from the pharmacist consultations. Some processes will likely change depending on the needs assessed during the discussion as well as the limitations of the clinic.

2.3.2. Marketing Your Skills and Services to the Medical Director and Clinic Manager

The pharmacist should describe the importance of the program, and the vision of progression of services, including both short and long-term goals during the meeting. Goals could include expanding the scope of the disease states managed, initiating group patient education classes, or regularly planning a short presentation with providers at the clinic for continuing education. General goals of the service should include delivery of comprehensive, integrated, and patient-centered care to improve patient health and reduce costs. As the climate regarding medical service reimbursement shifts from fee-for-service towards improving quality metrics, the efforts of the pharmacist can be focused to ensure that compensation is maximized. Within certain value-based reimbursement initiatives, achieving population health goals, such as a certain percentage of cardiovascular disease (CVD) patients receiving an appropriately dosed statin, can increase the rate of reimbursement to the clinic. Myriad examples of pharmacist-led initiatives in quality improvement exist, and it is recommended that the faculty member become familiar with current quality-based reimbursement models prior to meeting with the medical director and clinic manager [11,13,14]. In the authors' experience, improving just a few quality measures for the clinic often opens doors to a broader practice scope as the clinic management observes the positive impact the pharmacist has on patient care.

The faculty can consider discussing how pharmacists can help improve care by reducing medication errors, decreasing number of medications by discontinuing inappropriate medications, optimizing therapy to meet therapeutic goals, improving patient outcomes, improving patient satisfaction, increasing medication adherence, enhancing patient understanding, reducing patient and health-system costs, and decreasing hospitalizations [20–28]. The authors have found the Ambulatory Care Pharmacist's Survival guide to be a useful resource which highlights successful pharmacy practice initiatives, along with networking through national organizations, including the American Association of Colleges of Pharmacy (AACP), the American College of Clinical Pharmacy (ACCP), and the American Society of Health-Systems Pharmacists (ASHP) [6]. These organizations, and others like them, hold national and international meetings in which presenters highlight their practice initiatives and provide a platform for networking and establishing mentoring relationships with other practice faculty. Seeking out these mentoring relationships is recommended and can provide an excellent resource for academic pharmacists establishing ambulatory care practice sites.

2.3.3. Other Points of Discussion

Billing for pharmacy services may not be a requirement as a pharmacy practice faculty. However, inquiring about the billing structure may be important to consider if the site is amenable to billing patients for pharmacist services. Clinics participating in a split-funded faculty position may have a greater stake in ensuring revenue is generated from the pharmacy services. This revenue can aid the clinic in recuperating some of the cost of the pharmacist's salary, or can be used to provide more resources for the pharmacist to improve patient care. Although a discussion regarding billing practices are beyond the scope of this manuscript, many resources are available to practicing pharmacists regarding billing for clinical services [9,29–31]. Knowing the most common types of insurances that will be encountered at the site will also help to determine what medications are normally covered by insurance versus those that are unlikely to be covered.

The pharmacist should discuss the implementation of a collaborative practice agreement (CPA) in an effort to gain autonomy in decision making. As most providers may not be familiar with a CPA, providing a copy of one that was developed by the pharmacist or a sample copy that is available through resources may be helpful [6,7,20]. A collaborative practice may have a narrow or broad scope which will depend on state laws, as well as the comfort level of providers to allow a pharmacist to make clinical decisions regarding patient care. Discussion should focus on the benefits of a collaborative practice agreement [32–35]. In the authors' experiences, this includes easing care burden of providers, avoiding provider workflow interruptions to inquire about a patient, and improving the timeliness of patient care.

2.3.4. Keeping Faculty Responsibilities in Mind

A pharmacy practice faculty is likely required to precept pharmacy students and perhaps residents at the practice site; thus, it is important to discuss this role with the medical director and clinic manager. Explain that the learners, especially pharmacy residents, will operate as an extension of the pharmacist and will be able to closely monitor patients seen at the clinic under supervision. Learners can help coordinate in-services for providers, as well as complete projects that will improve care for patients and help to improve clinic functions [36,37]. Assess the clinic for opportunities where learners would be able to learn about, from, and with other healthcare professional learners [38]. Discuss how interprofessional education can allow for effective collaboration and allow all those involved to have a better understanding of their respective roles and responsibilities, develop a mutual respect for interprofessional practice, improve communication, and function more cohesively as a team to improve patient care. This has been identified as an essential component in maintaining ACPE accreditation and improving patient care [1,39].

An additional pharmacy practice faculty responsibility will likely be an expectation of research in an area of expertise. Clinical practice aligns with clinical research and provides an environment where new ideas may develop based upon scenarios in patient care. Inquire about the feasibility of research at the practice site, including the ability to collect patient information, availability of resources to help with data collection, the internal or external institutional review board (IRB) requirements at the site. Identifying opportunities early will help the pharmacist initiate research endeavors and plan for known obstacles.

2.4. Implementation

2.4.1. Recommendations for Starting Out

The pharmacist should request to attend provider meetings prior to starting services at the site even though he or he will have met with the medical director and the clinic manager. The pharmacist should provide an introduction, his or her integration and role within the healthcare team, and the services that can be provided. Additionally, determining areas where the HCPs feel that a pharmacist can provide value to the patients may help the HCPs buy into the new services, as it may directly help the patients.

The pharmacist should also consider attending staff meetings temporarily as they are getting started to become acquainted with the staff and help them understand the role of the pharmacist. Speaking with the staff may provide insight of the current systems and processes in place, and can also identify barriers and opportunities where the pharmacist might be able to help.

2.4.2. Evaluation

The pharmacist should regularly evaluate the success of current methods in achieving short and long-terms goals once clinical services have been established. Ask for feedback from either the medical director or HCPs at the site to determine if any changes need to be made to improve the integration of pharmacy services into the clinical workflow. Prior to starting services, it is important to identify some metrics which will define success for the ambulatory care pharmacist. These could include decrease in A1c, or blood pressure. Identify key personnel, such as an individual in the field of pharmacy informatics or information technology, who may be able to help navigate tracking data and designing reports with the desired outcomes. Learners can be helpful with tracking the clinical impact and sorting through data, which may be especially important for pharmacy practice faculty in their evaluations to achieve promotion and tenure. Showing the number of interventions the pharmacist and learners have made, care improvements that have occurred, and even estimating cost savings are all excellent ways to show that the contributions at the clinic are leading to positive outcomes for patients. This data can also be used for formalized research projects to be synergistic with the pharmacy practice faculty's goals and aspirations towards promotion.

3. Conclusions

Implementing a new clinical service at an ambulatory care site as a pharmacy practice faculty may be overwhelming but can also be exciting. Being aware of the appropriate information to gather prior to committing to a practice site is crucial in creating a valuable learning site. The pharmacist should ensure that an overview of the services that will be offered to the patients at the clinic has been provided, and inquire regarding the support and resources that can be expected from the site.

Open communication can increase the likelihood of success at the practice site and provide a great opportunity to showcase the importance of interprofessional practice in ambulatory care clinics without previous pharmacist services. Successful implementation will be essential to the education of our future pharmacists.

Key Considerations
• Have a clear vision of the pharmacist services at the practice site
• Be prepared prior to discussions with the medical director, other healthcare providers, and clinic manager, and anticipate questions that may arise
• Ensure that the key stakeholders have a clear understanding of the services that the pharmacist will provide to the patients at the clinic, and inquire regarding the support and resources that the pharmacist can expect from the site
• Prior to committing to a practice site, gather information regarding the feasibility of a successful clinic and seek mutually beneficial goals that will provide benefit and value to pharmacy students and residents, providers, patients, and to the pharmacy practice faculty
• Regular communication with the providers and staff will help identify barriers and help set up a thriving clinical practice site
• Recognize that establishing a new practice is a difficult process, and it may take a considerable amount of time for the pharmacist to become fully integrated into the clinic
• Determine needs versus wants and be prepared to negotiate to establish a successful learning environment
• Be flexible, but if a site is unable to accommodate basic needs to set up a successful practice, consider moving on to identify other sites

Author Contributions: Both authors were involved in all aspects of manuscript preparation.

Funding: The research received no external funding.

Conflicts of Interest: The authors have no conflicts of interest to disclose.

References

1. Accreditation Council for Pharmacy Education. Standards 2016. Available online: https://www.acpe-accredit.org/pdf/Standards2016FINAL.pdf (accessed on 14 April 2017).
2. Grabenstein, J.D. Trends in the Numbers of US Colleges of Pharmacy and Their Graduates, 1900 to 2014. *Am. J. Pharm. Educ.* **2016**, *80*, 25. [CrossRef] [PubMed]
3. Duke, L.J.; Staton, A.G.; McCullough, E.S.; Jain, R.; Miller, M.S.; Lynn Stevenson, T.; Fetterman, J.W.; Lynn Parham, R.; Sheffield, M.C.; Unterwagner, W.L.; et al. Impact of advanced pharmacy practice experience placement changes in colleges and schools of pharmacy. *Am. J. Pharm. Educ.* **2012**, *76*, 49. [CrossRef] [PubMed]
4. Hawes, E.M.; Misita, C.; Burkhart, J.I.; McKnight, L.; Deyo, Z.M.; Lee, R.A.; Howard, C.; Eckel, S.F. Prescribing pharmacists in the ambulatory care setting: Experience at the University of North Carolina Medical Center. *Am. J. Health Syst. Pharm.* **2016**, *73*, 1425–1433. [CrossRef] [PubMed]
5. Helling, D.K.; Johnson, S.G. Defining and advancing ambulatory care pharmacy practice: It is time to lengthen our stride. *Am. J. Health Syst. Pharm.* **2014**, *71*, 1348–1356. [CrossRef] [PubMed]
6. Westberg, S. *ACCP Ambulatory Care Pharmacist's Survival Guide*, 3rd ed.; American College of Clinical Pharmacy: Lenexa, KS, USA, 2013.
7. Kliethermes, M.A.; Brown, T.R. *Building a Successful Ambulatory Care Practice: A Complete Guide for Pharmacists*; American Society of Health-System Pharmacists: Bethesda, MA, USA, 2011.
8. Hammond, R.W.; Schwartz, A.H.; Campbell, M.J.; Remington, T.L.; Chuck, S.; Blair, M.M.; Vassey, A.M.; Rospond, R.M.; Herner, S.J.; Webb, C.E.; et al. Collaborative drug therapy management by pharmacists—2003. *Pharmacotherapy* **2003**, *23*, 1210–1225. [PubMed]

9.   McBane, S.E.; Dopp, A.L.; Abe, A.; Benavides, S.; Chester, E.A.; Dixon, D.L.; Dunn, M.; Johnson, M.D.; Nigro, S.J.; Rothrock-Christian, T.; et al. Collaborative drug therapy management and comprehensive medication management—2015. *Pharmacotherapy* **2015**, *35*, e39–e50. [PubMed]

10.   Pharmacy American College of Clinical Pharmacy. Standards of Practice for Clinical Pharmacists. Available online: https://www.accp.com/docs/positions/guidelines/standardsofpractice.pdf (accessed on 28 August 2018).

11.   Tan, E.C.; Stewart, K.; Elliott, R.A.; George, J. Pharmacist services provided in general practice clinics: A systematic review and meta-analysis. *Res. Soc. Adm. Pharm.* **2014**, *10*, 608–622. [CrossRef] [PubMed]

12.   Lee, J.K.; Alshehri, S.; Kutbi, H.; Martin, J. Optimizing pharmacotherapy in elderly patients: The role of pharmacists. *Integr. Pharm. Res. Pract.* **2015**, *4*, 101–111. [CrossRef] [PubMed]

13.   Giberson, S.; Yoder, S.; Lee, M. *Improving Patient and Health System Outcomes through Advanced Pharmacy Practice*; A Report to the US Surgeon General; US Public Health Service: Rockville, MD, USA, 2011.

14.   Chisholm-Burns, M.A.; Lee, J.K.; Spivey, C.A.; Slack, M.; Herrier, R.N.; Hall-Lipsy, E.; Graff Zivin, J.; Abraham, I.; Palmer, J.; Martin, J.R.; et al. US pharmacists' effect as team members on patient care: Systematic review and meta-analyses. *Med. Care* **2010**, *48*, 923–933. [CrossRef] [PubMed]

15.   Centers for Disase Control and Prevention. *Collaborative Practice Agreements and Pharmacists' Patient Care Services: A Resource for Pharmacists*; Centers for Disease Control and Prevention, US Department of Health and Human Services: Atlanta, GA, USA, 2013.

16.   Centers for Disase Control and Prevention. *Advancing Team-Based Care through Collaborative Practice Agreements: A Resource and Implementation Guide for Adding Pharmacists to the Care Team*; Centers for Disease Control and Prevention, US Department of Health and Human Services: Atlanta, GA, USA, 2017.

17.   Pharmacists' Patient Care Process. Joint Commission of Pharmacy Practitioners. Available online: https://www.pharmacist.com/sites/default/files/files/PatientCareProcess.pdf (accessed on 20 September 2018).

18.   Bonner, L. Pharmacists inch closer to accessing EHRs and HIEs. *Pharm. Today* **2016**, *22*, 44–47. [CrossRef]

19.   Nelson, S.D.; Poikonen, J.; Reese, T.; El Halta, D.; Weir, C. The pharmacist and the EHR. *J. Am. Med. Inform. Assoc.* **2016**, *24*, 193–197. [CrossRef] [PubMed]

20.   Martin, M.; Faber, D. Patient satisfaction with the clinical pharmacist and prescribers during hepatitis C virus management. *J. Clin. Pharm. Ther.* **2016**, *41*, 645–649. [CrossRef] [PubMed]

21.   Hadi, M.A.; Alldred, D.P.; Briggs, M.; Munyombwe, T.; Closs, S.J. Effectiveness of pharmacist-led medication review in chronic pain management: Systematic review and meta-analysis. *Clin. J. Pain.* **2014**, *30*, 1006–1014. [CrossRef] [PubMed]

22.   Woodall, T.; Landis, S.E.; Galvin, S.L.; Plaut, T.; Roth McClurg, M.T. Provision of annual wellness visits with comprehensive medication management by a clinical pharmacist practitioner. *Am. J. Health Syst. Pharm.* **2017**, *74*, 218–223. [CrossRef] [PubMed]

23.   Chisholm-Burns, M.; Zivin, J.G.; Lee, J.K.; Spivey, C.A.; Slack, M.; Herrier, R.N.; Hall-Lipsy, E.; Abraham, I.; Palmer, J. Economic effects of pharmacists on health outcomes in the United States: A systematic review. *Am. J. Health Syst. Pharm.* **2010**, *67*, 1624–1634. [CrossRef] [PubMed]

24.   Gallagher, J.; McCarthy, S.; Byrne, S. Economic evaluations of clinical pharmacist interventions on hospital inpatients: A systematic review of recent literature. *Int. J. Clin. Pharm.* **2014**, *36*, 1101–1114. [CrossRef] [PubMed]

25.   Touchette, D.R.; Doloresco, F.; Suda, K.J.; Perez, A.; Turner, S.; Jalundhwala, Y.; Tangonan, M.C.; Hoffman, J.M. Economic evaluations of clinical pharmacy services: 2006–2010. *Pharmacotherapy* **2014**, *34*, 771–793. [CrossRef] [PubMed]

26.   Yuan, Y.; Hay, J.W.; McCombs, J.S. Effects of ambulatory-care pharmacist consultation on mortality and hospitalization. *Am. J. Manag. Care* **2003**, *9*, 45–56. [PubMed]

27.   Cadman, B.; Wright, D.; Bale, A.; Barton, G.; Desborough, J.; Hammad, E.A.; Holland, R.; Howe, H.; Nunney, I.; Irvine, L. Pharmacist provided medicines reconciliation within 24 hours of admission and on discharge: A randomised controlled pilot study. *Br. Med. J.* **2017**, *7*, e013647. [CrossRef] [PubMed]

28.   Mekonnen, A.B.; McLachlan, A.J.; Jo-anne, E.B. Effectiveness of pharmacist-led medication reconciliation programmes on clinical outcomes at hospital transitions: A systematic review and meta-analysis. *Br. Med. J.* **2016**, *6*, e010003. [CrossRef] [PubMed]

29.   Scott, M.A.; Hitch, W.J.; Wilson, C.G.; Lugo, A.M. Billing for pharmacists' cognitive services in physicians' offices: Multiple methods of reimbursement. *J. Am. Pharm. Assoc.* **2012**, *52*, 175–180. [CrossRef] [PubMed]

30. Lenz, T.L.; Monaghan, M.S. Pay-for-performance model of medication therapy management in pharmacy practice. *J. Am. Pharm. Assoc.* **2011**, *51*, 425–431. [CrossRef] [PubMed]

31. Kliethermes, M.A. Understanding health care billing basics. *Pharm. Today* **2017**, *23*, 57–68. [CrossRef]

32. Adams, A.J.; Weaver, K.K. The continuum of pharmacist prescriptive authority. *Ann. Pharmacother.* **2016**, *50*, 778–784. [CrossRef] [PubMed]

33. Bingham, J.T.; Mallette, J.J. Federal Bureau of Prisons clinical pharmacy program improves patient A1C. *J. Am. Pharm. Assoc.* **2016**, *56*, 173–177. [CrossRef] [PubMed]

34. Klepser, M.E.; Adams, A.J.; Klepser, D.G. Antimicrobial stewardship in outpatient settings: Leveraging innovative physician-pharmacist collaborations to reduce antibiotic resistance. *Health Secur.* **2015**, *13*, 166–173. [CrossRef] [PubMed]

35. Sisson, E.M.; Dixon, D.L.; Kildow, D.C.; Van Tassell, B.W.; Carl, D.E.; Varghese, D.; Electricwala, B.; Carroll, N.V. Effectiveness of a Pharmacist-Physician Team-Based Collaboration to Improve Long-Term Blood Pressure Control at an Inner-City Safety-Net Clinic. *Pharmacotherapy* **2016**, *36*, 342–347. [CrossRef] [PubMed]

36. Rogers, J.; Pai, V.; Merandi, J.; Catt, C. Impact of a pharmacy student-driven medication delivery service at hospital discharge. *Am. J. Health Syst. Pharm.* **2017**, *74*, S24–S29. [CrossRef] [PubMed]

37. Melody, K.T.; Shah, C.J.; Patel, J.; Willey, V.J. Implementation of a Student Pharmacist-Run Targeted Medication Intervention Program. *J. Pharm. Pract.* **2017**, *30*, 109–114. [CrossRef] [PubMed]

38. Interprofessional Education Collaborative. *Core Competencies for Interprofessional Collaborative Practice: 2016 Update*; Interprofessional Education Collaborative: Washington, DC, USA, 2016.

39. Nester, J. The importance of interprofessional practice and education in the era of accountable care. *N. C. Med. J.* **2016**, *77*, 128–132. [CrossRef] [PubMed]

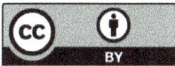

pharmacy

MDPI

Article

Measuring Adherence: A Proof of Concept Study for Multiple Medications for Chronic Conditions in Alternative Payment Models

Joel F. Farley [1,*], Arun Kumar [1] and Benjamin Y. Urick [2]

[1] Department of Pharmaceutical Care and Health Systems, College of Pharmacy, University of Minnesota, Minneapolis, MN 55455, USA

[2] Center for Medication Optimization, UNC Eshelman School of Pharmacy, University of North Carolina, Chapel Hill, NC 27599, USA

* Correspondence: farl0032@umn.edu; Tel.: +1-612-624-9624

Received: 30 May 2019; Accepted: 28 June 2019; Published: 2 July 2019

check for
updates

Abstract: Adherence to renin angiotensin system antagonists (RASA), non-insulin diabetes medications (NIDM) and statins has been included in the Medicare Star Ratings program since 2012. The long-term use of these measures emphasizes adherence to a limited number of chronic medications and may present opportunities for Part D plan sponsors to misuse the measures to influence their Medicare Part D Star Rating. It also does not capture the adherence needs of high-risk patients with multiple chronic conditions. The objective of this study was to describe the development of a new measure to capture adherence to multiple medications for chronic conditions (MMCC). The MMCC measure captures adherence to 71 different therapeutic categories of medication and was constructed using North Carolina Medicaid prescription claims data from 2015 to 2017. This measure was validated against the existing RASA, NIDM and statin adherence measures. This new measure was highly correlated with Star Rating measures, captured a greater number of eligible patients than these existing measures and had a lower proportion of patients meet the adherence threshold than the existing Star Ratings adherence measures. There is an opportunity to develop new measures, which include adherence to multiple medications in populations with multiple chronic conditions.

Keywords: medication adherence; quality measurement/benchmarking; multiple chronic conditions; CMS Star rating

---

1. Introduction

1.1. Medication Adherence and Multiple Chronic Conditions

Multiple chronic conditions (MCC), defined as the presence of two or more concurrent chronic conditions, presents a significant burden to the U.S. health care system. It is estimated that 50% of older adults have three or more concurrent chronic medical conditions [1]. The burden of MCC is felt by the health care system through increased health service utilization and expenditures. It is estimated that 66% of total U.S. health care spending is directly attributable to a disproportionally small number of approximately 27% of American's with MCC [2]. This burden is felt not only by the health care system, but also by patients through higher morbidity and mortality as well as reductions in patient reported quality of life [3] (p. 15).

The primary treatment modality for most chronic conditions comes in the form of prescription medication treatments. It is estimated that 60% of elderly patients are prescribed with three or more medications [4]. In reports from the U.S. Centers for Disease Control and Prevention (CDC), some 37% of older Americans are reported to use five or more prescription medications concurrently with this prevalence doubling since 1999 [5]. As the number of medications used by a patient to manage chronic conditions increases, so too does the risk of inappropriate medication use and adverse drug events [6,7].

Ensuring medications are used appropriately is imperative to reducing the burden of MCC. However, estimates of non-adherence to medications are reported to be as high as 50% for many chronic conditions [8,9]. Medication non-adherence is responsible for an estimated 33–69% of medication-related hospitalizations [10] and may result in an additional $300 billion in direct health care spending in the U.S annually [11]. Further evidence provided by the CDC suggests medication non-adherence is tied to approximately 50% of treatment failures in chronically ill patients and corresponds to approximately 125,000 deaths per year [12].

1.2. Adherence and Star Ratings

Given the importance of medication adherence to the quality of care provided to patients, a number of initiatives have been taken to improve rates of adherence to medications for chronic medical conditions. One initiative adopted by the Centers for Medicaid and Medicare Services (CMS) is to tie health plan payments and performance ratings to their population's medication adherence rates for a select number of chronic health conditions using the CMS Star Ratings program. Beginning in 2007, the Star Ratings program was implemented as a means for CMS and Medicare beneficiaries to assess and compare plans on their performance with a broad array of measures associated with the quality of care provided to patients. For standalone prescription drug plans (PDPs), these performance metrics provide a benchmark for patients to select health plans on the basis of the quality of care provided. For Medicare Advantage plans offering health and prescription drug benefits, these performance metrics have additional importance and have been tied to per member per month (PMPM) quality bonus payment rates since 2012 [13].

The metrics used to measure plan performance change from year to year with the 2018 Medicare Star Ratings including 48 different quality and performance measures, of which 14 involve ratings of prescription drug plan indicators [14]. Three of the 14 prescription drug plan indicators in the Star Ratings program measure medication adherence using a prescription claims-based measure of adherence termed the proportion of days covered (PDC). Under the Star Ratings program, patients are considered adherent to treatment if they have a PDC of 80% or higher and fill two or more prescriptions in a year for any of the following three chronic medication therapeutic categories: Renin angiotensin receptor antagonists (RASA) for hypertension, non-insulin diabetes medications (NIDM) and/or statin medications for hyperlipidemia. Each of these three medication adherence ratings is triple weighted in the Star Ratings program demonstrating their importance to achieving a summary Star Rating for the health plan, which can range anywhere from one to five Stars per plan year [15].

Although different metrics under the Star Ratings program churn over time, the three medication adherence measures used to evaluate plan performance have been in place in one form or another since 2012 [16]. The consistency of these measures in the Star Ratings program, as well as the heavy weights placed on these outcomes, leads to a heavy emphasis by health plans in achieving adherence targets. As a result, the trend in adherence to these medication therapeutic categories has increased significantly over time. From 2017 to 2019, an MAPD plan receiving five Star status for NIDM, RASA and statin medications saw an increase from 83% to 85%, 83% to 88% and 82% to 87% respectively [17]. Over the same time-period, a four star MAPD plan's targets increased for these same medication categories from 79% to 81%, 79% to 86% and 77% to 83% respectively.

1.3. Limitations of Star Ratings Adherence Measures

Improvements in medication adherence rates reported through the Medicare Star Ratings program are encouraging, but also raise a number of important questions. The trend in rates of adherence now exceeds what is commonly accepted as the true rate of medication adherence in the clinical literature. A recent study of more than 200,000 diabetic patients showed that only 69% or oral diabetes medication users are 80% or more adherent to their medication when measured using the medication possession ratio (MPR), which is a more liberal measure of adherence than the Star Ratings' PDC. [18]; another recent study, which including 238,372 patients using different oral anti-diabetes medications, suggested that 47.3%, 41.2% and 36.7% of patients were adherent to DPP4 inhibitors, sulfonylurea medications and thiazolidinedione therapies respectively when measured as a PDC of 80% or higher during a one year follow up period [19]. Similar findings are present when looking at other medication classes. Even in a large population of high-risk Medicare beneficiaries with a previous myocardial infarction (MI), the rate of adherence to statin medications as measured by a PDC of 80% or higher one year after their MI was only 59% at six months and 42% at two years in patients 66 to 75 years of age [20]. Combined, our review of the clinical literature suggest that the true rate of medication adherence to therapeutic classes included in the Star Ratings program is lower than that reported by CMS.

The discrepancy in Star Ratings-reported adherence rates and the rates commonly found in the clinical literature raise a number of important questions. The first question relates to the validity of the PDC as a measure of adherence when applied to performance-based value incentive models for payment. It is important to remember that the PDC measure does not measure actual consumption of medication by patients, but instead measures patterns of refills using prescription claims data. In essence, gaps between an actual fill date and an expected fill date, which is based on days supply from a prior fill, are counted as "uncovered" days in the PDC measurement. These gaps in coverage are compared to the length of time a person is observed to account for the proportion of days covered on treatment. Although the PDC has been validated against other commonly used measures of medication adherence such as patient self-report and medication electronic monitoring systems (MEMS) [21,22], they do not measure actual consumption of medication by patients and are imperfect metrics of actual adherence.

In addition, claims based adherence metrics may be subject to gaming by health plans attempting to improve Star Ratings and quality bonus payments. The use of automatic refill programs is one example of an early strategy employed by health plans to potentially gain higher PDC rates. Sending a refill to patients without their need to authorize the next fill reduces the risk that a patient will not fill their next medication from the pharmacy, but does not actually ensure in any way that once a patient receives their medication they will continue to use it. To reduce waste associated with shipping unneeded medication to patients, CMS implemented policies limiting this practice in 2013 [23,24] (p. 133).

The use of mail order programs and 90-day fills are other potential strategies to improve PDC rates even if not directly associated with improvements in patient medication consumption. Since the PDC relies on the need to identify gaps between fills to identify periods of non-adherence, reducing the number of potential gaps over a measurement period may artificially inflate PDC rates [25]. Over a 12-month period, the number of potential gaps is three with 90-day fills compared to eleven with 30-day fills. The use of 90 day fills, which are common in mail order programs, may result in artificial improvements in adherence that are not reflective of actual improvements in medication consumption patterns by patients.

Even if one assumes the PDC rates reported in the Star Ratings program reflects a valid rate of medication adherence in patients, the very high rates of adherence reported by health plans still raise concerns. First, the consistent use of the same measures over time means that health plans adopting programs to improve medication use in Medicare are focusing clinical efforts on a limited number of chronic conditions. As previously mentioned, it is estimated that 50% of older adults have three or more concurrent chronic conditions at any given time [1]. Focusing on a select number of these conditions does not address the entire scope of medical conditions a patient may have and may resulted in siloed clinical offerings by health plans in an attempt to improve plan ratings. In addition, the rates of adherence in four and five Star Plans are approaching the ceiling of the PDC measurement, which caps at 100%. This reduces the ability to differentiate high performing plans from low performing plans.

Given the potential limitations of the current medication adherence measures in the CMS Star Ratings program, opportunities to develop and validate new measures of medication adherence may be useful. The objective of this study is to describe the development of a measure of medication adherence for patients using multiple medications for chronic conditions. This measure was developed to incentivize payment to community pharmacies to improve medication adherence for a broad range of chronic conditions through the development and delivery of enhanced pharmacy services [26,27].

2. Materials and Methods

2.1. Setting

The development of a new measure designed to capture adherence to multiple medications for chronic conditions (MMCC) was used to support payment incentives under an alternative payment model (APM) in a network of community pharmacies providing enhanced services to Medicaid recipients in North Carolina. This program was supported by a CMS Innovations Award provided to Community Care of North Carolina, which serves as the primary care-based medical home for the state's Medicaid population. The specific aspects of this APM are described elsewhere [28]. In brief, the APM model included four different medication adherence metrics (RASA, NIDM, statin and MMCC) as well as three health service utilization measures (emergency department utilization, inpatient hospital visits and total cost of care) to measure the performance of each pharmacy relative to their peers. The MMCC measure described herein is one of the four adherence measures used to incentivize pharmacy performance.

2.2. Data

We constructed our measure of MMCC using North Carolina Medicaid prescription claims data from 2015 through 2017. As part of the APM, the measure was constructed on a quarterly basis with a rolling 12-month look back period to facilitate payment. Additional Medicaid claims data for outpatient and inpatient services as well as beneficiary enrollment data were also used to attribute patients to the network and facilitate payment. This study was not considered as human subjects research and was exempted from Institutional Review Board approval.

2.3. Sample

To be considered for inclusion into the MMCC measure, patients must first meet attribution criteria to the APM. Eligibility criteria included continuous Medicaid program enrollment for the entire calendar year (2015, 2016 or 2017). We further required that patients not be dually enrolled into the Medicare program to ensure we were able to fully capture all prescription drug claims. Finally, we limited the analysis to patients 18–64 years of age.

2.4. Medication Adherence Measurement

We used a list of 71 different therapeutic categories constructed by CCNC to identify therapeutic categories for inclusion in the MMCC measure. These categories were constructed by CCNC to identify high-risk chronic conditions effecting the Medicaid population. As seen in Table 1, the chronic conditions included in our measure spanned a wide variety of different therapeutic areas including chronic infectious conditions (e.g., hepatitis and HIV), diabetes, hypertension, additional cardiovascular conditions (e.g., diuretics, angina, anticoagulation), mental health conditions (depression, schizophrenia, bipolar disorder), osteoporosis, seizures and a number of other chronic conditions. This measure is much more inclusive of overall types of conditions patients might present with than the three Star Ratings adherence measures currently in use. Given that this list was constructed for purposes other than simply the construction of the MMCC adherence measure and applies specifically to a Medicaid population, which may require care management services, this study represents primarily a proof-of-concept exercise.

Table 1. Therapeutic categories included in initial multiple medications for chronic conditions (MMCC) adherence measurement.

Indication	Therapeutic Categories
Asthma	Anti-IgE Monoclonal Antibodies, Inhaled Corticosteroids, Leukotriene Modulators
Diabetes	Alpha-Glucosidase Inhibitors, Biguanides, Dipeptidyl Peptidase-4 (DPP-4) Inhibitors, Sulfonylureas, Thiazolidinediones
Hepatitis B	Hepatitis B agents
Hepatitis C	Inceivek, Interferon, Simeprevir, Ribavarin, Sofosbuvir, Boceprevir
HIV	Antiretrovirals (Entry inhibitors, integrase inhibitors, protease inhibitors, ritonavir) Antiretroviral Reverse Transcriptase Inhibitors (RTI) Non-nucleoside analogues, Antiretroviral RTI Nucleoside analogues (purine, pyrimidines, thymidines) Antiretroviral Nucleotide Analogues, Antiretroviral CMV agents, Cobicistat, Antiretroviral combination products
Hyperlipidemia	Antihyperlipidemics, Antihyperlipidemics-Bile Acid Sequestrants
Cardiovascular conditions	Antiadrenergic agents, Antianginal agents (non-nitrates), Antiarrhythmics, Antiplatelets
Hypertension	ACE Inhibitor, Alpha-beta blockers, Angiotensin II receptor antagonists, Beta-blockers, Calcium channel blockers, Renin inhibitors, Selective aldosterone receptor antagonists
Diuresis	Thiazide diuretics, Potassium sparing diuretics, Loop diuretics
ADHD	ADHD stimulants, ADHD miscellaneous
Dementia	Acetylcholinesterase inhibitors, NMDA receptor antagonists
Antidepressants	Alpha-2 Receptor Antagonists, Antidepressants-Combo, Antidepressants-Modified Cyclics, Serotonin-Norepinephrine Reuptake Inhibitors (SNRIs), Monoamine Oxidase Inhibitors (MAOIs), Selective Serotonin Reuptake Inhibitors (SSRIs)
Other Mental Health	Antipsychotics-Second Generation, Antipsychotic-First Generation, Antimanic Agents, Antiparkinson Agents
Seizures	Anticonvulsants misc.
Osteoporosis	Bone density Regulators-Bisphosphonates and Calcitonins, Bone density Regulators-Parathyroid Hormone, Vitamin D, Selective Estrogen Receptor Modulators
Contraception	Contraceptives misc.
Digestive Aids	Digestive enzymes misc.
Gout	Gout agents misc.
Thyroid Disorder	Hyperparathyroid Treatment-Vitamin D Analogs, Hypothyroid agents
Prostatic hypertrophy	Prostatic Hypertrophy Agents
Peptic ulcer	Peptic ulcer agents misc.

We measured adherence using PDC. A specific PDC was calculated for each of the 71 therapeutic categories of medications and followed the Star Ratings technical specifications. Hospitalized days were accounted for by crediting the patient for a medication believed to be given in the hospital if the patient was covered by the medication on the day they were admitted [29]. To be eligible for the MMCC measure, patients were required to use four or more of the 71 chronic therapeutic categories of medication from Table 1 over the 12 month calendar year period. In addition to the MMCC measure, we also constructed annual medication adherence rates for the three Star Ratings adherence measures (RASA, NIDM and statins) to evaluate correlations between the new measure and these established metrics. Patients were deemed adherent to the Star Ratings measures if their PDC was 80% or higher. To be considered adherent to the MMCC measure, we required patients to have a PDC of 80% or higher for at least 75% of the therapeutic categories used. For example, a patient using four specific therapeutic categories would be deemed adherent if they had a PDC of 80% or higher for at least three of the four therapeutic categories.

2.5. Criterion Validity Testing

We examined the potential criterion validity of the newly developed MMCC measure by correlating the measure with the three existing Star Ratings measures, which have gone through prior validation. This validity testing process assumes that adherence to Star Rating adherence measures and the MMCC measure are positively correlated. Given that the MMCC measure is constructed within each year (2015, 2016 and 2017) we first correlated the MMCC measure with each of the three Star Ratings measures using chi-square testing within the year of analysis. The chi-square comparison examines whether or not patients who were adherent to the MMCC measure (>75% of chronic medications used had a PDC ≥ 80%) were also categorized as adherent to the Star Ratings measure of interest (PDC ≥ 80%) Next, we assessed the correlation between MMCC and Star Ratings measures by running generalized estimating equations (GEE) models, which controlled for repeated observations for patients contributing adherence information across more than one single year of data to control for within subject variation. The GEE model specifies a binomial distribution with a log link. Data are converted to odds-ratios and are presented with corresponding 95% confidence intervals. All statistical analyses were deemed significant at $\alpha = 0.05$ and the analyses were run in SAS Version 9.4 (Cary, North Carolina, USA).

3. Results

Across the three-year period, more than 40,000 patients per year were eligible for the MMCC measure (Table 2). The number of patients eligible for the MMCC measure exceeded the approximate 10,000 patients a year eligible for the NIDM measure and more than 20,000 patients eligible per year for RASA and statin measures. The mean number of MMCC-eligible therapeutic categories was six with a range from four to 22. In 2017, the percent of patients eligible for adherence measures for NIDM, RASA and Statin medications that were adherent to treatment as defined by a PDC ≥ 80% (51.3%, 44.0% and 51.2%) was higher than the percent of patients adherent to the MMCC measure (34.6%). This trend was consistent across all years.

Table 2. Descriptive statistics of adherence measurement for full sample and MMCC [1] eligible patients.

	2015	2016	2017
Full Sample Eligible Population	N = 93,857	N = 96,824	N = 83,711
Eligible for NIDM [2] Adherence Measure	9681 (10.3%)	10,669 (11.0%)	9394 (11.2%)
Eligible for RASA [3] Adherence Measure	27,495 (29.3%)	28,853 (29.8%)	23,244 (27.8%)
Eligible for Statin Adherence Measure	23,201 (24.7%)	25,044 (25.9%)	21,565 (25.8%)
Adherent (≥ 80% PDC) NIDM Users	5101 (52.7%)	5988 (56.0%)	4821 (51.3%)
Adherent (≥ 80% PDC) RASA Users	15,030 (54.7%)	15,844 (54.9%)	10,242 (44.0%)
Adherent (≥ 80% PDC) Statin Users	12,996 (56.0%)	13,573 (54.2%)	11,030 (51.2%)
MMCC [1] Eligible Population	N = 43,712	N = 46,813	N = 40,001
Therapeutic Categories Defining Eligibility			
4 therapeutic categories	12,021 (27.5%)	12,520 (26.7%)	11,197 (28.0%)
5 therapeutic categories	9564 (21.9%)	10,194 (21.8%)	8899 (22.3%)
6 therapeutic categories	7192 (16.5%)	7747 (16.6%)	6680 (16/7%)
7 therapeutic categories	5353 (12.3%)	5849 (12.5%)	4787 (12.0%)
8 or more therapeutic categories	9582 (21.9%)	10,503 (22.4%)	8438 (21.1%)
Mean Count of Therapeutic Categories (SD)	6.1 (2.1)	6.1 (2.2)	6.1 (2.1)
Range of Therapeutic Categories	(4,21)	(4,22)	(4,21)
Also Eligible for Star Rating Adherence Measure	29,032 (66.4%)	31,343 (67.0%)	26,487 (66.2%)
Also Eligible for NIDM [2] Adherence Measure	8068 (18.5%)	8912 (19.0%)	7754 (19.4%)
Also Eligible for RASA [3] Adherence Measure	20,371 (46.6%)	21,651 (46.3%)	17,464 (43.7%)

Table 2. *Cont.*

	2015	2016	2017
Also Eligible for Statin Adherence Measure	19,460 (44.5%)	21,154 (45.2%)	18,063 (45.2%)
Adherent MMCC Users [4]	15,114 (34.6%)	15,133 (32.3%)	11,679 (29.2%)
MMCC Users Adherent to NIDM [2] (≥ 80% PDC)	4525 (56.1%)	5287 (59.3%)	4229 (54.9%)
MMCC Users Adherent to RASA [3] (≥ 80% PDC)	11,679 (57.3%)	12,387 (57.2%)	7998 (46.0%)
MMCC Users Adherent to Statin (≥ 80% PDC)	11,190 (57.5%)	11,722 (55.4%)	9515 (52.7%)

[1] MMCC = Multiple Medications for Chronic Conditions; [2] NIDM = Non-Insulin Diabetes Medications; [3] RASA = Renin Angiotensin System Antagonists; [4] MMCC Adherence Rate is defined as ≥ 75% of medications with ≥ 80% PDC.

Although unique from existing adherence measures, the three categories of medication that deem a patient eligible for inclusion into the Star Ratings program (RASA, NIDM and statins) were also common in patients eligible for the MMCC measure. Within each year, more than 66% of patients eligible for the MMCC measure were also eligible for inclusion into one or more of the Star Ratings adherence measurements. In 2017, 19.4%, 43.7% and 45.2% of patients eligible for MMCC measurement were also eligible for measurement of NIDM RASA, and statin medication adherence measures in the Star Ratings program respectively.

We hypothesized that among patients attributed to the MMCC measure who were also eligible for any of the three Star Ratings measures, adherence to the previously validated Star Ratings adherence measure would correlate with adherence to the new MMCC measure. Table 3 presents bivariate chi-square comparisons between each Star Ratings adherence measure and the MMCC measure. Overall, this correlation shows that among patients adherent to MMCC there is a higher likelihood of adherence to the three Star Ratings measures and similarly, among non-adherent MMCC patients there is a higher likelihood of non-adherence to Star Ratings measures. If a patient is not adherent to a Star Ratings PDC measure, they are unlikely to be adherent to the MMCC measure. For example, in 2017, only 6.9% of non-adherent NIDA users, 7.5% of non-adherent RASA users and 6.2% of non-adherent statin users were considered adherent for the MMCC measure. However, there were a significant number of patients deemed adherent to the Star ratings measures, which were not deemed adherent to the MMCC measure for each of the Star Ratings measures across each year. To illustrate, 50.7% of adherent NIDA users, 48.8% of adherent RASA users and 44.5% of adherent statin users were deemed not adherent to MMCC respectively in 2017.

Accounting for multiple observations across the three years, we further exaimine the relationship between adherence to the three existing Star Ratings measures and the probability of adherence to MMCC using GEE. Table 3 describes the odds-ratios and corresponding confidence intervals resulting from those tests. The odds ratio associated with MMCC adherence in adherent NIDA (Odds Ratio (OR) = 13.64: 95% CI: 12.6, 14.8), RASA (OR = 16.69: 95% CI: 15.8, 17.6) and Statin (OR = 21.32: 95% CI: 20.2, 22.6) users suggests a very strong correlation between the measures.

Table 3. Correlational testing between MMCC and existing Star Ratings adherence measurements.

		Chi-square Correlational Testing Between Star Ratings and MMCC Adherence Measures									Generalized Estimating Equation Testing Across All Years	
		2015		p-value	2016		p-value	2017		p-value		p-value
		MMCC[1] Adherence			MMCC Adherence			MMCC Adherence			Odds Ratio (95% CI)	
		<75%	≥75%		<75%	≥75%		<75%	≥75%			
NIDA[2] Adherence	<80%	3198 (39.6%)	345 (4.28%)	<0.001	3363 (37.7%)	262 (2.9%)	<0.001	3237 (42.2%)	238 (3.1%)	<0.001	13.64 (12.6, 14.8)	<0.001
	≥80%	1912 (23.7%)	2613 (32.4%)		2394 (26.9%)	2893 (32.4%)		2146 (27.9%)	2083 (27.0%)			
RASA[3] Adherence	<80%	8199 (40.3%)	493 (2.4%)	<0.001	8746 (40.4%)	518 (2.4%)	<0.001	8670 (49.9%)	706 (4.1%)	<0.001	16.69 (15.8, 17.6)	<0.001
	≥80%	5281 (25.9%)	6398 (31.4%)		5947 (27.5%)	6440 (29.7%)		3905 (22.5%)	4093 (23.6%)			
Statins Adherence	<80%	7775 (40.0%)	495 (2.5%)	<0.001	8763 (41.4%)	669 (3.2%)	<0.001	8016 (44.4%)	532 (3.0%)	<0.001	21.32 (20.2, 22.6)	<0.001
	≥80%	4140 (21.3%)	7050 (36.2%)		4736 (22.4%)	6986 (33.0%)		4238 (23.5%)	5277 (29.2%)			

[1] MMCC = Multiple Medications for Chronic Conditions;[2] NIDA = Non-Insulin Diabetes Adherence Measure;[3] RASA = Renin Angiotensin System Antagonists.

4. Discussion

Given the limitations associated with the three existing Star Ratings measures, we explored the implementation of a new MMCC measure of medication adherence. This measure captures more of the overall adherence needs of a patient by considering adherence to 71 different therapeutic categories of medication. This new measure has less opportunity for potential gaming by health plans, which are currently only required to emphasize adherence for a limited number of health conditions. As a more patient centered measure of medication adherence, the MMCC measure emphasizes more than a single chronic condition and is more reflective of the overall health needs of a patient. In addition, the focus on patients with multiple chronic conditions with the MMCC targets a high-risk population of patients with MCC who have higher than average health expenditures. Emphasizing adherence in this population is likely to pay greater dividends to actual health improvement than emphasizing adherence in patients with a single condition, some of which may be otherwise healthy.

The MMCC measures included more patients than any of the Star Ratings measures individually, and more than the total number across all Star Ratings measures combined. Additionally, there were many patients who were included in the traditional PDC measures who were not included in the MMCC measure. This suggests that the MMCC measure may target a different population than the traditional measures, and, because of larger denominators, be a more statistically reliable measure of medication adherence. Furthermore, the proportion of patients who met the adherence threshold for MMCC measure was substantially lower than the proportion of patients categorized as adherent to the traditional adherence measure. If confirmed in a Medicare population, this measure would solve some of the ceiling problems, which have been observed for four and five star plans.

To examine the criterion validity of this measure to previously validated adherence measurements, we correlated the MMCC measure with these three Star Ratings measures and found a very high correlation between them. However, we also found evidence that the criteria, which defined adherence to this new MMCC measure was more difficult to meet than the current criteria for NIDA, RASA or statin medication adherence. This suggests that the new measure may have less ceiling effect and provide better discriminative ability.

The results of this study should be interpreted in light of a number of important limitations. In many ways, this study represents a proof of concept investigation into the possibility of using an MMCC measure to capture medication adherence more broadly than that observed with limited therapeutic categories for single conditions. The therapeutic categories included in the measure were selected to support the needs of the state Medicaid program. This led to the inclusion of therapeutic categories that represent high-risk populations (e.g., HIV and Hepatitis) that might not represent the needs of commercially insured or Medicare plans to the same extent. For this measure to be accepted more broadly as a measure of plan performance, it is important to obtain the perspective of clinicians, patients and plans in the process of identifying which drug classes to include in an eventual MMCC measure. It should also undergo a formal validation process required of any new measure prior to implementation [30,31]. Finally, the proof of criterion validity in this study included the three Star Ratings measures, which we identified as having significant limitations in this article.

5. Conclusions

Given existing concerns associated with the use of medication adherence measures for limited therapeutic categories as part of the Star Ratings program in Medicare, opportunities for the development of new adherence performance measures exist. This proof of concept study shows the potential benefits associated with the development of a performance metric designed to capture adherence in patients with multiple chronic conditions. This measure correlated well with other validated adherence measures. Opportunities to develop and implement new quality metrics of medication adherence such as the MMCC should be explored.

Pharmacy **2019**, *7*, 81

Author Contributions: Conceptualization, J.F.F. and B.Y.U.; methodology, J.F.F. and B.Y.U.; software, J.F.F. and B.Y.U.; validation, J.F.F. and B.Y.U.; formal analysis, J.F.F. and B.Y.U.; investigation, J.F.F., B.Y.U., and A.K.; resources, J.F.F. and B.Y.U.; data curation, J.F.F. and B.Y.U.; writing (original draft preparation)—A.K. and J.F.F.; writing (review and editing)—J.F.F., B.Y.U. & A.K.; visualization, J.F.F. and B.Y.U.; supervision, J.F.F.; project administration, J.F.F. and B.Y.U.

Funding: The project described was supported by Grant Number 1C1CMS331338 from the Department of Health and Human Services, Centers for Medicare & Medicaid Services. The contents of this publication are solely the responsibility of the authors and do not necessarily represent the official views of the U.S. Department of Health and Human Services or any of its agencies. The research presented here was conducted by the awardee. Findings might or might not be consistent with or confirmed by the findings of the independent evaluation contractor.

Acknowledgments: The authors wish to acknowledge the following individuals who helped to develop the Multiple Medications for Chronic Conditions adherence measure while employed at Community Care of North Carolina: Troy Trygstad, Trista Pfeifenberger, David Wei, and Charles Shasky.

Conflicts of Interest: The authors declare no conflict of interest.

References

1. Ickowicz, E. Guiding principles for the care of older adults with multimorbidity: An approach for clinicians: American Geriatrics Society Expert Panel on the Care of Older Adults with Multimorbidity. *J. Am. Geriatr. Soc.* **2012**. [CrossRef]

2. Gerard, A. Chronic Care: Making the Case for Ongoing Care. Available online: https://folio.iupui.edu/bitstream/handle/10244/807/50968chronic.care.chartbook.pdf?sequence=1 (accessed on 21 March 2019).

3. Gerteis, J.; Izrael, D.; Deitz, D.; LeRoy, L.; Ricciardi, R.; Miller, T.; Basu, J. *Multiple Chronic Conditions Chartbook*; Agency For Healthcare Research and Quality: Rockville, MD, USA, 2010; p. 15.

4. Moore, K.L.; Patel, K.; Boscardin, W.J.; Steinman, M.A.; Ritchie, C.; Schwartz, J.B. Medication burden attributable to chronic co-morbid conditions in the very old and vulnerable. *PLoS ONE* **2018**, *13*, e0196109. [CrossRef] [PubMed]

5. Whitson, B. Managing Multiple Comorbidities. Available online: https://www.uptodate.com/contents/managing-multiple-comorbidities (accessed on 25 March 2019).

6. Cresswell, K.M.; Fernando, B.; McKinstry, B.; Sheikh, A. Adverse drug events in the elderly. *Br. Med. Bull.* **2007**, *83*, 259–274. [CrossRef] [PubMed]

7. Chrischilles, E.A.; VanGilder, R.; Wright, K.; Kelly, M.; Wallace, R.B. Inappropriate medication use as a risk factor for self-reported adverse drug effects in older adults. *J. Am. Geriatr. Soc.* **2009**, *57*, 1000–1006. [CrossRef] [PubMed]

8. Brown, M.T.; Bussell, J.K. Medication adherence: WHO cares? *Mayo. Clin. Proc.* **2011**, *86*, 304–314. [CrossRef] [PubMed]

9. Osterberg, L.; Blaschke, T. Adherence to Medication. *N. Engl. J. Med.* **2005**, *353*, 487–497. [CrossRef] [PubMed]

10. Oung, A.B.; Kosirog, E.; Chavez, B.; Brunner, J.; Saseen, J.J. Evaluation of medication adherence in chronic disease at a federally qualified health center. *Ther. Adv. Chronic Dis.* **2017**, *8*, 113–120. [CrossRef] [PubMed]

11. Neiman, A.B.; Ruppar, T.; Ho, M.; Garber, L.; Weidle, P.J.; Hong, Y.; George, M.G.; Thorpe, P.G. CDC grand rounds: improving medication adherence for chronic disease management—innovations and opportunities. *MMWR Morb. Mortal. Wkly. Rep.* **2017**, *66*, 1248. [CrossRef] [PubMed]

12. Why You Need to Take Your Medications as Prescribed or Instructed. Available online: https://www.fda.gov/drugs/resourcesforyou/specialfeatures/ucm485545.htm (accessed on 26 March 2019).

13. Yap, D. CMS Star Ratings; Compounding Bill Passes Senate, Heads to Obama. Available online: https://www.pharmacist.com/article/cms-star-ratings-compounding-bill-passes-senate-heads-obama?is_sso_called=1 (accessed on 26 March 2019).

14. CMS. Medicare 2018 Part C & D Star Ratings Technical Notes. Available online: https://www.cms.gov/Medicare/Prescription-Drug-Coverage/PrescriptionDrugCovGenIn/Downloads/2018-Star-Ratings-Technical-Notes-2017_09_06.pdf (accessed on 27 March 2019).

15. Chavez-Valdez, A.L. Request for Comments: Enhancements to the Star Ratings for 2018 and Beyond. Available online: https://www.cms.gov/Medicare/Prescription-Drug-Coverage/PrescriptionDrugCovGenIn/Downloads/Request-for-Comments-2018-Stars.pdf (accessed on 27 March 2019).

16. CMS. Part C and D Performance Data. Available online: https://www.cms.gov/medicare/prescription-drug-coverage/prescriptiondrugcovgenin/performancedata.html (accessed on 29 March 2019).

17. CMS. Trends in Part C & D Star Rating Measure Cut Points. Available online: https://www.cms.gov/Medicare/Prescription-Drug-Coverage/PrescriptionDrugCovGenIn/Downloads/2019_Cut_Point_Trend.pdf (accessed on 29 March 2019).

18. Kirkman, M.S.; Rowan-Martin, M.T.; Levin, R.; Fonseca, V.A.; Schmittdiel, J.A.; Herman, W.H.; Aubert, R.E. Determinants of Adherence to Diabetes Medications: Findings From a Large Pharmacy Claims Database. *Diabetes Care.* **2015**, *38*, 604–609. [CrossRef] [PubMed]

19. Farr, A.M.; Sheehan, J.J.; Curkendall, S.M.; Smith, D.M.; Johnston, S.S.; Kalsekar, I. Retrospective analysis of long-term adherence to and persistence with DPP-4 inhibitors in US adults with type 2 diabetes mellitus. *Adv. Ther.* **2014**, *31*, 1287–1305. [CrossRef] [PubMed]

20. Colantonio, L.D.; Huang, L.; Monda, K.L.; Bittner, V.; Serban, M.-C.; Taylor, B.; Brown, T.M.; Glasser, S.P.; Muntner, P.; Rosenson, R.S. Adherence to High-Intensity Statins Following a Myocardial Infarction Hospitalization Among Medicare Beneficiaries. *JAMA Cardiol.* **2017**, *2*, 890–895. [CrossRef] [PubMed]

21. Ailinger, R.L.; Black, P.L.; Lima-Garcia, N. Use of electronic monitoring in clinical nursing research. *Clin. Nurs. Res.* **2008**, *17*, 89–97. [CrossRef] [PubMed]

22. Hansen, R.A.; Kim, M.M.; Song, L.; Tu, W.; Wu, J.; Murray, M.D. Adherence: Comparison of Methods to Assess Medication Adherence and Classify Nonadherence. *Ann. Pharmacother.* **2009**, *43*, 413–422. [CrossRef] [PubMed]

23. Schweers, K. Medicare Addresses Mail Order Waste, Refill Synchronization for 2014. Available online: https://www.ncpanet.org/newsroom/ncpa\T1\textquoterights-blog---the-dose/2013/10/03/medicare-addresses-mail-order-waste-refill-synchronization-for-2014 (accessed on 20 April 2019).

24. CMS. Advance Notice of Methodological Changes for Calendar Year (CY) 2014 for Medicare Advantage (MA) Capitation Rates, Part C and Part D Payment Policies and 2014 Call Letter: Auto-Ship Refill Programs in Part D. Available online: https://www.cms.gov/Medicare/Health-Plans/MedicareAdvtgSpecRateStats/Downloads/Advance2014.pdf (accessed on 20 April 2019).

25. Farley, J.F.; Urick, B.Y.; Schondelemeyer, S.W. Community Pharmacy Versus Mail Order: An Uneven Comparison. *J. Manag. Care. Spec. Pharm.* **2019**, *25*, 724–725. [CrossRef] [PubMed]

26. Smith, M.G.; Shea, C.M.; Brown, P.; Wines, K.; Farley, J.F.; Ferreri, S.P. Pharmacy characteristics associated with the provision of medication management services within an integrated care management program. *J. Am. Pharm. Assoc.* **2017**, *57*, 217–221. [CrossRef] [PubMed]

27. Smith, M.G.; Ferreri, S.P.; Brown, P.; Wines, K.; Shea, C.M.; Pfeiffenberger, T.M. Implementing an integrated care management program in community pharmacies: A focus on medication management services. *J. Am. Pharm. Assoc.* **2017**, *57*, 229–235. [CrossRef] [PubMed]

28. Urick, B.Y.; Ferreri, S.P.; Shasky, C.; Pfeiffenberger, T.; Trygstad, T.; Farley, J.F. Lessons Learned from Using Global Outcome Measures to Assess Community Pharmacy Performance. *J. Manag. Care Spec. Pharm.* **2018**, *24*, 1278–1283. [CrossRef] [PubMed]

29. CMS. Medicare 2019 Part C & D Star Ratings Technical Notes. Available online: https://www.cms.gov/Medicare/Prescription-Drug-Coverage/PrescriptionDrugCovGenIn/Downloads/2019-Technical-Notes-preview-2.pdf (accessed on 29 March 2019).

30. PQA. Developing Measures That Matter. Available online: https://www.pqaalliance.org/measure-development (accessed on 20 April 2019).

31. NQF. How Endorsement Happens. Available online: https://www.qualityforum.org/Measuring_Performance/ABCs/How_Endorsement_Happens.aspx (accessed on 20 April 2019).

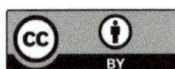

pharmacy

MDPI

Article

An Ethical Analysis of Pharmacy Benefit Manager (PBM) Practices

Jacob J. Drettwan and Andrea L. Kjos *

College of Pharmacy and Health Sciences, Drake University, Des Moines, IA 50311, USA;
jacob.drettwan@drake.edu
* Correspondence: andrea.kjos@drake.edu

Received: 29 April 2019; Accepted: 11 June 2019; Published: 14 June 2019

check for updates

Abstract: The high costs associated with pharmaceuticals and the accompanying stakeholders are being closely evaluated in the search for solutions. As a major stakeholder in the U.S. pharmaceutical market, the practices of pharmacy benefit manager (PBM) organizations have been under increased scrutiny. Examples of controversial practices have included incentives driving formulary status and prohibiting pharmacists from disclosing information on lower-cost prescription alternatives. Ethical investigations have been largely omitted within the debate on the responsibilities of these organizations in the health care system. Ethical analysis of organizational practices is justified based on the potential impact during health care delivery. The objective of this study was to analyze several specific PBM practices using multiple ethical decision-making models to determine their ethical nature. This study systematically applied multiple ethical decision-making models and codes of ethics to a variety of practices associated with PBM-related dilemmas encountered in the pharmaceutical environment. The assessed scenarios resulted in mixed outcomes. PBM practices were both ethical and unethical depending on the applied ethical model. Despite variation across applied models, some practices were predominately ethical or unethical. The point of sale rebates were consistently determined as ethical, whereas market consolidation, gag clauses, and fluctuation of pharmacy reimbursements were all predominantly determined as unethical. The application of using provider codes of ethics created additional comparison and also contained mixed findings. This study provided a unique assessment of PBM practices and provides context from a variety of ethical perspectives. To the knowledge of the authors, these perspectives have not been previously applied to PBM practices in the literature. The application of ethical decision-making models offers a unique context to current health care dilemmas. It is important to analyze health care dilemmas using ethics-based frameworks to contribute solutions addressing complexities and values of all stakeholders in the health care environment.

Keywords: pharmacy benefit manager (PBM); ethics; pharmaceutical regulation; health care policy; decision-making; organizations; ethical models; code of ethics; pharmacist

1. Introduction

The costs of pharmaceuticals as a portion of health care spending has continued to vex the United States (U.S.) as well as the rest of the world for several decades [1]. This issue has prompted vigorous discussion from a variety of stakeholders in the attempt to find agreeable solutions to a seemingly insolvable problem [2]. Discussions with experts and stakeholders have included government payers, health insurance organizations and pharmaceutical manufacturers. The most common frameworks considered in solutions are economic and legal rationales [3]. Economic defense of high costs often point towards the capitalistic free market and hence, theory of supply and demand. Further, legal considerations rely on explanations related to intellectual property rights, patents, proprietary information, obligations to shareholders, as well as complexities of government policies, regulation and oversight [1,2]. As an example of legal complexities, the United States health care practices (including health insurance law) are regulated at the state level (e.g., New York will differ from California), in contrast to uniformity at a national level [4]. This results in a variety of co-existing regulations depending on the regional location of the organization, the care provider, or the patient. Even beyond the U.S., legally sanctioned intellectual property rights and patent laws for pharmaceuticals are not always consistent across countries, resulting in complexities in the world-wide market [5].

In the U.S., the fiduciary issue of high spending on pharmaceuticals is one that involves specific interrelated stakeholder organizations including manufacturers, wholesalers, pharmacies, pharmacy benefit managers (PBMs), and plan sponsors (i.e., health insurance organizations) [6,7]. Briefly, these organizations and their relationships include the following: Pharmaceuticals are developed and made by manufacturers, delivered to pharmacies by wholesale distributors, obtained by patients at pharmacies where there is often reduced pricing according to coverage by plan sponsors [6,7]. PBMs are organizations that developed to provide added value and reduced costs by specifically managing the pharmaceutical benefit on behalf of a plan sponsor. In addition to using formularies and utilization requirements to control cost and incentivize cost-effective medication use, PBMs also negotiate lower prices from manufacturers [8]. This practice is commonly known as rebating. Although ideally a cost-saving tool, rebate levels are confidential and the actual cost savings is unknown. Under normal market conditions this would not be problematic, however, there is evidence to suggest that the most cost-effective pharmaceuticals are not being incentivized due to how PBMs sometimes place higher-priced pharmaceuticals as the preferred status on formularies and patients may spend more than they would for lower cost, equally effective alternatives [8]. Recently, PBM business practices such as rebating have begun to receive public scrutiny as the U.S. looks for solutions to the problem of high costs of pharmaceuticals [9–13]. Additional business practices undergoing scrutiny include exclusion lists, gag clauses, rapid fluctuation in pharmacy reimbursement rates, market consolidation and point of sale rebates [14]. In brief, exclusion lists are a way to specify non-coverage of certain medications, that is, it is a list of prescription medications that are excluded from any plan sponsor coverage. It has been noted that these exclusion lists are growing longer, in particular, for new or more expensive prescription medications [15]. A lesser-known policy referred to as gag clauses are in reference to a commercial contract between a PBM and pharmacies prohibiting a pharmacist's ability to inform a patient whether or not a prescription has alternative purchasing options [16]. Another concern with PBMs has been the fluctuation of reimbursements through the use of redirect and indirect remuneration (DIR) fees assessed to pharmacies, retrospectively, dependent upon pharmacy performance or upon changes in market prices [17]. The practice known as point of sale rebates refers to PBM contracts with a discount program to offer cash-paying consumers an ability to purchase prescription medications at prices lower than a pharmacy's list price of the medication [18] and circumvents the effectiveness of utilization incentives towards lower cost alternatives. Finally, as in many industries, the market consolidation of PBMs with other types of organization in the form of vertical integration challenge the intent of legal anti-trust statutes [7] (pp. 30–32), further attracting public scrutiny.

Health providers often find themselves as reluctant mediators between patients and high cost pharmaceuticals. Generally, provider involvement includes prescribing, educating, dispensing, and even administration of pharmaceuticals pursuant to laws regulating the scope of practice for various types of health professions. Specific to physicians, it has been argued that "physicians often neglect, or are simply unaware of, their role as economic agents for patients. Physicians play a crucial role in controlling prices and enabling patients to access affordable therapies" [19] (p. 9). In contrast, many community pharmacists are well versed in advocating for patient access to medications in the commercial environment of high costs [20].

It is pertinent that the experts and researchers continue work to find agreeable solutions to the problem of high costs of pharmaceuticals. To frame these discussions, an ethical framework would stand in contrast to the use of an economic or legal framework. Although there are a number of ethical theories worthy of consideration, in comparison to other frameworks, the ethical dialog uses concepts such as avoiding harm, duty to patients, virtues, justice, or the common good. Interestingly, stakeholder organizations and their corresponding practices described above, have remained largely uncriticized in the ethical literature, with the only exception being pharmaceutical manufacturers [19,21]. However, PBMs have been showing signs of increased scrutiny by private nonprofit health foundations [8], the U.S. government [7,14], professional pharmacy organizations [20,22] and in the economic literature [23,24]. The increased scrutiny directed toward PBMs has resulted from shielded business practices that may raise ethical concerns. For example, the literature has debated whether the reduced prices for some result in increased prices for others [13,19]. More specifically, PBMs may be causing a form of price-shifting between stakeholders, resulting in increased profits for manufacturers and PBMs, reduced revenues for pharmacies, reduced prices for some patients and plan sponsors, and increased prices for other patients and plan sponsors [23].

An ethical-oriented framework is one that is easily relatable to the case-based decisions of health care providers (e.g., pharmacists or physicians) [25]. Ethical principles are used in health care to provide a moral grounding for the day to day work of providers. The study of ethics remains an important part of education and culture for nearly all care providers charged with supporting the health of individuals in society [26,27]. Codes of ethics exist for clinical health professionals, and are intended to guide decision-making in the face of competing interests, social dilemmas, or conflicts encountered during the provision of care [28]. Although the study and application of ethics remain at the core of health professionals' conduct, some have begun to question the degree to which the application of ethical principles may be in conflict with daily work requirements within the health care system, especially when balancing fiscal considerations [29]. Some base a growing concern for physician burnout and failing mental health on a kind of moral crisis [30]. Further, an application of a concept previously used for combat veterans known as moral injury has been used in the context of health care and posited as resulting from providers feeling as if their work is dissonant with their own moral and ethical principles [31].

Although there is an abundance of literature in the application of ethics in health care related to the provider-patient interactions, there has been substantially less attention on how health care organizations impact providers during the delivery of care [32]. In fact, organizational ethics is considered as an adjacent field to more typical bioethics applications in health care. However, some ethical theory work has shown new approaches using contextual differences to shape discussion when a dilemma includes both clinical and organizationally ethical standpoints [33]. As the dilemma of the high costs of pharmaceuticals is situated most prominently at an organizational level, it has been rarely considered through the more common bioethical (i.e., provider-patient focused) lens in the health care literature. Arguments to address this gap have used organizational ethics to demonstrate that stakeholder organizations can make decisions from a moral point of view in cooperation with the broader health care environment [21]. In addition, some have discussed a need for a cross-over between ethics and other fields, such as economics, to avoid economic-based solutions that inadvertently compound ethical concerns [19].

Specific to the field of pharmacy, a comprehensive review of the theory of pharmacy ethics found the existence of very little formal literature on philosophical values or frameworks specific to pharmacy [34]. Rather, this review found application of traditional medically-based bioethical concepts to pharmacy-oriented practice scenarios, as well as the application of professional codes to direct the behavior of pharmacists. Therefore, research on pharmacy ethics presents an area ripe for investigation due to the constant balance of the clinical aspects of patient care with commercial aspects of practice, especially in the community pharmacy settings [34]. Some limited theory-based research in this area found health care organizations do shape the ethical decision-making of pharmacists [35]. For example, some research has found that professional hierarchies, closeness (or distance) from patient care, or daily gatekeeping (i.e., roles balancing clinical care with fiscal responsibility) can require a great deal of provider moral contemplation [36]. Further, this literature has discussed that intensification of commercial pressures in the profession of pharmacy are resulting in pharmacists feeling pressure to make unethical decisions that may be in conflict with their moral values [36]. This evidence only serves to strengthen the argument of growing moral injury distress in health care providers. With the growing concern over the moral crisis faced by providers, the authors were interested in how questionable practices by key organizations undergoing public scrutiny would stand through a framework more commonly aligned with the decision-making of providers, that of an ethical analysis.

When considering potential economic and legal solutions, an ethical analysis would provide a novel and grounded framework for understanding the potential ethical considerations by providers as well as broader context for stakeholders. Moreover, there exists a gap in the literature relating to how such organizational practices in health care, and those of PBMs in particular, might fare under ethical examination. Therefore, as a first step towards bridging this gap, this study sought to investigate the ethical nature of PBM practices using ethical decision-making models.

Ethical issues in health care, including pharmacy, are commonly discussed using four core bioethical principles of beneficence, non-maleficence, autonomy and justice [37,38] as well as with professional codes of ethics [34]. In addition, some pharmacy specific texts have included fidelity and truthfulness as newer ethical principles with application and relevance [39]. However, work by Cooper et. al. described that much previous empirical ethical work in pharmacy commonly used these principles solely due to normative consideration rather than because these values are reported by pharmacists themselves. These authors observed pharmacists used a range of ethical values during the reasoning process, and that various ethical approaches may have relevance to pharmacy dilemmas. Moreover, research has found that even when provided a four-stage process guideline, pharmacists displayed limited abilities in ethical reasoning [39]. Cooper and colleagues' open-ended empirical approach hoped to capture the complexity and nuance in pharmacist decision-making, however, it was found that pharmacists frequently reasoned dilemmas in legal terms and lacked ethical awareness. Therefore, given the overall lack of literature on ethical theory in pharmacy combined with the possibility of criticism on the application of normative ethical theory (i.e., the four major bioethical principles), it is prudent to take a comprehensive approach.

There is some ethical theory literature which proposes the use of multiple frameworks to compare contextual differences from a clinical versus an organizational standpoint [28,33]. Further, this work argues complexities of health care rarely allow one model to capture value differences among all stakeholders. Thus, it would be of interest to use multiple ethical models in order to compare potential value differences encased in various ethical scenarios. The literature suggests that pharmacists may need additional guidance for ethical decision-making in practice [39] and that there have been calls for integration of novel ethical schemas for grappling with complex and especially commercial aspects of health care [34]. As a result, the authors chose to use established decision-making models based upon a diversity of ethical theories and principles.

Philosophical decision-making models assist with debate and identification of action steps given an ethical issue. Work by Hammaker and Knadig, have summarized eight decision-making models based on the major philosophers cited by the U.S. Supreme Court, the U.S. Court of Appeals, and the state Supreme Courts since 2010 [40]. These models comprehensively cover teachings and writings of philosophers that included: Kant, Rawls, Dworkin, Bentham, Mill, Confucius, Socrates/Plato/Aristotle, Bradley, Epictetus, and Sartre [40] (p. 8). These decision-making models were appealing to use as a framework in this study because they have been used extensively in the U.S. legal system, which the literature has shown is important to pharmacists [39]. They include principles from deontology, teleology, and utilitarianism as well as others. Regarding the eight accepted decision-making models, this study chose six to use for analysis. After consideration, two models were excluded from the final analysis due to inapplicability and ambiguity of context when attempting to create a consistent assessment. In place of the two excluded decision-making models, the authors chose to examine how two professional codes of ethics might assess each of the issues. Provider codes of ethics are also referenced in the literature as ways health care providers are taught and therefore utilize ethical values in practice [19,34].

In sum, because there has been a lack of ethically-based work surrounding organizations involved in the high costs of drugs and that a gap remains in ethics-based pharmacy research, this study used scrutinized PBM practices to comprehensively consider these issues within an ethical framework. Therefore, the objective of this study was to systematically apply multiple ethical decision-making models to specific PBM practices and determine their ethical nature.

2. Methods

2.1. Conceptualization

In this study, several types of controversial PBM practices were chosen for evaluation. PBM practices were chosen based those receiving evaluation in U.S. government issued reports [7,14]. First, this study identified if the practice was receiving scrutiny and a potential cause for increasing drug pricing [14] (pp. 32–38). Second, the authors assessed if the practice could stimulate changes in the drug supply chain [7] (pp. 26–32). And finally, the authors predicted if this practice or related changes in the drug supply chain could present ethical concerns to providers. If a PBM practice was able to sufficiently meet all elements for inclusion, it was evaluated using a systematic approach to determine its ethical nature. This study was limited to a maximum of five ethical scenarios to ensure a thorough analysis. The scenarios considered the market environment, including the purpose of the organization, typical goals (i.e., cost-effectiveness and profit-maximization) and motivations of the involved stakeholders. The scenarios considered in this study were purposely hypothetical and therefore did not use actual cases, or details from any specific organization or company. The models have differences in value considerations, yet all of which are considered a reputable means of determining an ethical decision with health care and the legal systems [40]. This comprehensive approach provides a framework for future work. The chosen ethical scenarios are detailed in Table 1.

Table 1. Ethical Scenarios.

Gag Clauses	A commercial contract between a pharmacy benefit manager and a network of pharmacies prohibiting a pharmacist from informing a patient of alternative prescription purchasing options [16]
Fluctuation of Pharmacy Reimbursement Rate	PBM determined redirect and indirect remuneration (DIR) fees assessed to pharmacies retrospectively dependent upon incentive-based performance [17] (p. 33)
Exclusion Lists	List of branded prescription medications to be excluded from insurance coverage [15]
Market Consolidation	Large mergers and acquisitions have been increasing between pharmacy benefit management organizations and other organizations within health care [7] (pp. 30–32)
Point-of-Sale Rebates	A commercial contract between pharmacy benefit manager and discount card providers offering cash-paying patients discounted prescription pricing [18]

2.2. Analytical Approach

This study used a systematic ethical analysis of PBM practices utilizing decision-making models [40] (pp. 4–35) based upon a foundation of ethical philosophies. The six decision-making models were applied to all five selected PBM practices in a detailed step-wise assessment. The foundational ethical philosophies that comprise the six models are fully described in chapter one of the Hammaker and Knadig text [40]. These were the utility model (utilitarianism), exceptions model, choices model, justice model, common good model, and virtue model. In the utility model, maximizing good and minimizing harm are the foci of this ethical determination. The exceptions model is a unique framework to consider the ethical nature if an individual exception became the standard or norm for all. The choices model places a focus on how decisions are made, with an emphasis being placed on moral respect for individual choices. The justice model, commonly applied in health care, involves the consideration of the distribution of limited resources. The common good model is similar to the utility model, but rather than focus on benefits to individuals, it asks to focus on how a decision might benefit everyone. Finally, the virtue model focuses on core values aspired to by the decider, and determinations whether a given scenario helps or hinders one towards reaching these values. Examples of core values of health professionals may include characteristics of compassion, honesty, or self-control. Complete descriptions of the specific step-wise framework for application of the models were included in Table S1A–F, in the Supplemental

Materials. More specific details about the foundational ethical theory and foundational philosophies for each of the models can be found the Hammaker and Knadig text.

To demonstrate reproducibility, the following outlines an example of how a step-wise application of each ethical model would be conducted. These steps and application responses were applied to the five chosen ethical scenarios. They were determined by the authors separately, and then together through detailed discussion until a consensus for each scenario was reached. In this application, the steps outlined for the justice model (Table S1D, Supplementary Materials) were applied to the PBM practice known as exclusion lists.

The justice model contains five steps: (Step 1) Define the distribution of resources by determining who is getting the benefits and burdens in the situation. Should those who get benefits also share burdens? (Application Response 1) The purpose of the PBM's formulary cost structure is to fairly distribute prescription benefits and burdens (i.e., costs) across all plan members, assuming reasons for any inequality are fair and just. (Step 2) Once the distribution is known, establish which criterion for distribution would be the fairest and justify why it would be most fair in the situation. (Application Response 2) The fairest distribution is typically through PBM authorized prescription cost structures based on medication tiering and copayment agreements with plan members. The use of these structures and formularies allows for fair distribution based on principles of cost-effectiveness medication use. (Step 3) Select a framework to decide what is fair if disagreement persists over which outcome is fair or over which criterion for inequality is best in the situation, then choose a framework to decide what is fair. (Application Response 3) The framework used to determine fairness has been built into the PBM authorized formulary structure and plan sponsor pricing. Factors such as employment, premiums, maximum out-of-pocket expenses, exclusion lists, etc. all have a role in pricing and payment. Following agreed upon terms of the authorized formulary will most consistently produce a fair outcome. (Step 4) Make an ethical decision. Decide whether an action will produce a fair distribution and why. (Application Response 4) This practice is deemed ethical. Exclusion lists are applied to prevent inconsistencies within authorized cost structures to maximize cost-effectiveness for plan members. (Step 5) Monitor and reassess when applicable.

Ethical scenarios were also assessed using the Pharmacist Code of Ethics and the Physician Code of Ethics [41,42]. These two professional codes of ethics were chosen because of the potential impact of these health care providers as fiduciary advocates in the pharmaceutical market. For the analysis with the professional codes, the authors added the total number of sections (i.e., Section I, Section II.) finding the practice as ethical, to the total number finding the practice as unethical, to calculate the overall ethical determination. In other words, the authors assessed whether each section would call the practice ethical or unethical. Inclusion of other health provider's codes of ethics was beyond the scope of the study's objective. There was no weighting assigned to these assessments, each model or code section stood on its own merits. Once an ethical nature was determined using each model and an individual code of ethics, the resulting ethical determinations were totaled.

3. Results

The PBM practice that was most likely to be found ethical by the models included point of sale rebates. Exclusion lists were equally found to be both ethical and unethical, depending on the model applied. In contrast, a clear majority of ethical models found market consolidation and gag clauses to be unethical. Additionally, all ethical models unanimously found that the fluctuation of pharmacy reimbursement rates to be unethical.

The ethical models found different results for each PBM practice, with the exception of the common good and choices models, which made identical ethical assessments. Further, the codes of ethics applied also found differing assessments. The Physician Code of Ethics aligned most closely with the utility and the justice models. In contrast, the Pharmacist Code of Ethics aligned most closely with the choices and common good models.

A complete summary and cross-tabulation of ethical assessments for the models and codes of ethics can be found in Table 2, below.

Pharmacy **2019**, *7*, 65

Table 2. Ethical Analysis.

Scenario & Model	Market Consolidation	Pharmacy Reimbursement Rate	Gag Clauses	Exclusion Lists	Point of Sale Rebates	Totals
Utility	Ethical	Unethical	Ethical	Ethical	Ethical	Ethical: 4 Unethical: 1
Exceptions	Unethical	Unethical	Ethical	Ethical	Unethical	Ethical: 2 Unethical: 3
Choices	Unethical	Unethical	Unethical	Unethical	Ethical	Ethical: 1 Unethical: 4
Justice	Unethical	Unethical	Unethical	Ethical	Ethical	Ethical: 2 Unethical: 3
Common Good	Unethical	Unethical	Unethical	Unethical	Ethical	Ethical: 1 Unethical: 4
Virtue	Ethical	Unethical	Unethical	Unethical	Ethical	Ethical: 2 Unethical: 3
Pharmacist	Unethical	Unethical	Unethical	Unethical	Ethical	Ethical: 1 Unethical: 4
Physician	Unethical	Unethical	N/A	Ethical	Ethical	Ethical: 2 Unethical: 2
Totals	Ethical: 2 Unethical: 6	Ethical: 0 Unethical: 8	Ethical: 2 Unethical: 5	Ethical: 4 Unethical: 4	Ethical: 7 Unethical: 1	Ethical: 15/39 Unethical: 24/39

4. Discussion

This study systematically applied multiple ethical decision-making models to a variety of PBM practices. The results showed a novel assessment of ethically questionable PBM practices with mixed findings on their ethical nature. The PBM practices were determined to be simultaneously ethical and unethical depending on the varied considerations for each applied model. The application of the codes of ethics of pharmacists or physicians further created comparisons for these results.

In consideration of the PBM practices, exclusion lists produced the most varied findings when the ethical models were applied. More consistent results were established with all other PBM practices, which were predominately deemed unethical. Point-of-sale rebates were the only PBM practice with a consistent ethical determination. This practice has been more recently scrutinized and more information will develop with changes in the market that could change results [43]. Future assessment is warranted for this ethically questionable scenario.

The majority of PBM practices resulted in an unethical determination. These results can be attributed, in part, to the ethical philosophies in which the decision-making models are based. Generally, philosophical renderings consist strictly of a two-sided pendulum, one beneficence (i.e., ensuring welfare) and the other maleficence (i.e., opposes welfare). When applying the theories or models, a decision must be made with little acceptance or consideration of an ethical spectrum. However, the context does matter and could change the decision. It has also been noted that vagueness of ethical codes is also a cause of conflict for a consensus of interpretation [19] (pp. 4–35). Many PBM actions were simultaneously ethical and unethical dependent on the applied philosophical model. However, unethical results are more prevalent because greater significance tends to be placed on acts of beneficence or maleficence with a direct effect on individuals rather than societies. Whereas, the objective of PBM organizations is the cost-effective management of medication use for an entire covered group of people, or a population, and therefore more closely align with the needs of a broader society than an individual.

More specifically, the common good model and the choices model produced identical ethical determinations for all PBM practices under ethical assessment. The models, although different in structure and application, produced identical results due to a shared emphasis on the individual within a society. The common good model determines ethical nature through the distribution of benefits and burdens of individuals within a society, as well as the sustainability of the distribution. The choices model requires individuals to be given an individualized determination of their life outcome via specific choices and values. The choices model and the common good model both ethically assess society through an individualized perception. The two models strongly favor an unethical determination of recently scrutinized PBM practices.

The utility model and common good model produced the most contradicting results among the ethical models. Regarding the five practices assessed, three showed disagreement. The utility model and the common good model are nearly identical in their structure and application, however found different results. The models assess foreseeable benefits and burdens resulting from an action. Then, the models determine the most beneficial option available as an ethical decision. However, the important distinction is the utility model only considers those immediately affected by an action, whereas the common good model considers the benefit and burden to all of society and also accounts for unintentional and non-immediate benefits and burdens. The subtle difference is significant when determining results. An example of such disagreement is also demonstrated when assessing gag clauses. The utility model determines gag clauses to be justified and therefore ethical because they produce the best overall outcome and the greatest long-term benefit to those affected. The common good model determines gag clauses to conflict with the pharmacist's ethical obligation, which prioritizes the importance of maintaining a beneficial and truthful relationship with patients. The ideologies upheld by a pharmacist's ability to communicate transparently to patients contribute more common good to society than any common good deriving from the PBM's gag clause. In this scenario, the common good is the general condition that all patients have equal access to a quality relationship with their pharmacist.

The differences among the models for the ethical scenario of market consolidation further demonstrate how subtle philosophical orientation can provide context to an ethical determination. Both the utility model and virtue model supported market consolidation but for different reasons. For example, the utility model supported market consolidation as ethical because of the potential effect on the distribution of benefits and burdens of those immediately affected by the action. Those immediately affected are likely to already hold a prescription benefit plan within the established system. The consolidation of entities within the pre-established market will further benefit plan holders due to increased access to affordable care through plan participation. Those who do not hold plans within the system will not have any direct benefit and are likely burdened by a decreased supply within the market upon entry. However, the utility model does not take those individuals into consideration when making an ethical determination due to a lack of immediate effect. The virtue model focuses primarily on the aspirations of a professional and secondarily on the action itself. More specifically, the virtue model emphasizes a health care professional's ability to deliver high-quality and equitable care to the patient population. This emphasis on delivery of care supports the consolidation of the market. Consolidation allows for near universal availability, coverage, and access to prescription benefits, which benefits both the health care professionals and patients financially and clinically. However, the patient must have sufficient resources to gain access to the market in order to experience the added benefits consolidation offers. The common good and choices models place emphasis on individual assessment. In general, consolidation usually places importance on the benefit to a population or society rather than an individual perception.

The Physician's Code of Ethics, virtue model, justice model, and exceptions model produced mixed results. In contrast, the utility model, choices model, common good model and Pharmacist's Code of Ethics were more consistent. An interesting finding was a lack of alignment between the Pharmacist's Code of Ethics and the Physician's Code of Ethics. This could be due to specificities within each code of ethics. The physician's code appears to have a broadened perspective, emphasizing the value of societal health as well as the individual patient. For example, Sections VII and IX (Table S2B, Supplementary Materials) are both pointing towards the broader community and societal issues of health care access to all and to public health. Whereas, the pharmacist's code has an emphasis focused more specifically on individual patients. For example, the only mention of broader society is in Section VIII (Table S2A) and this section speaks of a balance towards the broader societal distribution of resources with individual patients. The similar but differing ethical values could be viewed as a system of checks and balances between types of care providers or could be viewed as a way to better understand the foundational values of each unique profession. It would be of further interest to compare ethical codes for additional health professions.

The future success of quality care relies on providers who are willing to actively assess the changing landscape of the health care system and confront potentially unethical practices. Grass-roots advocacy by health providers have had, and continue to have, the potential to make changes in health care both from a regulatory and organizational standpoint. Therefore, it is critical for providers to be knowledgeable about current practices impacting foundational values that guide their work. Despite the multiplicity of theory-based ethical models as well as ethical codes among the health professions, it is important that providers are supported when complex problems in health care infringe on their moral values. Further, ethical models and professional codes can assist in guidance, but should be used cautiously if applied singularly or in a simplified dichotomous (i.e., ethical/unethical) or authoritative way. Therefore, this study provides an example of how to use theory-based models and multiple professional codes to deepen the understanding of current ethical problems in practice. Finally, in pharmacy as in other health professions, ethical standards can have important legal implications and thus, make practical application essential.

5. Limitations

The limitations of this study can be categorized into a few areas. Despite a structured step-wise process, there remains subjectivity in decision-making application and the rationales for determinations. Others following a similar assessment may or may not have greater insight and exposure to the actions and therefore may conclude alternative findings compared to those found in this study. Second, there is an inherent lack of certainty in organizational assumptions based on cost-effectiveness information and actuarial analysis as to whether or not a specific practice brings greater benefits or burdens to a population. The authors propose the assessment in this study to be value-neutral but remains hypothetical, nonetheless. For example, many of these determinations were made under the assumption that both PBMs and plan sponsor organizations value efforts to lower the cost of health care delivery in the U.S. while maintaining profit expectations of both employees and investors. These assumed values are an area of ambiguity, differ between organizations, and may undergo fluctuation based on environmental factors in the marketplace. For example, exclusion lists were initially expected to decrease pharmaceutical expenditures by limiting market availability to drug manufactures. However, further market development revealed exclusion lists do not always produce decreased expenditures [15].

Additionally, fundamental assumptions were made of both PBMs and the closely linked organization of plan sponsors. A fundamental concept of PBM organizations is to increase purchasing power when negotiating with manufacturers to provide discounted drug pricing. This discount is passed to the plan sponsor via rebates. PBMs can, therefore, produce savings on behalf of the plan sponsor from these negotiated rebates. In theory, the plan sponsor uses the rebates to reduce the costs to all of the plan members. However, some PBMs have openly claimed all rebates are retained, with no distribution to plan members in any way [44] (p. 12). Rebates are assumed to be retrospectively applied to future pricing. However, it is possible that these rebates are not accounted for in pricing models. The potential for organizational variations must be considered when assessing the ethical nature of organizational practices [23]. Recent policy proposals in the U.S.'s Centers for Medicare and Medicaid Services (CMS) have furthered market uncertainty. Recent analyses have been unable to accurately predict potential financial outcomes of developed regulations due to irregular responses from manufacturers, plan sponsors, and PBMs [45]. However, supply chain transparency and point-of-sale rebates are considered market trends that could benefit the overall population.

6. Conclusions

This analysis fills a gap in the literature to use ethically-based frameworks to assess organizations involved in the high costs of pharmaceuticals. To the knowledge of the authors, an ethical perspective has not been previously applied to scrutinized organizational PBM practices. Theory-based ethical decision-making models provided a variety of perspectives that offer practical context to current dilemmas in health care. Depending on the applied model, the assessed scenarios resulted in a mix of ethical and unethical determinations. Despite variation across applied models, some practices were predominately ethical or unethical. Point of sale rebates were consistently determined as ethical, whereas market consolidation, gag clauses, and fluctuation of pharmacy reimbursements were all predominantly determined as unethical. The application using provider codes of ethics created additional and diverse comparison for the analysis. The codes of ethics were different in their overall assessment for ethical determination with the physician's code aligning more closely with values of societal benefit, whereas the pharmacist's code aligned more closely with patient-centric values.

This approach can be applied across many areas of health care as a mechanism allowing for the productive analysis and open-minded deliberations of health care issues. The systematic assessment of ethical dilemmas help guide providers towards grounds for concrete argumentation when applied with a fundamental understanding of involved stakeholders and realistic solutions. It remains imperative that health care professionals retain accountability towards addressing difficult ethical questions in practice. Moreover, given the potential moral distress encountered as professionals closely tied with both the clinical and fiduciary aspects of medication use, it is essential that pharmacists remain committed to ethical reasoning amidst a rapidly evolving pharmaceutical market.

Supplementary Materials: The following are available online at http://www.mdpi.com/2226-4787/7/2/65/s1, Table S1A: Utility Model, Table S1B: Exceptions Model, Table S1C: Choices Model, Table S1D: Justice Model, Table S1E: Common Good Model, Table S1F: Virtue Model, Table S2A: Pharmacist Code of Ethics (American Pharmacists Association), Table S2B: Physician Code of Ethics (American Medical Association).

Author Contributions: Conceptualization, J.J.D. and A.L.K.; methodology, A.L.K.; validation, J.J.D. and A.L.K.; formal analysis, J.J.D. and A.L.K.; investigation, J.J.D. Resources, J.J.D. and A.L.K.; data curation, J.J.D. and A.L.K. writing—original draft preparation, J.J.D.; writing—review and editing, J.J.D. and A.L.K.; visualization, J.J.D. and A.L.K.; supervision, A.L.K.; project administration, A.L.K.; funding acquisition, A.L.K.

Funding: This study was funded by Drake University College of Pharmacy and Health Sciences and the Harris Research Endowment.

Acknowledgments: The authors would like to express sincere gratitude to Erin Ulrich and Stacy Gnacinski for conceptualization support and their valuable insights on application of ethics in the health professions. This work was presented at the 18th Midwest Social and Administrative Pharmacy Conference, August 2018, in Madison, Wisconsin, USA. Finally, the authors are grateful to the reviewers for their constructive comments.

Conflicts of Interest: The authors declare no conflict of interest.

References

1. Kesselheim, A.S.; Avorn, J.; Sarpatwari, A. The High Cost of Prescription Drugs in the United States: Origins and Prospects for Reform. *JAMA* **2016**, *316*, 858–871. [CrossRef] [PubMed]

2. Califf, R.M.; Slavitt, A. Lowering Cost and Increasing Access to Drugs without Jeopardizing Innovation. *JAMA* **2019**, *321*, 1571–1573. [CrossRef] [PubMed]

3. De George, R.T. Intellectual property and pharmaceutical drugs: An ethical analysis. *Bus. Ethics Q.* **2005**, *15*, 549–575. [CrossRef] [PubMed]

4. Gaynor, M. Competition policy in health care markets: Navigating the enforcement and policy maze. *Health Aff.* **2014**, *33*, 1088–1093. [CrossRef] [PubMed]

5. Vogler, S.; Haasis, M.; Dedet, G.; Lam, J.; Pedersen, B.K.; World Health Organization. Medicines Reimbursement Policies in Europe. 2018. Available online: http://www.euro.who.int/__data/assets/pdf_file/0011/376625/pharmaceutical-reimbursement-eng.pdf?ua=1 (accessed on 6 June 2019).

6. Schulman, K.A.; Dabora, M. The relationship between pharmacy benefit managers (PBMs) and the cost of therapies in the US pharmaceutical market: A policy primer for clinicians. *Am. Heart J.* **2018**, *206*, 113–122. [CrossRef]

7. U.S. Senate Committee on Finance, Minority Staff. A Tangled Web. 2018. Available online: https://www.finance.senate.gov/imo/media/doc/A%20Tangled%20Web.pdf (accessed on 31 May 2019).

8. Seeley, E.; Kesselheilm, A.S.; Commonwealth Fund. Pharmacy Benefit Managers: Practices, Controversies, and What Lies Ahead. 2019. Available online: https://www.commonwealthfund.org/publications/issue-briefs/2019/mar/pharmacy-benefit-managers-practices-controversies-what-lies-ahead (accessed on 31 May 2019).

9. Carter, E.L. PBM Practices Drive Up Costs for Rx Drugs. *Wall Street Journal*. 24 February 2019, p. A.16. Available online: https://www.wsj.com/articles/pbm-practices-drive-up-costs-for-rx-drugs-11551039255?mod=searchresults&page=2&pos=2 (accessed on 24 April 2019).

10. Schneider, C. Legislation makes drug costs more transparent. *Des Moines Register* **2019**, X.6. Available online: https://www.desmoinesregister.com/story/news/local/community/2019/04/13/charles-schneider-legislation-makes-drug-costs-more-transparent/3451783002/ (accessed on 24 April 2019).

11. U.S. Department o Health and Human Services, Assistant Secretary for Public Affairs (ASPA). Trump Administration Proposes to Lower Drug Costs by Targeting Backdoor Rebates and Encouraging Direct Discounts to Patients. 2019. Available online: https://www.hhs.gov/about/news/2019/01/31/trump-administration-proposes-to-lower-drug-costs-by-targeting-backdoor-rebates-and-encouraging-direct-discounts-to-patients.html (accessed on 17 May 2019).

12. Werble, C. Health Policy Brief: Pharmacy Benefit Managers. *Health Aff.* **2017**. Available online: https://www.healthaffairs.org/do/10.1377/hpb20171409.000178/full/ (accessed on 13 June 2019).

13. Dusetzina, S.B.; Bach, P.B. Prescription Drugs—List Price, Net Price, and the Rebate Caught in the Middle. *JAMA* **2019**, *321*, 1563–1564. [CrossRef]

14. U.S. Department of Health and Human Services. American Patients First: The Trump Administration Blueprint to Lower Drug Prices and Reduce Out-of-Pocket Costs. 2018. Available online: https://www.hhs.gov/sites/default/files/AmericanPatientsFirst.pdf (accessed on 20 May 2019).

15. Cohen, J.P.; Khoury, C.E.; Milne, C.; Peters, S.M. Rising Drug Costs Drives the Growth of Pharmacy Benefit Managers Exclusion Lists: Are Exclusion Decisions Value-Based? *Health Serv. Res.* **2017**, *53*, 2758–2769. [CrossRef]

16. National Academy for State Health Policy. State Health Policy Blog, State Legislation that Bans Pharmacy Benefit Managers' "Gag Clauses.". 2018. Available online: https://nashp.org/trending-now-state-legislation-that-bans-pharmacy-benefit-managers-gag-clauses/ (accessed on 24 April 2019).

17. Gabay, M. Direct and Indirect Remuneration Fees: The Controversy Continues. *Hosp. Pharm.* **2017**, *52*, 740–741. [CrossRef]

18. Express Scripts. Cross-Industry Partnership Reduces the Cost of Popular Diabetes, Asthma and Other Brand Name Drugs. 2017. Available online: https://www.prnewswire.com/news-releases/cross-industry-partnership-reduces-the-cost-of-popular-diabetes-asthma-and-other-brand-name-drugs-300453059.html (accessed on 24 April 2019).

19. Parker-Lue, S.; Santoro, M.; Koski, G. The Ethics and Economics of Pharmaceutical Pricing. *Annu. Rev. Pharmacol. Toxicol.* **2015**, *55*, 191–206. [CrossRef] [PubMed]

20. Millonig, M.K.; Wolters Kluwer. Financial Strain Leads to Pharmacy Closures, and That Leads to Medication Nonadherence. 2019. Available online: https://www.wolterskluwercdi.com/blog/pharmacy-closures-nonadherence/ (accessed on 31 May 2019).

21. Spinello, R. Ethics, pricing and the pharmaceutical industry. *J. Bus. Ethics* **1992**, *11*, 617–626. [CrossRef]

22. National Community Pharmacy Association. Pharmacy Associations Urge Senate Judiciary Committee to Hold Hearing on PBMs. 2018. Available online: https://www.ncpanet.org/newsroom/news-releases/2018/04/09/pharmacy-associations-urge-senate-judiciary-committee-to-hold-hearing-on-pbms (accessed on 27 April 2019).

23. Lyles, A. Pharmacy Benefit Management Companies: Do They Create Value in the US Healthcare System? *Pharmacoeconomics* **2017**, *35*, 493–500. [CrossRef]

24. Danzon, P.M. Pharmacy Benefit Management: Are Reporting Requirements Pro- or Anticompetitive? *Int. J. Econ. Bus.* **2015**, *22*, 245–261. [CrossRef]

25. Veatch, R.M.; Haddah, A. *Case Studies in Pharmacy Ethics*; Oxford University Press: New York, NY, USA, 1999; pp. 3–15.

26. Dahnke, M.D. Utilizing codes of ethics in health professions education. *Adv. Health Sci. Educ.* **2014**, *19*, 611–623. [CrossRef] [PubMed]

27. Buerki, R.A.; Vottero, L.D. *Pharmacy Ethics: A Foundation for Professional Practice*; American Pharmacists Association: Washington, DC, USA, 2013.

28. Breen, G.M.; Littleton, V.; Loyal, M.; Meemon, N.; Paek, S.C.; Seblega, B. An ethical analysis of professional codes in health and medical care. *Ethics Med.* **2010**, *26*, 25–48.

29. Howe, E.G. How Should Physicians Respond When the Best Treatment for an Individual Patient Conflicts with Practice Guidelines about the Use of a Limited Resource? *AMA J. Ethics* **2017**, *19*, 550–557. [PubMed]

30. Cole, T.R.; Carlin, N. The suffering of physicians. *Lancet* **2009**, *374*, 1414–1415. [CrossRef]

31. Talbot, S.G.; Dean, W. Physicians aren't 'Burning Out'. They're Suffering from Moral Injury. *STAT*. 26 July 2018. Available online: https://www.statnews.com/2018/07/26/physicians-not-burning-out-they-are-suffering-moral-injury/ (accessed on 25 April 2019).

32. Fox, R.C. Is Medical Education Asking Too Much of Bioethics? *Daedalus* **1999**, *128*, 1–25.

33. Bean, S. Navigating the murky intersection between clinical and organizational ethics: A hybrid case taxonomy. *Bioethics* **2011**, *25*, 320–325. [CrossRef]

34. Wingfield, J.; Bissell, P.; Anderson, C. The Scope of pharmacy ethics—An evaluation of the international research literature, 1990–2002. *Soc. Sci. Med.* **2004**, *58*, 2383–2396. [CrossRef]

35. Chiarello, E. How organizational context affects bioethical decision-making: Pharmacists' management of gatekeeping processes in retail and hospital settings. *Soc. Sci. Med.* **2013**, *98*, 319–329. [CrossRef]

36. Vuković Rodríguez, J.; Juričić, Ž. Perceptions and attitudes of community pharmacists toward professional ethics and ethical dilemmas in the workplace. *Res. Soc. Adm. Pharm.* **2018**, *14*, 441–450. [CrossRef]
37. Beauchamp, T.L. *Principles of Biomedical Ethics*, 5th ed.; Oxford University Press: New York, NY, USA, 2001.
38. Cooper, R.J.; Bissell, P.; Wingfield, J. A new prescription for empirical ethics research in pharmacy: A critical review of the literature. *J. Med. Ethics* **2007**, *33*, 82–86. [CrossRef]
39. Cooper, R.J.; Bissell, P.; Wingfield, J. Ethical decision- making, passivity and pharmacy. *J. Med. Ethics* **2008**, *34*, 441–445. [CrossRef]
40. Hammaker, D.K.; Knadig, T.M.; Tomlinson, S.J. *Health Care Ethics and the Law*; Jones & Bartlett Learning: Burlington, MA, USA, 2017.
41. American Pharmacists Association. Code of Ethics. 1994. Available online: https://www.pharmacist.com/code-ethics (accessed on 24 April 2019).
42. American Medical Association. Code of Medical Ethics Overview. Available online: https://www.ama-assn.org/delivering-care/ethics/code-medical-ethics-overview (accessed on 24 April 2019).
43. Minemyer, P.; Fierce Healthcare. UnitedHealth to Expand Use of Point-of-Sale Drug Discounts. 2019. Available online: https://www.fiercehealthcare.com/payer/unitedhealth-to-further-expand-use-point-sale-drug-discounts (accessed on 24 April 2019).
44. Wellmark Health Plan of Iowa Inc. Group Insurance Policy. 2017. Available online: http://www.lemars.k12.ia.us/wp-content/uploads/2018/07/10-17-IA-WHPI-L-SG-FI-SS-101-Print-Master.pdf (accessed on 25 April 2019).
45. Sachs, R. Trump Administration Releases Long-Awaited Drug Rebate Proposal. *Health Aff.* **2019**. Available online: https://www.healthaffairs.org/do/10.1377/ (accessed on 13 June 2019).

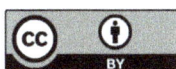

pharmacy

MDPI

Article

Opportunities for Outpatient Pharmacy Services for Patients with Cystic Fibrosis: Perceptions of Healthcare Team Members

Olufunmilola Abraham * [ID] **and Ashley Morris**

Social and Administrative Sciences Division, University of Wisconsin-Madison School of Pharmacy, Madison, WI 53705, USA; amorris4@wisc.edu
* Correspondence: olufunmilola.abraham@wisc.edu; Tel.: +1-(608)-263-4498

Received: 27 February 2019; Accepted: 27 March 2019; Published: 3 April 2019

check for
updates

Abstract: Cystic fibrosis (CF) is one of the most common life-threatening, genetic conditions. People with CF follow complex, time-consuming treatment regimens to manage their chronic condition. Due to the complexity of the disease, multidisciplinary care from CF Foundation (CFF)-accredited centers is recommended for people with CF. These centers include several types of healthcare professionals specializing in CF; however, pharmacists are not required members. The purpose of this study was to identify the outpatient care needs of people living with CF that pharmacists could address to improve their quality of care. Healthcare members from a CFF accredited center and pharmacists were recruited to participate in semi-structured, audio-recorded interviews. Prevalent codes were identified and data analysis was conducted, guided by the systems engineering initiative for patient safety (SEIPS) model. The objective was to understand the medication and pharmacy-related needs of patients with CF and care team perspectives on pharmacists providing support for these patients. From the themes that emerged, pharmacists can provide support for people living with CF (medication burden, medication access, medication education) and the CF care team (drug monitoring and adherence, prior authorizations and insurance coverage, refill history). Pharmacists are well-positioned to address these difficulties to improve quality of care for people living with cystic fibrosis.

Keywords: cystic fibrosis; pharmacists; pharmacy services, medication management; medication use burden

1. Introduction

Cystic fibrosis (CF) is one of the most prevalent chronic and fatal genetic diseases, affecting approximately 70,000 people worldwide and 30,000 in the United States alone [1,2]. CF is a progressive, multisystem disease that primarily affects the respiratory and digestive systems as well as the pancreas, liver, and reproductive system [1]. CF is an incurable autosomal recessive disorder caused by mutations in the CF transmembrane conductance regulator (CFTR) [3]. The CFTR transports chloride and sodium ions in and out of epithelial cells which controls the movement of water in tissues of the body [4]. Mutations in the CFTR cause thick secretions of mucus to line several organs in the body such as the lungs, pancreas, digestive system, and reproductive system [4]. Consequently, the thick mucus production puts patients with CF at risk of developing bacterial infections in the lungs [1]. Although advances in treatment and knowledge of CF have extended the median predicted survival age to 47.7 years for individuals born in 2016 (compared to age 42.7 years for those born between 2012 and 2016), patients manage complex, time-consuming, and lifelong treatment regimens [1,5].

Medication management with CF is challenging and burdensome. Patients often use eight or more medications daily with lengthy treatments, such as inhaled antibiotics, that can range 1–3 h each day [1]. CF medications include CFTR modulators, mucus thinners, bronchodilators, antibiotics, anti-inflammatories, and pancreatic enzymes [6]. Patients with CF also need to perform airway clearance techniques which may include the use of a vest and nebulizer treatments [6]. Vest treatment is a high-frequency chest wall compression therapy that loosens mucus in the lungs and can be performed in 30-min sessions two to four times per day. Treatment of comorbidities such as depression, anxiety, and diabetes further complicate CF management [4]. Consequently, CF medication adherence can be as low as 50%, particularly among children and adolescents [1,7]. Poor adherence can lead to negative health outcomes such as exacerbations, hospitalizations, and increased healthcare costs [7].

The complexity of managing CF warrants a multidisciplinary healthcare team. The CF Foundation (CFF) recommends that patients visit accredited centers with specialized healthcare professionals at least four times annually [8]. The CFF requires accredited centers to include healthcare team members such as physicians, nurses, respiratory therapists, dietitians, social workers, and program coordinators [9]. Pharmacists are only listed as recommended healthcare team members [9]. However, CF standards of care in countries such as Australia and Britain consider pharmacists to be vital healthcare team members [10–13]. There has been limited research exploring how pharmacists in outpatient settings can support people living with CF, which is a missed opportunity to improve the care of these patients. There is an urgent need to increase access to pharmacist-provided outpatient care for people with CF to improve their treatment adherence, medication self-management, and overall health-related quality of life. This study aims to describe works system characteristics for the pharmacists' role in caring for patients with cystic fibrosis.

2. Materials and Methods

2.1. Theoretical Framework

The systems engineering initiative for patient safety (SEIPS) 2.0 Model was applied to guide our understanding of medication management and interactions between pharmacists and other members of CF healthcare team [14]. The SEIPS model is the most widely used systems engineering framework for patient and healthcare research and embraces three important principles: (1) A holistic systems-based approach, (2) person-centeredness, and (3) design-driven improvement needs to be person-centered to enhance and improve outcomes. The framework proposes the following components of the work system: Person, organization, tools and technology, environment, and tasks. To explore a collaborative process in which patients, pharmacists, and other members of the CF healthcare team can actively engage in medication discussions, it is necessary to understand the activities (or "work") that each of these individuals carries out with regard to CF medications.

In the SEIPS framework, person(s) are professional or non-professional individuals and characteristics of those individuals, like age and expertise. Tasks are specific actions within larger work processes, with characteristics such as difficulty, complexity, variety, ambiguity, and sequence. Organizations, in the SEIPS framework, are thought of as structures external to a person put in place by people that organize time, space, resources, and activity. Tools and technologies are objects that people use to do work or that assist people in doing work, and is described by usability, accessibility, familiarity, etc. The SEIPS framework separates environment into two factors: The internal environment (the physical environment—lighting, noise, temperature, etc.,) and the external environment, which are economic, ecological, and policy factors outside an organization.

2.2. Setting, Sample, and Recruitment

CF healthcare team member participants were recruited from a CFF-accredited center in an urban city hospital in Western Pennsylvania. Pharmacists were purposefully recruited from independent, inpatient, outpatient, and small-chain pharmacies in an urban city in Western Pennsylvania. The research team worked with the center director to identify study participants. CF healthcare member participants declined compensation and pharmacist participants received a $50 incentive. Verbal consent was obtained from study participants. This study was approved by the University of Pittsburgh Institutional Review Board.

2.3. Data Collection

We conducted key informant interviews with stakeholders integral to the CF medication management process. The research team developed semi-structured interview guides using open-ended questions to understand the medication and pharmacy-related issues for people living with CF. Two members of the research team assessed the interview guides and provided feedback to ensure content validity. Appendix A contains the guides used to conduct study interviews with pharmacists and other healthcare team members (such as physicians, nurses, dieticians). A research assistant conducted 20-min, in-person, and audio-recorded interviews with study participants from July to September 2016. Participant demographic characteristics such as age, sex, ethnicity, and race were collected. Interviews were conducted until data saturation was achieved. All interviews were professionally transcribed verbatim. To ensure study rigor and trustworthiness, pilot-tested interview guides were used, and reflective journaling and peer debriefing were completed after each interview.

2.4. Data Analysis

The research team reviewed the transcripts for accuracy. Interview transcripts were analyzed to develop a list of codes that represented the main conceptual categories within the data. An initial draft of the codebook was developed by members of the research team. The codebook was later simplified and refined based on the results of the first two rounds of coding. Coding was carried out using NVivo10 (QSR International, Melbourne, Australia), a qualitative data analysis software program that enables multi-coder projects. Interviews were coded by at least one of the coders, with the two coders overlapping on 12 of the interviews. Disagreements in coding were adjudicated jointly by the principal investigator and coders. The interview transcripts were coded to identify prevalent themes. Bi-weekly coding meetings were held to review all codes and resolve any discrepancies. Two coders coded the interviews to ensure interrater reliability and had an average Kappa score of 0.60. After the initial coding process, AM conducted deductive content analysis using the categories described in the work system components of the SEIPS 2.0 theoretical framework. Interview transcripts were reviewed using the SEIPS 2.0 Model by searching for key words, such as "pharmacist", "benefit", "patient", "medication", or "management". Responses were classified according to the corresponding work system components of the SEIPS 2.0 model. Within those components, similar topics and ideas were aggregated into constructs. OA reviewed the application of the SEIPS 2.0 model to the data to validate the coding. Any discrepancies or differences in opinion were resolved and consensus was researched before final results were obtained.

3. Results

A total of 22 participants were interviewed, including 8 pharmacists, 6 pulmonologists, 6 nurses, and 2 dietitians. Of the 22 participants, 12 (55%) were female, 12 (55%) were aged 50 years or older, 21 (95%) were non-Hispanic and White, 7 (32%) had worked 0–10 years, and 7 (32%) had worked 21–30 years (Table 1). The predominant themes that emerged from this study are discussed within each of the work system components of the SEIPS 2.0 model [14]. Additional verbatim quotes from study participants which elaborate on each construct beyond what is provided in the results section is available in Appendix B.

Table 1. Participant Demographics (n = 22).

Characteristics	No. (%) [1] n = 22
Gender	
Women	12 (55)
Men	10 (45)
Age	
<30 years	3 (14 1)
30–49 years	7 (32 1)
≥50 years	12 (55 1)
Race	
White/Caucasian, Non-Hispanic	21 (95)
White, Hispanic	1 (5)
Role	
Nurse	6 (27 1)
Pulmonologist	6 (27 1)
Registered Dietician	2 (9 1)
Pharmacist	8 (36 1)
Years Worked	
0–10 years	7 (32)
11–20 years	4 (18)
21–30 years	7 (32)
30+ years	4 (18)

[1] Because of rounding, percentage may not total 100.

3.1. Person

Most members of the CF healthcare team have thorough experience working with people with CF. Pharmacists have variable levels of expertise in CF and in providing services for people with CF. There is also variation in the setting in which these pharmacists had experience providing service to people with CF.

Experience and Expertise Caring for People with CF

Pharmacists experience with CF varied: Two pharmacists described providing pharmacy services to only one to two patients with CF, while three pharmacists reported working with patients with CF for many years. As pharmacists' experience working with CF varied, so did their understanding of the disease. All pharmacists understood healthcare services for patients with CF to be complex, robust, and requiring of multidisciplinary care, no matter the amount of experience they reported.

> *"I've dealt with [CF] for like 30 years ... From the medication standpoint I think I know pretty much a lot of what their needs are, for the medications they need, and also the insurance coverage and everything that I try to do."—Pharmacist 8*

3.2. Tasks

Tasks that participants identified for pharmacists to perform include medication management, medication education, and medication access.

3.2.1. Medication Management Burden

Any tasks that must be done by patients, members of the CF care team, or pharmacists to maintain patient compliance to their individual medication regimen or treatment plan are considered in medication management. All members of the healthcare team and most pharmacists identified a high treatment burden in people with CF, describing medication management as complex, time-demanding, confusing, and difficult for the patients in their care. Nurses and pharmacists described additional medication management burden for the pediatric CF population.

> *"I think adherence, treatment burden. I mean, our patients can have like an hour and a half of inhale antibiotics twice to three times a day. Plus, enzymes with each meal and every snack."—Nurse 1*

> *"I think a lot of them struggle because they have so many meds to take. I think sometimes it can be difficult for them to necessarily be motivated to take all their medications."—Dietician 1*

3.2.2. Medication Education

All healthcare professionals rely on and advocate for verbal education between a patient with CF and each member of the care team. Pharmacists highlight the importance of specialized, one-on-one counseling, but the frequency by which they believe this counseling should occur and the topics that should be covered by pharmacists varied. Physicians verbally educate people with CF, but primarily rely on nurse educators to supplement initial educational conversations. Nurses educate verbally and provide written materials for people with CF, but describe CF education as a team effort, including dieticians and respiratory therapists as educators. Nurse educators do not rely on community pharmacist involvement to educate patients with CF on their medicines. Members of the existing CF healthcare team highlighted additional educational efforts that needed to be in place for transition from child to adult care.

> *"great benefit comes from one on one counseling. We will, as pharmacists here, we will actually get to a patient's home, counsel them on how to actually use their medication."—Pharmacist 3*

> *"we, the [doctors] may introduce the medication to the patient … but then that gets followed up by our nurse educators … I think they sort of try to reinforce our initial educational efforts."—Physician 3*

Many physicians stated they were aware that patients and their families want to hear information from the doctor, not other members of the healthcare team. Nurses also felt that patients wanted to hear information from the physician.

> *"Parents and patients—I think, want to hear it from the doc, but I think giving them a different perspective from somebody else has some real power."—Physician 2*

There was unanimous agreement amongst the healthcare providers that verbal counseling should be supplemented by additional education materials. There was a split opinion about the effectiveness of this material, as this content was currently offered as written paper pamphlets. Dieticians also employ pre- and post-testing material during verbal counseling.

> *"I think that combined with some of the technology and certainly as I said, the handouts, the pamphlets, paperwork, things like that. Something tangible."—Pharmacist 5*

> *"I think most of the pamphlets go in the garbage."—Nurse 5*

3.2.3. Medication Access and Insurance Challenges

All healthcare professionals discussed the challenges people with CF face regarding insurance. Prior authorizations were described as a major challenge by the healthcare team, and nurses and pharmacists identified this was something in which pharmacist could assist.

> *"definitely access. A lot of the times, patients struggle with getting prior authorization or letters of medical necessity, which oftentimes can delay therapy. Or even maybe as simple as their insurance will only cover the medication if it's coming from a specialty pharmacy"—Pharmacist 1*

"If we could get more of a pharmacist, we would ... I would love for some of the higher-level prior authorizations to be taken over, too, by the pharmacist."—Nurse 2

Physicians and nurses also discussed financial burden for people with CF because of the high cost of medications. Pharmacists also identified medication access challenges regarding the need for one patient with CF to rely on multiple pharmacies (including specialty pharmacy) to obtain all their medications.

"I think they have challenges in terms of expense, they have challenges in terms of getting them through their insurance, and they have challenges just keeping up with the compliance intake."—Physician 6

3.3. Organization

The organizational impact on pharmacist involvement in the CF care team was highlighted by study participants.

3.3.1. Awareness of Pharmacy Services

Physicians unanimously reported that they rarely interacted with community pharmacies, and many physicians identified that nurses were the primary point of contact with pharmacists. Most nurses reported they communicate with outpatient pharmacies daily via telephone conversations. Dieticians also report working with pharmacists daily, primarily to overcome insurance barriers.

"I don't always necessarily think their knowledge of CF is as vast as it could be, I mean I know it's a very specialized disease. But most of the time, if you provide them with an explanation, they're willing to work with you ... I'd say I deal with them pretty regularly though. Daily."—Dietician 1

Existing communication between the CF care team and pharmacists was described as minimal by physicians. The healthcare team members had some ideas by which this communication could be improved, such as including pharmacists on rounds.

"It isn't much. I mean, I'm not going to be judgmental and say the communication is poor. I would just say that there tends not to be much."—Physician 5

"I think it's not even the pharmacists that we need to improve communication with, but the layers that exist before the pharmacist ... when you finally get to that pharmacist, they understand, they know what you're talking about and it's a little easier."—Nurse 4

3.3.2. Benefits and Drawbacks of Pharmacist Involvement

Pharmacists identified several areas in which they could be helpful, including medication education and discharge counseling, relieving other care team members' workload by handling drug-related issues, and providing private counseling in community pharmacies to improve adherence.

"we can provide a different aspect of monitoring care that the physicians then don't need to do. So all the drug level monitoring, some of the compliance monitoring, some of trying to figure out how to make things taste better, or how to fit them down a G-tube, or how to avoid drug interactions by spacing certain meds away from each other."—Pharmacist 6

"I think the most important benefit is—would be number one, education."—Pharmacist 3

The healthcare team members identified several ways in which pharmacists could contribute to overall care for patients with CF, including insurance coverage and drug acquisition, refill history, medication safety, and patient education.

"It would be particularly useful if there were pharmacists always available who could be doing the tracking and the, making sure that the flow of medications continues through the paperwork and other hurdles."—Physician 6

"As the medication regimens are getting more and more complex, we need the expertise of a pharmacist to help do some of those higher prior authorizations that require a little more knowledge and data to defend"—Nurse 3

Pharmacists anticipated only a few drawbacks of being a member of the healthcare team that cares for people with CF. The primary concern discussed by several pharmacists was care coordination and the increased complexity required to uphold good communication practices between the care team. Pharmacists also mentioned increased costs for the healthcare system, as pharmacists were not included in the hospital's existing financial model.

"I think bringing all parties together so that we're all working cohesively is probably the biggest challenge."—Pharmacist 4

"If you don't have robust communication with the nursing staff as well as the physician or collaboration between the three of them, then that can create a serious issue ... "—Pharmacist 3

"So not any drawbacks that I can think of other than, possibly, I guess, increased cost of the health care system. But in the hopes of the program, or the hopes of the CF pharmacist is to reduce costs elsewhere."—Pharmacist 1

Members of the CF care team also identified increased financial burden on the hospital to support pharmacists providing care but were primarily concerned with patients feeling overwhelmed by having to visit with another member of the healthcare team. The care team was also concerned that community pharmacists' knowledge about CF may be limited to properly support people with CF.

"Our patients meet with four or five team members in every visit, so inserting yet another person that extends their hours long visit, they just might get tired of seeing so many people."—Physician 6

"The barriers will include, education. Not every pharmacist is trained in CF ... and so, there's issues around patient populations, and disease frequency"—Physician 5

"Predominantly money ... Resources, limited resources! Space and money. Yeah, and time"—Nurse 3

3.4. Tools and Technologies

Participants discussed the potential for a mobile application to be used as a tool to improve medication adherence for people with CF. Pharmacists also identified the use of social media as a tool to communicate with people with CF.

Technologies That Influence Adherence and Prescribing

All healthcare professionals perceived benefit to offering a mobile application for use by people with CF, though there were differing opinions about the content and purpose of the app. In general, pharmacists described the app as a tool to support existing medication management techniques. Physicians thought an app could be helpful for self-management or compliance.

"I always feel that some sort of knowledge center with that has a wealth of videos, a video library that would be able to, number one show people how to use their medication. Number two, go through the clinical aspects of the medication. Side effects, storage, and stability."—Pharmacist 3

"I think it could be very helpful for, perhaps, keeping them on track for when they're supposed to take them ... as a reminder function, I think it could be very valuable."—Physician 3

"We've had different nutrition apps and we've asked people to go home and look at things and that doesn't really happen."—Dietician 1

There were some concerns to offering a mobile application, including effectiveness of a mobile app as an educational tool, and how the app could be safely offered in clinic, using a communal device.

"Well, in the clinic setting that's hard to do on a pad because it has to be sterilized between patients. And so, we think it's easier to hand out papers."—Nurse 2

"In terms of whether they would take the time to actually learn the details of the medicines through an app, I'm a little skeptical but it might work."—Physician 6

Participants were also concerned that a mobile application may not be appropriate for all ages of people with CF. Pharmacists believe medication education is only successful if patients were reached in their environment, providing education through blog posts or social media, or preparing them to explain CF in their own way.

"I think that is targeted—it would definitely be for adolescents, and not necessarily our older patients."—Physician 4

"I mean if I'm looking at how old the average patient is, you know, we gotta look where they are. So you would use the data to suggest, 'Hey they're probably on Facebook' . . . you scroll and you're watching and it's like, everything is in a video. It's all video digesting content."—Pharmacist 2

In terms of other medication adherence tools, there was interest among physicians to implement compliance-tracking devices to install on the patient's vest.

"We are now instituting a way of determining whether patients are using their vest. There are some devices that you can plug the vest into, and so you can tell from the electrical current use whether the device has been turned on or not."—Physician 5

3.5. Environment

Participants solely discussed external environment factors, including collaborative practice agreements for pharmacists and issues with care team access to complete refill histories.

3.5.1. Collaborative Practice Agreements

Pharmacist participants advocated for their CF care team involvement as decision-makers through collaborative practice agreements. Pharmacists had several ideas about what the partnership between pharmacists and other healthcare professionals could look like, and identified many reasons this would be beneficial to improve health care for people with CF.

"I think that pharmacists have an opportunity to even go further and be—take part in collaborative practice agreements . . . where pharmacists could change the therapy without having direct physician oversight."—Pharmacist 1

"We would be a physician extender. So the physician is billing for the services that the pharmacist provides . . . we touch these patients multiple times a month."—Pharmacist 2

3.5.2. Refill History Access

All members of the CF care team rely on refill and dispense histories as their primary method to tracking medication adherence, and supplement refill history knowledge by discussing medication adherence with the patient. Physicians also evaluated lung function tests to supplement refill history and improve their understanding of patient compliance.

"No, not one particular method ... you often can tell by their nonverbals, by the look on their face when you ask them a question ... and we have patient fill histories that we can look at."—Nurse 3

"I always discuss it with the patient to see what barriers there are between them adhering to the medication and non-adherence ... I think it's very individual."—Dietician 1

4. Discussion

Despite the benefits that inpatient pharmacists have made in the care of patients with CF, pharmacists are not required members of the healthcare team at CFF-accredited centers [15–17]. The perceptions of CF care team participants about where pharmacists could contribute were reported within the components of the SEIPS model (person, tasks, organization, tools and technologies, and environment) [14]. This study identified specific opportunities for pharmacists to assist with medication challenges experienced by people living with CF, including poor medication adherence, medication counseling, and limited medication access because of barriers such as prior authorizations or insurance coverage. Though pharmacists can provide benefit to CF patient care, members of the CF care team may not fully appreciate the value and contributions pharmacists can provide. Establishing a team of pharmacists with advanced CF expertise may improve care coordination with the CF care team and eliminate some of the issues people with CF face regarding medication management and treatment burden.

Medication adherence due to high medication burden is a serious concern for all members of the CF care team. Study findings identified several medication challenges for people with CF, with the CF care team and pharmacists describing treatment management as burdensome, time-consuming, and complex. The typical medication regimen requires multiple medications in different forms (i.e., inhaled, oral, intravenous) to be taken two to three times each day [1,4,6]. Consequently, medication adherence can be difficult, which has been shown in other studies [1,7]. A recent study found that recognizing the importance of CF medications is a predominant barrier to patient adherence to treatment regimens [18]. The pediatric and adolescent population is especially vulnerable. Previous research has shown that adolescents with CF in particular have low adherence rates which can be attributed to forgetfulness, being too busy, feeling that treatments give them less freedom, and believing that skipping treatment is acceptable [19,20]. To monitor adherence, members of the CF care team frequently consult a patient's medication refill history, a log that community pharmacists are responsible for maintaining. Results show the CF care team is aware of pharmacist involvement in refill history maintenance.

Further complicating medication adherence, medication access is a significant issue experienced by people with CF; study findings show members of the CF care team are burdened by tasks to improve access for patients in their care. Some insurance providers will only cover medications from specialty pharmacies, which do not always stock CF medications. Insurance companies may also only cover specific medications causing patients with CF to not receive the medications they were prescribed. In addition, medication cost was an identified concern. Participants stated that some CF medications from specialty pharmacies cost thousands of dollars and even those covered by insurance have high copays. The high cost of these medications (i.e., Orkambi®, Kalydeco®) limits access to patients with CF [21]. In handling medication access challenges, study participants explained that issues with prior authorizations were time consuming and caused delays in patients receiving their CF medications. A previous study found that insurance prominently impacts the health of patients with CF, where patients who had Medicaid or public insurance had a higher risk of death while waiting for a lung transplant than those who had private or Medicare insurance [22]. A previous study shows pharmacists are well-positioned to address prior authorization and insurance coverage challenges that burden existing CF care team workload [23]. Study findings show the CF care team identified pharmacist assistance with this task as a perceived benefit to the organization.

The study identified challenges in care coordination and transitions of care for patients with CF. Pharmacist participants revealed that they are often not included by other healthcare members in the care of patients with CF even though they see the patients more frequently. The coordination of care is often difficult due to the many pharmacies that patients with CF use for their medications. CF care team participants reported they do not expect community pharmacists to have the level of expertise required to properly educate people with CF, knowing that many community pharmacists have little contact or opportunity to experience providing care for a patient with CF. This suggests a community pharmacist's level of expertise and interaction with nurses and dieticians impacts CF care team awareness of pharmacy services they can provide. Consequently, as shown in a previous study, medication reconciliation needs to be prioritized [24]. Pharmacists are easily accessible medication experts that can provide clinical services to people with chronic conditions such as CF more frequently than other healthcare professionals [25–27].

Pharmacists are in the community and can provide counseling and education to people living with CF about their medications or address any barriers. Previous research has shown that pharmacists involved in CF care have provided patient education on medications and treatment management, monitored drug-drug interactions, and detected appropriate medication dosing [15]. Other benefits of pharmacists included in CF care in the inpatient setting include improving medication monitoring, communication with the multidisciplinary healthcare team, and efficient use of resources when caring for patients [16,17]. Due to the complexity of CF treatment regimens, participants recommended that it would be beneficial for the pharmacist to create medication schedules for patients with CF to avoid drug interactions. Participants also stated that pharmacists could assess adherence in people with CF by reviewing their medication list and addressing any issues that arise. In addition, participants recommended that pharmacists address insurance issues encountered by patients with CF. Outpatient pharmacists within CFF-accredited centers will be well-positioned to assist patients to navigate insurance issues with prior authorizations, medication access, and cost. Consequently, this would relieve the burden from the healthcare members at the CFF accredited center and patients with CF. Pharmacists can also provide medication education to CF patients. Results from this study suggest that CF patients prefer online learning materials or interactive technology such as tablets or mobile applications. Previous studies have used smartphone applications and telehealth to improve adherence in patients with CF and were shown to be feasible and acceptable [28,29]. Consequently, innovative methods using technology should be implemented to deliver education to patients with CF.

Limitations

Healthcare members were recruited from one CFF-accredited center, so the results may not generalizable to all regions. Pharmacists who were knowledgeable about CF were also recruited to participate in interviews which creates selection bias and cannot be generalizable to all pharmacists.

5. Conclusions

People living with CF experience many medication and pharmacy-related challenges such as high medication burden, medication access, cost, insurance coverage, and care coordination. Although pharmacists are not required members of the healthcare team for CFF accredited centers, this study identified many benefits of having outpatient pharmacists support patients with CF. Pharmacists can help relieve the medication burden for patients with CF by creating schedules that avoid drug interactions. Additionally, pharmacists can assist with assessing drug monitoring and adherence, and assist with insurance issues.

Author Contributions: Conceptualization, O.A.; methodology, O.A.; validation, O.A.; formal analysis, O.A. and A.M.; investigation, O.A.; resources, O.A.; data curation, O.A.; writing—original draft preparation, O.A. and A.M.; writing—review and editing, O.A. and A.M.; visualization, O.A.; supervision, O.A.; project administration, O.A.

Funding: This research received no external funding.

Acknowledgments: Daniel Weiner for helping to facilitate data collection and Alison Feathers for assisting in data collection and analysis.

Conflicts of Interest: The authors declare no conflict of interest.

Appendix A

Appendix A.1 Pharmacist Interview Guide

A. Introductory Questions about Cystic Fibrosis (CF)

1. Can you describe what do you know about CF?
2. What do you know about the healthcare services needed for patients with CF?
3. Have you had experiences providing pharmacy services for patients with CF?

   If Yes:

   a. Please describe the pharmacy services that were provided.
   b. Were there specific medication use challenges that these patients experienced?
   c. Were there specific pharmacy-related problems they experienced? (i.e., access to medication, insurance, etc.)
   d. Were these able to be addressed?

   If No:

   a. Describe the pharmacy-related needs or problems of CF patients. (May probe for issues related to access to medications, insurance issues, etc.)
   b. What recommendations do you have for addressing these pharmacy-related issues?

4. What do you think are the benefits or drawbacks of pharmacist involvement in the care of patients with CF?
5. Can you describe how pharmacists could potentially partner with other healthcare professionals to improve care for patients with CF?

B. Support for People Living with CF
We would like to know more about how pharmacists can support people living with CF.

1. From your experience, what common difficulties do patients have when taking medications for chronic conditions?
2. Can you describe possible ways pharmacists could assist patients with CF?
   (How do you think pharmacists could be equipped to support patients with CF?)

   a. Do you think pharmacists can support people living with CF? If so, how?
   In what ways can community pharmacists uniquely support people with CF?

C. Preferences for Medication Education
We would like to know more about how you think people living with CF should be educated about their medications.

1. How do you think a patient using medication for CF should be educated on his/her condition and medication regimen?

   a. How often do you think a patient using medication for CF should be educated about taking his/her medications correctly?

2. If you have provided medication education for patients with CF, what types of educational materials have you used?
   If No: What types of education materials have you used with patients with other types of chronic conditions?

3. What types of education materials do you think would be most helpful for providing medication education for patients with CF?
4. Assuming patients want information about their medications, how do you think patients prefer to receive education about their medications?
   Probe for different educational methods (one-on-one counseling with the pharmacist, written materials/pamphlets, interactive technology like on an iPad, videos on the Internet or TV, using an app on a smartphone or tablet)
5. Do you think patients with CF would be interested in using an app, like on a smartphone or tablet, to learn about his/her medicines and self-management? If so, why?

   If Yes:

   a. How do you think an app could help patients with CF to learn about their medicines and self-management?
   b. What features and content do you think would be beneficial to the app design?

6. Of the methods we discussed, which do you believe is the most effective method for delivering education to patients at a community pharmacy?

D. Pharmacist Counseling
We will now ask you about providing medication counseling for people living with CF.

1. How do you feel about talking to patients with CF about their medications?
2. Can you describe potential ways that pharmacists could be better equipped to provide medication counseling for people living with CF?
3. How do the elements of the pharmacy (waiting area, space) facilitate or impede counseling to patients with CF?
   (If not discussed) Please describe any changes you believe would help.
4. Can you describe other ways to engage younger CF patients in medication use discussions?
   Do you have anything you'd like to add before we end?

Appendix A.2 Other Healthcare Team Members Interview Guide

A. Introductory Questions

1. Tell me about what you do in your CF care center.
2. Describe the pharmacy-related needs or problems of CF patients. (May probe for issues related to access to medications, insurance issues, etc.)
3. What kinds of challenges do you think that CF patients face regarding the use of CF medications?
4. What types of medications or treatments seem to be especially hard for CF patients to administer or adhere to correctly?
5. What method(s) do you use to assess if patients are adhering to their medication regimens?
6. What recommendations do you have for addressing these medication or pharmacy-related issues?

B. Medication Education
We would like to ask you about providing adolescent or young adults (AYA) with CF information about their medicines.

1. Have you provided any form of medication education to patients with CF?

   a. If Yes: Please describe what information was provided (i.e., drug information, dosing, side effects, etc.) and how often you provided medication education.
   b. What steps do you take to make sure the patient with CF has understood the medication information you provided?

2. How well do you think that patients with CF are educated on their medications?

    a. How can their knowledge about medicines be improved?

3. Who do you think should be educating patients with CF on their medications? (Probe for doctor, pharmacist, nurse, etc.)

4. Assuming patients want to learn about their medications, how do you think patients with CF prefer to learn about their medications? (Probe for one-on-one counseling with the pharmacist/doctor/nurse, written materials/pamphlets, interactive technology like on an iPad, videos on the Internet or TV, using an app on a smartphone or tablet)

5. Do you think patients with CF would be interested in using an app, like on a smartphone or tablet, to learn about his/her medicines and self-management? If so, why?

    a. If Yes: How do you think an app could help patients with CF to learn about their medicines and self-management?

    b. What features and content do you think would be beneficial to the app design?

6. Are there any other ways that you can think of that would be helpful for patients with CF to learn about their medicines?

C. Experiences with Outpatient, Specialty, and Community Pharmacists

We would now like to ask you some questions about your experiences with outpatient and community pharmacists.

1. How often and in what practice setting (i.e., in-patient, outpatient, community pharmacies such as Giant Eagle, Rite Aid, CVS, Walgreen's, etc.) do you interact with pharmacists involved in the care of patients with CF?

2. How would you describe the communication between pharmacists and other CF healthcare team members?

3. Can you describe any possible ways to improve communication between the healthcare team members and pharmacists?

4. How do you think pharmacists can support the other members of the healthcare team providing care for people with CF?

5. What challenges with treatment and medications do you think pharmacists could possibly address for patients with CF?

6. Do you think there are any barriers to pharmacist involvement in the care of patients with CF?

    a. If so, what kinds of barriers?

7. Do you think there would be any benefits by implementing outpatient pharmacy services in your CF center?

    a. If so, what benefits?

8. Do you think there are there any barriers to implementing outpatient pharmacy services?

    a. If so, what kinds of barriers?

9. Do you think community pharmacists can uniquely support patients with CF? (Pharmacists practicing at Giant Eagle, Rite Aid, CVS, Walgreen's, etc.) If so, how?

Do you have anything you'd like to add before we end?

Appendix B

Table A1. Themes, subthemes, and verbatim quotes from participant interviews.

Work System Components and Themes	Additional Verbatim Quotes
Person(s)	
Experience and Expertise Caring for People with CF	*"CF is an autosomal recessive disorder essentially where, in a nutshell, you have these CFTR mutations where secretions in different mutli-organ systems become thick … oftentimes leading to lung transplant later on down the road. But it also affects the liver, pancreas, and then also male reproductive systems. So it's multi-organ disease."—Pharmacist 1* *"I've been able to provide probably only to about two patients that we've had with CF—well actually, one with CF"—Pharmacist 3* *"I do cover the pulmonology service on the floors. I do all their pharmacokinetics for all their levels, I help them pick the antibiotics, I make sure all their meds are right, I help with their prescriptions, writing them and whatever, if they ever need me to go in and talk to them about something, I certainly would be able to do so"—Pharmacist 6*
Tasks	
Medication Management Burden	*"the challenging administration options for the administration options for the medications as most of them are inhaled, oftentimes have to do them 3 times a day—to 2 times a day … so it takes up a large portion of these patients' time"—Pharmacist 1* *"I think Cayston® … but it's a three time a day medication. So, I think even though it only takes three minutes to nebulize, it's three times a day. I find that patients don't do medications three times a day. Tobi tends to take between twenty minutes and a half an hour to nebulize … even though it's only every other month, they tend to struggle in those months because it's an added medication to their day. They seem to be able to get Pulmozyme® in, although when they travel it's hard because it's a refrigerated medication. And then HyperSal® is twice a day and it makes you cough, so—and it tastes bad, so some of the patients don't want to use the Hyper-Sal because it makes you cough."—Nurse 4* *"I think that one of the main difficulties is just remembering to take the medication … a lot of times patients can get busy and forget to take those dosing of the medications. I think sometimes too, particularly with antibiotics, patients start feeling really well and they decide not to take their medications after they start feeling well. And then on the flip side of things, you can also have patients feel not so well, and they think that their medications are contributing to their poor state and decide not to take their medications."—Pharmacist 1* *"I know that there are medication use challenges that they do experience because they are children. They are not as familiar with how to use a nebulizer. It can be challenging to them."—Pharmacist 3*
Medication Education	*"We don't necessarily expect any local pharmacy, brick and mortar I'm referring to, to do patient teaching for their meds. It's too complex, too specialized."—Nurse 3* *"I think most people learn best from one on one counseling. If you give someone written materials, it's more likely than not that they will not be read … we're very careful about education in our clinic. And we have a dedicated person call a nurse educator … and they tend to meet with the families and go over the finer points about the medications."—Physician 5* *"For our end, with the kind of quiz that we're doing, that's actually geared more towards our transition patients, so patients going from teens to adults. I think it's really important"—Dietician 1*
Medication Access and Insurance Challenges	*"So, the pharmacy said the medication was denied, then we have to reach out to the insurance company and do a prior auth … if the auth is denied, then we do the appeal … if we can't get the appeal, then we have to have our physician reach out. We don't handle the enzyme authorizations or the supplements. We have a dietician that does those."—Nurse 1* *"The drugs can be astonishingly expensive. Some as much as $306,000 a year for Kalydeco for example."—Physician 5* *"coordinating all the prescriptions, right? There's a lot of fragmentation, right? They're going to maybe two, three, four pharmacies to get their medicine. And just managing that is a burden."—Pharmacist 2*
Organization	
Awareness of Pharmacy-Related Needs	*"They can help with anti-microbial management looking at past cultures and … helping physicians and nurses decide which anti-microbial regiments would be best for the patient to—as to not limit our options for future use based on antimicrobial resistance."—Pharmacist 1*

Table A1. *Cont.*

Work System Components and Themes	Additional Verbatim Quotes
Benefits and Drawbacks of Pharmacist Involvement	*"It's just infuriating to find out that we think we gave a patient an antibiotic, which was prescribed, and find out eight days later that they haven't gotten it yet because of insurance hoops, prior authorizations ... They're little snags, but they result in devastating consequences. So, those are all things that a pharmacist can help us with."—Nurse 3* *"more education, maybe more safety for the patients, better outcomes for the patient."—Dietician 2* *"Sometimes we go in and we review their medications when they first come into clinic and we go over what they're taking. I think if there was a more in-depth conversation."—Nurse 1* *"I think that our nutritionist would like him [the pharmacist] to help in ... helping with patients who are interested in our herbal remedies. And what are the food and drug interactions."—Nurse 5*
Tools and Technologies	
Technologies that Influence Adherence and Prescribing	*"we used to call all the pharmacists and order them, so we had more interaction than we do now. Now with the electronic medical record and electronic e-prescribing, we have much less interaction. And I find that we probably have, maybe some or more delays to patients getting their meds because of that."—Nurse 2* *"I think that video presentations with graphics followed by a quiz is probably the best way to do it so that they learn and then have to self-reflect and then spit out what the answers are."—Physician 1* *"I think—specifically for young people, videos, apps ... some sort of content like that, they can watch it at their own time, rewatch to understand a missing point. And then make notes and reach out to us like, 'Hey I watched this, and these are the questions I have.'"—Pharmacist 4* *"I think that we have a lot online now and we have iPads ... that's what kids really like. They want to see something online"—Nurse 3*
Environment	
Collaborative Practice Agreements	*"I think that we can help them to streamline some of their therapies, or make adjustments, additions and subtractions, like discontinuations of things as they progress through."—Pharmacist 7*
Refill History Access	*"Well a lot of the pharmacies are set up, especially with the expensive drugs, it seems they try to track them more because they have a vested interest to do so. So, we'll get reminder calls."—Nurse 2* *"[the pharmacists] call us—I think that's a generous—you know, for refills, they'll call us, or fax for refills and I think that helps families. Some of the pharmacists call for medication lists because they are kind of keeping an eye on what the family is getting and sending automatic refills to the family."—Nurse 4* *"The most effective test we have right now is lung function testing. And lung function testing is kind of the final common pathway for all therapies. To say if your lungs are good then you must be doing the right thing."—Physician 5*

References

1. Sawicki, G.S.; Tiddens, H. Managing treatment complexity in cystic fibrosis: Challenges and opportunities. *Pediatr. Pulmonol.* **2012**, *47*, 523–533. [CrossRef] [PubMed]
2. Cystic Fibrosis Foundation: About Cystic Fibrosis. Available online: https://www.cff.org/What-is-CF/About-Cystic-Fibrosis/ (accessed on 1 December 2018).
3. Autosomal Recessive Inheritance | My46. Available online: https://www.my46.org/intro/autosomal-recessive-inheritance (accessed on 25 February 2019).
4. Quittner, A.L.; Saez-Flores, E.; Barton, J.D. The psychological burden of cystic fibrosis. *Curr. Opin. Pulm. Med.* **2016**, *22*, 187–191. [CrossRef] [PubMed]
5. Cystic Fibrosis Foundation: 2016 Patient Registry Reports. Available online: https://www.cff.org/Research/Researcher-Resources/Patient-Registry/2016-Patient-Registry-Reports/ (accessed on 1 December 2017).
6. Cystic Fibrosis Foundation: Treatments and therapies. Available online: https://www.cff.org/Life-With-CF/Treatments-and-Therapies/ (accessed on 1 December 2017).
7. Goodfellow, N.A.; Hawwa, A.F.; Reid, A.J.; Horne, R.; Shields, M.D.; McElnay, J.C. Adherence to treatment in children and adolescents with cystic fibrosis: A cross-sectional, multi-method study investigating the influence of beliefs about treatment and parental depressive symptoms. *BMC Pulm. Med.* **2015**, *15*, 43. [CrossRef] [PubMed]
8. Cystic Fibrosis Foundation: Care Centers. Available online: https://www.cff.org/Care/Care-Centers/ (accessed on 1 December 2017).

9.   Cystic Fibrosis Foundation: Your CF Care Team. Available online: https://www.cff.org/Care/Your-CF-Care-Team/ (accessed on 1 December 2017).

10.   Kerem, E.; Conway, S.; Elborn, S.; Heijerman, H. Standards of care for patients with cystic fibrosis: A European consensus. *J. Cyst. Fibros.* **2005**, *4*, 7–26. [CrossRef] [PubMed]

11.   Geiss, S.K.; Hobbs, S.A.; Hammersley-Maercklein, G.; Kramer, J.C.; Henley, M. Psychosocial factors related to perceived compliance with cystic fibrosis treatment. *J. Clin. Psychol.* **1992**, *48*, 99–103. [CrossRef]

12.   Cystic Fibrosis Trus: Consensus Documents. Available online: https://www.cysticfibrosis.org.uk/en/theworkwedo/clinicalcare/consensusdocuments (accessed on 24 February 2019).

13.   Bell, S.C.; Robinson, P.J.; Fitzgerald, D.A. *Cystic Fibrosis Standards of Care, Australia*; Johns Hopkins University: Baltimore, MA, USA, 2008; p. 76.

14.   Holden, R.J.; Carayon, P.; Gurses, A.P.; Hoonakker, P.; Hundt, A.S.; Ozok, A.A.; Rivera-Rodriguez, A.J. SEIPS 2.0: A human factors framework for studying and improving the work of healthcare professionals and patients. *Ergonomics* **2013**, *56*. [CrossRef] [PubMed]

15.   Sterner-Allison, J.L. Management of adolescent and adult inpatients with cystic fibrosis. *Am. J. Health Syst. Pharm.* **1999**, *56*, 158–160. [CrossRef] [PubMed]

16.   Redfern, J.; Webb, A.K. Benefits of a dedicated cystic fibrosis pharmacist. *J. R. Soc. Med.* **2004**, *97*, 2–7. [PubMed]

17.   Cies, J.J.; Varlotta, L. Clinical pharmacist impact on care, length of stay, and cost in pediatric cystic fibrosis (CF) patients. *Pediatr. Pulmonol.* **2013**, *48*, 1190–1194. [CrossRef] [PubMed]

18.   Lewis, K.L.; John, B.; Condren, M.; Carter, S.M. Evaluation of Medication-related Self-care Skills in Patients With Cystic Fibrosis. *J. Pediatr. Pharmacol. Ther.* **2016**, *21*, 502–511. [CrossRef] [PubMed]

19.   Modi, A.C.; Quittner, A.L. Barriers to Treatment Adherence for Children with Cystic Fibrosis and Asthma: What Gets in the Way? *J. Pediatr. Psychol.* **2006**, *31*, 846–858. [CrossRef] [PubMed]

20.   Dziuban, E.J.; Saab-Abazeed, L.; Chaudhry, S.R.; Streetman, D.S.; Nasr, S.Z. Identifying barriers to treatment adherence and related attitudinal patterns in adolescents with cystic fibrosis. *Pediatr. Pulmonol.* **2010**, *45*, 450–458. [CrossRef] [PubMed]

21.   Ferkol, T.; Quinton, P. Precision Medicine: At What Price? *Am. J. Respir. Crit. Care Med.* **2015**, *192*, 658–659. [CrossRef] [PubMed]

22.   Krivchenia, K.; Tumin, D.; Tobias, J.D.; Hayes, D. Increased Mortality in Adult Cystic Fibrosis Patients with Medicaid Insurance Awaiting Lung Transplantation. *Lung* **2016**, *194*, 799–806. [CrossRef] [PubMed]

23.   Abraham, O.; Li, J.S.; Monangai, K.E.; Feathers, A.M.; Weiner, D. The pharmacist's role in supporting people living with cystic fibrosis. *J. Am. Pharm. Assoc.* **2018**, *58*, 246–249. [CrossRef] [PubMed]

24.   Horace, A.E.; Ahmed, F. Polypharmacy in pediatric patients and opportunities for pharmacists' involvement. *Integr. Pharm. Res. Pract.* **2015**, *4*, 113–126. [CrossRef] [PubMed]

25.   McInnis, T. *Get the Medications Right: A Nationwide Snapshot of Expert Practices—Comprehensive Medication Management in Ambulatory/Community Pharmacy*; Health2 Resources: Vienna, VA, USA, 2016.

26.   Giberson, S.; Yoder, S.; Lee, M. *Improving Patient and Health System Outcomes through Advanced Pharmacy Practice: A Report to the U. S. Surgeon General*; U.S. Public Health Service: Washington, DC, USA, 2011.

27.   National Center for Chronic Disease Prevention and Health Promotion: A Program Guide for Public Health: Partnering with the Pharmacist in the Prevention and Control of Chronic Diseases. Available online: https://www.cdc.gov/dhdsp/programs/spha/docs/pharmacist_guide.pdf (accessed on 24 February 2019).

28.   Wood, J.; Jenkins, S.; Putrino, D.; Mulrennan, S.; Morey, S.; Cecins, N.; Hill, K. High usability of a smartphone application for reporting symptoms in adults with cystic fibrosis. *J. Telemed. Telecare* **2018**, *24*, 547–552. [CrossRef] [PubMed]

29.   Gur, M.; Nir, V.; Teleshov, A.; Bar-Yoseph, R.; Manor, E.; Diab, G.; Bentur, L. The use of telehealth (text messaging and video communications) in patients with cystic fibrosis: A pilot study. *J. Telemed. Telecare* **2017**, *23*, 489–493. [CrossRef] [PubMed]

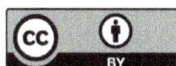

pharmacy

MDPI

Article

Health Workers' Perceptions and Expectations of the Role of the Pharmacist in Emergency Units: A Qualitative Study in Kupang, Indonesia

Laila Safitrih [1], Dyah A. Perwitasari [1,*], Nelci Ndoen [2] and Keri L. Dandan [3]

[1] Faculty of Pharmacy, University of Ahmad Dahlan, Yogyakarta 55166, Indonesia; lsafitrih18@gmail.com
[2] Pharmacy Unit, Prof. Dr. W.Z. Johannes Hospital, Kupang 85112, Indonesia; nelci.ndoen1975@gmail.com
[3] Faculty of Pharmacy, University of Padjajaran, Bandung 45363, Indonesia; lestarikd@unpad.ac.id
* Correspondence: dyah.perwitasari@pharm.uad.ac.id; Tel.: +62-274563515

Received: 15 February 2019; Accepted: 19 March 2019; Published: 22 March 2019

check for updates

Abstract: Background. An essential way to ensure patient safety in the hospital is by applying pharmacy services in emergency units. This strategy was implemented in Indonesia several years ago, with the aim of ensuring that adequate pharmacy services are given to patients in hospitals. To achieve this, pharmacists are required to cooperate with other health workers via inter-professional teamwork. This study intended to identify the perceptions and expectations of health workers with respect to pharmacy services in emergency units. **Methods**. This was a qualitative study, using a phenomenological approach with a semi-structured interview technique to obtain data. This study was performed at the Prof. Dr. W.Z. Johannes Hospital Kupang from June to September 2018. The results of the interviews were thematically analyzed using QSR NVivo software 11. **Results**. The themes identified in this study included: (1) The positive impact of pharmacists in service; (2) Badan Penyelenggara Jaminan Sosial (BPJS) influence; (3) Acceptance of health workers; (4) Medication administration information; and (5) Expectations of health workers. Various perceptions were conveyed by participants regarding the emergency unit services in the hospital's pharmaceutical department. Data obtained proved that the existence of a pharmacist increased the efficiency of time for services and prevented human error. **Conclusion**. Pharmacists and policy-makers play a significant role in providing appropriate pharmaceutical services in emergency units. Pharmacists also need to improve their quality of practice in accordance with their competence. They must review the patient medical history and physician's prescriptions, educate the patients and other health workers, so that the workload and service time will be reduced.

Keywords: pharmacy; emergency unit; health workers

1. Introduction

One essential way to ensure patient safety in hospitals is by ensuring the presence of pharmacists in emergency rooms. One measure, based on the decision of Accreditation Commission for Hospital (KARS: Komisi Akreditasi Rumah Sakit) in 2012 and 2016 Number 72, aims at ensuring that adequate pharmacy services are given to patients in hospitals. To ensure adequate patient safety in hospitals, pharmacists collaborate with other health workers via inter-professional teamwork. Unfortunately, the relationship between pharmacists and other health personals in developing and developed countries is not cordial [1]. For instance, one study conducted in Canada revealed that a main obstacle to pharmacists in working in hospitals is inadequate support from other health workers [2].

Studies about health workers' perceptions of the role of pharmacists in emergency units have not been conducted in Indonesia. Clinical pharmacist development in Indonesia is still in its infancy.

However, problems in emergency units related to medications are increasing, and these can result in medication error. This study aims at identifying the perceptions and expectations of health workers with respect to the emergency pharmacy units in hospitals located in the city of Kupang.

2. Methods

2.1. Study Design

Qualitative research was undertaken, with a phenomenological approach using a semi-structured interview technique to obtain data. The research was conducted at the Regional General Hospital Prof. Dr. W.Z. Johannes Kupang between June and September 2018.

2.2. Guidelines of the Interview

The questions, which were designed during the study, followed the open-ended question rule. Open-ended questions were purposed to explore the perception of health providers about the pharmacy service in emergency units. The interview guide followed previous studies [3]. However, some questions were designed with the purpose of understanding the impact of pharmacist services on patients' safety, the cost control, the behavior of health professionals toward pharmacists with respect to high-alert medications, and health professional's expectations toward pharmacy services in the ward.

2.3. Recruitment Strategy

We used purposive and convenience sampling technique with variations of age, profession, and employment duration. The researcher found information on the participants by contacting a key informant working in the hospital. The researcher directly met the participants at the emergency unit. An informed consent process was conducted by the researcher. Anonymity was used to maintain confidentiality. The interview was conducted directly and recorded based on the permission of the participants. There were two groups of participants: physicians and nurses. Health workers who were willing to take part in the study filled out a form stating their willingness to participate. The researcher ensured that confidentiality was maintained. A face-to-face interview method was conducted using a purposive sampling technique. The interview was held in a closed emergency unit area within the participants' working hours.

2.4. Data Analysis

Data was analyzed using the QSR NVivo 11 software. The examined data were theoretical, which enabled the researcher to determine pre-themes from the research questions. The code was developed from information that was specific or relevant to the research question.

The interview transcript was analyzed by NVivo 11 codebook. The themes were designed based on theoretical thematic analysis, where the codes associated with the research questions were arranged. The themes were arranged based on the Standard of Pharmacy services and the interview. We used open coding without pre-setting and we did not use code from every list; however, we modified the codes during the coding process.

2.5. Ethical Consideration

This research received approval from the Research Ethics Commission of the Ahmad Dahlan University (N: 011803044, ED 19.07.2019).

2.6. Trustworthiness

This study conducted by researchers with the expertise of lecturers, practitioners, and master's students. The pharmacy services disclosed in this study were based on the perspectives of physicians and nurses. To minimize study bias, we involved hospital workers to check the data interpretation. An endeavor was made to achieve transferability by explaining the study in more detail. Confirmability was conducted by reflexivity, involving an explanation of the motive, background, perspective, and study finding implications. The themes were designed by LS and reviewed by DA and one external reviewer. Data credibility was guaranteed using member check with transferability used to give a detailed description [4].

3. Results

We present our study results according to themes, using narratives and tables with examples of direct quotes from the participants. The narratives of the quotes from physicians and nurses are presented according to the themes. Some narratives are separated with respect to physicians and nurses because of the different perspectives between them, especially in terms of the theme of acceptability of the pharmacist's role among other health workers. We encoded the physician as "P" and the nurse as "N".

Participant:

A total of eight participants consisting of medical practitioners and nurses participated in the research. The participants' characteristics are shown in Table 1. The themes identified in this study are presented in Table 2.

Table 1. Participants' Characteritics.

Characteristics	N	%
Age		
<30	2	25
30–40	3	37.5
40–50	3	37.5
Gender		
Male	4	50
Female	4	50
Profession		
General physician	4	50
Nurse	4	50
Working (Mean 7.4 years)		
<10 years	4	50
>10 years	4	50

Table 2. Theme classifications and participant quotes.

Major Themes	Examples
Positive impact of pharmacists in service	*When a pharmacist comes across a problem associated with wrong dosage, he will review it. Luckily for me, mine was very careful, we could not just take medicine without his assistance—N1.*
Effect of National Insurance (Badan Penyelenggara Jaminan Sosial:BPJS)	*We are more flexible with BPJS patients because certainty is guaranteed, but in the case of accident victims, we sometimes ask them to pay upfront, most times they ask us to treat them with the guarantee of paying up later. However, sometimes they do not redeem these bills. So it's wrong too—P4*
Acceptance of health workers	*It's just a matter of language, if communication is good, ok, if for example the communication is insistent, it doesn't depend on the doctor—P4*
Drug information	*Same is applicable with medicine. All who understand the medicine are pharmacists. It never goes down to the patient—P2.*
Expectations of health workers	*If we had the slightest idea that this drug would be finishing soonest, we would have made adequate provision for it. Since it hasn't been replaced till now, we are assuming it must have run out of production—N2.* *It is expected that more drugs are purchased, especially if there is an emergency—N4.* *It is not only about the pharmacist. Pharmacists are all good, and they ensure the availability of medicine in hospitals—P1.* *Pharmacists must understand that the drugs are fast moving, so they can do the planning of the procurement better—N2.* *Pharmacists have to increase their effort in planning the procurement of drug in the emergency unit—P4.*

3.1. Positive Impact of Pharmacists on Services

3.1.1. Time Efficiency

The presence of pharmacists in emergency units has a positive impact on patients and health workers and it is an essential contextual factor for health workers. The efficient of pharmacy services can improve the time efficiency. With the presence of the pharmacist, faster service is provided to patients.

For example: a patient with heart failure, will need furosemide to lower their breathing rate. But what will happen a situation where there is no pharmacist to prescribe the drug, will the patient be left to die?-P1

We have to wait for a moment, when we have to get the medicine from the pharmacy—N3.

3.1.2. Medication Error Prevention

Installing an emergency medical system is essential in order to prevent human errors associated with medication. Pharmacist has competency in reviewing the prescription, including to recalculate the dosage based on the patients' condition. This competency is expected by the nurse to be applied in the Emergency unit.

Giving the wrong prescription, can endanger the lives of patients, and the effect can be very fatal—N2

Participants realized that they could make a medication error both in the prescription and administration phases. Participants opined that the presence of pharmacists in the emergency department influences patient's safety as they tend to review and re-check a prescription to ensure the drugs received are safe and appropriate for consumption.

In my opinion, pharmacists have a huge influence on drug prescription, because drugs need to be properly checked and given with the right prescription—P2

Patient safety at the emergency department is crucial. Human error can occur and it is possible for the pharmacist to make mistakes. Therefore, it is important to crosscheck all prescriptions given to avoid human error.

I tried digging it again, by asking him if he was sure the prescription was ok—P3

We are already accustomed to double checking our prescriptions. Whenever I give out prescription it is cross checked by the pharmacist and if ok, given to the nurse, who also checks and issues according to instructions. Hence, it must be safe—P4

3.2. Effect of National Health Insurance

3.2.1. Drug Supply Limitation

In this research the participants expressed the influence of the health financing system on medicine management and the availability of medication in hospitals. There tend to be many issues related to the unavailability of drugs, especially those guaranteed by insurance. Participants stated that one of the administrative barriers which was related to pharmacist work was insurance. When the patients visit the hospital, the pharmacist checks the insurance of the patients as a guarantee. After that, the medicine is delivered to the patients. According to the participants, this situation can hold up service. Thus, insurance is a barrier to services.

Usually the BPJS drugs sometimes run out in government hospitals. That's the problem, so we ask them first—P1

Sometimes, when the drugs are not available, we have to buy the drugs outside of the hospital—N2

3.2.2. Dilemma

BPJS can influence the service system in the emergency unit. Before delivering the medicine to the patients, the pharmacist should make sure that the patients is under the guarantee of BPJS. This situation should not become the obstacle in the delivery of medicine.

> *Actually it doesn't violate the standard operating procedure (SOP) defined by BPJS, however, in the most of the patient's times, they opt for payment immediately they step into a medical facility. So these conditions has been shown to prevent such actions—P3*

In contrast to this perception, this system is more of a dilemma for other participants where they cannot sue the pharmacist. This is because most times after the drug is given, the guarantee requested is not available and the patient fails to pay. This can be detrimental to the hospital. According to one respondent, services can be more flexible for patients with insurance because health workers do not need to think about their patient's medication costs.

With respect to costs, one of the roles of pharmacists is to ensure that patients make full payment at the hospital; however, this research reveals the existence of a BPJS (national insurance) system, in which participants fail to notice any form of reduction in health costs owing to the presence of a pharmacist in the emergency unit.

In terms of costs, the pharmacist controls the hospital, but this research revealed that with the existence of a BPJS system, participants failed to witness a reduction in health costs. By using BPJS, patients paid nothing, so the reduction of the costs due to the pharmacist' role was not clear.

> *If it's here because the general hospital costs are usually not too big, then the patient can afford for the costs—N1*

> *Most of the patients are BPJS members, so money is not the problem for them, because everything is free?—N1*

3.3. Acceptance of Health Workers

In terms of therapy selection, the data showed the diverse behavior between doctors and pharmacists. One participant revealed that there was a communication hierarchy which made the pharmacist's advice difficult to accept. Pharmacist intervention is expected with the expectation that the service can run smoothly without any form of dispute.

> *In the emergency room, we also collided with hierarchy of the health professional. Sometimes the specialists ask for particular medicines. The pharmacist can discuss with the doctor for a change in medication if he runs out of medicine—P1.*

Meanwhile, other participants could accept the pharmacist's intervention as long as it was under the pharmacist's confirmation, especially for narcotics with serious adverse drug reactions. Pharmacists have also confirmed that drugs that contain narcotics have side effects capable of endangering the life of patients.

> *I often get angry when someone changes medicine without confirmation if the drugs have some side effects that can endanger them—P2*

In addition, other participants stated that the doctor was the decision maker and the person responsible for patient therapy. All decisions regarding therapy need to be properly communicated.

> *It's just a matter of language, if communication is good, ok, if for example the communication is unclear, it doesn't depend on the doctor—P4*

In terms of medicine information services, one of the participants who happened to be a doctor stated that patients rarely asked them questions because they felt more comfortable asking someone who had similar knowledge and professional experience.

It was not a problem I did not bother asking them because I had a friend with similar professional knowledge—P3

3.4. Drug Information

The action of giving the drug information by pharmacists in emergency units is still limited. This is still often performed by other nurses and doctors and considered to be a waste of time, creating a greater workload. Pharmacists are still passive in dealing directly with patients. According to the participants, pharmacists are the most appropriate health workers and are competent with respect to drug information.

Actually, the activity of counseling, education and information to patients is suboptimal. The problem is that we ordered medication, which means that we are in the emergency unit and no pharmacists here. Clarifying prescriptions to patients will mean doubling the effort, so it will be better for me to give the medicine already explained by the pharmacy—P4.

So far communication is usually between pharmacists and nurses, and sometimes with patients which is most times rare—N2.

3.5. Expectations of Health Workers

3.5.1. Drug Availability

Health workers expect pharmacists to do the drug procurement, thus avoiding shortages of medicine.

Other participants stated that drug supply was not the responsibility of other hospital personnel but rather that of the pharmacy. Other participant said that the drug supply is not only the responsibility of the pharmacist, but also other staff. Participants expected pharmacists to perform optimal drug planning, avoiding the unavailability of drugs. There are some techniques for the drug procurement, such as epidemiologic, consumption and the combination of epidemiologic-consumption. Pharmacists have competencies in this area, so that the other health professionals expect the best effort for the drug procurement.

3.5.2. Drug Utilization Review

Overall, pharmacy services are also expected to be applied at the emergency department. According to participants, pharmacists do not only manage medicines and medical devices but also ensure the safety of patients. The pharmacy service should be in the emergency unit, especially when taking into account drug management, information, and patient safety. Collaboration with other health workers is expected to be focused on patient safety. It is also important that the pharmacist is given the responsibility of keeping track of a patient's medical history. This will support inter professional communication between doctors and pharmacists. In giving therapeutic advice, one doctor stated that the pharmacist also needs to know the history of the drug so as to give the right advice that fits the needs of the individual.

The history of the treatment should be known to the pharmacist. So he can have an idea of the patients' eligibility to take the drug. Yes, those are things that I think are necessary for adequate collaboration between doctors and pharmacists. Not all of the cases in the emergency unit are new—P2.

Pharmacist can remind us about the patient's history, such as drug allergy—P4

Some doctors revealed that a detailed medical history can provide a good understanding of the patient's condition and treatment. Not only is it beneficial, but it can also reduce workload and save service time.

We need it, maybe the pharmacists are more active in directing services to patients, and those who must be served. It is not right with us. Direct service means medicament delivery—P2.

3.5.3. Drug Information and Education

Drug information was expected to be delivered to the patients. This activity can decrease the workload of other health professionals, since currently, they also have to give information and education to the patients.

We need the pharmacist to give direct service to the patients, such as information and education—N2

Just give the drug information and education to the patients—P4

On the other hand, the nurses also expected the pharmacist to give the education about drug admixture. The nurses need more education about the incompatibility of drugs in the case of admixture.

Sometimes, we do not understand about how to admixture the drugs. In the past, we also did not learn about it—N2.

Training on how to admixture the drugs is given; however, it is necessary to increase the frequency and carry out routine checkups.

A few months ago there was but lately there is no such training—N4

The working environment and the large number of patients should be considered in order to reduce medication errors.

This means that many patients come into the emergency room, sometimes we also can't blame human error because it can be tiring—P4

If the patients are few, it's ok. But if there are many patients coming to ask for this, we get confused. Hassle—N3

4. Discussion

Medical information needs to be given in the emergency unit, covering a wide range of aspects including medicine selection, dosage and administration, medicine reactions that harm intravenous compatibility, drug interactions, and identification of unknown medicines. Pharmacists stationed at the emergency unit must ensure that appropriate access is provided at the primary, secondary, and tertiary levels to ensure the smooth and prompt respond to medical requests [5]. Simone et al. reported that almost 66% of nurses expected a protocol or informative brochure in the emergency room on how to admixture intravenous drugs [6]. Inadequate pharmacological knowledge and fatigue caused by high workload for nurses are some of the managerial and human factors that lead to medication error [7]. Another qualitative study revealed that the main factors that contribute in reducing drug safety problems include sustainable education for health workers, the development of a culture that encourages awareness for reporting medication errors, the use of technology, and the promotion and implementation of policies related to patient safety [8].

One of the impacts associated with the implementation of national health insurance is regulation and medical supply, which ultimately affect the availability of drugs. Lack of medication is mostly caused by high demand for certain types of needs such as cancer treatment and dialysis. The budgets for the purchase of medicines are routinely being siphoned to meet the shortage of cancer drugs [9]. According to Prabowo, one of the factors that influences the availability of medicine in the BPJS era is the inability of the pharmacist to procure adequate medicine [10]. A method to anticipate drug unavailability is substitution of drugs with other trade names that meet the criteria. More factors must be involved by the pharmacist in the drug procurement process, so that drug unavailability could be avoided.

A study about implementing a comprehensive pharmacist program in emergency unit, the department pharmacist program revealed an increase in cost efficiency, with 76.7% of respondents stating that the role of pharmacists could reduce the cost of healthcare [3,11]. According to a recent study, with pharmacy program in emergency unit, cost of efficiency reached 74.03%. This type of intervention can be said to be quite significant in terms of cost-saving. In that study, the health costs were not a concern for participants, and no significant cost savings were made by the pharmacists [12]. According to other research, the opportunity for cost savings in many countries is limited where the average cost for each patient per treatment represents only a small part of the total cost. Thus, it is difficult to justify the result [13].

In a study conducted by Keller et al. using a qualitative research approach, one participant stated hierarchy as one of the obstacles between doctors and nurses, and expressed relief that they could communicate outside the hospital with ease [14]. A similar study revealed that doctors might think that making prescriptions and ensuring the patient follows the instructions or orders is better than participating in decision-making. Differences in the educational level and knowledge between professions can impact members' ability to exchange ideas and interpret patient health problems, thereby affecting the quality of treatment provided. This level of education and knowledge gap will hinder the process of effective communication [15]. A qualitative study conducted by Pun et al. revealed one of the problems of inter professional communication in the emergency unit as being the transfer of medical information to inadequate staff. Owing to the fact that patients often enter the emergency unit without medical records, a comprehensive understanding of the patient's condition and treatment history should be made to support quality health services [16]. A drug utilization review should be conducted precisely in the emergency unit because of the inconsistency in the patient's medical records. The pharmacist has the competence to perform drug reconciliation and to prevent medication errors during patient visits to the emergency unit [17,18].

Some pharmacy services can be developed at the emergency unit and this service involves creditors, regulators, and administrators of health care facilities [5]. For the clinical pharmacy practice in the hospital ward, normally one pharmacist must undertake prescription review, monitoring of treatment, giving of drug information, and education and counseling for 30 patients. For outpatient services, one pharmacist must perform prescription screening and drug administration, and provide information, education, and counseling for 50 patients [19]. According to this situation, ideally, one pharmacist must be placed in the emergency unit.

For clinical practice, the pharmacy service in the emergency unit is still related to drug supply management. The national standard should be developed to increase the quality of the pharmacist services. The interprofessional relationship concept should be accepted and applied by all health professionals. This concept must be introduced in undergraduate education.

Health workers' perceptions of the pharmacist's role in the emergency unit include not only services but also the patients' safety in the emergency unit. This perception brings up expectations about patient safety. On the other hand, the national health insurance system may influence perceptions and expectations. To the best of our knowledge, this study is the first qualitative study conducted in Indonesia on the topic of health workers' perceptions of the pharmacist's role in emergency units. Currently there is no national standard for the pharmacy services in emergency units. Our findings can be used as a consideration to develop the standard of the pharmacist's role in the emergency unit. Physicians and nurses perceive that delivering the drug information is an important job of the pharmacist in the emergency unit. However, the pharmacist's role can be limited by national health insurance due to the limited medications available in the emergency unit. During emergency situations, the physician and the nurse need medications appropriate to the patients' conditions. The pharmacist is responsible for the availability of the medications.

This study has the limitation due to the use of only one method, which was the semi structured interview method. Thus, we cannot generalize the results. The results of study were more focused on drug supply management and drug information. In these cases, the small number of participants can support the validity of the study findings. Furthermore, data analysis was only carried out by the researcher to clarify the efficiency of the data obtained.

5. Conclusions

Various perceptions are conveyed by participants regarding the pharmacy service in emergency units. The existence of a pharmacist may increase the efficiency of service time and prevent human error. The national health insurance service is in charge of the role played by health workers and pharmacists. Communication, information, and adequate medical education are still insufficient in emergency units. Participants expect that pharmacists and policy makers make adequate provisions for drugs in the emergency units. Pharmacists need to enhance the quality of practice in accordance with their competence, especially in tracking the patient's drug history and in terms of drug education for both patients and health workers. These expectations are intended reduce the workload of participants, save time, and improve the quality of communication among medical personnel.

Author Contributions: Conceptualization, D.A.P. and K.L.D.; Data curation, L.S. and N.N.; Formal analysis, D.A.P.; Funding acquisition, L.S.; Investigation, N.N.; Methodology, L.S., D.A.P. and N.N.; Project administration, K.L.D.; Resources, D.A.P.; Software, K.L.D.; Supervision, D.A.P., N.N., K.L.D.; Validation, N.N. and K.L.D.; Writing—original draft, L.S. and D.A.P.; Writing—review and editing, D.A.P., N.N., K.L.D.

Funding: This research received no external funding.

Acknowledgments: The authors thank the staff of the RSUD WZ Johannes, Kupang, Indonesia.

Conflicts of Interest: The authors declare no conflict of interest.

References

1. Rayes, I.K.; Abduelkarem, A.R. A qualitative study exploring physicians' perceptions on the role of community pharmacists in Dubai. *Pharm. Pract. (Granada)* **2016**, *14*, 738. [CrossRef] [PubMed]
2. Abdalla, A.A.; Adwi, G.M.; Al Mahdy, A.F. Physicians' Perception About The Role Of Clinical Pharmacists And Potential Barriers To Clinical Pharmacy. *World J. Pharm. Pharm. Sci.* **2015**, *4*, 61–72.
3. Fahmy, S.A.; Rasool, B.K.A.; Abdu, S. Health-care professionals' perceptions and expectations of pharmacists' role in the emergency department, United Arab Emirates. *East. Mediterr. Health J.* **2013**, *19*, 794–801. [CrossRef]
4. Cohen, D.; Crabtree, B. Qualitative Research Guidelines Project. Available online: http://www.qualres.org/HomeLinc-3684.html (accessed on 26 March 2018).
5. ASHP Guidelines on Emergency Medicine Pharmacist Services. *Am. Soc. Health-Syst. Pharm.* **2011**, *68*, e81–e95. [CrossRef]
6. Di Simone, E.; Giannetta, N.; Auddin, F.; Cicotto, A.; Grilli, D.; Di Muzio, M. Medication errors in the emergency department: Knowledge, attitude, behavior, and training needs of nurses. *Indian J. Crit. Care Med.* **2018**, *22*, 346–352. [CrossRef] [PubMed]
7. Ehsani, S.R.; Cheragi, M.A.; Nejati, A.; Salari, A.; Esmaeilpoor, A.H.; Nejad, E.M. Medication errors of nurses in the emergency department. *J. Med. Ethics Hist. Med.* **2013**, *6*, 11. [PubMed]
8. Aljadhey, H.; Mahmoud, M.A.; Hassali, M.A.; Alrasheedy, A.; Alahmad, A.; Saleem, F.; Sheikh, A.; Murray, M.; Bates, D.W. Challenges to and the future of medication safety in Saudi Arabia: A qualitative study. *Saudi Pharm. J.* **2014**, *22*, 326–332. [CrossRef]
9. Tani, A. NTT Often Experienced Lack of Medication in Public Health Facilities. Available online: http://rri.co.id/kupang/post/berita/347846/daerah/ntt_sering_alami_kekurangan_obat_pada_fasilitas_kesehatan_masyarakat.html (accessed on 6 December 2018).
10. Prabowo, P.; Satibi; Pamudji, G.W. Analysis of Factors Affecting the Availability of Drugs at the BPJS Era in Rsud Dr. Soedono Madiun. *J. Manag. Pharm. Pract.* **2016**, *6*, 213–218.
11. Aldridge, V.E.; Park, H.K.; Bounthavong, M.; Morreale, A.P. Implementing a comprehensive, 24-hour emergency department pharmacy program. *Am. J. Health Syst. Pharm* **2009**, *66*, 1943–1947. [CrossRef]
12. Gunawan, C.A.; Pribadi, F.; Risdiana, I. Analisis Efisiensi Biaya Obat Setelah Dilakukan Telaah Resep Dan Intervensi Apoteker Dalam Pelayanan Farmasi Pasien BPJS Rawat Jalan Di Rs Pku Muhammadiyah Yogyakarta. *Proc. Health Archit.* **2017**, *1*, 35–44.
13. Roman, C.; Edwards, G.; Dooley, M.; Mitra, B. Roles of the emergency medicine pharmacist: A systematic review. *Am. J. Health Syst. Pharm.* **2018**, *75*, 796–806. [CrossRef]

14. Kathryn, B.K.; Terry, L.E.; Julia, B.; Mira, S.; Amalinnette, R.Z. Implementing Successful Interprofessional Communication Opportunities In Health Care Education: A Qualitative Analysis. *Int. J. Med. Educ.* **2013**, *4*, 253–259. [CrossRef]

15. Fatalina, F.; Sumartini; Widyandana; Sedyowinarso, M. Perception and Acceptance of Interprofessional Collaborative Practice in the Field of Maternity in Health Workers. *Pendidik. Kedokt. Indones.* **2015**, *1*, 28–36.

16. Pun, J.K.; Matthiessen, C.M.; Murray, K.A.; Slade, D. Factors affecting communication in emergency departments: Doctors and nurses' perceptions of communication in a trilingual ED in Hong Kong. *Int. J. Emerg. Med.* **2015**, *8*, 48. [CrossRef] [PubMed]

17. De Winter, S.; Vanbrabant, P.; Laeremans, P.; Foulon, V.; Willems, L.; Verelst, S.; Spriet, I. Developing a decision rule to optimise clinical pharmacist resources for medication reconciliation in the emergency department. *Emerg. Med. J.* **2017**, *34*, 502–508. [CrossRef]

18. De Winter, S.; Spriet, I.; Indevuyst, C.; Vanbrabant, P.; Desruelles, D.; Sabbe, M.; Gillet, J.B.; Wilmer, A.; Willems, L. Pharmacist- versus physician-acquired medication history: A prospective study at the emergency department. *Qual. Saf. Health Care* **2010**, *19*, 371–375. [CrossRef] [PubMed]

19. Anonymous. *Regulation of the Minister of Health of Republic Indonesia concerning Phnarmaceutical Service Standards in Hospitals*; Minister of Health of Republic Indonesia. Available online: http://jdih.bumn.go.id/baca/PP%20NOMOR%2072%20TAHUN%202016.pdf (accessed on 2 March 2019).

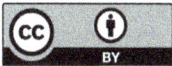

pharmacy

MDPI

Brief Report

Innovative Collaboration between a Medical Clinic and a Community Pharmacy: A Case Report

William R. Doucette

College of Pharmacy, University of Iowa, Iowa City, IA 52242, USA; william-doucette@uiowa.edu

Received: 10 May 2019; Accepted: 11 June 2019; Published: 14 June 2019

check for
updates

Abstract: As value-based payments become more common in healthcare, providers can develop collaborative relationships to support performance. A medical clinic and community pharmacy worked together to deliver collaborative medication management services to targeted patients in an accountable care organization. The community pharmacy was paid by the clinic to conduct comprehensive medication reviews (CMRs) for 116 patients. The CMRs initially were delivered to patients taking at least 10 medications and to patients rated as high cost/risk by the clinic. The most common medication-related problem types were Needs additional therapy (38.8%) and Suboptimal therapy (19.0%). The most common pharmacist actions were to Change medication (18.1%) and Initiate new therapy (13.8%). Financial analyses showed net savings in annual patient out-of-pocket expenses just over $15,000 for the cohort of patients, and net annual direct cost savings from a payer perspective of about $70,000. This innovative partnership between a medical clinic system and a regional pharmacy chain built upon initial discussions and planning. The partners were able to address problems that arose with their collaboration, changing their approach as needed. The outcomes were positive for the clinic and pharmacy, their patients and the payer(s). Interested providers are encouraged to pursue similar collaborations, which could be key to success in today's healthcare environment.

Keywords: comprehensive medication review; community pharmacy; collaboration

1. Introduction

The current healthcare environment has made value-based payments a popular approach [1,2]. Under such programs, providers often can benefit from closer coordination with each other across the continuum of care. An important provider dyad, especially for managing chronic conditions, is the medical clinic–community pharmacy. Both of these providers are involved with helping patients achieve positive outcomes from medication therapy while working to limit total costs of care [2,3].

Though some clinic–pharmacy coordination is occurring, few detailed descriptions have been published about successful collaboration between clinics and community pharmacies under the evolving value-based payment environment [4,5]. Over the past five years, the Iowa Department of Public Health has worked with a team at the University of Iowa College of Pharmacy to foster team care among clinic–community pharmacy partners to improve management of hypertension and diabetes. This work has stimulated some clinic–community pharmacy collaboration. The objective of this case report is to describe the development, operations, and outcomes of an innovative clinic–community pharmacy collaborative care model for providers facing value-based payments.

McFarland Clinic has been a leading multispecialty clinic organization in Iowa for over 70 years. It is Iowa's largest physician-owned multispecialty clinic. The McFarland Clinic provider network serves patients through about 20 locations in central Iowa, delivering over 1 million patient visits annually, involving more than 280 providers and 1000 staff members. McFarland Clinic embraces innovation which enables excellence in clinical practice. Given the presence of value-based payment programs by accountable care organizations (ACOs), McFarland Clinic leaders were considering ways to successfully apply a population health management model to support their value-based performance.

NuCara Pharmacy is a full-service regional pharmacy chain with more than 20 locations in four states. NuCara strives to provide the best products, the best service, and latest innovations to benefit their patients and customers. Their pharmacists work with patients and other providers to optimize medication therapy, in addition to delivering a range of pharmacy services. Their services include compounding custom prescription medications, medication management, immunizations, medication synchronization, medication packaging, infusion services, and sales of home medical equipment. They participate in a value-based pharmacy program operated by a large payer, which made closer coordination with clinics of interest to them.

2. Materials and Methods

To gather data about this case study, a key informant from both the participating clinic and the participating pharmacy was interviewed, using semi-structured questions. The set of interview questions was developed from an initial description of the clinic-community pharmacy joint activities by a participating pharmacist. The questions asked about having the pharmacy conduct comprehensive medication reviews for patients using a lot of medications, a pharmacy medication management service for high risk/high cost patients, and the start of medication adherence management service provided by the pharmacy. The interviews were audiotaped, transcribed verbatim, and then analyzed. The responses were coded for the topics describing how the partners developed their joint activities, as well as how they operated. In addition, some documents describing the partnership were shared with the investigator.

In addition, a financial analysis was conducted by the pharmacy to estimate the net benefit associated with the joint activities. A conservative approach was followed, focusing on cost savings resulting from changes in medication therapy made in response to the CMRs, primarily from brand or non-formulary medications to generic formulary medications. Such savings were estimated for 12 months, from a payer perspective and for patient out-of-pocket expenses. Medication costs were calculated using insurance payment formulas for the insurance the patients had, or a cash formula used for that medication. Estimated actual acquisition costs for the pharmacy were used for product costs. No related cost estimates for reduced clinic visits, ER visits or hospitalizations were included in the financial analysis.

3. Results

Initial Teamwork: Both of these providers have locations in Ames, Iowa that participated in an initial effort at team management of patients with diabetes, working with a team at the University of Iowa. For this first effort, representatives of the McFarland Clinic and NuCara Pharmacy met with personnel from the University of Iowa and the Iowa Department of Public Health to discuss how the team approach could work between their organizations. Though these providers worked to collaborate, this initial effort was limited by having few targeted patients not meeting diabetes goals (e.g., hemoglobin a1c target, BP target). Thus, this coordinated work on team management of medications for patients with diabetes did not persist. However, it did lay the groundwork for later collaboration, as the providers were able to better understand each other's practices, appreciate their respective expertise and establish a working rapport.

Medication Management for High Medication Use Patients: One approach pursued by the clinic to try to improve ACO performance metrics was to optimize medication therapy for their patients who were taking at least ten different medications and were covered by an insurer's ACO program. The clinic approached NuCara Pharmacy in Ames about providing a comprehensive medication review (CMR) service for a panel of patients with high medication use. The primary discussions occurred between the physician and pharmacist who had worked together in the initial team management for patients with diabetes. After a mutually agreeable plan had been outlined, each provider worked with their own organization's leadership to get support to proceed. The pharmacy was willing to provide a comprehensive medication management service, for which the clinic paid the pharmacy using a fee for service approach. The physician leader talked with the clinic's providers about the program to gain their support and feedback. No formal agreement was signed initially, to allow flexibility to adjust the collaboration, though one was signed later.

To begin the service, the clinic identified a list of about 200 patients in the Ames area to receive a comprehensive medication review (CMR) by one of the pharmacy's pharmacists. These patients were taking at least ten different medications, which was considered high medication use. Some of these patients got their medications dispensed from the participating pharmacy, while most did not. The clinic sent an initial letter to each patient that described the program and encouraged them to work with the pharmacy to receive a CMR. After the letters were sent out, the pharmacy phoned the patients on the list to determine their willingness to participate in the program and to schedule CMRs for interested patients. There was a low response rate from patients initially. To address this issue, the clinic revised the patient letter and added the patient's provider's signature. Also, the NuCara pharmacist tweaked the telephone contact script. Together, these changes improved the patient participation in this CMR program. The pharmacy provided collaborative comprehensive medication management services to 85 patients in this first phase.

Most of the CMRs were conducted over the telephone, though some were completed in the pharmacy. The pharmacist first gathered patient information from the available patient records (either from the pharmacy or from the clinic EMR) to get an initial view of the patient's medication regimen and labs. Then, the pharmacist talked with the patient to collect additional information about how the medications were being taken, and if likely adverse effects were present. While on the call with the patient the pharmacist discussed a medication plan to address any identified problems. The plan was implemented by working with the patient and/or the involved provider(s). Communication with providers used multiple modes, including secure text through the EMR, faxing the clinic, and phoning the clinic.

Another obstacle was limited responses by clinic providers to clinical notes sent by the pharmacist. It was typical that the pharmacist identified either a question or a potential medication-related problem when reviewing a patient's medications. In such instances the pharmacist sent a note to the involved provider(s) asking them to clarify the situation or to adjust medication therapy. Unfortunately, since this was the first time many of the clinic providers were collaborating closely with a community pharmacist on medication management, the providers hesitated to respond to pharmacist notes/queries. The pharmacist and physician leader discussed this situation, and the physician leader communicated with the clinic providers to clarify the objectives of the collaboration, asking them to be responsive to the pharmacist's notes/queries.

The pharmacist worked with the patients' dispensing pharmacies to get their medication lists and/or dispensing records, which were used for the CMRs. It required considerable effort to get other pharmacies to provide medication information, but some did eventually provide patient medication information requested by the pharmacist. To get more complete clinical information about the listed patients, the pharmacist worked with the clinic to get access to the clinic's EMR. The EMR provided the pharmacist with clinical information that allowed more efficient and effective CMRs to be conducted. In addition, the pharmacist was able to use a secure texting feature in the EMR. However, its effectiveness in communicating with the clinic providers was variable because not all of them used it.

Medication Management for High Risk Patients: After the success of the initial teamwork to address patients with high medication use, the clinic and pharmacy developed another joint effort focused on patients with high risk and/or high cost. From a list of high risk patients from the clinic, 31 patients received comprehensive medication review services from the pharmacy in the second phase of this collaboration. The clinic continued to pay the pharmacy to provide the collaborative CMR service. As with the previous teamwork, the clinic notified the patients that the pharmacy would be contacting them about the CMR service. The same collaborative CMR service was delivered to this second group of patients, who typically had multiple chronic conditions or were taking high cost medications. As with the first group, not many of these patients were getting their medications dispensed at NuCara Pharmacy. Though the communication processes were smoother than during the initial phase, some patients declined to have the CMR service. Similarly, the responsiveness of providers was somewhat better with this second group, after having the processes improved during the work with the first group of patients.

The partners conducted an aggregate evaluation of the collaborative comprehensive medication review services for the two groups. This work provided CMRs for a total of 116 patients. One component of their assessment was to characterize the medication-related problems identified by the pharmacist when conducting the CMRs. The most frequent types of medication-related problems were "Needs additional therapy" (38.8% of patients) and "Suboptimal therapy" (19.0%) (Table S1).

In addition, the pharmacist's actions were summarized. The most common pharmacist action was to work with the provider and patient to change a medication (18.1%) (Table S2). The pharmacist also worked to initiate new drug therapy (13.8%) and helped to discontinue unnecessary or problematic medications (12.9%). The pharmacist also educated patients to improve their medication administration technique (e.g., use of inhaler) (11.2%).

For the financial analysis, the net cost savings associated with pharmacist services under the partnership were calculated from a patient perspective and a payer perspective. The estimated 12-month direct cost savings for the 116 patients totaled $15,483. Also, direct cost savings on medications for a payer were estimated to be $70,513.74 over 12 months. Based on a variable fee amount for the different patient groups, the cost to the clinic for paying the pharmacist to conduct the CMRs totaled $13,150.

Current State of Collaborative Medication Management: The partners have built on the success of the comprehensive medication review service by implementing a service targeted at improving medication adherence, which is a common challenge for chronic medication therapy. This step was an initiative raised by the pharmacy to work together to improve medication adherence for shared patients: Adherence Services Referral Program. The adherence program can help the pharmacy perform well on metrics in a value-based pharmacy program in which it is participating. For this adherence program NuCara Pharmacy worked together with Medicap, another regional pharmacy chain who also has a pharmacy in Ames and others in central Iowa. Together these pharmacies are working with McFarland Clinics in their communities to identify and address medication nonadherence for only their own dispensing patients. Building on the success of the collaborative CMRs with one NuCara Pharmacy, McFarland Clinics is working with over a dozen pharmacies between NuCara and Medicap pharmacies–with all of the pharmacies participating in a value-based pharmacy program that includes adherence-based metrics. A progressive aspect of this newer program is that McFarland has allowed these pharmacy partners to access their EMRs through the web-based EpicCare Links. Such a connection creates efficiencies for the pharmacists caring for mutual patients of McFarland Clinics, while eliminating some phone calls to the clinic. Though it is too early to evaluate this adherence program, it is promising.

4. Discussion

This case report describes collaboration that occurred primarily over about 18 months between McFarland Clinic and NuCara Pharmacy. These partners built on an initial team-based project to implement collaborative comprehensive medication review services, delivered by a pharmacist working with clinic providers and patients. There were several innovative components of this collaboration, including: a clinic paying a community pharmacy to improve patient care under an ACO model, the clinic actively engaging patients and providers to participate with the pharmacy services, and the clinic connecting with the pharmacy via its EMR. Given the widespread presence of ACOs, and the many clinics that do not employ pharmacists, this model could be useful to a large number of providers. Progressive clinics and pharmacies that want to succeed under the value-based payment programs being used more commonly today should explore the feasibility of implementing a similar approach in their communities [6].

Facilitators and obstacles of this collaborative approach can be identified. An important facilitator is having a trusted, motivated partner [7–9]. In this case, the partners gained familiarity by working on a small project facilitated by the Iowa Department of Public Health and the University of Iowa. Other prospective partners can identify opportunities to work together to address a problem in their community or among mutual patients. Perhaps it is finding a way to improve medication adherence, or in coordinating to better manage a key chronic condition, such as diabetes or hypertension, represented in performance metrics. Working together will give the partners an opportunity to get to know each other better, which is a starting point for developing a working rapport and trust [10].

A related facilitator for establishing successful clinic-pharmacy collaboration is to start small [10]. Both of the key practitioners from the clinic and pharmacy partners in this case identified starting in a limited way as an important factor in their progress. The clinic approached the pharmacy about providing some type of service that could help with their patients who were the highest medication users. The pharmacy had some experience with providing comprehensive medication reviews, and offered that as a viable option. Upon discussion, the partners agreed that the clinic would send a list of patients using at least ten medications, who became the targets for the first phase of the medication review service. This relatively narrow focus allowed the clinic and pharmacy to work through issues that arose as the new program was implemented, including communications with patients, responsiveness of clinic providers to pharmacist notes and pharmacy access to the clinic EMR. Potential partners seeking to pursue a similar collaborative model would benefit from discussing patient groups or issues to get their collaboration started. Then, spend time clarifying roles of the parties involved, including what services are to be performed, how communication will be conducted, and details for any payments or revenue sharing. Starting small, but with a clear plan, should support positive results on innovative collaboration for pharmacy services.

A third factor that can contribute to a successful collaborative working relationship is to collect data that track performance on key variables or metrics [6]. In this case, the parties tracked the number and type of medication-related problems identified and managed through the comprehensive medication review service. In addition, they examined finances associated with the program. It takes some planning and effort to determine which data to collect, how it will be collected, and then how it will be analyzed. Each of these partners had some resources and experience in evaluating new services or programs, which helped them make a feasible evaluation plan for their collaboration. In addition, they worked with Telligen, the CMS quality improvement organization (QIO) that serves Iowa. While Telligen did not have data for the commercial ACO, they did have data for the small number of Medicare beneficiaries who received a CMR. Partners should prospectively plan for some type of evaluation of their efforts at collaboration. Such an assessment can be used internally to build support for the program (e.g., among providers), as well as externally (e.g., to talk with payers or other potential partners).

An obstacle encountered by these partners was limited responsiveness by clinic providers to pharmacist notes sent either by fax or via the clinic EMR. This likely occurred since many of the providers were not used to receiving clinical notes from pharmacists. Rather, their communications with pharmacists tended to focus on renewing prescription orders or clarifying questions on new orders. For the CMR service, the pharmacist had to communicate with the providers about potential problems with the medications, sometimes with suggested changes in therapy. Again, the clinic providers may not have wanted to receive such feedback at first and ignored it. The lead clinic physician spent more time communicating with his colleagues about the collaboration, and the responsiveness of the providers improved. Prospective partners, especially within a clinic or system, should have discussions beforehand about what types of communications they could receive and how they should respond to them. Having clear expectations about communication should smooth out some of the progress when implementing a new collaborative program.

Patient acceptance was a challenge for the collaborative comprehensive medication review service delivered to the two patients groups identified at the clinic. This mostly arose because not all of the patients were regular patients at the partner pharmacy. Rather, the pharmacy was serving as the provider for the CMR services for the clinic's patients. Though the clinic sent letters to the patients before the pharmacy telephoned them, over half of the patients initially declined the CMR service. An adjustment in the letter from the clinic, incorporating their physician's agreement, helped the providers and patients both have more confidence in that particular patient receiving the CMR service. The pharmacy also made helpful changes in their phone script when contacting the patients. The latest service, focused on medication adherence, is directed only at current patients of the clinic and pharmacy. Thus, the difficulty of not having a relationship with the patient will not be present for the pharmacy. Prospective partners can address this issue by limiting their collaboration to only mutual patients. In addition, having an announcement about any collaborative program initiated by the clinic would be vital to informing patients about a new service opportunity.

5. Conclusions

In conclusion, this case report describes an innovative partnership between a medical clinic system and a regional pharmacy chain. Both organizations are innovative, and were willing to work together. Their collaboration built upon initial discussions and planning. They were able to continue to communicate to address problems that arose with their collaborative program. The outcomes were positive for both the clinic and pharmacy, their patients and the payer(s). The clinic improved performance associated with ACO metrics and received helpful clinical input from a pharmacist. The pharmacy expanded its services and generated new revenue. Patients received more coordinated care, which supported some cost savings for the patients and payers. Interested clinics, health systems and pharmacies are encouraged to pursue similar collaborations, which could be key to success in today's healthcare environment.

Supplementary Materials: The following are available online at http://www.mdpi.com/2226-4787/7/2/62/s1, Table S1: Medication-related problems identified during comprehensive medication reviews (CMRs) (N = 116), Table S2: Pharmacist actions for medication-related problems (N = 116).

Funding: This project was funded by the Iowa Department of Public Health.

Acknowledgments: The author would like to acknowledge Donald Skinner and Ashley Loeffelholz for their participation in the interviews for this study.

Conflicts of Interest: The author declares no conflict of interests. The funder had no role in the design of the study; in the collection, analyses, or interpretation of data; in the writing of the manuscript; or in the decision to publish the results.

References

1. Burwell, S.M. Setting value-based payment goals–HHS efforts to improve U.S. health care. *N. Engl. J. Med.* **2015**, *372*, 897–899. [CrossRef] [PubMed]
2. Maddox, K.E.J.; Sen, A.P.; Samson, L.W.; Zuckerman, R.B.; DeLew, N.; Epstein, A.M. Elements of program design in Medicare's value-based and alternative payment models: a narrative review. *J. Gen. Intern. Med.* **2017**, *32*, 1249–1254. [CrossRef] [PubMed]
3. Community Care of North Carolina. Community Pharmacy Enhanced Services Network. Available online: http://www.communitycarenc.org/what-we-do/supporting-primary-care/pharmacy/cpesn (accessed on 5 May 2019).
4. Parekh, N.; McClellan, M.; Shrank, W.H. Payment reform, medication use, and costs: can we afford to leave out drugs? *J. Gen. Intern. Med.* **2019**, *34*, 473–476. [CrossRef] [PubMed]
5. Luder, H.R.; Shannon, P.; Kirby, J.; Frede, S.M. Community pharmacist collaboration with a patient-centered medical home: Establishment of a patient-centered medical neighborhood and payment model. *J. Am. Pharm. Assoc.* **2018**, *58*, 44–50. [CrossRef] [PubMed]

6. Cowart, K.; Olson, K. Impact of pharmacist care provision in value-based care settings: How are we measuring value-added services? *J. Am. Pharm. Assoc.* **2019**, *59*, 125–128. [CrossRef] [PubMed]

7. Snyder, M.E.; Earl, T.R.; Gilchrist, S.; Greenberg, M.; Heisler, H.; Revels, M.; Matson-Koffman, D. Collaborative drug therapy management: Case studies of three community-based models of care. *Prev. Chron. Dis.* **2015**, *12*, 140504. [CrossRef] [PubMed]

8. Zillich, A.J.; Doucette, W.R.; Carter, B.L.; Kreiter, C.D. Development and initial validation of an instrument to measure physician-pharmacist collaboration from the physician perspective. *Value Health* **2005**, *8*, 59–66. [CrossRef] [PubMed]

9. Geonnotti, K.; Taylor, E.F.; Peikes, D.; Schottenfeld, L.; Burak, H.; McNellis, R.; Genevro, J. *Engaging Primary Care Practices in Quality Improvement Strategies for Practice Facilitators*; AHRQ: Rockville, MD, USA, 2015.

10. McDonough, R.P.; Doucette, W.R. Developing collaborative working relationships between pharmacists and physicians. *J. Am. Pharm. Assoc.* **2001**, *41*, 682–692.

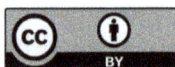

pharmacy

MDPI

Article

A Primer on Quality Assurance and Performance Improvement for Interprofessional Chronic Kidney Disease Care: A Path to Joint Commission Certification

Linda Awdishu [1,2,*], Teri Moore [2], Michelle Morrison [2], Christy Turner [2] and Danuta Trzebinska [2]

1   School of Pharmacy and Pharmaceutical Sciences, University of California, San Diego, CA 92093, USA
2   Nephrology Department, School of Medicine, University of California, San Diego, CA 92093, USA
*   Correspondence: lawdishu@ucsd.edu; Tel.: +1-858-534-3919

Received: 14 February 2019; Accepted: 27 June 2019; Published: 3 July 2019

check for updates

Abstract: Interprofessional care for chronic kidney disease facilitates the delivery of high quality, comprehensive care to a complex, at-risk population. Interprofessional care is resource intensive and requires a value proposition. Joint Commission certification is a voluntary process that improves patient outcomes, provides external validity to hospital administration and enhances visibility to patients and referring providers. This is a single-center, retrospective study describing quality assurance and performance improvement in chronic kidney disease, Joint Commission certification and quality outcomes. A total of 440 patients were included in the analysis. Thirteen quality indicators consisting of clinical and process of care indicators were developed and measured for a period of two years from 2009–2017. Significant improvements or at least persistently high performance were noted for key quality indicators such as blood pressure control (85%), estimation of cardiovascular risk (100%), measurement of hemoglobin A1c (98%), vaccination (93%), referrals for vascular access and transplantation (100%), placement of permanent dialysis access (61%), discussion of advanced directives (94%), online patient education (71%) and completion of office visit documentation (100%). High patient satisfaction scores (94–96%) are consistent with excellent quality of care provided.

Keywords: chronic kidney disease; interprofessional care; quality assurance

---

1. Introduction

Interprofessional (IP) care for chronic kidney disease (CKD) facilitates the delivery of comprehensive care to a complex, at-risk population. Evidence based strategies for slowing progression of CKD are well described but not consistently applied to the individual patient. Interprofessional teams focus on implementing evidenced based care to slow down the progression of CKD, educating patients about their disease and streamlining the transition to end stage renal disease (ESRD). This comprehensive care has been shown to reduce hospitalizations [1–6] lower mortality [1,3,4,7–9], slow the progression of CKD [1–3,10,11] and prepare patients for transitions in care [4,7,8]. Despite these benefits, IP CKD programs are difficult to implement because of resources. Advocates of IP care should provide evidence of value to justify the additional cost since CKD consumes a disproportionate share of healthcare funding globally [12,13]. The Joint Commission (TJC) certification is a voluntary process that can improve patient outcomes, provides external validity to hospital administration and enhances visibility to patients and referring providers. In this paper, we describe the development of an IP CKD program and the pathway to TJC disease specific certification in CKD care.

2. Materials and Methods

This is a retrospective, single center study of all adult patients receiving care in the IP CKD Program from July 2011–2016. We included all adult patients with CKD receiving IP care. Patients with less than 3 months of follow up in the program were excluded from the analysis. Clinical data including patient demographics, comorbidities, laboratory results, vital signs measured during clinic visits, medications, process of care measures as well as outcomes of dialysis initiation, transplantation or death were extracted from the electronic health record (EHR). To analyze patient demographics and performance measures for each recertification cycle, we used descriptive statistics including mean and standard deviation (SD) or median and range for continuous data when appropriate, frequency counts and percentage for categorical data. Descriptive statistics were calculated using R version (3.4.2). The institutional review board (IRB) for human subjects approved this study with a waiver of consent.

2.1. Program Description

The pharmacist wrote the proposal for the IP CKD Program and obtained funding from the health system. This program was set up as its own cost center and the pharmacist funding is supported by the health system for direct patient care and administration of the CKD program. The nephrologist and pharmacist created the infrastructure for the program including a mission statement, clinic schedules, job descriptions, template notes and standard orders. Our institutional IP CKD Program opened in 2007 and provides comprehensive care to patients with CKD stage 2 through 5. Patients are referred for IP care by a nephrologist or through direct referral from other disciplines. The program does not have specific referring criteria; rather any patient who the referring physician feels would benefit from IP CKD care is eligible. The program consists of two half-day clinics, which operate in the same physical space as other nephrology clinics. Patients are seen every 1 to 6 months depending on disease severity. Visits are approximately 90 and 45 min for new and return patients, respectively. The core IP team consists of a nephrologist/medical director, pharmacist/program administrator, nurse, dietitian, social worker and patient education coordinator. Interprofessional care is provided based on institutional CKD guidelines and documented in the EHR. Chronic kidney disease guidelines were developed using Kidney Disease Improving Global Outcomes (KDIGO) guidelines, Kidney Disease Outcomes Quality Initiative (KDOQI), Joint National Commission hypertension guidelines, American Diabetes Association diabetes care guidelines, American Heart Association guidelines as well primary and tertiary references [14–69]. These were approved by our institutional Pharmacy and Therapeutics Committee and updated annually.

Patients receive many services in addition to the traditional nephrology care such as cardiovascular risk assessment, dietary counseling on CKD diet, weight loss, vaccinations, smoking cessation, medication reconciliation and management, personalized medication schedules, assistance with insurance and transportation issues as well as assistance with transition of care to transplant, dialysis or hospice (Appendix A). Patient education is provided during each visit on an individual basis, through online educational videos (https://www.youtube.com/playlist?list=PLp5o_4MxOoYRJ_zYObvWzC-O0VE7wFqaG) and in a classroom setting. Educational topics include introduction to CKD, medications and CKD, diet, social support networks, renal replacement modalities and transplantation.

Each team member has defined roles and responsibilities to optimize patient care. All members of the IP team receive orientation to the program and institutional CKD guidelines. Team members are evaluated for competency initially and must demonstrate continuing competency and education annually. Competency is assessed verbally and through the demonstration of skills where appropriate. Team members answer questions about mini case scenarios to test their knowledge of CKD staging, overall goals of care based on CKD stage, laboratory parameters and foods high in phosphorus and potassium. Skills such as blood pressure measurement or administration of medications are evaluated by demonstration. Contemporary topics in CKD care are reviewed during a mandatory monthly journal club. The Medical Director and Program Administrator conduct annual performance reviews for all team members incorporating 360-degree feedback from team members.

2.2. Design of Quality Assessment and Performance Improvement Program (QAPI) and CKD Registry

The IP team determined appropriate quality indicators consisting of clinical, process and financial measures such as blood pressure (BP) control, prevalence of permanent vascular access at dialysis initiation, vaccination rates, patient education among others (Table 1). These measures were chosen on the basis of their importance for delaying CKD progression, streamlining transitions in care, improving patient experience and applicability to the majority of the program population. Each quality indicator was defined, baseline and targets established and strategies were developed to achieve target goals. For example, we defined BP control as the percentage of patients achieving the target BP per Joint National Committee guidelines. We established our baseline rate of control and set a target for improvement. Strategies to achieve the target included medical assistant education on performing a BP measurement, providing home BP monitors and logs to patients for home monitoring, patient education and nursing telephone follow up for patients with uncontrolled hypertension.

We developed a CKD registry in the EHR enabling the automated reporting of CKD outcomes. Data is electronically extracted and presented in a QAPI dashboard, which is reviewed on a monthly basis by the IP team and submitted to TJC. All outliers are reviewed in detail during the monthly team meeting and new strategies to achieve targets are developed on an as needed basis.

Table 1. Summary of performance measures.

Indicators	Type/Definition	Target Goal	Rationale	Time Period of Implementation
Systolic and diastolic blood pressure	Clinical Median SBP and DBP values.	SBP < 130 DBP < 80	The control of blood pressure in the United States continues to be suboptimal. Among adults with hypertension, 48% were at goal [70]. Control of blood pressure is associated with a reduction in cardiovascular morbidity and mortality and slower CKD progression.	2009–2011
BP Control	Clinical Percentage of office visits with systolic blood pressure at goal according to national guidelines.	Positive trend		2011–2015
Hemoglobin	Clinical Median hemoglobin value.	10.5–12 g/dL	The target hemoglobin in CKD is controversial [17,38]. Studies have demonstrated that normalizing the hemoglobin value with erythropoietin stimulating agents results in increased risk of cardiovascular morbidity and mortality.	2009–2011
Pneumococcal vaccinations	Clinical/Percentage of patients with documented vaccination with Prevnar 13® and Pneumovax 23®.	Positive trend	Patients with CKD are at increased risk of pneumococcal infection and vaccination is recommended by the Centers for Disease Prevention and Control [71].	2011–2013
Fistula at time of dialysis initiation	Clinical/Percentage of patients starting hemodialysis with arteriovenous fistula (AVF) in place.	Positive trend	AVF use for hemodialysis is associated with improved morbidity and mortality and lower costs compared to the use of a central venous catheter. Despite this, use of CVC nearly exceeds 80% in patients initiating hemodialysis. In 2006, the Centers for Medicare and Medicaid set a 66% national prevalent AVF goal, resulting in improvements in prevalent but not incident hemodialysis patients [72,73].	2013–2017

Table 1. *Cont.*

Indicators	Type/Definition	Target Goal	Rationale	Time Period of Implementation
Vascular access and kidney transplant referral	Process of Care/Percentage of medically appropriate patients with eGFR < 20 mL/min/1.73 m^2 with referral to vascular access and/or transplantation. Not all patients are transplant candidates and we use criteria from the transplant program to screen for referral (i.e., age less than 70 years, no active cancer in the past 5 years and adherent to therapies). Patients who decline dialysis and/or chose palliative care are not referred to vascular surgery.	Positive trend	Standardizing the referral process for vascular access and transplantation using specific criteria would improve rates of timely and appropriate referrals.	2009–2011
Advanced Directives	Process of Care/Percentage of patients with whom advanced directives were discussed.	Positive trend	Nephrologists caring for CKD patients are in a position to discuss transitions in care and patient preferences.	2011–2013
Patient Education	Process of Care/All new patients receiving education on CKD within 3 months of entering the program.	Positive trend	Patient education can increase knowledge of CKD progression and complications with the goal of increasing patient engagement.	2009–2011
	Process of Care/Online education viewing.			2015–2017
Testing of Hemoglobin A1c	Process of Care/All patients with DM and CKD stage 2–5 with HgA1c tested in last 6 months.	90%	Tight control of glucose is associated with a reduction of microvascular and macrovascular complications. Patients with controlled diabetes should have HgA1c checked every 6 months and if uncontrolled every 3 months [61].	2015–2017
Access to care	Process of Care/Median days to first appointment.	Negative trend	Two half day clinics limits the number of visits. Patients experienced long waiting periods from referral to first appointment.	2013–2015
ASCVD risk estimation	Process of Care/Percentage of patient visits with ASCVD risk estimated and documented.	Positive trend	Cardiovascular disease is the leading cause of death in patients with CKD. The ASCVD risk calculator provides an estimate of a patient's risk for a cardiovascular event with the goal of reducing the risk with medical management and lifestyle modification [74].	2015–2017
Cancellation rate	Financial/Percentage of office visits cancelled by patients.	Negative trend	Patients with CKD have numerous barriers to their access to care. Evaluating the clinic cancellation rate and reasons may improve the appointment process and access to CKD care.	2011–2013
Encounter documentation	Financial/Percentage of office visit encounters with complete documentation within 48 h.	Positive trend	Complete encounter documentation is required to effectively bill for services.	2013–2015

BP = blood pressure, SBP = systolic blood pressure, DBP = diastolic blood pressure, CKD = chronic kidney disease, AVF = arteriovenous fistula, CVC = central venous catheter, eGFR = estimated glomerular filtration rate, DM = diabetes mellitus, ASCVD = atherosclerotic cardiovascular disease.

3. Results

A total of 440 patients currently receive care in the IP CKD program. The demographics are summarized in Table 2.

Table 2. Patient demographics.

Characteristic	n = 440
Age, years (mean ± SD)	64.2 ± 14.5
Gender, Male (%)	55
Ethnicity, Hispanic (%)	24
CKD Stage (%)	
1–2	8
3	51
4	24
5	17
Urine protein to creatinine ratio, mg/mg (median, range)	325 (0–31,552)
Co-morbidities (%)	
Diabetes	50
Hypertension	92

The mean age of the population is 64.2 ± 14.5 years, 55% are male and the majority are White with 24% Hispanic patients as the second largest ethnicity. The majority of patients are in CKD stage 3 (51%) followed by stage 4 (24%) and stage 5 (17%). Approximately half of the patients have diabetes and 92% have hypertension.

Prior to the first certification in 2010, we chose the following quality indicators: (1) blood pressure control (median systolic and diastolic blood pressure, percent of patients with SBP ≤ 130 mmHg, percent of patients with SBP ≤ 140 mmHg), (2) median hemoglobin, (3) screening for appropriate patient referrals to vascular surgery and transplant and (4) percent of patients with education about CKD within 3 months of clinic enrollment (Table 3).

Table 3. Performance measurement report: 2009–2011.

	Reporting Year 1				Reporting Year 2			
Performance Indicators	Jul-Sep	Oct-Dec	Jan-Mar	Apr-Jun	Jul-Sep	Oct-Dec	Jan-Mar	Apr-Jun
All patients (N)	190	219	198	199	191	199	208	216
Median SBP (mmHg)	136	137	135	132	127	131	133	131
Median DBP (mmHg)	73	74	74	70	70	72	73	72
Median Hemoglobin (g/dL)	11	11	12	11	12	11	11	11
Patients with Referral to Vascular Surgery (%)	96	100	96	100	100	100	91	100
Patients with Referral to Transplant Program (%)	88	100	100	100	100	100	81	100
Patients Attending Patient Education Classes (%)	29	33	50	50	100	100	100	100

CKD = chronic kidney disease; DBP = diastolic blood pressure; SBP = systolic blood pressure.

We collected 6 months of data on those measures for the initial certification. The range of median systolic blood pressure was 127–137 mmHg, 36–44% of patients had SBP ≤ 130 mmHg, and 56–76% of patients had SBP ≤ 140 mmHg. Eighty-eight to 100% of patients had an appropriate referral to vascular surgery or transplantation. The percentage of patients who received in classroom CKD education within the first 3 months of joining the clinic steadily rose from 33% to 50%. We received Disease Specific Certification for CKD with no findings for improvement and were noted to be the first program in the United States with this designation. After receiving our certification, our surveyor invited us to present our program outcomes to the Quality Net Conference for the Centers for Medicare and Medicaid.

In the first recertification cycle 2011–2013, we chose the following indicators: (1) SBP ≤ 130 mmHg (2) pneumococcal vaccination rate (3) discussion of advanced directives (4) office visit cancellation rate (Table 4).

Table 4. Program performance measurement report: 2011–2013.

Performance Indicators	Reporting Year 1				Reporting Year 2			
	Jul-Sep	Oct-Dec	Jan-Mar	Apr-Jun	Jul-Sep	Oct-Dec	Jan-Mar	Apr-Jun
All patients (N)	209	210	223	227	228	214	211	225
Patients with SBP ≤ 130 mmHg (%)	57	54	51	51	45	47	49	58
Patients with SBP ≤ 140 mmHg (%)	79	88	79	85	75	74	79	82
Patients with Pneumococcal Vaccine (%)	49	61	69	84	88	89	93	93
Patients with Advanced Directive Addressed (%)	29	75	94	93	94	93	93	89
Office Visit Cancellation Rate (%)	-	28	25	19	23	22	25	21

SBP = systolic blood pressure.

Tight control of SBP ≤ 130 mmHg was achieved in 47–58% of patients and SBP ≤ 140mmHg was obtained in 74–85% of patients. Pneumococcal vaccination included Prevnar 13 and Pneumovax 23 and the rate rapidly rose from 49% in the first quarter to 93% in the last quarter of the cycle, as did the percentage of patients who discussed advanced directives with our social worker, from 29% to 94% over a two-year period. We were not able to sustain a decrease in the rate of cancellation of office visits after an initial drop from 28% to 19%.

In the second recertification cycle 2013–2015, we chose the following quality indicators: (1) SBP ≤ 130 and 140 mmHg (2) percentage of patients starting hemodialysis (HD) with AVF or arteriovenous graft (AVG), (3) median days from referral to first appointment in CKD clinic and (4) percent of office notes closed in EHR within 48 h (Table 5).

Table 5. Performance measurement report: 2013–2015.

Performance Indicators	Reporting Year 1				Reporting Year 2			
	Jul-Sep	Oct-Dec	Jan-Mar	Apr-Jun	Jul-Sep	Oct-Dec	Jan-Mar	Apr-Jun
All patients (N)	240	234	241	156	256	259	223	136
Patients w/SBP ≤ 130 mm Hg (%)	53	56	55	55	-	-	-	-
Patients w/SBP ≤ 140 mm Hg (%)	81	84	82	85	85	79	82	83
Patients w/AVF or Graft at Dialysis Start (%)	100	100	100	100	60	25	75	50
Median Days from Referral to First Appointment	17	13	7	7	9	37	12	14
Notes Closed within 48 h (%)	45	98	96	99	92	95	98	100

AVF = arteriovenous fistula, SBP = systolic blood pressure.

In December 2013, the Joint National Commission released new guidelines recommending a blood pressure goal of ≤140 mmHg and we decided to stop tracking the SBP goal ≤130 mmHg. We achieved SBP control to ≤140 mmHg in 79–85% of patients. The percentage of patients starting dialysis with AVF or AVG varied from 25 to 100% in different quarters with overall average of 77%. The median wait time from referral to first CKD clinic appointment varied from 7 to 37 days. The percentage of note closure within 48 h improved from 45% to 100%.

In the third recertification cycle 2015–2017, the following quality indicators were chosen: (1) patient viewing of online education videos, (2) continuation of permanent dialysis access indicator, (3) ordering of hemoglobin A1c every 6 months for patients with diabetes and (4) estimation and documentation of atherosclerotic cardiovascular disease (ASCVD) risk (Table 6).

Table 6. Performance measurement report: 2015–2017.

Performance Indicators	Reporting Year 1				Reporting Year 2			
	Jul-Sep	Oct-Dec	Jan-Mar	Apr-Jun	Jul-Sep	Oct-Dec	Jan-Mar	Apr-Jun
All patients (N)	216	252	219	247	224	225	212	243
% Patients w/AVF or Graft at Dialysis Start	100	89	50	100	0	44	56	50
% Patients w/Online Patient Education	0	10	25	35	48	55	64	71
% Patients w/DM and HgA1c Order within 6 mo	90	94	90	93	89	91	97	98
% Patients w/ASCVD Risk Documentation	82	100	99	100	98	99	100	100

ASCVD=atherosclerotic cardiovascular disease; AV = arteriovenous fistula, DM = diabetes mellitus, HgA1c = glycated hemoglobin, mo = months.

Fifteen patient education videos were created to improve treatment adherence, self-care, and clinical outcomes for CKD patients. CKD team members, including the nephrologist, pharmacist, dietitian, and social worker, each created several 5–15 min videos on specific topics related to CKD patient care that were peer reviewed by all team members. The videos were filmed in English at a production studio located on the main university campus. The entire process of video planning and filming took three months. After production of videos was complete, a CKD playlist of videos was created and published on YouTube (https://www.youtube.com/playlist?list=PLp5o_4MxOoYRJ_zYObvWzC-O0VE7wFqaG). A link to the videos was shared through e-mail, EHR patient messaging and posted on the CKD program website. A brochure advertising the videos was created and distributed to patients in clinic and through mail. For patients without computers, internet access, or mobile phones, a DVD was distributed in clinic or the video was played for the patient on clinic computers. Each patient was asked about video views during the office visit and this was documented in the EHR using smart fields for electronic data extraction. There was a steep and consistent increase in the percentage of patients viewing our online education videos from 0 to 71%. The 15 videos received a total of 284,808 views and the total number of views per videos ranged from 276 to 132,710 far surpassing our patient population. Videos with the highest views included content on: (1) symptoms of kidney disease (132,710 views), (2) stages of kidney disease (91,265 views), and (3) laboratory values of kidney disease (18,615 views).

For the other quality indicators, the percentage of permanent dialysis access at dialysis initiation was 0–100% (median 61%), and, the number of patients starting dialysis was low ranging from 0–3 per month. Hemoglobin A1c testing was high at baseline at 90% and remained consistently high with a range of 89–98%. ASCVD risk was not routinely documented in office visit notes at baseline. After implementation of an automated ASCVD risk estimate calculator in the EHR, we demonstrated an immediate increase in documentation to 82% in the first quarter of implementation and subsequent increase to 100% documentation. We received re-certification with no findings for improvement and positive feedback on the successful development of online education for patients with CKD.

Patient satisfaction was measured using The Consumer Assessment of Health Providers and Systems surveys administered by Press Ganey and collected for each certification and recertification cycle. From 2012 to present, the percentage of surveys where patients reported "yes, definitely" on a 3-point scale for their likelihood to recommend the program and the physician communication domain were approximately 94% and 96%, respectively.

4. Discussion

In this study, we demonstrated that IP care for CKD could be implemented and sustained over a long time period at an academic institution. The process of obtaining TJC certification is educational and rewarding. It provides opportunity to examine program performance and identify gaps in care. TJC certification ensures an ongoing process of quality measure development, implementation of interventions to achieve program goals and measurement of outcomes. In contrast to other regulatory agencies, TJC certification provides flexibility for programs to determine their own meaningful measures of performance. Over the past eight years, we have defined and measured 13 quality indicators for CKD care. Overall, we were able to improve performance on the majority of quality indicators or at least maintain the high performance. Most indicators were retired at the end of the recertification cycle. Some were considered critical to CKD care and were continued in additional cycles.

4.1. Blood Pressure Control

Blood pressure control remained a performance measure for 3 cycles of recertification since it is essential to preventing CKD progression and we found opportunity for performance improvement. On average, blood pressure control was achieved in 81% of patients. When we targeted a more stringent goal (<130/80 mmHg), between 53–67% of our patients were able to achieve that target. Despite a drop in control with implementation of more stringent targets, we still achieved higher rates of control compared to the literature. Thanamayooran and colleagues demonstrated that 40% of patients achieved a target blood pressure of <130/80 mmHg when receiving IP CKD care [75]. Surveys of the general population have demonstrated that 13.2–37% of patients with CKD achieve a target blood pressure [76,77].

Achieving a target clinic blood pressure proved to be challenging. To improve blood pressure control, the entire IP team was engaged in numerous aspects. Our medical assistants have yearly competency evaluation on accurate blood pressure measurement and ensure elevated blood pressure measurements are repeated and recorded. The dietitian counsels on dietary sodium restriction and educates patients on how to read food labels. The pharmacist assesses medication adherence, adverse effects of antihypertensives and optimizes therapy. Nurses perform routine telephone follow up on home blood pressure measurements for patients whose clinic measurements are not at goal. The social worker assesses financial resources and addresses barriers to medication access and provides a free blood pressure monitor to patients in need. The physician reviews the team recommendations, summarizes a plan that optimizes the antihypertensive regimen and includes principles of healthy lifestyle (regular exercise, low sodium diet, limiting alcohol intake, etc.). Over 90% of our patients monitor and log home blood pressure, which facilitates medication adjustment based on home readings. A significant number of patients have a white coat hypertension, so the use of clinic readings underestimates true blood pressure control [28,70]. With the implementation of and increased patient engagement in the EHR, it may become possible to report performance based on home readings. Future initiatives for blood pressure control include having patients enter their home readings into the MyChart portal of the EPIC EHR using their mobile device or laptop so values are recorded and actionable. We have not yet implemented this blood pressure initiative due to a lack of educational materials and resources to educate patients on this electronic reporting.

4.2. Education

Education on CKD is critical in empowering patients to be active participants in their care and has been associated with decrease in hospitalizations and mortality [1,3–5,7,8,11]. In a prospective, randomized, controlled trial of an IP CKD educational intervention, the IP care group showed a significant delay in initiation of dialysis therapy compared to the usual care group ($p < 0.0001$) [78]. Pre-dialysis education is important in assuring a smooth transition to dialysis including placement of permanent access and/or transition to transplantation [79]. Peritoneal dialysis (PD) and home hemodialysis (HD) are underutilized in the United States with ~90% of patients receiving in-center HD [80]. We believe that extensive education provided to our patients was the reason for a relatively high percent of our patients starting renal replacement therapy with PD (30%) compared to in-center HD (70%). This is consistent with other studies that showed that CKD education is associated with increased selection of home HD and PD modalities as opposed to in center HD [81]. In a survey of practicing nephrologists, over 90% of the nephrologists would choose home dialysis for themselves, yet few CKD patients are on home dialysis therapy [82]. Clinicians should apply the same standards for taking care of patients that they would desire for themselves or family members, should they develop ESRD. Various medical programs are increasingly adopting technology solutions to support self-management practices [83,84]. We were able to educate many more patients with online videos than group classes (70% vs. 33% respectively). Online education provides the solution to several barriers faced with in-person education including transportation to the facility, scheduling, learning pace (i.e., patients can watch videos at their convenience and pace), and frequent physician visits or hospitalization. One major limitation is the production of videos in different languages. Due to limited resources, we did not translate the education videos into Spanish; consequently, not every patient benefited from the videos.

4.3. Vascular Access

Timely permanent access creation for chronic dialysis is complicated by numerous clinical and psychosocial factors making this an important but challenging quality metric. Use of AVF for HD is associated with improved mortality and morbidity and lower cost compared to the use of a central venous catheter [10,72,85]. Over the last decade, the rate of AVF use in prevalent dialysis patients has improved significantly from approximately 35% to 65% [80]. However, at dialysis initiation, AVF use continues to be very low with over 80% of patients initiating dialysis using a tunneled catheter [80]. Emergent start of dialysis continues to be too common and likely contributes to high mortality and morbidity in the first 6 months of starting dialysis, especially in patients over 65 years of age [80].

Early in our program development, we experienced significant delays from patient referral to vascular surgery to the actual visit and/or placement of permanent vascular access. In order to address this problem, we created a joint CKD-vascular surgery clinic, scheduled once a month, where patients who had advanced CKD could see the nephrologist and surgeon during the same visit. This coordination of care resulted in timely vascular access evaluation and surgery. On average, 77% of patients started HD with a functional AVF in the first 2-year cycle and 61% in the second cycle. One challenge we encountered with this quality indicator is the small number of patients who transition from CKD stage 5 to HD making it difficult to compare and trend month-to-month data or to demonstrate significant improvement. Our results are similar to other studies demonstrating higher AVF rates of 45.2–68.4% in patients receiving IP CKD care compared to 4.8–58.8% in the usual care groups [1,4,86,87]. Despite receiving comprehensive education and IP care, there are patients who will start HD with a tunneled catheter for multiple reasons including: (1) late referral of patients with advanced CKD and low socioeconomic status, (2) emergent dialysis for acute kidney injury in patients who previously had moderate (not advanced) CKD at baseline and (3) patients who initially choose peritoneal dialysis, yet start with HD due to unforeseen acute deterioration in health. We are developing and implementing a protocol for urgent start PD (within 24–48 h after placement of PD catheter) to address the latter problem.

4.4. Transplantation

Survival rates for patients with ESRD are much better for those undergoing kidney transplantation compared to those receiving chronic dialysis [80]. Our program ensures timely referral of appropriate candidates to the transplant program once the GFR approaches 20 mL/min/1.73 m^2. Our experience is that patients from our CKD IP program have better health related outcomes (i.e., health maintenance, self-monitoring of health outcomes and medication adherence) and experience a higher likelihood of placement on the transplant waiting list (not reported). However, we have not measured and compared our referral to listing ratios to that of usual nephrology care. Some patients receive preemptive kidney transplantation while others start accruing waiting time prior to initiation of dialysis (i.e., once the GFR is below 20 mL/min/1.73 m^2). To facilitate transplant referral, we have worked with the transplant program and informatics team to enable the clear and visible display of transplant listing status in each patient's EHR.

4.5. Vaccinations

Vaccinations are one of the most beneficial health prevention strategies to reduce morbidity and mortality associated with communicable infections. Patients with CKD should receive an annual influenza vaccine, pneumococcal and hepatitis B vaccinations [71]. We focused on pneumococcal rather than hepatitis B vaccination since our baseline rate for hepatitis B vaccination was high whereas there was an opportunity for improvement in pneumococcal vaccination rate. To improve this measure, we ensured accurate documentation of vaccination history by the pharmacist for every patient and we streamlined the vaccination ordering process. We experienced a robust increase in pneumococcal vaccine administrations from a baseline of less than 50% to over 90% patients at the end of the reporting cycle.

4.6. Advanced Directives

During the re-certification process, there is opportunity to discuss the retirement of measures and adoption of new quality measures. Our Joint Commission surveyor felt that providers in IP CKD clinic are in a unique position to discuss transitions in care and patient preferences and suggested we start tracking discussions about advanced directives with our patients. Discussion of advanced directives can be uncomfortable especially in an ambulatory care setting and with younger patients. Our social worker felt best prepared and positioned to lead the discussions with patients. Despite our perceived concerns around this measure, we were able to initiate conversations about advanced directives in 90% patients, which was a significant improvement from a baseline value of less than 30%. In 2015, Medicare spending exceeded $64 billion for beneficiaries with CKD and $34 billion for ESRD costs totaling over $98 billion [80]. The cost is disproportionally high for dialysis patients in the last year of their life. Discussing advanced directives with pre-dialysis and dialysis patients is critical to select medical interventions that are aligned with patient preferences, while reducing unnecessary cost to society.

4.7. Cardiovascular Disease Risk

Cardiovascular disease (CVD) remains the leading cause of death in the United States and most other developed countries [88]. Among patients with CKD, death from CVD is far more common than progression to ESRD. CKD has been identified as an independent risk factor for CVD, even after adjustment for usual comorbid conditions [74]. The risk for CVD increases as GFR declines [80,89]. Assessing the risk is critical given high prevalence and poorer prognosis after a CV event in patients with CKD compared to general population (i.e., adjusted two-year survival of patients with acute myocardial infarction is 81% in general population, compared to 56% for CKD Stage 4–5 [80]. Estimating risk for CVD in patients with CKD is complicated due to the presence of traditional and non-traditional cardiac risk factors. Online and smart phone risk calculators have been developed by the American College of Cardiology, available: http://tools.acc.org/ASCVD-Risk-Estimator-Plus/#!/calculate/estimate/ (Last Accessed: 6/25/18). We worked with the informatics team to implement an electronic ASCVD risk calculator in the EHR, resulting in a quick and steep increase in documentation of this important risk from zero to 100% by the end of the reporting cycle. Patients with high ASCVD risk receive additional attention in terms of education on the importance of lifestyle modifications, appropriate medical management and referrals to cardiology.

4.8. Other Indicators

For other indicators, we were successful in improving the rate of completion of office visit documentation in the EHR within 48 h of the office visit from below 50% to approximately 100%. We ensured that over 90% of diabetic patients had HgA1C checked at least every 6 months. We did not make much improvement in some process measures like clinic cancellation rate or access to care due to numerous factors outside of our control.

4.9. Challenges

Upfront cost of an IP team is the biggest challenge to implementing and maintaining IP CKD care. The standard fee-for-service model in the United States does not reimburse many team members other than physicians or advanced practice professionals (physician extenders). Dieticians are reimbursed by Medicare for evaluating patients with CKD stage 4, though we encountered logistical challenges with scheduling patients for two separate visits (with the physician and dietician) during the same CKD visit, obtaining insurance authorization for each visit with the dietitian and placing a physician referral to the dietician for each subsequent visit. Medicare provides reimbursement for 6 educational sessions on dialysis modalities, but these sessions must be of at least 30 minutes duration and provided by a physician or physician extender. Medication therapy management services provided by the pharmacist are not reimbursable under the current Medicare structure since the CKD visit is done in conjunction with the physician. Social worker services are not reimbursable unless counseling is provided for a mental health condition. However, IP CKD programs have a potential for creating downstream or indirect revenues by increase in outpatients starts of dialysis, more patients starting dialysis with a permanent access, more PD utilization, improved referrals for living kidney donor transplantation and in turn higher rates of transplantation. All of those help to offset the cost of IP care or even make IP CKD programs cost effective.

In 2015, Medicare ESRD expenditure/person/year was $88,750 for a HD patient, $75,140 for a PD patient and $34,084 for a transplant patient [80]. Patients who receive dialysis with AVF have a lower total cost/member/year compared to those with HD catheters [80]. More recently, Lin and colleagues evaluated the cost-effectiveness of a theoretical IP CKD program compared to usual CKD care in U.S. Medicare beneficiaries with stage 3 and 4 CKD between the age of 45 and 84 years. The results of the model showed that a Medicare-funded IP CKD program could be cost effective by decreasing the need for RRT and prolonging life [13].

Space may also pose a challenge when developing a new program. We initially secured space by sharing the same clinic space and time allocation as the general nephrology clinics. This was not as challenging compared to securing new space as part of our goals to expand the program. We struggle with obtaining new space to add additional clinics in other geographic locations to better serve our diverse patient population.

4.10. Limitations of Our Study

There are several limitations to our study. This is an observational, descriptive study evaluating the impact of Joint Commission certification and recertification on clinical and process of care outcomes for patients with CKD. Since there was no control group in this study, it is possible that clinical outcomes achieved in this program could be achieved in a physician-based clinic. However, various team members led many of the quality improvement projects (i.e., vaccination rates by pharmacist, advanced directives by social worker, permanent dialysis access by a nephrologist) and it is unlikely that one team member alone could do all of it. This shared approach was critical to our success and this degree of quality improvement would not likely be sustained over a long period of time in a physician-based clinic. Secondly, some of the patients referred to our program received care in the general nephrology clinic prior to referral and it is possible the previous care had impacted their outcomes, but this bias may have been in both directions for the outcomes of interest. Lastly, the results may not be generalizable to non-academic programs given differences in the informatics resources, patient population and IP team members. Additional research is needed to compare the outcomes and cost-effectiveness of IP care to usual CKD care and to evaluate the feasibility of disseminating this model of care to other institutions.

5. Conclusions

Joint Commission certification requires the development and implementation of robust quality assurance and performance improvement plans. CKD care delivery involves a set complex processes and improvement in outcome measures are best achieved using a team-based approach where high quality care is a priority for all IP team members. Achieving certification is not a simple task, it requires strong leadership, dedication, time commitment and institutional support with the reward of nationally recognized, external validation of the excellence in care to the patients we serve.

Author Contributions: Conceptualization, L.A. and D.T.; methodology, L.A. and D.T.; formal analysis, L.A. and D.T.; investigation, L.A., T.M., M.M., C.T., D.T.; data curation, L.A., T.M.; writing—original draft preparation, L.A., T.M., M.M., C.T., D.T.; writing—review & editing, L.A., M.M., C.T., D.T.

Funding: This research received no external funding.

Conflicts of Interest: The authors declare no conflict of interest.

Appendix A

Table A1. Chronic kidney disease program team roles and responsibilities.

Medical Director	1. Medical history 2. Physical exam 3. Orders for encounter (lab tests, referrals, medications, follow-up) 4. Documentation of visit in EPIC 5. Supervises nephrology fellow and medical residents 6. Supervises interprofessional team 7. Plan and present classes on kidney disease 8. Oversees medical management for CKD population 9. Strategic planning with respect to program growth, outcomes 10. Participate in staff evaluations 11. Attend and direct team meetings
Pharmacist and Program Administrator	1. Medication history and medication reconciliation 2. Medication therapy management (evaluate doses for renal function, etc.) 3. Assist with orders for encounter (lab tests, referrals, medications, follow-up) 4. Counsel patient on new medications, medication changes and provide a current list of their medications 5. Documentation of visit in EPIC 6. Supervises pharmacy residents and students 7. Supervises interprofessional team 8. Plan and present classes on kidney disease 9. Responsible for analyzing and presenting program outcomes 10. Staff recruitment and performance appraisal 11. Lead team meetings 12. Strategic planning with respect to program growth, outcomes 13. Prepare budget annually
Dietitian	1. Evaluate nutritionally relevant information 2. Assess diet and make recommendations for changes in diet or dietary supplements 3. Document assessment, care plan and education in EPIC 4. Plan and present classes in nutrition 5. Create meal plans for individual needs 6. Monitor dietary change and provide feedback 7. Attend CKD team meetings
Case Manager	1. Brief psychosocial assessment on all new patients and document in EPIC 2. Assess for changes on return visits 3. Address any insurance and community resource needs with patients as appropriate 4. For patients in CKD IV or higher, begin discussing dialysis plans, preference for PD versus HD and location 5. Assist in teaching Modalities (Kidney Treatment Options) class to new patients and document their attendance and preference in EPIC progress notes 6. Refer patients anticipated to need dialysis for insurance verification 7. Assisting with transition to dialysis 8. Assist with placement in long term facilities or communication with outside facilities 9. Facilitate communication between patients, CKD team members and other medicine/surgical disciplines (example vascular access, interventional radiology) 10. For any unfunded or partially funded patients; notify dialysis administrator and clinical service chief and request temporary acceptance until funding is secured 11. Attend CKD team meetings

Table A1. *Cont.*

Nurse	1. Schedules patients into the CKD clinic 2. Triages new referrals to CKD clinic 3. Reviews clinic schedule every week to ensure appropriate numbers of patients 4. Prints out the after visit summary and discharges patient from the visit 5. Reviews next appointment, lab work needed for appointment, procedures, referrals and medication changes/prescriptions 6. Confirms patients understanding of care plan 7. Administers erythropoietin stimulating agents in clinic when prescribed 8. Administers vaccinations in clinic when prescribed 9. Documents in EPIC 10. Receives patient calls and requests for refills from call center and triages these to appropriate individuals 11. Attend CKD team meetings
Medical Assistant	1. Takes vital signs on patient (blood pressure, pulse height and weight) 2. Puts the patient into the rooms 3. Notifies CKD team of patient arrival 4. Triages late appointments with Medical Director or Program Administrator
Patient Education Coordinator/ Administrative Assistant	1. Schedule team meetings, create agendas and attend meeting 2. Maintain SharePoint site for communications 3. Coordinates all aspects of patient education classes (mailings, patient outreach, coordinate logistics for rooms, audio-visual, and refreshments, speakers, handouts) 4. Maintains database of all clinic patients 5. Prepare and mail new patient education packets 6. Collect patient data for quality indicators database 7. Maintain office and educational material supplies 8. Program coordinator for 10-week Wellness Program. Responsible for brochure, mailings, patient outreach, scheduling logistics for rooms, audio-visual, and refreshments, speakers, handouts

References

1. Chen, Y.R.; Yang, Y.; Wang, S.C.; Chiu, P.F.; Chou, W.Y.; Lin, C.Y.; Chang, J.M.; Chen, T.W.; Ferng, S.H.; Lin, C.L. Effectiveness of multidisciplinary care for chronic kidney disease in Taiwan: A 3-year prospective cohort study. *Nephrol. Dial. Transplant.* **2013**, *28*, 671–682. [CrossRef] [PubMed]

2. Chen, Y.R.; Yang, Y.; Wang, S.C.; Chou, W.Y.; Chiu, P.F.; Lin, C.Y.; Tsai, W.C.; Chang, J.M.; Chen, T.W.; Ferng, S.H.; et al. Multidisciplinary care improves clinical outcome and reduces medical costs for pre-end-stage renal disease in Taiwan. *Nephrology* **2014**, *19*, 699–707. [CrossRef] [PubMed]

3. Shi, Y.; Xiong, J.; Chen, Y.; Deng, J.; Peng, H.; Zhao, J. The effectiveness of multidisciplinary care models for patients with chronic kidney disease: A systematic review and meta-analysis. *Int. Urol. Nephrol.* **2018**, *50*, 301–312. [CrossRef] [PubMed]

4. Goldstein, M.; Yassa, T.; Dacouris, N.; McFarlane, P. Multidisciplinary predialysis care and morbidity and mortality of patients on dialysis. *Am. J. Kidney Dis.* **2004**, *44*, 706–714. [CrossRef]

5. Levin, A.; Lewis, M.; Mortiboy, P.; Faber, S.; Hare, I.; Porter, E.C.; Mendelssohn, D.C. Multidisciplinary predialysis programs: Quantification and limitations of their impact on patient outcomes in two Canadian settings. *Am. J. Kidney Dis.* **1997**, *29*, 533–540. [CrossRef]

6. Yu, Y.J.; Wu, I.W.; Huang, C.Y.; Hsu, K.H.; Lee, C.C.; Sun, C.Y.; Hsu, H.J.; Wu, M.S. Multidisciplinary predialysis education reduced the inpatient and total medical costs of the first 6 months of dialysis in incident hemodialysis patients. *PLoS ONE* **2014**, *9*, e112820. [CrossRef] [PubMed]

7. Wang, S.M.; Hsiao, L.C.; Ting, I.W.; Yu, T.M.; Liang, C.C.; Kuo, H.L.; Chang, C.T.; Liu, J.H.; Chou, C.Y.; Huang, C.C. Multidisciplinary care in patients with chronic kidney disease: A systematic review and meta-analysis. *Eur. J. Intern Med.* **2015**, *26*, 640–645. [CrossRef]

8. Hemmelgarn, B.R.; Manns, B.J.; Zhang, J.; Tonelli, M.; Klarenbach, S.; Walsh, M.; Culleton, B.F. Association between multidisciplinary care and survival for elderly patients with chronic kidney disease. *J. Am. Soc. Nephrol.* **2007**, *18*, 993–999. [CrossRef]

9. Curtis, B.M.; Ravani, P.; Malberti, F.; Kennett, F.; Taylor, P.A.; Djurdjev, O.; Levin, A. The short- and long-term impact of multi-disciplinary clinics in addition to standard nephrology care on patient outcomes. *Nephrol. Dial. Transplant.* **2005**, *20*, 147–154. [CrossRef]

10. Chen, P.M.; Lai, T.S.; Chen, P.Y.; Lai, C.F.; Yang, S.Y.; Wu, V.; Chiang, C.K.; Kao, T.W.; Huang, J.W.; Chiang, W.C.; et al. Multidisciplinary care program for advanced chronic kidney disease: Reduces renal replacement and medical costs. *Am. J. Med.* **2015**, *128*, 68–76. [CrossRef]

11. Bayliss, E.A.; Bhardwaja, B.; Ross, C.; Beck, A.; Lanese, D.M. Multidisciplinary team care may slow the rate of decline in renal function. *Clin. J. Am. Soc. Nephrol.* **2011**, *6*, 704–710. [CrossRef] [PubMed]

12. Fluck, R.J.; Taal, M.W. What is the value of multidisciplinary care for chronic kidney disease? *PLoS Med.* **2018**, *15*, e1002533. [CrossRef] [PubMed]

13. Lin, E.; Chertow, G.M.; Yan, B.; Malcolm, E.; Goldhaber-Fiebert, J.D. Cost-effectiveness of multidisciplinary care in mild to moderate chronic kidney disease in the United States: A modeling study. *PLoS Med.* **2018**, *15*, e1002532. [CrossRef] [PubMed]

14. Hebert, L.A.; Bhardwaja, B.; Ross, C.; Beck, A.; Lanese, D.M. Effects of blood pressure control on progressive renal disease in blacks and whites. Modification of Diet in Renal Disease Study Grou. *Hypertension* **1997**, *30*, 428–435. [CrossRef] [PubMed]

15. Gerstein, H.; Yusuf, S.; Mann, J.F.E.; Hoogwerf, B.; Zinman, B.; Held, C.; Fisher, M.; Wolffenbuttel, B.H.R.; Pagans, J.B.; Richardson, L.; et al. Effects of ramipril on cardiovascular and microvascular outcomes in people with diabetes mellitus: Results of the HOPE study and MICRO-HOPE substudy. Heart Outcomes Prevention Evaluation Study Investigators. *Lancet* **2000**, *355*, 253–259.

16. Syrjanen, J.; Mustonen, J.; Pasternack, A. Hypertriglyceridaemia and hyperuricaemia are risk factors for progression of IgA nephropathy. *Nephrol. Dial. Transplant.* **2000**, *15*, 34–42. [CrossRef]

17. IV. NKF-K/DOQI Clinical Practice Guidelines for Anemia of Chronic Kidney Disease: Update 2000. *Am. J. Kidney Dis.* **2001**, *37*, S182–S238. Available online: https://www.ajkd.org/article/S0272-6386(01)70008-X/fulltext (accessed on 2 July 2019). [CrossRef]

18. III. NKF-K/DOQI Clinical Practice Guidelines for Vascular Access: Update 2000. *Am. J. Kidney Dis.* **2001**, *37*, S137–S181. Available online: https://www.ajkd.org/article/S0272-6386(01)70007-8/fulltext (accessed on 2 July 2019).

19. Kopple, J.D. National kidney foundation K/DOQI clinical practice guidelines for nutrition in chronic renal failure. *Am. J. Kidney Dis.* **2001**, *37*, S66–S70. [CrossRef]

20. Parving, H.H.; Lehnert, H.; Bröchner-Mortensen, J.; Gomis, R.; Andersen, S.; Arner, P. The effect of irbesartan on the development of diabetic nephropathy in patients with type 2 diabetes. *N. Engl. J. Med.* **2001**, *345*, 870–878.

21. Svensson, P.; de Faire, U.; Sleight, P.; Yusuf, S.; Ostergren, J. Comparative effects of ramipril on ambulatory and office blood pressures: A HOPE Substudy. *Hypertension* **2001**, *38*, E28–E32. [CrossRef] [PubMed]

22. National Kidney Foundation. K/DOQI clinical practice guidelines for chronic kidney disease: Evaluation, classification, and stratification. *Am. J. Kidney Dis.* **2002**, *39*, S1–S266.

23. DaRoza, G.; Loewen, A.; Djurdjev, O.; Love, J.; Kempston, C.; Burnett, S.; Kiaii, M.; Taylor, P.A.; Levin, A. Stage of chronic kidney disease predicts seroconversion after hepatitis B immunization: Earlier is better. *Am. J. Kidney Dis.* **2003**, *42*, 1184–1192. [CrossRef] [PubMed]

24. Hermida, R.C.; Calvo, C.; Ayala, D.E.; Dominguez, M.J.; Covelo, M.; Fernandez, J.R.; Mojon, A.; Lopez, J.E. Administration time-dependent effects of valsartan on ambulatory blood pressure in hypertensive subjects. *Hypertension* **2003**, *42*, 283–290. [CrossRef]

25. Kidney Disease Outcomes Quality Initiative (K/DOQI) Group. K/DOQI clinical practice guidelines for management of dyslipidemias in patients with kidney disease. *Am. J. Kidney Dis.* **2003**, *41*, S1–S91.

26. National Kidney Foundation. K/DOQI clinical practice guidelines for bone metabolism and disease in chronic kidney disease. *Am. J. Kidney Dis.* **2003**, *42*, S1–S201.

27. De Zeeuw, D.; Remuzzi, G.; Parving, H.H.; Keane, W.F.; Zhang, Z.; Shahinfar, S.; Snapinn, S.; Cooper, M.E.; Mitch, W.E.; Brenner, B.M. Proteinuria, a target for renoprotection in patients with type 2 diabetic nephropathy: Lessons from RENAAL. *Kidney Int.* **2004**, *65*, 2309–2320. [CrossRef]

28. Kidney Disease Outcomes Quality Initiative (K/DOQI) Group. K/DOQI clinical practice guidelines on hypertension and antihypertensive agents in chronic kidney disease. *Am. J. Kidney Dis.* **2004**, *43*, S1–S290.

29. Rayner, H.C.; Besarab, A.; Brown, W.W.; Disney, A.; Saito, A.; Pisoni, R.L. Vascular access results from the Dialysis Outcomes and Practice Patterns Study (DOPPS): Performance against Kidney Disease Outcomes Quality Initiative (K/DOQI) Clinical Practice Guidelines. *Am. J. Kidney Dis.* **2004**, *44*, 22–26. [CrossRef]

30. Ruggenenti, P.; Fassi, A.; Ilieva, A.P.; Bruno, S.; Iliev, I.P.; Brusegan, V.; Rubis, N.; Gherardi, G.; Arnoldi, F.; Ganeva, M.; et al. Preventing microalbuminuria in type 2 diabetes. *N. Engl. J. Med.* **2004**, *351*, 1941–1951. [CrossRef]

31. Snyder, R.W.; Berns, J.S. Use of insulin and oral hypoglycemic medications in patients with diabetes mellitus and advanced kidney disease. *Semin. Dial.* **2004**, *17*, 365–370. [CrossRef] [PubMed]

32. Aranda, P.; Segura, J.; Ruilope, L.M.; Aranda, F.J.; Frutos, M.A.; Lopez, V.; de Novales, E.L. Long-term renoprotective effects of standard versus high doses of telmisartan in hypertensive nondiabetic nephropathies. *Am. J. Kidney Dis.* **2005**, *46*, 1074–1079. [CrossRef] [PubMed]

33. Hermida, R.C.; Ayala, D.E.; Calvo, C. Administration-time-dependent effects of antihypertensive treatment on the circadian pattern of blood pressure. *Curr. Opin. Nephrol. Hypertens.* **2005**, *14*, 453–459. [CrossRef] [PubMed]

34. Moe, S.M.; Chertow, G.M.; Coburn, J.W.; Quarles, L.D.; Goodman, W.G.; Block, G.A.; Drüeke, T.B.; Cunningham, J.; Sherrard, D.J.; McCary, L.C.; et al. Achieving NKF-K/DOQI bone metabolism and disease treatment goals with cinacalcet HCl. *Kidney Int.* **2005**, *67*, 760–771. [CrossRef] [PubMed]

35. Noordzij, M.; Korevaar, J.C.; Boeschoten, E.W.; Dekker, F.W.; Bos, W.J.; Krediet, R.T.; Netherlands Cooperative Study on the Adequacy of Dialysis (NECOSAD) Study Group. The Kidney Disease Outcomes Quality Initiative (K/DOQI) Guideline for Bone Metabolism and Disease in CKD: Association with mortality in dialysis patients. *Am. J. Kidney Dis.* **2005**, *46*, 925–932. [PubMed]

36. Epstein, M.; Williams, G.H.; Weinberger, M.; Lewin, A.; Krause, S.; Mukherjee, R.; Patni, R.; Beckerman, B. Selective aldosterone blockade with eplerenone reduces albuminuria in patients with type 2 diabetes. *Clin. J. Am. Soc. Nephrol.* **2006**, *1*, 940–951. [CrossRef] [PubMed]

37. Gennari, F.J.; Hood, V.L.; Greene, T.; Wang, X.; Levey, A.S. Effect of dietary protein intake on serum total CO_2 concentration in chronic kidney disease: Modification of Diet in Renal Disease study findings. *Clin. J. Am. Soc. Nephrol.* **2006**, *1*, 52–57. [CrossRef] [PubMed]

38. KDOQI; National Kidney Foundation. KDOQI Clinical Practice Guidelines and Clinical Practice Recommendations for Anemia in Chronic Kidney Disease. *Am. J. Kidney Dis.* **2006**, *47*, S11–S145.

39. Uribarri, J. Phosphorus homeostasis in normal health and in chronic kidney disease patients with special emphasis on dietary phosphorus intake. *Semin. Dial.* **2007**, *20*, 295–301. [CrossRef]

40. Mann, J.F.; Schmieder, R.E.; McQueen, M.; Dyal, L.; Schumacher, H.; Pogue, J.; Wang, X.; Maggioni, A.; Budaj, A.; Chaithiraphan, S.; et al. Renal outcomes with telmisartan, ramipril, or both, in people at high vascular risk (the ONTARGET study): A multicentre, randomised, double-blind, controlled trial. *Lancet* **2008**, *372*, 547–553. [CrossRef]

41. Parving, H.H.; Persson, F.; Lewis, J.B.; Lewis, E.J.; Hollenberg, N.K. Aliskiren combined with losartan in type 2 diabetes and nephropathy. *N. Engl. J. Med.* **2008**, *358*, 2433–2446. [CrossRef] [PubMed]

42. Spinowitz, B.; Germain, M.; Benz, R.; Wolfson, M.; McGowan, T.; Tang, K.L.; Kamin, M.; Epoetin Alfa Extended Dosing Study Group. A randomized study of extended dosing regimens for initiation of epoetin alfa treatment for anemia of chronic kidney disease. *Clin. J. Am. Soc. Nephrol.* **2008**, *3*, 1015–1021. [PubMed]

43. Burgess, E.; Muirhead, N.; Rene de Cotret, P.; Chiu, A.; Pichette, V.; Tobe, S. Supramaximal dose of candesartan in proteinuric renal disease. *J. Am. Soc. Nephrol.* **2009**, *20*, 893–900. [CrossRef] [PubMed]

44. De Brito-Ashurst, I.; Varagunam, M.; Raftery, M.J.; Yaqoob, M.M. Bicarbonate supplementation slows progression of CKD and improves nutritional status. *J. Am. Soc. Nephrol.* **2009**, *20*, 2075–2084. [CrossRef] [PubMed]

45. Hsu, C.Y.; Iribarren, C.; McCulloch, C.E.; Darbinian, J.; Go, A.S. Risk factors for end-stage renal disease: 25-year follow-u. *Arch. Intern. Med.* **2009**, *169*, 342–350. [CrossRef] [PubMed]

46. Khosla, N.; Kalaitzidis, R.; Bakris, G.L. Predictors of hyperkalemia risk following hypertension control with aldosterone blockade. *Am. J. Nephrol.* **2009**, *30*, 418–424. [CrossRef] [PubMed]

47. Madero, M.; Sarnak, M.J.; Wang, X.; Greene, T.; Beck, G.J.; Kusek, J.W.; Collins, A.J.; Levey, A.S.; Menon, V. Uric acid and long-term outcomes in CKD. *Am. J. Kidney Dis.* **2009**, *53*, 796–803. [CrossRef]

48. Mann, J.F.; Schmieder, R.E.; Dyal, L.; McQueen, M.J.; Schumacher, H.; Pogue, J.; Wang, X.; Probstfield, J.L.; Avezum, A.; Cardona-Munoz, E.; et al. Effect of telmisartan on renal outcomes: A randomized trial. *Ann. Intern. Med.* **2009**, *151*, 1–10. [CrossRef]

49. Navaneethan, S.D.; Nigwekar, S.U.; Sehgal, A.R.; Strippoli, G.F. Aldosterone antagonists for preventing the progression of chronic kidney disease: A systematic review and meta-analysis. *Clin. J. Am. Soc. Nephrol.* **2009**, *4*, 542–551. [CrossRef]

50. Dowling, T.C.; Matzke, G.R.; Murphy, J.E.; Burckart, G.J. Evaluation of renal drug dosing: Prescribing information and clinical pharmacist approaches. *Pharmacotherapy* **2010**, *30*, 776–786. [CrossRef]

51. Phisitkul, S.; Khanna, A.; Simoni, J.; Broglio, K.; Sheather, S.; Rajab, M.H.; Wesson, D.E. Amelioration of metabolic acidosis in patients with low GFR reduced kidney endothelin production and kidney injury, and better preserved GFR. *Kidney Int.* **2010**, *77*, 617–623. [CrossRef] [PubMed]

52. Riddle, M.C.; Ambrosius, W.T.; Brillon, D.J.; Buse, J.B.; Byington, R.P.; Cohen, R.M.; Goff, D.C., Jr.; Malozowski, S.; Margolis, K.L.; Probstfield, J.L.; et al. Epidemiologic relationships between A1C and all-cause mortality during a median 3.4-year follow-up of glycemic treatment in the ACCORD trial. *Diabetes Care* **2010**, *33*, 983–990. [PubMed]

53. ACCORD Study Group; Gerstein, H.C.; Miller, M.E.; Genuth, S.; Ismail-Beigi, F.; Buse, J.B.; Goff, D.C., Jr.; Probstfield, J.L.; Cushman, W.C.; Ginsberg, H.N.; et al. Long-term effects of intensive glucose lowering on cardiovascular outcomes. *N. Engl. J. Med.* **2011**, *364*, 818–828.

54. Haller, H.; Ito, S.; Izzo, J.L., Jr.; Januszewicz, A.; Katayama, S.; Menne, J.; Mimran, A.; Rabelink, T.J.; Ritz, E.; Ruilope, L.M.; et al. Olmesartan for the delay or prevention of microalbuminuria in type 2 diabetes. *N. Engl. J. Med.* **2011**, *364*, 907–917. [CrossRef] [PubMed]

55. Maione, A.; Navaneethan, S.D.; Graziano, G.; Mitchell, R.; Johnson, D.; Mann, J.F.; Gao, P.; Craig, J.C.; Tognoni, G.; Perkovic, V.; et al. Angiotensin-converting enzyme inhibitors, angiotensin receptor blockers and combined therapy in patients with micro- and macroalbuminuria and other cardiovascular risk factors: A systematic review of randomized controlled trials. *Nephrol. Dial. Transplant.* **2011**, *26*, 2827–2847. [CrossRef] [PubMed]

56. Nyman, H.A.; Dowling, T.C.; Hudson, J.Q.; Peter, W.L.; Joy, M.S.; Nolin, T.D. Comparative evaluation of the Cockcroft-Gault Equation and the Modification of Diet in Renal Disease (MDRD) study equation for drug dosing: An opinion of the Nephrology Practice and Research Network of the American College of Clinical Pharmacy. *Pharmacotherapy* **2011**, *31*, 1130–1144. [CrossRef]

57. Tsioufis, C.; Andrikou, I.; Thomopoulos, C.; Petras, D.; Manolis, A.; Stefanadis, C. Comparative prognostic role of nighttime blood pressure and nondipping profile on renal outcomes. *Am. J. Nephrol.* **2011**, *33*, 277–288. [CrossRef]

58. Tsioufis, C.; Andrikou, I.; Thomopoulos, C.; Syrseloudis, D.; Stergiou, G.; Stefanadis, C. Increased nighttime blood pressure or nondipping profile for prediction of cardiovascular outcomes. *J. Hum. Hypertens.* **2011**, *25*, 281–293. [CrossRef]

59. Liu, W.C.; Hung, C.C.; Chen, S.C.; Yeh, S.M.; Lin, M.Y.; Chiu, Y.W.; Kuo, M.C.; Chang, J.M.; Hwang, S.J.; Chen, H.C. Association of hyperuricemia with renal outcomes, cardiovascular disease, and mortality. *Clin. J. Am. Soc. Nephrol.* **2012**, *7*, 541–548. [CrossRef]

60. Parving, H.H.; Brenner, B.M.; McMurray, J.J.V.; de Zeeuw, D.; Haffner, S.M.; Solomon, S.D.; Chaturvedi, N.; Persson, F.; Desai, A.S.; Nicolaides, M.; et al. Cardiorenal end points in a trial of aliskiren for type 2 diabetes. *N. Engl. J. Med.* **2012**, *367*, 2204–2213. [CrossRef]

61. American Diabetes Association. Standards of medical care in diabetes—2013. *Diabetes Care* **2013**, *36*, S11–S66. [CrossRef] [PubMed]

62. Chertow, G.M.; Parfrey, P.S. Cinacalcet for cardiovascular disease in patients undergoing dialysis. *N. Engl. J. Med.* **2013**, *368*, 1844–1845. [PubMed]

63. James, P.A.; Oparil, S.; Carter, B.L.; Cushman, W.C.; Dennison-Himmelfarb, C.; Handler, J.; Lackland, D.T.; LeFevre, M.L.; MacKenzie, T.D.; Ogedegbe, O.; et al. 2014 evidence-based guideline for the management of high blood pressure in adults: Report from the panel members appointed to the Eighth Joint National Committee (JNC 8). *JAMA* **2014**, *311*, 507–520. [CrossRef] [PubMed]

64. Stone, N.J.; Robinson, J.G.; Lichtenstein, A.H.; Merz, C.N.B.; Blum, C.B.; Eckel, R.H.; Goldberg, A.C.; Gordon, D.; Levy, D.; Lloyd-Jones, D.M.; et al. 2013 ACC/AHA guideline on the treatment of blood cholesterol to reduce atherosclerotic cardiovascular risk in adults: A report of the American College of Cardiology/American Heart Association Task Force on Practice Guidelines. *Circulation* **2014**, *129*, S1–S45. [CrossRef] [PubMed]

65. Wanner, C.; Tonelli, M. Kidney Disease: Improving Global Outcomes Lipid Guideline Development Work Group Members. KDIGO Clinical Practice Guideline for Lipid Management in CKD: Summary of recommendation statements and clinical approach to the patient. *Kidney Int.* **2014**, *85*, 1303–1309. [CrossRef] [PubMed]

66. Cooper, M.E.; Perkovic, V.; McGill, J.B.; Groop, P.H.; Wanner, C.; Rosenstock, J.; Hehnke, U.; Woerle, H.J.; von Eynatten, M. Kidney Disease End Points in a Pooled Analysis of Individual Patient-Level Data From a Large Clinical Trials Program of the Dipeptidyl Peptidase 4 Inhibitor Linagliptin in Type 2 Diabetes. *Am. J. Kidney Dis.* **2015**, *66*, 441–449. [CrossRef] [PubMed]

67. The SPRINT Research Group A Randomized Trial of Intensive versus Standard Blood-Pressure Control. *N. Engl. J. Med.* **2015**, *373*, 2103–2116. Available online: https://www.nejm.org/doi/full/10.1056/nejmoa1511939 (accessed on 2 July 2019). [CrossRef]

68. Wong, M.G.; Perkovic, V.; Chalmers, J.; Woodward, M.; Li, Q.; Cooper, M.E.; Hamet, P.; Harrap, S.; Heller, S.; MacMahon, S.; et al. Mancia GLong-term Benefits of Intensive Glucose Control for Preventing End-Stage Kidney Disease: ADVANCE-ON. *Diabetes Care* **2016**, *39*, 694–700. [CrossRef]

69. Isakova, T.; Nickolas, T.L.; Denburg, M.; Yarlagadda, S.; Weiner, D.E.; Gutiérrez, O.M.; Bansal, V.; Rosas, S.E.; Nigwekar, S.; Yee, J.; et al. KDOQI US Commentary on the 2017 KDIGO Clinical Practice Guideline Update for the Diagnosis, Evaluation, Prevention, and Treatment of Chronic Kidney Disease-Mineral and Bone Disorder (CKD-MBD). *Am. J. Kidney Dis.* **2017**, *70*, 737–751. [CrossRef]

70. Fryar, C.D.; Ostchega, Y.; Hales, C.M.; Zhang, G.; Kruszon-Moran, D. Hypertension Prevalence and Control Among Adults: United States, 2015–2016. *NCHS Data Brief.* **2017**, *289*, 1–8.

71. Kausz, A.; Pahari, D. The value of vaccination in chronic kidney disease. *Semin. Dial.* **2004**, *17*, 9–11. [CrossRef] [PubMed]

72. Lee, T. Fistula First Initiative: Historical Impact on Vascular Access Practice Patterns and Influence on Future Vascular Access Care. *Cardiovasc. Eng. Technol.* **2017**, *8*, 244–254. [CrossRef] [PubMed]

73. Greenberg, J.; Jayarajan, S.; Reddy, S.; Schmieder, F.A.; Roberts, A.B.; van Bemmelen, P.S.; Lee, J.; Choi, E.T. Long-Term Outcomes of Fistula First Initiative in an Urban University Hospital—Is It Still Relevant? *Vasc. Endovasc. Surg.* **2017**, *51*, 125–130. [CrossRef] [PubMed]

74. Gargiulo, R.; Suhail, F.; Lerma, E.V. Cardiovascular disease and chronic kidney disease. *Dis. Mon.* **2015**, *61*, 403–413. [CrossRef] [PubMed]

75. Thanamayooran, S.; Rose, C.; Hirsch, D.J. Effectiveness of a multidisciplinary kidney disease clinic in achieving treatment guideline targets. *Nephrol. Dial. Transplant.* **2005**, *20*, 2385–2393. [CrossRef] [PubMed]

76. Olives, C.; Myerson, R.; Mokdad, A.H.; Murray, C.J.; Lim, S.S. Prevalence, awareness, treatment, and control of hypertension in United States counties, 2001–2009. *PLoS ONE* **2013**, *8*, e60308. [CrossRef] [PubMed]

77. Sarafidis, P.A.; Li, S.; Chen, S.C.; Collins, A.J.; Brown, W.W.; Klag, M.J.; Bakris, G.L. Hypertension awareness, treatment, and control in chronic kidney disease. *Am. J. Med.* **2008**, *121*, 332–340. [CrossRef]

78. Devins, G.M.; Mendelssohn, D.C.; Barré, P.E.; Binik, Y.M. Predialysis psychoeducational intervention and coping styles influence time to dialysis in chronic kidney disease. *Am. J. Kidney Dis.* **2003**, *42*, 693–703. [CrossRef]

79. Cavanaugh, K.L.; Wingard, R.L.; Hakim, R.M.; Elasy, T.A.; Ikizler, T.A. Patient dialysis knowledge is associated with permanent arteriovenous access use in chronic hemodialysis. *Clin. J. Am. Soc. Nephrol.* **2009**, *4*, 950–956. [CrossRef]

80. Saran, R.; Robinson, B.; Abbott, K.C.; Agodoa, L.Y.C.; Bhave, N.; Bragg-Gresham, J.; Balkrishnan, R.; Dietrich, X.; Eckard, A.; Eggers, P.W.; et al. US Renal Data System 2017 Annual Data Report: Epidemiology of Kidney Disease in the United States. *Am. J. Kidney Dis.* **2018**, *71*, A7. [CrossRef]

81. Goovaerts, T.; Jadoul, M.; Goffin, E. Influence of a pre-dialysis education programme (PDEP) on the mode of renal replacement therapy. *Nephrol. Dial. Transplant.* **2005**, *20*, 1842–1847. [CrossRef] [PubMed]

82. Merighi, J.R.; Schatell, D.R.; Bragg-Gresham, J.L.; Witten, B.; Mehrotra, R. Insights into nephrologist training, clinical practice, and dialysis choice. *Hemodial. Int.* **2012**, *16*, 242–251. [CrossRef] [PubMed]

83. Ong, S.W.; Jassal, S.V.; Porter, E.; Logan, A.G.; Miller, J.A. Using an electronic self-management tool to support patients with chronic kidney disease (CKD): A CKD clinic self-care model. *Semin. Dial.* **2013**, *26*, 195–202. [CrossRef] [PubMed]

84. Saxena, N.; Rizk, D.V. The interdisciplinary team: The whole is larger than the parts. *Adv. Chronic Kidney Dis.* **2014**, *21*, 333–337. [CrossRef] [PubMed]

85. Malas, M.B.; Canner, J.K.; Hicks, C.W.; Arhuidese, I.J.; Zarkowsky, D.S.; Qazi, U.; Schneider, E.B.; Black, J.H.; Segev, D.L.; Freischlag, J.A. Trends in incident hemodialysis access and mortality. *JAMA Surg.* **2015**, *150*, 441–448.

86. Fenton, A.; Sayar, Z.; Dodds, A.; Dasgupta, I. Multidisciplinary care improves outcome of patients with stage 5 chronic kidney disease. *Nephron. Clin. Pract.* **2010**, *115*, c283–c288.

87. Wei, S.Y.; Chang, Y.Y.; Mau, L.W.; Lin, M.Y.; Chiu, H.C.; Tsai, J.C.; Huang, C.J.; Chen, H.C.; Hwang, S.J. Chronic kidney disease care program improves quality of pre-end-stage renal disease care and reduces medical costs. *Nephrology* **2010**, *15*, 108–115. [CrossRef]

88. Xu, J.; Murphy, S.L.; Kochanek, K.D.; Bastian, B.A. Deaths: Final Data for 2013. *Natl. Vital. Stat. Rep.* **2016**, *64*, 1–119.

89. Go, A.S.; Chertow, G.M.; Fan, D.; McCulloch, C.E.; Hsu, C.Y. Chronic kidney disease and the risks of death, cardiovascular events, and hospitalization. *N. Engl. J. Med.* **2004**, *351*, 1296–1305. [CrossRef]

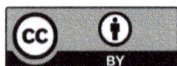

pharmacy

MDPI

Commentary

Preparing Pharmacists for Collaborative/Integrated Health Settings

Frank J. Ascione

UM Center for Interprofessional Education, University of Michigan College of Pharmacy, Ann Arbor, MI 48109, USA; fascione@umich.edu; Tel.: +1-734-763-0100

Received: 24 April 2019; Accepted: 16 May 2019; Published: 20 May 2019

check for updates

Abstract: Pharmacy practice is changing to accommodate the need for pharmacists to be better team members in newly emerging collaborative care and integrated health systems. Pharmacy schools could lead this change by educating students to be effective participants in these relatively new models of care. Schools are encouraged to follow the approach outlined in the recent guidance published by the Health Professions Accreditors Collaborative (HPAC) for interprofessional practice and education ("the new IPE"). This approach includes articulating an IPE plan, establishing goals, assessing student achievement of the necessary IPE competencies, developing educational plans that are multi-faceted and longitudinal, and modifying the existing assessment/evaluation process to ensure the quality of the IPE effort. These curricular decisions should be based on existing and new research on the effectiveness of IPE on student's attitudes, knowledge, skills, and behavior. A key decision is how to create effective interactions between pharmacy students and those of other professions. Educational emphasis should be directed toward team building skills, not just individual competencies. The pharmacy faculty probably need to enhance their teaching abilities to accommodate this change, such as learning new technology (e.g., simulations, managing online exchanges) and demonstrating a willingness to teach students from other professions.

Keywords: pharmacists; pharmacy education; interprofessional practice and education

1. Introduction

An integrative/collaborative approach to health care services is needed to create a more efficient workforce and positive health outcomes [1,2]. Collaborative care is defined as occurring "when multiple health workers from different professional backgrounds provide comprehensive services by working with patients, their families, and communities to deliver the highest quality of care across settings." Integrative Health Care is described as "bringing together inputs, delivery, management and organization of services related to diagnosis, treatment, care, rehabilitation and health promotion. Integration is a means to improve services in relation to access, quality, user satisfaction and efficiency." Both approaches require enhanced cooperation among all levels of caregivers to ensure optimal service [1,3].

The call for more cooperation is not new and neither is the potential role of pharmacists in this effort [4,5]. Despite those historical appeals, there was limited local, national, and international effort to vigorously promote this approach for many years. That apathy began to change with the publication of the Institute of Medicine (IOM) report in 1999 entitled To Err Is Human [6]. This report suggested that as many as 98,000 hospital deaths per year were due to medical errors. A key finding of the report was the observation that these deaths likely arose "from the decentralized and fragmented nature of the health care delivery system—or "non-system," to some observers."

The 1999 IOM report created a more concentrated effort of health professional collaboration, particularly around patient safety. However, other problems of the health care system, such as fragmented care, poor access, suboptimal patient outcomes, dissatisfied patients, and a frustrated work force, were still present. These issues were later highlighted in two key reports. The World Health Organization (WHO) noted in a 2010 report entitled that interprofessional collaboration connected with shared education would strengthen health care delivery and improve outcomes [1]. At the same time, an international commission of professional and academic leaders published a report in the Lancet calling for a new direction in health professional workforce education that emphasizes more interprofessional education and collaboration [7].

The result of these calls for action is an international movement toward reform of health professional education and practice [8–10]. This effort presents a great opportunity for pharmacy, which is recognized by many health professionals for its expertise in drug products and medication management [11–13]. However, pharmacy suffers the same barriers to team practice as other professions: a fractionated health system, scope of practice restrictions, hierarchical order of decision-making, and an insufficient educational focus on the skills needed to be an effective multi-professional team member or leader [14,15]. The purpose of this paper is to address the lack of educational focus and offer suggestions for curricular changes that support greater implementation of interprofessional practice and education (known as the "new IPE" [10]) principles in pharmacy education.

2. Approach

Pharmacy education traditionally focused on the "shaping" of student learners to become pharmacists. That identity revolves around teaching the skills needed to become drug product and medication management experts [16]. Like all health professions education, this "uni-professional" approach can be a barrier to preparing learners to function effectively in collaborative/integrative care practice settings, which could prevent them from providing high quality care to patients. Instead, a multi-professonial approach is needed with a shift toward inclusion of more interprofessional experiences, resulting in the development of a dual identity as both a pharmacist and as a key participant of collaborative care teams or as members of integrated health systems [9,17].

The idea of the dual or multi-professional approach of educating students to become pharmacists and effective members of the health care team has been discussed extensively in the past few years. The 2004 report on Educational Outcomes by the Center for the Advancement of Pharmacy Education (CAPE) mentions the need to educate pharmacy students to become effective members of interprofessional health care teams [18]. This focus was expanded in the 2013 CAPE guidelines which identified the "collaborator" role of pharmacy [19]. The 2013 report suggested that learning objectives for pharmacy students should include establishing a climate of shared values, defining clear roles and responsibilities, communicating effectively with other professions, and promoting joint problem solving. The 2013 CAPE report generated a number of research papers on desirable approaches to promoting IPE in pharmacy education in such areas as Integrative Health Education [20], Advanced Pharmacy Practice Experiences [21], and Entrustable Professional Activities [22].

The CAPE guidelines identified the need for IPE in pharmacy curricula and subsequent research identified possible strategies. These efforts were the basis for the Accreditation Council for Pharmacy Education (ACPE) Standard 11, which identifies key elements desired in a pharmacy curriculum to prepare students to become contributing members of an interprofessional team [23].

None of the efforts to date have provided a universally accepted plan for appropriate integration of IPE in pharmacy curricula. Fortunately, a recent guidance published by the Health Professions Accreditors Collaborative (HPAC), which is a collaboration among at least 25 of the accrediting agencies (including pharmacy), offers a template for developing that approach [9]. It suggests that every educational plan include the following characteristics:

A. Rationale: Articulate a vision, framework, and justification for the IPE plan.
B. Outcome-based Goals: State in terms that will allow the assessment of students' achievement of objectives and interprofessional competencies for collaborative practice.

C.   Deliberate Design: Intentionally design and sequence a series of classroom, extracurricular, and clinical learning activities integrated into the existing professional curriculum that are longitudinal in nature, spanning the entire length of the program and including content and instructional formats appropriate to the level of the learner and to the outcome-based goals.

D.   Assessment and Evaluation: Use methods to assess individual learners' mastery of interprofessional competencies and to evaluate the IPE plan for quality improvement purposes; and if appropriate, education and practice outcomes, research and scholarship.

These are general guidelines for all health professions educational programs. The specifics for each health profession have not been developed yet. However, possible applications to pharmacy education are offered in the following paragraphs:

Rationale. Pharmacy educators have a solid rationale for the development of pharmacists as drug product and medication therapy experts, especially applied to areas such as improved therapeutic outcomes, patient adherence, drug safety, and transitions of care [24–26]. The expansion of this professional role to becoming effective participants in collaborative/integrative care is not as clear. The HPAC guidelines suggest that a conceptual model is needed to provide an overview of how collaborative activities are linked to better health outcomes. The example in the guidance is the Institute of Medicine Interprofessional Learning Continuum Model that illustrates the continuum of IPE through all levels of learners (undergraduate, graduate, and current practitioners) and how the learning process is affected by factors such as culture and the availability of needed resources [2]. Another useful model is the one developed by WHO, which suggests a positive relationship between IPE, collaborative care, and positive health outcomes [1].

These models imply that the pharmacist's expert knowledge of drug products and medication management would be a necessary but not a sufficient factor in ensuring better health outcomes. To be more effective contributors, pharmacy education would need to go beyond teaching drug product/medication expertise to a more expansive instruction on factors such as the social determinants of health, the principles of human behavior, and non-medication strategies to improve health [19,27–30].

Outcome-based goals. Pharmacy educational programs already have a clear set of learning outcomes identified through the standards set ACPE and promoted by CAPE [19,23]. These outcomes include a strong foundational knowledge in the sciences, understanding of the principles of pharmacy practice, demonstration of the skills needed to manage medication therapy and medication use systems, and awareness of the best pathways to promoting health wellness in improving population-based care.

The HPAC guidance suggests that a related but broader set of competencies are needed to effectively cooperate with other health professionals. The competencies created by the Interprofessional Education Collaborative (IPEC) [31] was the suggested starting point for dual interprofessional development of students. They are:

Competency 1, Values/Ethics for Interprofessional Practice: Work with individuals of other professions to maintain a climate of mutual respect and shared values.

Competency 2, Roles/Responsibilities: Use the knowledge of one's own role and those of other professions to appropriately assess and address the health care needs of patients and to promote and advance the health of populations.

Competency 3, Interprofessional Communication: Communicate with patients, families, communities, and professionals in health and other fields in a responsive and responsible manner that supports a team approach to the promotion and maintenance of health and the prevention and treatment of disease.

Competency 4, Teams and Teamwork: Apply relationship-building values and principles of team dynamics to perform effectively in different team roles to plan, deliver, and evaluate patient/population-centered care and population health programs and policies that are safe, timely, efficient, effective, and equitable.

ACPE has already addressed some of these competencies under its interprofessional education standard (standard 11). This standard focuses on demonstrating competence in three key elements:

Interprofessional team dynamics, interprofessional team education, and interprofessional team practice [23]. The newness of the standard means that there are very few examples of successful strategies performed by Colleges of Pharmacy to meet those criteria.

Deliberate Design. Pharmacy education programs already need to be intentionally designed and sequenced to meet accreditation [23] and licensing standards [32]. The design for IPE preparation would emphasize the same approach but would focus on a progression based, multifaceted, longitudinal integration of the IPEC interprofessional competencies into the full length of the existing pharmacy curriculum [31].

A key aspect of an IPE educational program is the focus on pharmacy students learning about, from, and with students from other professions regarding how to collaborate and improve health outcomes, which is consistent with the WHO definition of IPE [1]. In order to achieve this goal, traditional methods of teaching pharmacy students (e.g., lecture or classroom discussions) need to change.

Approaches need to be multifaceted and include student-to-student IPE learning activities that go beyond courses, such as one-time gatherings of many different professions to address an issue (e.g., disaster preparedness events), online exchanges, and IPE simulations. Formally designed team based learning exercises with students from other professions need to be emphasized. Clinical rotations that highlight multi-professional teamwork supervised by faculty from multiple professions are needed to demonstrate the full value of collaborative care [28,33–35].

Assessment and Evaluation. Pharmacy accreditation already focuses on the key elements of student assessment, the quality of the mentoring process, and the value of the strategic educational plan [23]. IPE assessment builds on that foundation by focusing on student abilities to function as effective team members; emphasizing supervision and mentoring by a multi-professional faculty in team care environments; and strategic planning that includes the dual process of professional and interprofessional socialization. Assessment of the pharmacy student should include measures of changes in perceptions and knowledge of the capabilities of other professions, understanding of teamwork, and the demonstration/performance of collaborative behaviors in simulations and health practice settings [2,9,31].

3. Discussion

Pharmacy faculty are always confronted with challenges to update the curriculum to prepare students for the constantly changing health care environment. Moving toward a more interprofessional focus is especially challenging because of the need to engage other professional schools in the process. Here are some useful suggestions, based on my long time experience as a pharmacy educator (and Dean) and as a Director of a University-wide Interprofessional Center, that may assist in ensuring that the IPE curricular goals are met.

A. The curricular decisions on IPE should be based on research that identifies the best educational strategies. This information is lacking in many areas because the IPE movement is still new, which means that more scholarship is required in this area. Many questions need to be resolved through thoughtful research and vigorous assessment of the various efforts. For example, what will be the typical practice models in the future and what would be the key roles of the various health professions? What are the specific skills needed to become an effective team member? Who are the important individuals that pharmacists need to interact with in the collaborative/integrative care environment? Does the nature of the pharmacist team role change in different practice settings (e.g., institutions vs ambulatory care)? What are the proper links between learner education, effective collaborative/integrative practice, and positive health outcomes? Resolution of these questions are needed before a valued based IPE curriculum can be successfully implemented.

B. Despite our knowledge gaps, a crucial ingredient to any IPE curriculum is the level of discourse with students from other professions. The WHO definition of IPE emphasizes intense interaction of learners from different professions directed toward joint problem solving exercises [1]. The key for pharmacy curricular planners is deciding the priority of formal contact with a multitude of professions given the inherent logistical challenges. ACPE's standard 11 states that the "curriculum prepares all students to provide entry-level, patient-centered care in a variety of practice settings as a contributing member of an interprofessional team. In the aggregate, team exposure includes prescribers as well as other healthcare professionals" [23]. This standard is helpful because it recognizes the medication management focus of pharmacy practice. However, it does not address the value of interactions with professionals who are not prescribers e.g., social work). These interactions should be based on their value to enhancing the perspective/knowledge of pharmacy students, not simply their educational accessibility. Co-location of these schools on the same campus is desirable but not necessary; it is appropriate to meet with students from other professions through specific collaborating institutions or through regional networks [9,36,37].

C.   The IPE emphasis should be on team building skills not just individual competencies [38]. The models used to support the rationale for interprofessional education emphasize the value of health professional teamwork in creating positive health outcomes [1,2,27]. Thus, popular team building techniques such as TeamSTepps [39] or the Interprofessional Collaborator Assessment Rubric (ICAR) [40] should be used extensively in the teaching process in order to emphasize group development. The focus is on educating pharmacy students to engage in shared decision making, joint accountability for patient care and population health [41].

D.   Pharmacy educators need to accept, endorse, and participate in a multi-professional approach to teaching their students. These actions may consist of acquiring a new set of teaching skills. These skills include effective facilitation of formal team based learning, use of technology such as simulations, or creating/managing online multi-professional forums. There also must be a willingness to teach non-pharmacy learners and to encourage other professionals to instruct pharmacy students [28,31,35,41,42].

4. Conclusions

Pharmacists are moving toward more active participation in collaborative/integrative models of care. This involvement emphasizes teamwork skills, more extensive interaction with other health professionals, and a broader understanding of the patient's health needs. Implementing IPE in pharmacy education is necessary in order for students to be successful in this new practice model. The approach to implementation of IPE discussed in this paper is endorsed and supported in the HPAC Guidance [9]. However, implementation will only be effective if it is not viewed as a supplemental addition but rather a full integration into the curriculum. There are many examples of productive new attempts at curricular implementation in pharmacy schools [43–47]. These strategies are likely to expand in the future.

The focus of this paper is on the implementation of IPE in the United States, but these academic and practice issues are prevalent throughout the world [48]. In fact, the WHO report promoting IPE viewed the movement as an important strategy to mitigate the global workforce crises [1]. The International Pharmaceutical Federation (FIP), the major international pharmacy organization, has promoted interprofessional education and practice for many years. Its 2016 report entitled: "Global Vision for Education and Workforce" emphasizes that pharmacy must develop a care model that is based on collaboration with other health professionals [49].

The need for pharmacists to be educated to be more collaborative is universal but the strategies are more likely to vary by country due to different pharmacy educational requirements, regulation of the scope of pharmacy practice, payer systems, and the availability of other health professionals [50,51]. Nevertheless, examples of successful implementation of IPE within pharmacy education and practice exist outside the United States, many of which set the standard for the whole world [52–57].

Successful integration globally of IPE principles into pharmacy curricula is extensive and will continue to grow in the future. These efforts will increase the educational shift necessary to ensure pharmacists are essential members of the future collaborative teams and full participants in the integrative health approaches needed to ensure better health outcomes to the patients we serve.

Funding: This research received no external funding.

Conflicts of Interest: The author declares no conflict of interest.

References

1. *World Health Organization: Framework for Action on Interprofessional Education & Collaborative Practice*; Department of Human Resources for Health: Geneva, Switzerland, 2010.
2. *Institute of Medicine: Measuring the Impact of Interprofessional Education on Collaborative Practice and Patient Outcomes*; National Academies Press: Washington, DC, USA, 2015.
3. Gröne, O.; Garcia-Barbero, M. *Trends in Integrated Care—Reflections on Conceptual Issues*; World Health Organization: Copenhagen, Denmark, 2002.
4. University of Michigan. *Conference on Health Education*; University of Michigan Press: Ann Arbor, MI, USA, 16–18 February 1967.
5. *Institute of Medicine: Educating for the Health Team*; National Academy of Sciences: Washington, DC, USA, 1972.
6. *Institute of Medicine: To Err is Human: Building a Safer Health System*; National Academy of Sciences: Washington, DC, USA, 1999.
7. Frenk, J.; Chen, L.; Bhutta, Z.A.; Cohen, J.; Crisp, N.; Evans, T.; Fineberg, H.; Garcia, P.; Ke, Y.; Kelley, P.; et al. Health professionals for a new century: Transforming education to strengthen health systems in an interdependent world. *Lancet* **2010**, *376*, 1923–1958. [CrossRef]
8. Interprofessional Education Collaborative (IPEC). Available online: https://www.ipecollaborative.org/ (accessed on 28 March 2019).
9. Health Professions Accreditors Collaborative (HPAC). Available online: http://healthprofessionsaccreditors.org (accessed on 15 April 2019).
10. National Center for Interprofessional Practice and Education. Available online: https://nexusipe.org/ (accessed on 11 April 2019).
11. Williams, C.R.; Woodall, T.; Gilmore, C.; Griffen, W.R.; Galvin, S.L.; LaValleee, L.A.; Roberts, C.; Ives, T.J. Physician perceptions of integrating advanced practice pharmacists into practice. *J. Am. Pharm. Assoc.* **2018**, *58*, 73–78. [CrossRef] [PubMed]
12. Kozminski, M.; Busby, R.; McGivney, M.S.; Klatt, P.M.; Hackett, S.R.; Merenstein, J.H.; Hackett, S.R. Pharmacist integration into the medical home. *J. Am. Pharm. Assoc.* **2011**, *51*, 173–183. [CrossRef] [PubMed]
13. Fay, A.E.; Ferreri, S.P.; Shepherd, G.; Lundeen, K.; Tong, G.L.; Pfeiffenberger, T. Care team perspectives on community pharmacy enhanced services. *J. Am. Pharm. Assoc.* **2018**, *58*, S83–S88. [CrossRef]
14. Hogue, M.D.; Bugdalski-Stutrud, C.; Smith, M.; Tomecki, M.; Burns, A.; Kliethermes, M.A.; Beatty, S.; Beiergrohslein, M.; Trygstad, T.; Trewet, C. Pharmacist engagement in medical home practices: Report of the Apha–AppM Medical Home Workgroup. *J. Am. Pharm. Assoc.* **2013**, *53*, 118–124. [CrossRef]
15. Lounsbery, J.L.; Green, C.G.; Bennett, M.S. Evaluation of pharmacists' barriers to the implementation of medication therapy management services. *J. Am. Pharm. Assoc.* **2009**, 51–58. [CrossRef]
16. American Association Colleges of Pharmacy (AACP). Available online: https://www.aacp.org/about-aacp (accessed on 30 March 2019).
17. Hossein, K.; Orchard, C.; Spence-Laschinger, H.K.; Farah, R. An interprofessional socialization framework for developing an interprofessional identity among health professions students. *J. Interprof. Care Volume* **2013**, *27*, 448–453. [CrossRef]
18. American Association of Colleges of Pharmacy (AACP). Educational Outcomes 2004. Available online: https://www.aacp.org/about-aacp (accessed on 7 May 2019).
19. Medina, M.S.; Plaza, C.M.; Stowe, C.D.; Robinson, E.T.; Delander, G.; Beck, D.; Melchert, R.B.; Supernaw, R.B.; Roche, V.F.; Gleason, B.L.; et al. Center for the Advancement of Pharmacy Education 2013 Educational Outcomes. *Am. J. Pharm. Educ.* **2013**, *77*, 162. [CrossRef]

20. Lee, J.K.; Hume, A.L.; Willis, R.; Boon, H.; Lebensohn, P.; Brooks, A.; Kligler, B. Pharmacy Competencies for Interprofessional Integrative Health Care Education. *Am. J. Pharm. Educ.* **2018**, *82*, 6302. [CrossRef]

21. Dennis, V.C.; May, D.W.; Kanmaz, T.J.; Reidt, S.L.; Serres, M.L.; Edwards, H.D. Pharmacy Student Learning During Advanced Pharmacy Practice Experiences in Relation to the CAPE 2013 Outcomes. *Am. J. Pharm. Educ.* **2016**, *80*, 127. [CrossRef] [PubMed]

22. Haines, S.T.; Pittenger, A.; Plaza, C. Describing Entrustable Professional Activities Is Merely the First Step. *Am. J. Pharm. Educ.* **2017**, *81*, 18. [CrossRef] [PubMed]

23. Accreditation Council for Pharmacy Education (ACPE): Accreditation Standards and Key Elements for the Professional Program in Pharmacy Leading to the Doctor of Pharmacy Degree. Available online: https://www.acpe-accredit.org/pdf/Standards2016FINAL.pdf (accessed on 20 April 2019).

24. American Pharmacist Association. Available online: https://www.pharmacist.com/?is_sso_called=1 (accessed on 11 April 2019).

25. American College of Clinical Pharmacy (ACCP). Available online: https://www.accp.com/ (accessed on 11 April 2019).

26. American Society of Health Systems Pharmacists (ASHP). Available online: https://www.ashp.org/ (accessed on 11 April 2019).

27. *Institute of Medicine: A Framework for Educating Health Professionals to Address the Social Determinants of Health*; National Academies Press: Washington, DC, USA, 2016.

28. Sweet, B.V.; Madeo, A.; Fitzgerald, M.; House, J.B.; Pardee, M.; Zebrack, B.; Sweier, D.; Hornyak, J.; Arslanian-Engoren, C.; Mattison, D.; et al. Moving from Individual Roles to Functional Teams: A semester-long course in case-based decision making. *J. Interprof. Educ. Pract.* **2017**, *7*, 11–16. [CrossRef]

29. O'Reilly, C.L.; Bell, J.S.; Chen, T.F. Consumer-led Mental Health Education for Pharmacy Students. *Am. J. Pharm. Educ.* **2010**, *74*, 67. [CrossRef]

30. Vogt, E.M.; Finley, P.R. Heart of Pharmacy: A Course Exploring the Psychosocial Issues of Patient Care. *Am. J. Pharm. Educ.* **2009**, *73*, 149. [CrossRef]

31. Interprofessional Education Collaborative (IPEC): Core Competencies for Interprofessional Collaborative Practice: 2016 Update. Available online: https://nebula.wsimg.com/2f68a39520b03336b41038c370497473?AccessKeyId=DC06780E69ED19E2B3A5&disposition=0&alloworigin=1 (accessed on 28 March 2019).

32. The National Association of Boards of Pharmacy (NABP): PCOA School Outcomes for Students Nearing the End of Their Didactic Curriculum. Available online: https://nabp.pharmacy/wp-content/uploads/2018/11/ACPE-PCOA-Report-2018.pdf (accessed on 30 March 2019).

33. Hammick, M.; Freeth, D.; Koppel, I.; Reeves, S.; Barr, H. A best evidence systematic review of interprofessional education: BEME Guide no. 9. *Med. Teach.* **2007**, *29*, 735–751. [CrossRef]

34. Reeves, S.; Fletcher, S.; Barr, H.; Birch, I.; Boet, S.; Davies, N.; Kitto, S.A. BEME systematic review of the effects of interprofessional education: BEME Guide No. 39. *Med. Teach.* **2016**, *38*, 656–668. [CrossRef]

35. Team Based Learning Collaborative. Available online: http://www.teambasedlearning.org/ (accessed on 10 May 2019).

36. Ascione, F.J.; Sick, B.; Karpa, K.; McAuley, J.; Nickol, D.R.; Weber, Z.A.; Pfeifle, A.L. The Big Ten IPE Academic Alliance: A regional approach to developing Interprofessional Education and practice. *J. Interprof. Educ. Pract.* **2019**, *15*, 9–14. [CrossRef]

37. Nagelkirk, J.; Coggin, P.J.; Pawl, B.; Thompson, M.E. The Midwest Interprofessional, Education, and Research Center: A regional approach to innovations in interprofessional education and practice. *J. Interprof. Educ. Pract.* **2017**, *7*, 47–52. [CrossRef]

38. Ginsburg, S.; Regehr, G.; Hatala, R.; Mcnaughton, N.; Frohna, A.; Hodges, B.; Lingard, L.; Stern, D. Context, Conflict, and Resolution: A New Conceptual Framework for Evaluating Professionalism. *Acad. Med.* **2000**, *75*, S6–S11. [CrossRef] [PubMed]

39. Agency for HealthCare Research and Quality (AHRQ): TeamStepps Discussion. Available online: https://www.ahrq.gov/teamstepps/index.html (accessed on 15 April 2019).

40. American Council of Academic Physical Therapy (ACAPT): Interprofessional Collaborator Assessment Rubric in NIPEC Assessment Resources and Tools. Available online: https://acapt.org/docs/default-source/consortium-(nipec)/nipec-resources/icar-1.pdf?sfvrsn=0&sfvrsn=0 (accessed on 12 April 2019).

41. University of Michigan Center for Interprofessional Education: IPE Course Adaptor Toolkit. Available online: http://ipetoolkit.umich.edu/ (accessed on 19 April 2019).

42. Cameron, A.; Ignjatovic, M.; Langlois, S.; Dematteo, D.; DiProspero, L.; Wagner, S.; Reeves, S. An Interprofessional Education Session for First-Year Health Science Students. *Am. J. Pharm. Educ.* **2009**, *73*, 4. [CrossRef]

43. Smith, K.M.; Scott, D.R.; Barner, J.G.; DeHart, R.M.; Scott, J.D.; Martin, S.J. Interprofessional Education in Six US Colleges of Pharmacy. *Am. J. Pharm. Educ.* **2009**, *73*, 4. [CrossRef]

44. Remington, T.L.; Foulk, M.A.; Williams, B.C. Evaluation of Evidence for Interprofessional Education. *Am. J. Pharm. Educ.* **2006**, *70*, 3. [CrossRef]

45. Truong, H.; Gorman, M.J.; East, M.; Klima, D.W.; Hinderer, K.A.; Hogue, G.L.; Brown, V.; Joyner, R.L. The Eastern Shore Collaborative for Interprofessional Education's Implementation and Impact over Five Years. *Am. J. Pharm. Educ.* **2018**, *82*, 4. [CrossRef] [PubMed]

46. Nagge, J.; Lee-Poy, M.F.; Richard, C.L. Evaluation of a Unique Interprofessional Education Program Involving Medical and Pharmacy Students. *Am. J. Pharm. Educ.* **2017**, *81*, 10. [CrossRef] [PubMed]

47. Jones, K.M.; Blumenthal, D.K.; Burke, J.M.; Condren, M.; Hansen, R.; Holiday-Goodman, M.; Peterson, C.D. Interprofessional Education in Introductory Pharmacy Practice Experiences at US Colleges and Schools of Pharmacy. *Am. J. Pharm. Educ.* **2012**, *76*, 5. [CrossRef] [PubMed]

48. El-Awaisi, A.; Barr, H. East meets West: Working together in interprofessional education and practice. *J. Interprof. Educ. Pract.* **2017**, *7*, 72–74. [CrossRef]

49. International Pharmaceutical Federation: Global Vision for Education and Workforce 2016. Available online: https://www.fip.org/files/fip/PharmacyEducation/Global_Conference_docs/FIP_global_vision_online_version.pdf (accessed on 9 May 2019).

50. International Pharmaceutical Federation: Research, Development and Evaluation Strategies for Pharmaceutical Education and the Workforce: A Global Report 2017. Available online: https://www.fip.org/files/fip/publications/RDES_FIPEd.pdf (accessed on 8 May 2019).

51. International Pharmaceutical Federation: Pharmacy Workforce Intelligence: Global Trends 2018. Available online: https://www.fip.org/files/fip/PharmacyEducation/Workforce_Report_2018.pdf (accessed on 8 May 2019).

52. El-Awaisi, A.; Awaisu, A.; El Hajj, M.S.; Alemrayat, B.; Al-Jayyousi, G.; Wong, N.; Verjee, M.A. Delivering Tobacco Cessation Content in the Middle East Through Interprofessional Learning. *Am. J. Pharm. Educ.* **2017**, *81*, 91. [CrossRef]

53. Grace Frankel, G.; Louizos, C.; Austin, Z. Canadian Educational Approaches for the Advancement of Pharmacy Practice. *Am. J. Pharm. Educ.* **2014**, *78*, 143. [CrossRef]

54. Fløystad, E.T.; Elfrid, M.; Atle, O. Investigating the utility of medication reviews amongst elderly home care patients in Norway—An interprofessional perspective. *J. Interprof. Educ. Pract.* **2018**, *13*, 83–89. [CrossRef]

55. Wang, J.; Hu, X.; Liu, J.; Li, L. Pharmacy students' attitudes towards physician-pharmacist collaboration: Intervention effect of integrating cooperative learning into an interprofessional team-based community service. *J. Interprof. Care* **2016**, *30*, 591–598. [CrossRef]

56. Monash University College of Pharmacy and Pharmaceutical Sciences. Interprofessional Offerings. Available online: https://www.monash.edu/search?f.Faculties%7C38=Pharmacy+and+Pharmaceutical+Sciences&form=matrix&query=interprofessional&profile=_default&collection=monash-main-search (accessed on 10 May 2019).

57. University of Toronto Leslie Dan Faculty of Pharmacy. Interprofessional Education. Available online: https://pharmacy.utoronto.ca/programs-and-admissions/pharmd/current-students/interprofessional-education-ipe/ (accessed on 10 May 2019).

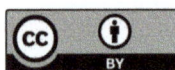

pharmacy

MDPI

Article

Advancing Pharmacist Collaborative Care within Academic Health Systems

Linda Awdishu [1,2,*], Renu F. Singh [1,2], Ila Saunders [1,2], Felix K. Yam [1,3], Jan D. Hirsch [1,4], Sarah Lorentz [1], Rabia S. Atayee [1,2], Joseph D. Ma [1,2], Shirley M. Tsunoda [1,2], Jennifer Namba [1,2], Christina L. Mnatzaganian [1,2], Nathan A. Painter [1,2], Jonathan H. Watanabe [1], Kelly C. Lee [1,2], Charles D. Daniels [1,2] and Candis M. Morello [1,3]

[1] San Diego Skaggs School of Pharmacy and Pharmaceutical Sciences, University of California, La Jolla, CA 92093, USA; rfsingh@ucsd.edu (R.F.S.); isaunders@ucsd.edu (I.S.); fyam@ucsd.edu (F.K.Y.); jdhirsch@uci.edu (J.D.H.); slorentz@ucsd.edu (S.L.); ratayee@ucsd.edu (R.S.A.); jdma@ucsd.edu (J.D.M.); smtsunoda@ucsd.edu (S.M.T.); jnamba@ucsd.edu (J.N.); cmnatzaganian@ucsd.edu (C.L.M.); npainter@ucsd.edu (N.A.P.); Jhwatanabe@ucsd.edu (J.H.W.); kellylee@ucsd.edu (K.C.L.); cdaniels@ucsd.edu (C.D.D.); candismorello@ucsd.edu (C.M.M.)
[2] San Diego Health System, University of California, La Jolla, CA 92093, USA
[3] Veterans Affairs San Diego Healthcare System, La Jolla, CA 92093, USA
[4] Irvine School of Pharmacy and Pharmaceutical Sciences, University of California, Irvine, CA 92697, USA
[*] Correspondence: lawdishu@ucsd.edu

Received: 1 May 2019; Accepted: 5 October 2019; Published: 11 October 2019

check for updates

Abstract: Introduction: The scope of pharmacy practice has evolved over the last few decades to focus on the optimization of medication therapy. Despite this positive impact, the lack of reimbursement remains a significant barrier to the implementation of innovative pharmacist practice models. **Summary**: We describe the successful development, implementation and outcomes of three types of pharmacist collaborative care models: (1) a pharmacist with physician oversight, (2) pharmacist–interprofessional teams and (3) physician–pharmacist teams. The outcome measurement of these pharmacist care models varied from the design phase to patient volume measurement and to comprehensive quality dashboards. All of these practice models have been successfully funded by affiliated health systems or grants. **Conclusions**: The expansion of pharmacist services delivered by clinical faculty has several benefits to affiliated health systems: (1) significant improvements in patient care quality, (2) access to experts in specialty areas, and (3) the dissemination of outcomes with national and international recognition, increasing the visibility of the health system.

Keywords: collaborative practice; clinical pharmacy; advanced practice pharmacist provider

1. Introduction

Collaborative care between pharmacists and physicians has been recognized to improve pharmacotherapeutic outcomes and provide increased value and efficiency to the health care system [1]. Models for collaborative drug therapy management have been designed with a focus on the most studied chronic diseases including hypertension (HTN) and type 2 diabetes (T2D). Numerous studies have demonstrated the positive impact that physician–pharmacist collaborative management can have on blood pressure and glycosylated hemoglobin (A1C) among patients with HTN and DM [2–4]. Additionally, this positive impact has been demonstrated for other chronic diseases [5,6]. More recently, Matzke and colleagues demonstrated that pharmacists integrated in a patient-centered medical home reduce hospitalizations by 23.4%, resulting in estimated cost savings of $2619 per patient [7]. Despite the overwhelmingly positive impact of pharmacist services on patient outcomes, the integration of pharmacists in ambulatory care programs is not widespread. A survey conducted by Hattingh and colleagues identified three major themes as factors that impacted the provision of pharmacist services: (1) pharmacist characteristics, (2) local needs, structures and support, and (3) an enabling practice framework [8,9]. In this paper, we describe the program development, successful implementation and outcomes of pharmacist collaborative care models provided by the University of California, San Diego Skaggs School of Pharmacy and Pharmaceutical Sciences (SSPPS) faculty in two affiliated academic health systems.

Setting

For decades, the scope of pharmacy practice in the United States (US) has expanded to optimize medication use to achieve patient health-related goals. More recently, the passage of California Senate Bill 493 allows all pharmacists to administer drugs and biologics when ordered by a prescriber, furnish oral contraceptives, travel medications and nicotine replacement products for smoking cessation, as well as administer vaccinations. This bill established an Advanced Practice Pharmacist (APP) recognition and authorizes APPs to perform patient assessments, order and interpret drug therapy–related tests, refer patients to other health care providers, initiate, adjust, and discontinue drug therapy upon referral from a patient's treating prescriber and in accordance with established protocols, and participate in the evaluation and management of diseases and health conditions in collaboration with other health care providers. The APP recognition requires a separate APh licensure application, review and approval from the California Board of Pharmacy.

At UC San Diego Health (UCSDH) and the Veteran's Affairs San Diego Healthcare System (VASDHS), comprehensive collaborations were developed in which pharmacists provide patient care under collaborative practice agreements (CPA) in the inpatient and ambulatory care settings. The positive impact of pharmacist services has been established using various models of care for chronic disease management [10–12]. However, recognition of pharmacists as providers has been challenged, and reimbursement for services has been limited. The lack of reimbursement for services creates a barrier to the implementation of new pharmacist care models in health systems [13].

2. Health System Overview

UCSDH is a comprehensive health system with an average daily census of approximately 600 patients and over 580,000 ambulatory care visits per year. Approximately 12 faculty from SSPPS provide collaborative care within the health system. Since 2010, the UCSDH pharmacy department developed a program expanding the role of the pharmacist in inpatient and ambulatory care and affiliated clinic settings. VASDHS provides care to more than 249,594 Veterans in the San Diego and Imperial Valley counties. In addition to the main facility in San Diego, VASDHS has six community-based outpatient clinics. Two faculty from SSPPS provide patient care within VASDHS. Faculty partner with staff pharmacists within each affiliated health system to develop new services. CPAs were developed and implemented for practice areas including chronic kidney disease (CKD), diabetes, family medicine, heart failure (HF), oncology, pain and palliative care, psychiatry, solid organ transplantation (SOT), and transitions of care (TOC). Collaborative care is delivered using three main care models: (1) pharmacists with physician oversight, (2) pharmacist–interprofessional teams, and (3) physician–pharmacist teams.

2.1. Needs Assessment and Proposal Development

Each program arose from a clinical need identified by the health system or through a needs assessment conducted by individual faculty with subspecialty expertise. Some needs were based on regulatory requirements (e.g., solid organ transplant), gaps identified by a physician champion, or grant funding available for novel clinical services. Initial steps include proposal development, identified gaps in care, proposed outcome measures, and a business case for return on investment. All pharmacist practices were successfully funded by affiliated health systems or grants.

2.2. Implementation

A multi-professional, collaborative approach involving pharmacists, physicians, nurses and administration personnel was required to establish and streamline the patient care process for the target population. Clinical program development included creating a scope of practice and credentialing, clinical guidelines or protocols, clinic schedules and space, referral criteria and documentation templates in the electronic health record (EHR). In each affiliated practice setting, the pharmacist–physician team determined the pharmacist scope of practice. Within the scope of practice, prescribing authorities were defined for specific diseases or conditions. These authorities include the initiation, adjustment and discontinuation of medications according to program-specific clinical guidelines or health system policies, where appropriate. Pharmacists have the authority to order medication-related tests (i.e., laboratory, pharmacogenomic and radiographic tests) to monitor therapy outcomes and make referrals to other providers. The CPA is not limited to specific medications (with the exception of controlled substances, where this is required by the Drug Enforcement Agency), providing prescribing flexibility. All pharmacists who wished to establish a CPA with a physician must have been licensed in California and demonstrate experience and competence treating patients within their specialty in order to be credentialed through their respective health system.

2.3. Outcome Measurement

EHRs enable the measurement of patient care clinical and process outcomes. Each program is responsible for defining, measuring and reporting care outcomes. Collaborative practice outcome measurements are in different phases, with some at the design phase and others using comprehensive dashboards. Dashboards are useful tools for tracking outcome measures and identifying areas for performance improvement. However, this approach is largely retrospective and dependent on the frequency of outcome trending. EHR disease registries are used to capture, manage and provide access to condition-specific information for a specified group of patients to support organized clinical care [14,15]. Registries enable point of care integration with clinical practice guidelines, outreach to patients between visits to address care gaps and periodic evaluation of aggregate data and performance to manage a population [16]. Several registries have been developed at UCSDH and VASDHS for patients with conditions such as CKD, T2D and thrombotic disorders.

3. Collaborative Care Models

3.1. Pharmacist with Physician Oversight Care Model

3.1.1. VASDHS Diabetes Intense Medical Management "Tune Up" Clinic

In 2009, a needs assessment identified over 9600 Veteran patients had a diabetes diagnosis and A1C values > 9% (per internal VASDHS VISN 22 Registry Data). In May 2009, the Diabetes Intense Medical Management (DIMM) "Tune Up" Clinic was created as a collaborative pharmacist–endocrinologist clinic to manage complex T2D patients and help them achieve clinical goals (e.g., A1C, blood pressure, lipid, weight goals) within 6 months. The clinical pharmacist specialist employs a short-term model that couples personalized clinical care with patient-specific diabetes education during an average of three 60 min visits over 6 months. After achieving goals, patients are referred back to their primary care provider (PCP). This allows a collaborative effort between the PCP and the pharmacist, frees up time during PCP visits to address other patient disorders, and provides patients with lifelong skills to manage their T2D and related metabolic disorders. The intended outcomes were to help PCPs and the medical center to achieve performance measures, avoid health system costs to treat diabetes complications, and prevent or delay patients from experiencing costly long-term complications of diabetes. Prior to implementation, the DIMM "Tune Up" clinic was reviewed, approved, and supported by key decision makers at the medical center: the Chief of Pharmacy, the Chief of Endocrinology, and the Chief of Internal Medicine, representing the PCPs.

Clinical issues, comorbidities, complications, socioeconomic and behavioral issues are integrated and assessed using the MTM Spider Web©, a visual tool developed for systematically creating a patient-centered clinical care plan [17]. The comprehensive nature of the tool helps ensure completeness and accuracy, as well as aiding patients to participate in shared decision-making while improving awareness and knowledge to assist in self-advocacy in their care. Strong emphasis is placed on adherence and educating and empowering patients to take control of their own diabetes without hypoglycemic events. Patients receive an individualized action plan and a personal medication record at each visit.

DIMM clinic outcomes demonstrate a 2.4% reduction in A1C compared to 0.8% in a PCP control group within 6 months, and glycemic control was achieved without significantly impacting medication regimen complexity [18,19]. A pharmacoeconomic analysis demonstrated that DIMM Clinic care resulted in $5287 savings per patient compared to usual PCP care, translating to a $9 to $1 return on investment [20]. Cost savings to the institution and reimbursement from insurance, as well as the strong metabolic outcomes, have justified continued clinic funding.

3.1.2. UCSDH Diabetes Self-Management

The Diabetes Self-Management Program is an ambulatory care clinic providing diabetes self-management education for up to 350 patients annually with pre-diabetes or T2D. This program was developed, implemented and led by two pharmacists and a physician champion. Subsequently, it was accredited by the Diabetes Education Accreditation Program enabling insurance billing. The pharmacists are funded by the medical group and provide care following a CPA. Patients are referred by their UCSDH provider for group classes or individual visits at four different UCSDH outpatient clinics. The group education classes consist of two core, two-hour classes, each 1–2 weeks apart, covering seven diabetes self-management topics. For patients with cognitive deficits, hearing or visual impairment, a language barrier, or those requiring insulin initiation, individual 60 min visits are preferred. Services provided include medication reconciliation and the assessment of adherence, nutrition habits, and glucose meter results, with education tailored to patient's specific needs. All patients set specific behavioral goals for themselves. Pharmacist recommendations are electronically sent to the referring provider after the visit. Telephone follow-up occurs 1–2 weeks following the classes or visits.

Annually, the program has over 500 office visits and 300 telephone follow ups. For group education, 45.8% patients attended one or two group meetings, and 13.2% attended three or four group meetings; the remaining patients were seen individually [21]. The mean decrease in A1C at 6 months was −0.6% compared to usual care −0.2%, $p < 0.001$, with no significant change in body mass index [21]. The program has also demonstrated a reduction in the number of patients with A1C > 8%, resulting in 55% achieving A1C <8% after 3 months and improved screening for A1C, with 57% of patients receiving two or more screenings per year. The outcomes have enabled continued funding of the program and the addition of a dietician (0.1 FTE) and scheduler (0.2 FTE).

3.1.3. VASDHS Heart Failure Medication Management Clinic

Established in 2012, the HF medication management clinic objective was to reduce HF readmissions and improve outcomes in collaboration with the VA Advanced HF Team comprising cardiologists, nurse practitioners and nurses. The pharmacists' scope of practice includes prescribing HF-related medications and ordering relevant laboratory and diagnostic studies. The advanced HF team establishes a diagnosis and initiates treatment, then referring patients for 30 to 60 min visits focused on medication management and follow-up. The pharmacist evaluates volume overload and worsening signs of congestion, titrates neurohormonal blockade to target doses, adjusts diuretics, assesses medication adherence and adverse effects. Typical medication titration visits can occur every 2–4 weeks, whereas patients requiring frequent diuretic adjustment may be seen weekly. The pharmacist works with the VASDHS quality improvement team to improve HF care and reduce hospital readmissions.

3.1.4. SSPPS Partners in Medication Therapy (PMT)

PMT was established to provide medication therapy management services to self-insured employers, medical groups, and health plans. Services include optimizing medications and patient education on medication therapy for chronic diseases such as T2D, asthma, and cardiovascular disease. Partnerships with large third-party health plans generated opportunities for SSPPS APPs to work with different PCPs in Independent Practice Associations to provide telehealth visits. Patients were identified and referred to the APP based on gaps in therapy, adherence problems, or lack of treatment goal attainment detected by the health plan pharmacy claims data or the EHR. Clinical protocols were developed for chronic conditions such as HTN and T2D as well as therapeutic interchange to reduce drug costs. Under a CPA, APPs were authorized to initiate, modify, substitute, or discontinue agreed-upon medications according to the protocol and to authorize refills.

Using individual medical group EHR remote access, four APPs performed one-hour phone sessions to provide comprehensive medication management, order labs, document recommendations and communicate with PCP as needed. Each patient received an updated medication list and action plan. Follow up frequency was determined by patient-specific needs. Patients were discharged after goal attainment or failure to have detectable improvement after 6 to 12 months. In an initial four-month pilot program with St. Joseph Heritage Healthcare (Orange County, CA, USA), 756 patients were referred and screened with 61 resulting appointments.

3.2. Interprofessional (IP) Care Model

3.2.1. UCSDH Chronic Kidney Disease (CKD)

In 2007, the CKD program was developed as an ambulatory clinic providing evidence-based IP care to delay CKD progression for approximately 400 patients with CKD Stages 2–5. UCSDHS funded the program as a separate cost center allowing financial outcomes including office visit volumes, medication revenue and expenses to be measured. The team consists of a nephrologist, pharmacist, nurse, dietitian and social worker. Patients see all team members at each visit, with new visits lasting approximately 90 min and return visits 60 min.

Under a CPA, the pharmacist conducts medication reconciliation, adherence assessment, and comprehensive medication management, facilitates access to medications, and provides patient education on changes to the medication therapy plan as well as the patient's progress towards their health-related outcomes. The pharmacist optimizes medication therapy for hypertension, diabetes, proteinuria, hyperlipidemia, anemia, bone disease, hyperkalemia, metabolic acidosis and vaccinations. The pharmacist estimates kidney function and adjusts the doses of medications. The pharmacist orders prescriptions to the community pharmacy, medications to be administered in clinic, vaccinations and medications to be administered in the infusion centers. Patients receive one-on-one education during their clinic visit, are provided links to online education videos (developed by the CKD Program), and can attend a group class on dialysis modalities and kidney transplantation.

Implementation barriers included the expense of an IP team and low insurance reimbursement rates. Additionally, the pharmacist, social worker, and dietitian could not bill the insurers for their individual services, and the physician could not bill more complex office visits for services provided by the team. To minimize facility overhead expenses, the CKD program operates clinics in the same physical space as general nephrology clinics. Clinic volumes are at capacity, and the expansion of the program has been limited due to cost and available space. Despite challenges with expansion, this program has been sustained with a steady stream of new referrals.

This program was the first in the US to receive disease-specific certification in CKD from the Joint Commission, demonstrating high-quality care to patients [22]. Clinical and process outcomes routinely measured include but are not limited to blood pressure control, non-steroidal anti-inflammatory drug (NSAID) usage and counseling on avoidance, sick day management with angiotensin converting enzyme inhibitors or angiotensin receptor blockers, and referral for vascular access and transplantation as well as vaccination rates. With over 1000 office visits per year, the team achieved systolic blood pressure control in 58% of patients, with 0% of patients prescribed NSAIDs, 98% counselled to avoid NSAID products, and 64% viewing online CKD educational videos [23].

3.2.2. UCSDH Oncology

Moores Cancer Center, the only National Cancer Institute-designated Comprehensive Cancer Center in San Diego, provides over 56,000 cancer patient visits annually including approximately 200 autologous and allogeneic hematopoietic stem cell transplants.

In 2014, the clinical pharmacy program was developed and implemented by a pharmacist in collaboration with a physician champion. Funding was provided by the cancer center for clinical services for two full days per week. The pharmacist initially developed a clinical practice in the thoracic medical oncology and the blood and marrow transplant departments. After one year of practicing, the pharmacist collaborated with leadership to expand the clinical pharmacy program by one full-time equivalent clinical pharmacy specialist in the head and neck/thoracic medical oncology ambulatory clinics.

The IP teams consist of oncologists, pharmacists, nurse case managers, mid-level providers (nurse practitioners and physician assistants), and medical assistants with the support of a social worker and a nutritionist on an as-needed basis. Clinical services provided by the pharmacist include medication management under a CPA, conducting medication reconciliation, oral chemotherapy adherence assessment, symptom management, immunization screening and ordering, therapeutic drug monitoring, oncology stewardship, and chemotherapy order preparation. The pharmacist provides literature support for the off-label utilization of cancer treatments. In addition, patients receive one-on-one education with the pharmacist or attend a group class focused on Chemotherapy and Immunotherapy Treatment that was developed and implemented by the pharmacist.

3.2.3. UCSDH Pain and Palliative Care

The ambulatory and inpatient palliative care IP consult team is comprised of physicians, pharmacists, social workers, nurse practitioners and a chaplain. A description of the CPA development has been previously published [24]. In accordance with California code 4052, UCSDH palliative care pharmacists have independent prescriptive authority, with Drug Enforcement Agency (DEA) licensure and National Provider Index (NPI) status. Reasons for pharmacist consultation included physical symptom management, including but not limited to cancer-related pain, constipation, nausea and vomiting, fatigue, and insomnia.

Initial studies evaluating palliative care pharmacist contributions in the ambulatory care and inpatient settings have been positive [25–27]. Patients seen in clinic by a palliative care pharmacist versus patients who received standard of care showed trends for better pain control and health-related quality of life and function [26]. Medication prescribing changes by palliative care pharmacists commonly include a change in dose and/or the initiation of a new medication [27]. Positive trends were observed in pain control for patients with cancer over subsequent clinic visits [27]. Analgesic efficacy was improved by 17% and non-adherence was reduced by 13% [27].

Additionally, in the inpatient setting, the palliative care pharmacist provides opioid stewardship and guideline development for safe and effective analgesia. Prescribing trends are evaluated for safety and efficacy. Areas of focus include but are not limited to the prescription of fentanyl patches, patient-controlled analgesia, gabapentinoids, ketamine oral and intravenous infusion, lidocaine intravenous infusion, mexiletine, methadone, and naloxone [23,28–36]. Guidelines for the appropriate use of end-of-life opioids were developed [37]. Early access to the inpatient palliative care pharmacist resulted in a shortened length of stay, shortened length from admission to palliative care consult, and a positive impact on time from consult to discharge or death [25].

3.2.4. UCSDH Solid Organ Transplantation

The Solid Organ Transplant program is a comprehensive IP center that provides evidenced-based, full-spectrum care from pre-transplant evaluation to post-transplant management for patients needing a kidney, pancreas, liver, lung, or heart transplant. The teams consist of transplant physician specialists (i.e., nephrologist, hepatologist, cardiologist, etc.), transplant surgeons, pharmacists, nurses, dietitians, and social workers. In 2004, the bylaws of the United Network for Organ Sharing were amended to include pharmacists as necessary providers on the transplant team [38]. There are eight dedicated transplant pharmacists, including two faculty pharmacists who each devote 15% effort to ambulatory patient care and receive salary support from the UCSDHS Center for Transplantation. Revenue generated by improving patient utilization of discharge and ambulatory UCSDH pharmacies has led to expansion and continued salary support for transplant pharmacists.

Similar to other services in the health system, transplant pharmacists initiate, discontinue, change, and monitor drug therapy under a CPA. Working closely with transplant physicians and surgeons, pharmacists manage a patient's immunosuppressive therapies, as well as treatments for complications of immunosuppression, other associated medical conditions, and preventative therapies. The pharmacists conduct medication reconciliation, adherence assessment, a focused assessment of immunosuppression, MTM for various complications of transplantation, order laboratory tests, immunizations, facilitate access to medications and provide comprehensive patient education. In 2018, approximately 95 kidney, 41 liver, 56 heart, and 23 lung transplants were performed, and long-term follow-up was provided.

3.2.5. UCSDH Transitions of Care (TOC)

The TOC program aims to optimize care and reduce hospital readmissions by providing hospital and ambulatory care continuity services for approximately 7800 high-risk patients within UCSDH. Funding support for the TOC program was initially driven by Medicare incentive programs such as Delivery System Reform Incentive Payment (DSRIP) and the Community-Based Care Transitions Program (CCTP) to improve care transitions for high-risk patients. The TOC pilot program was implemented by a pharmacist to target patients with advanced stages of HF. Following the conclusion of the DSRIP and CCTP projects, funding from UCSDH was justified with documented interventions from the pilot programs. The TOC pharmacist service has since expanded to include other populations (e.g., HIV) and select groups of managed care patients. An SSPPS faculty member joined the TOC program with UCSDH funding support of 40% in an effort to assist with the increased breadth of patient services.

TOC pharmacists work under a CPA with prescribing authority to initiate, adjust, monitor, or discontinue medication therapy for HF and related conditions in hospital and ambulatory clinics. Inpatient TOC pharmacists make rounds daily with an IP team, conduct admission and discharge medication reconciliation, assess adherence, collaborate with the medical team on medication therapy, facilitate access to medications, and provide comprehensive patient education. Ambulatory TOC pharmacists perform phone-call follow-up and focus on post-discharge patients in-clinic to conduct medication reconciliation, assess adherence, perform MTM for HF and related conditions, facilitate medication access, and provide patient education.

Given the expense of pharmacist salaries and the inability to bill insurers for pharmacist services, funding remains the primary barrier to expanding the TOC program. Funding for pharmacy technicians and longitudinal TOC introductory pharmacy practice experiences for pharmacy students have been implemented to maximize budget resources. Approximately 70% of patients require a pharmacist intervention, with an average of two interventions per patient.

3.3. Pharmacist-Physician Team Care Model

3.3.1. UCSDH Family Medicine Clinics

The UCSDH Family Medicine Clinics provide services at three locations throughout San Diego County to patients from pre-conception to end-of-life care. Since 2010, two clinical pharmacists have provided chronic disease management under a CPA. Patients are identified by the PCP and are referred for a "shared" collaborative visit with a pharmacist and a family medicine physician. During each visit, the pharmacist conducts medication reconciliation and reviews the patient's past medical history, relevant family and social histories, risk factors, allergies, medications, and lab results. Pharmacists manage anticoagulation, diabetes, HTN, hyperlipidemia, tobacco cessation, and immunizations. A care plan is developed with the patient that includes treatment goals and education. The plan is communicated with the physician, who also meets with the patient to address any further questions or health problems. Based on the complexity of the visit, insurance is billed with the physician signing off on the care plan. The PCP is also notified of the care plan. Patients are seen in 30 min appointments with regular follow-up, accounting for over 1000 annual office visits.

Ongoing and regular physician referrals remain a challenge. Patients may also be identified through EHR registries or dashboards and then scheduled for a pharmacist visit, although patients are more likely to attend visits when suggested by their PCP. Additionally, since the physician paired with each pharmacist is different at each session, it is not always guaranteed that a patients' own PCP will be the physician during their shared visit. The physician sees his/her own limited set of patients for the session, and so challenges arise with respect to timing and visit duration, impacting the patient and provider experience. While these types of visits do increase IP collaboration and allow for more complex visits and reimbursement, there have been discussions about moving toward a more independent-pharmacist model within the clinics.

Clinical outcome measures being implemented include improved A1C, anticoagulation time in the therapeutic range, the achievement of goal blood pressure, and the primary and secondary prevention of coronary artery disease and stroke. This particular program was selected as one of three in 2018 by the Centers for Disease Control and Prevention for an evaluability assessment site visit as a program routinely using innovative strategies in hypertension care [39].

3.3.2. Geriatric Community Partnerships

In 2015, UCSDH was awarded a grant from the federal Health Resources Services Administration Geriatrics Workforce Enhancement Program (GWEP) of the Department of Health and Human Services to train and research novel approaches to providing older adult care. One particular focus of this proposal was the incorporation of a clinical pharmacist in a primary care clinic to provide direct-patient care for underserved populations via a partnership with the Medicare–Medicaid-funded Program of All-Inclusive Care for the Elderly (PACE) Clinic in San Ysidro, CA, and to train and embed a pharmacist fellow in the clinic to perform comprehensive medication management under a CPA [40]. The funding also supported a part-time student pharmacist to assist with clinic provider education on potentially inappropriate medications, polypharmacy, medication regimen complexity, program development, and participation in required rapid-cycle quality improvement projects [41]. The patient population was 90% percent Spanish-speaking, with limited health literacy and, as Medicaid qualifiers, they were low-income patients with an average of 14 medications per patient. The pharmacist conducts transitions of care medication reconciliation, manages anticoagulant dosing, initiates immunizations, reduces the use of inappropriate medication and high-cost medications, and provides medication usage recommendations to center management [42]. The clinic has continued its funding of a full-time clinical pharmacist.

3.3.3. UCSDH Psychiatry

UCSDH Outpatient Psychiatry Services include general psychiatry and specialty clinics in mental health such as college mental health, child and teen psychiatry, addiction treatment, treatment-resistant depression, women's reproductive mental health, sexual health, early psychosis, and senior behavioral health. The clinics employ numerous health professionals to provide a full range of outpatient psychiatric services, including intakes, individual and group psychotherapy, pharmacotherapy, and psychoeducation. Established in 2008 [43], the pharmacist clinic has experienced between approximately 150–300 annual office visits [43]. The patient population varies from county-funded patients with severe mental illness to public and private funding for mood disorders, anxiety disorders, PTSD, and ADHD. The Department of Psychiatry provides funding for 10% work for the psychiatric pharmacist's clinic time.

During each visit, the psychiatric pharmacist spends approximately 30–45 min providing psychotropic medication management under a CPA. The pharmacist conducts medication reconciliation, assesses medication adherence and adverse effects, evaluates medication dosing, assists with refills and insurance authorizations, and makes referrals to other services. The pharmacist and attending psychiatrist develop the therapeutic plan and then discuss the plan with the patient. The pharmacist has a DEA license, which allows the initiation and modification of controlled and non-controlled medications. Recently, the pharmacist coordinated the initiation of a new, long-acting, injectable antipsychotic program to improve patient access and continuity of care.

Implementation challenges include funding for the pharmacist's work, insurance billing, shared visit scheduling, and regulatory requirements for documentation. Program outcomes include patient encounter volumes, top patient diagnosis, and pharmacist interventions. Future program outcomes will include symptom improvement using standard rating scales and required medication monitoring documentation.

4. Discussion

In this paper, we describe collaborative pharmacist–physician practice models that provide clinical care to patients with complex disease states. The pharmacists not only focus on the optimization of care for their respective specialties but also provide comprehensive care for comorbid conditions and complications. Notably, the pharmacists provide a large scope of services which encompass medication therapy management, including but not limited to medication reconciliation, initiating and adjusting medications, the ordering and monitoring of laboratory tests, performing physical examination, assessing and optimizing adherence, promoting healthy lifestyles, and providing education. These services were delivered using different care models integrating the pharmacist within IP teams or partnering with physicians.

The type of practice model chosen was based on the disease state, patient complexity, needs assessment, strategic goals, and financial viability. We summarized the advantages and disadvantages for the described care models (Table 1). For example, the DIMM clinic model is a pharmacist with physician oversight model since evidence-based medication optimization to improve glycemic control could be most efficiently delivered by the pharmacist provider. However, in psychiatry, the pharmacist–physician team care model was chosen due to patient complexity and the need for an individualized approach to management that considers numerous patient factors.

Table 1. Advantages and disadvantages of different pharmacist care models.

Care Model	Advantages	Disadvantages
Pharmacist with physician oversight	Autonomy in clinical decision making. Efficient model for optimizing medication management using evidence-based guidelines. Improves public recognition of advanced pharmacist provider roles.	Can only be applied to patients with established diagnosis who mainly require optimization of medications. Complex patients requiring additional diagnostic testing may not be appropriate. Pharmacist may feel a disconnect from physician collaborator. Dependent on referrals from physician collaborators. Low reimbursement on visits in the United States.
Interprofessional	Best suited for complex disease states or patients with numerous comorbidities. Patient convenience-comprehensive care delivered in one single office visit. Greater ability to achieve target clinical outcomes with multi-prong management (e.g., lifestyle modification, medications, social interventions) Higher reimbursement since physician provider bills for visits.	Requires greater coordination of team members during visits to ensure efficiency. Less time for each health professional to spend with patient. Longer visit duration for patients. Longer visits may result in lower patient volumes. Interprofessional team is resource intensive.
Pharmacist-Physician Team	Can manage established and newly diagnosed patients who may require additional diagnostic testing. Enhances care provided in physician only visits due to optimization of drug therapy. Easier to coordinate team members. Higher reimbursement since physician provider bills for visits.	Less pharmacist autonomy Longer visits Dependent on referrals for patient volume.

Importantly, the majority of these care models have been funded by the affiliated health systems, and a few are funded by grant mechanisms. This was made possible by creating goals that align with the health system priority initiatives and recruiting faculty whose expertise could help to achieve these goals. A business case was developed by reviewing published literature, identifying potential quality outcomes and direct and indirect financial metrics. Several studies have been published demonstrating the financial benefit of pharmacist care services in a variety of care environments from community pharmacy to ambulatory care clinics and to hospital acute care environments. In a study examining the impact of the community pharmacist-initiated management of uncomplicated urinary tract infections, pharmacist care was associated with lower costs ($72.47) when compared to family ($141.53) and emergency ($368.16) physician-initiated care, estimated to result in significant long-term net total savings of $51 million [44]. Ourth and colleagues conducted a cost-effectiveness study of clinical pharmacists managing diabetes and found a negative cost per quality of life adjusted years after 3 years, suggesting that it is cost-effective to incorporate pharmacists into diabetes care teams [45]. Similarly, studies of transitions of care programs have demonstrated significant cost savings. Ni and colleagues documented average cost savings of $2139 in the first 180 days after discharge [46].

The practices described in this paper proved to be sustainable with continued funding for long periods of time despite cessation of grant funding. Moore and colleagues found that after initially funding pharmacist services through grant mechanisms and demonstrating quality care, the services could be continued and expanded through funding by accountable care organizations [47]. We demonstrate that clinical faculty can effectively provide comprehensive pharmacist services to a large breadth of complex patient populations across multiple practice settings in affiliated health systems. Our programs position pharmacists to obtain APP status in the future given their collaborative practice meets necessary criteria for APh licensure.

We stated that the outcome measurement of these pharmacist care models varies with some practices in the design phase and others measuring patient volume to robust clinical and process outcome dashboards. Successful programs measure meaningful outcomes that demonstrate the return on investment for the health system. Many of our programs have developed significant improvements in clinical and process outcomes. We demonstrated that pharmacist-delivered diabetes care resulted in A1c reductions of 2.4%, compared to 0.8% for standard of care, with significant cost savings. The pharmacist within the IP CKD care team focused on reducing the number of patients prescribed an NSAID to 0% and counseling over 98% patients on NSAID avoidance. In palliative care, pharmacist interventions resulted in 17% improved medication efficacy and a reduction in non-adherence by 13%. Transitions of care pharmacists demonstrated a significant reduction in hospital readmissions with cost savings to the institution. These clinical and process outcomes have been revised as needed for continuous quality improvement, with the retirement of outcomes at goal and new outcomes identified. In some instances, new outcomes or strategies were developed for financial sustainability. These results have been disseminated at national and international IP conferences, or published in journals with broad readership. This dissemination is critical to allow for these care models to be easily replicated at other institutions.

The value of pharmacist services we described has received notable recognition from government agencies, accreditation bodies, and professional societies. From these various models of pharmacist services, we identified some common facilitators. These included a gap in care that could be met with pharmacist services, a linkage between clinical and financial outcomes, a physician champion to support proposals, and the strategic recruitment of faculty with expertise in these growth areas at affiliated health systems.

Program design and implementation always comes with challenges; space and funding are well-recognized resource barriers. However, our collective approach has been to share our faculty experiences and to brainstorm funding mechanisms and develop successful space propositions such as colocation. The colocation of interprofessional team members in a shared work space and elimination of private physician work offices has been shown to improve team communication, cohesiveness, and team primacy [48]. An important facilitator of funding challenges is the joint appointment of the UCSDH Chief Pharmacy Officer as a clinical faculty member that provides a critical advantage for the development of new clinical services at UCSDH. Our future directions include the development of new clinical faculty practice settings in geriatrics and infectious disease within the affiliated health systems.

5. Conclusions

In conclusion, the expansion of pharmacist services delivered by clinical faculty has several benefits to affiliated health systems: (1) significant improvements in patient care quality, (2) access to experts in specialty areas, and (3) the dissemination of outcomes and national and international recognition, increasing the visibility of the health system.

Author Contributions: Conceptualization, L.A., C.L.M., R.F.S., I.S.; Writing—Original Draft Preparation, L.A., C.L.M., R.F.S., I.S., J.D.H., S.L., R.S.A., J.D.M., S.M.T., J.N., C.L.M., N.A.P., J.H.W., F.K.Y., K.C.L., C.D.D.; Writing—Review & Editing, L.A., C.L.M., R.F.S., I.S., J.D.H., S.L., R.S.A., J.D.M., S.M.T., J.N., C.L.M., N.A.P., J.H.W., F.K.Y., K.C.L., C.D.D.; Project Administration, L.A.

Funding: This research received no external funding.

Conflicts of Interest: The authors declare no conflict of interest.

References

1. American College of Clinical Pharmacy; Hammond, R.W.; Schwartz, A.H.; Campbell, M.J.; Remington, T.L.; Chuck, S.; Blair, M.M.; Vassey, A.M.; Rospond, R.M.; Herner, S.J.; et al. Collaborative drug therapy management by pharmacists—2003. *Pharmacotherapy* **2003**, *23*, 1210–1225. [PubMed]
2. Carter, B.L.; Ardery, G.; Dawson, J.D.; James, P.A.; Bergus, G.R.; Doucette, W.R.; Chrischilles, E.A.; Franciscus, C.L.; Xu, Y. Physician and pharmacist collaboration to improve blood pressure control. *Arch. Intern. Med.* **2009**, *169*, 1996–2002. [CrossRef] [PubMed]
3. Carter, B.L.; Bergus, G.R.; Dawson, J.D.; Farris, K.B.; Doucette, W.R.; Chrischilles, E.A.; Hartz, A.J. A cluster randomized trial to evaluate physician/pharmacist collaboration to improve blood pressure control. *J. Clin. Hypertens. (Greenwich)* **2008**, *10*, 260–271. [CrossRef]

4. Hirsch, J.D.; Steers, N.; Adler, D.S.; Kuo, G.M.; Morello, C.M.; Lang, M.; Singh, R.F.; Wood, Y.; Kaplan, R.M.; Mangione, C.M. Primary care-based, pharmacist-physician collaborative medication-therapy management of hypertension: A randomized, pragmatic trial. *Clin Ther.* **2014**, *36*, 1244–1254. [CrossRef] [PubMed]

5. Greer, N.L.; Minneapolis, V.A. *Pharmacist-Led Chronic Disease Management: A Systematic Review of Effectiveness and Harms Compared to Usual Care*; Department of Veterans Affairs Health Services Research & Development Service: Washington, DC, USA, 2015.

6. McAlister, F.A.; Stewart, S.; Ferrua, S.; McMurray, J.J. Multidisciplinary strategies for the management of heart failure patients at high risk for admission-A systematic review of randomized trials. *J. Am. Coll. Cardiol.* **2004**, *44*, 810–819.

7. Matzke, G.R.; Moczygemba, L.R.; Williams, K.J.; Czar, M.J.; Lee, W.T. Impact of a pharmacist-physician collaborative care model on patient outcomes and health services utilization. *Am. J. Health Syst. Pharm.* **2018**, *75*, 1039–1047. [CrossRef]

8. Hattingh, L.; Sim, T.F.; Sunderland, B.; Czarniak, P. Successful implementation and provision of enhanced and extended pharmacy services. *Res. Soc. Adm. Pharm.* **2019**, in press. [CrossRef]

9. Sim, T.F.; Wright, B.; Hattingh, L.; Parsons, R.; Sunderland, B.; Czarniak, P. A cross-sectional survey of enhanced and extended professional services in community pharmacies: A pharmacy perspective. *Res. Soc. Adm. Pharm.* **2019**, in press. [CrossRef]

10. Jeong, S.; Lee, M.; Ji, E. Effect of pharmaceutical care interventions on glycemic control in patients with diabetes: A systematic review and meta-analysis. *Ther. Clin. Risk Manag.* **2018**, *14*, 1813–1829. [CrossRef]

11. Lee, J.K.; Slack, M.K.; Martin, J.; Ehrman, C.; Chisholm-Burns, M. Geriatric patient care by U.S. pharmacists in healthcare teams: Systematic review and meta-analyses. *J. Am. Geriatr. Soc.* **2013**, *61*, 1119–1127. [CrossRef]

12. Houle, S.K.; Chuck, A.W.; McAlister, F.A.; Tsuyuki, R.T. Effect of a pharmacist-managed hypertension program on health system costs: An evaluation of the Study of Cardiovascular Risk Intervention by Pharmacists-Hypertension (SCRIP-HTN). *Pharmacotherapy* **2012**, *32*, 527–537. [CrossRef] [PubMed]

13. Smith, M. Primary Care Pharmacist Services Align With Payment Reform and Provider "Joy of Practice". *Ann. Pharmacother.* **2019**, *53*, 311–315. [CrossRef] [PubMed]

14. Schmittdiel, J.A.; Gopalan, A.; Lin, M.W.; Banerjee, S.; Chau, C.V.; Adams, A.S. Population Health Management for Diabetes: Health Care System-Level Approaches for Improving Quality and Addressing Disparities. *Curr. Diabetes Rep.* **2017**, *17*, 31. [CrossRef] [PubMed]

15. Mendu, M.L.; Ahmed, S.; Maron, J.K.; Rao, S.K.; Chaguturu, S.K.; May, M.F.; Mutter, W.P.; Burdge, K.A.; Steele, D.J.; Mount, D.B.; et al. Development of an electronic health record-based chronic kidney disease registry to promopulation health management. *BMC Nephrol.* **2019**, *20*, 72. [CrossRef] [PubMed]

16. Foundatiote pon, C.H.-C. Using Computerized Registries in Chronic Disease Care. 2004. Available online: https://www.chcf.org/publication/using-computerized-registries-in-chronic-disease-care/ (accessed on 10 October 2019).

17. Morello, C.M.; Hirsch, J.D.; Lee, K.C. Navigating complex patients using an innovative tool: The MTM Spider Web. *J. Am. Pharm. Assoc. (2003)* **2013**, *53*, 530–538. [CrossRef] [PubMed]

18. Morello, C.M.; Christopher, M.L.; Ortega, L.; Khoan, J.; Rotunno, T.; Edelman, S.V.; Henry, R.R.; Hirsch, J.D. Clinical Outcomes Associated With a Collaborative Pharmacist-Endocrinologist Diabetes Intense Medical Management "Tune Up" Clinic in Complex Patients. *Ann. Pharmacother.* **2016**, *50*, 8–16. [CrossRef] [PubMed]

19. Morello, C.M.; Rotunno, T.; Khoan, J.; Hirsch, J.D. Hirsch, Improved Glycemic Control With Minimal Change in Medication Regimen Complexity in a Pharmacist-Endocrinologist Diabetes Intense Medical Management (DIMM) "Tune Up" Clinic. *Ann. Pharmacother.* **2018**, *52*, 1091–1097. [CrossRef]

20. Hirsch, J.D.; Bounthavong, M.; Arjmand, A.; Ha, D.R.; Cadiz, C.L.; Zimmerman, A.; Ourth, H.; Morreale, A.P.; Edelman, S.V.; Morello, C.M. Estimated Cost-Effectiveness, Cost Benefit, and Risk Reduction Associated with an Endocrinologist-Pharmacist Diabetes Intense Medical Management "Tune-Up" Clinic. *J. Manag. Care Sp. Pharm.* **2017**, *23*, 318–326. [CrossRef]

21. Singh, R.F.; Kelly, P.; Tam, A.; Bronner, J.; Morello, C.M.; Hirsch, J.D. Evaluation of a short, interactive diabetes self-management program by pharmacists for type 2 diabetes. *BMC Res. Notes* **2018**, *11*, 828. [CrossRef]

22. Commission, T.J. A Multidisciplinary Approach to Improvement in Chronic Kidney Disease Care. *Source* **2019**, *17*, 1–4.

23. Awdishu, L.; Moore, T.; Morrison, M.; Turner, C.; Trzebinska, D. A Primer on Quality Assurance and Performance Improvement for Interprofessional Chronic Kidney Disease Care: A Path to Joint Commission Certification. *Pharmacy* **2019**, *7*, 83. [CrossRef] [PubMed]

24. Atayee, R.S.; Best, B.M.; Daniels, C.E. Development of an ambulatory palliative care pharmacist practice. *J. Palliat. Med.* **2008**, *11*, 1077–1082. [CrossRef] [PubMed]

25. Atayee, R.S.; Sam, A.M.; Edmonds, K.P. Patterns of Palliative Care Pharmacist Interventions and Outcomes as Part of Inpatient Palliative Care Consult Service. *J. Palliat. Med.* **2018**, *21*, 1761–1767. [CrossRef] [PubMed]

26. Hansen, P.R.; Ma, J.D.; Atayee, R.S. Preliminary analysis of midlevel practitioners on pain and health-related quality of life and function for a palliative care service at a comprehensive cancer center. *J. Palliat. Med.* **2012**, *15*, 388–389. [CrossRef] [PubMed]

27. Ma, J.D.; Tran, V.; Chan, C.; Mitchell, W.M.; Atayee, R.S. Retrospective analysis of pharmacist interventions in an ambulatory palliative care practice. *J. Oncol. Pharm. Pract.* **2016**, *22*, 757–765. [CrossRef] [PubMed]

28. Amin, P.; Roeland, E.; Atayee, R. Case report: Efficacy and tolerability of ketamine in opioid-refractory cancer pain. *J. Pain Palliat. Care Pharmacother.* **2014**, *28*, 233–242. [CrossRef]

29. Hakim, R.C.; Edmonds, K.P.; Atayee, R.S. Case Report: Utility of Ketamine, Lidocaine, and Mexiletine as Nonopioid Adjuvants in Complex Cancer-Associated Pain. *J. Pain Palliat. Care Pharmacother.* **2018**, *32*, 15–19. [CrossRef]

30. Jahansouz, F.H.J.; Dhillon, K.; Helmons, P.; Lamott, J.A.; Kolan, S.; Atayee, R.S. Evaluation of fentanyl patch orders in an academic medical center. *Hosp. Pharm.* **2011**, *46*, 854–863.

31. Jahansouz, F.R.S.; Lamott, J.; Chu, F.; Atayee, R. Impact of smart infusion pump implementation on intravenous patient-controlled analgesia medication errors. *Calif. J. Health-Syst. Pharm.* **2013**, *25*, 145–150.

32. Karimian, P.; Atayee, R.S.; Ajayi, T.A.; Edmonds, K.P. Methadone Dose Selection for Treatment of Pain Compared with Consensus Recommendations. *J. Palliat. Med.* **2017**, *20*, 1385–1388. [CrossRef]

33. Ryan, A.J.; Lin, F.; Atayee, R.S. Ketamine mouthwash for mucositis pain. *J. Palliat. Med.* **2009**, *12*, 989–991. [CrossRef] [PubMed]

34. Savelloni, J.; Gunter, H.; Lee, K.C.; Hsu, C.; Yi, C.; Edmonds, K.P.; Furnish, T.; Atayee, R.S. Risk of respiratory depression with opioids and concomitant gabapentinoids. *J. Pain Res.* **2017**, *10*, 2635–2641. [CrossRef] [PubMed]

35. Sexton, J.; Atayee, R.S.; Bruner, H.C. Case Report: Ketamine for Pain and Depression in Advanced Cancer. *J. Palliat. Med.* **2018**, *21*, 1670–1673. [CrossRef] [PubMed]

36. Yung, L.; Lee, K.C.; Hsu, C.; Furnish, T.; Atayee, R.S. Patterns of naloxone use in hospitalized patients. *Postgrad. Med. J.* **2017**, *129*, 40–45. [CrossRef] [PubMed]

37. Lin, K.J.; Ching, A.; Edmonds, K.P.; Roeland, E.J.; Revta, C.; Ma, J.D.; Atayee, R.S. Variable Patterns of Continuous Morphine Infusions at End of Life. *J. Palliat. Med.* **2015**, *18*, 786–789. [CrossRef]

38. United Network for Organ Sharing. Attachment 1 to Appendix B of the UNOS Bylaws; Designated Transplant Program Criteria. 2004. Available online: https://unos.org/wp-content/uploads/unos/Appendix_B_AttachI_XIII.pdf (accessed on 10 October 2019).

39. Centers for Disease Control and Prevention. University of California San Diego Pharmacy Program Field Notes. 2018. Available online: https://www.cdc.gov/dhdsp/docs/UCSD_Field_Notes-508.pdf (accessed on 10 October 2019).

40. Park, P.E.; Watanabe, J.H. Empowering the interdisciplinary care team for improving care in seniors via clinical pharmacy: The San Diego Geriatrics Workforce Enhancement Program. *J. Contemp. Pharm. Pract.* **2017**, *64*, 24–31.

41. Tam, S.H.Y.; Hirsch, J.D.; Watanabe, J.H. Medication Regimen Complexity in Long-Term Care Facilities and Adverse Drug Events-Related Hospitalizations. *Consult. Pharm.* **2017**, *32*, 281–284. [CrossRef]

42. Watanabe, J.H.; Chau, D.L.; Hirsch, J.D. Federal and Individual Spending on the 10 Costliest Medications in Medicare Part D from 2011 to 2015. *J. Am. Geriatr. Soc.* **2018**, *66*, 1621–1624. [CrossRef]

43. Tallian, K.B.; Hirsch, J.D.; Kuo, G.M.; Chang, C.A.; Gilmer, T.; Messinger, M.; Chan, P.; Daniels, C.E.; Lee, K.C. Development of a pharmacist-psychiatrist collaborative medication therapy management clinic. *J. Am. Pharm. Assoc. (2003)* **2012**, *52*, e252–e258. [CrossRef]

44. Sanyal, C.; Husereau, D.R.; Beahm, N.P.; Smyth, D.; Tsuyuki, R.T. Cost-effectiveness and budget impact of the management of uncomplicated urinary tract infection by community pharmacists. *BMC Health Serv. Res.* **2019**, *19*, 499. [CrossRef]

45. Ourth, H.; Nelson, J.; Spoutz, P.; Morreale, A.P. Development of a Pharmacoeconomic Model to Demonstrate the Effect of Clinical Pharmacist Involvement in Diabetes Management. *J. Manag. Care Spec. Pharm.* **2018**, *24*, 449–457. [CrossRef] [PubMed]
46. Ni, W.; Colayco, D.; Hashimoto, J.; Komoto, K.; Gowda, C.; Wearda, B.; McCombs, J. Reduction of healthcare costs through a transitions-of-care program. *Am. J. Health. Syst. Pharm.* **2018**, *75*, 613–621. [CrossRef] [PubMed]
47. Moore, G.D.; Kosirog, E.R.; Vande Griend, J.P.; Freund, J.E.; Saseen, J.J. Expansion of clinical pharmacist positions through sustainable funding. *Am. J. Health Syst. Pharm.* **2018**, *75*, 978–981. [CrossRef] [PubMed]
48. Stroebel, R.J.; Obeidat, B.; Lim, L.; Mitchell, J.D.; Jasperson, D.B.; Zimring, C. The impact of clinic design on teamwork development in primary care. *Health Care Manag. Rev.* Available online: https://www.ncbi.nlm.nih.gov/pubmed/31385829 (accessed on 10 October 2019). [CrossRef] [PubMed]

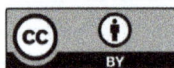

MDPI

Brief Report

Development of a Unique Student Pharmacist Internship in a Primary Care Provider System

Norman E. Fenn III [1], Natalie R. Gadbois [2], Gwen J. Seamon [2], Shannon L. Castek [2] and Kimberly S. Plake [2,*]

[1] Fisch College of Pharmacy, The University of Texas at Tyler, Tyler, TX 75799, USA; nfenn@uttyler.edu
[2] College of Pharmacy, Purdue University, West Lafayette, IN 47907, USA; ngadbois@purdue.edu (N.R.G.); gjseamon@gmail.com (G.J.S.); scastek@gmail.com (S.L.C.)
* Correspondence: kplake@purdue.edu; Tel.: +1-765-494-5966

Received: 6 March 2019; Accepted: 9 April 2019; Published: 13 April 2019

check for updates

Abstract: Purpose: To describe a unique pharmacy intern program in a group of federally qualified health center (FQHC) outpatient primary care provider clinics. Summary: A pharmacy intern program was created at the North Central Nursing Clinics in Indiana, a group of four FQHC outpatient primary care provider facilities. Intern-performed tasks included: Prior authorization (PA) requests, medication assistance program (MAP) applications, sample procurement and inventory, and contraceptive devices for implantation inventory management. Interns interacted with clinic administration, nurse practitioners, and medical staff to complete their assigned responsibilities. Over a one-year period, the interns completed documentation on more than 2000 charts during a combined 12 h a week. Interns identified the interprofessional interactions as the most beneficial experience, while providers acknowledged no difference in the processing of paperwork during the transition of duties from pharmacy fellow to intern. Conclusion: This unique pharmacy intern program was successfully created and implemented in a primary care provider office, resulting in learning opportunities for pharmacy interns, as well as operational efficiencies to fellows, providers, and the organization.

Keywords: pharmacy intern; student pharmacist; primary care; interprofessional; federally qualified health center

1. Introduction

Pharmacy interns have a variety of different roles and responsibilities and typically work in community and hospital pharmacy environments [1–6]. Student pharmacists, serving as interns, contribute to their educational process and professional development as they gain practical experiences related to the pharmacy curriculum. While there is evidence of student pharmacist involvement in direct patient care activities through student-run free clinics, these students operate on a volunteer basis or are participating as part of a required pharmacy practice experience, compared to intern positions that are paid [7–10]. Currently, there are no descriptions of the role of pharmacy interns in the literature beyond those in hospital or community pharmacy settings. In this manuscript, a unique pharmacy intern program in a rural outpatient primary care facility is described.

The North Central Nursing Clinics (NCNC) in Indiana consist of four primary care provider offices in rural communities. Affiliated with the Purdue University School of Nursing and College of Pharmacy, the clinics are led by nurse practitioners whose specialties include pediatrics, family medicine, and women's health. Other integral members of the healthcare team include support staff (e.g., front office personnel, billing, insurance navigators), social workers, medical assistants, and nurses. The clinics are federally qualified health centers (FQHC), and all four sites are considered

Level 2 Patient-Centered Medical Homes. As part of the FQHC requirements, no patient is denied care based on their ability to pay for healthcare services. The patient population served at each of the clinics varies, with 42–45% of patients enrolled in Medicaid and/or Medicare and 22–23% of patients being uninsured. Roughly 10% of the clinics' patients are native Spanish speakers, requiring translational and interpretive services.

Pharmacy fellows are licensed pharmacists who serve as the sole provider of clinical pharmacy services at the clinics as part of the Purdue University College of Pharmacy Academia and Ambulatory Care Fellowship program. Fellows spend approximately 50% of their time in clinic and perform multiple roles in the clinics, including: conducting patient visits for chronic diseases under collaborative practice agreements (CPAs), precepting student pharmacists on advanced pharmacy practice experiences (APPEs), and providing cost-effective medication recommendations. Fellows are also responsible for completing prior authorizations (PAs), assisting patients in obtaining medication through medication assistance programs (MAPs), and drug inventory management. Completion of a postgraduate year one residency is a prerequisite for the fellowship program, as the fellows are required to operate independently at these clinics. Two of the clinics serve as the fellows' primary practice sites, with one fellow based at each clinic. In addition, each fellow provides remote pharmacy services for the clinics not staffed by the fellowship program.

2. Pharmacy Internship Program Description and Review

In August 2016, pharmacy services expanded, which resulted in increased direct patient care activities and the need for assistance with administrative tasks. As a response to this need, the pharmacy internship program was created. Two interns were hired for a total of 12 h per week. Described duties included completing PAs, coordinating MAP applications, and tracking contraceptive device prescription processing for each of the four clinics, as well as managing inventory of medication samples at the main clinic. It was decided by all involved parties that students recruited for the intern positions would have completed at least their first year of the professional program. Both interns are supervised by the on-site fellow and communicate any issues or questions to them. The interns each work primarily out of one clinic site location, but assist with administrative responsibilities for patients from all of the clinics. All documentation by the interns is submitted to both the responsible provider and the fellow for review. Interns also perform follow-up phone calls with the patient and the pharmacy as necessary to ensure timely processing of medications and expedite patient care. When processing PAs, if an adjustment can be made due to a formulary requirement or therapeutically equivalent medication, the fellow is authorized to change the medication order, either through a CPA or with verbal authorization from the provider.

From October 2017 to October 2018, pharmacy interns completed in excess of 2000 documented tasks (Table 1). Interns initially worked a combined 12 h a week at the clinic. For quality assessment, interns were instructed to document their daily workload processes, recording the number of PAs, MAPs, contraceptive devices, inventory and other assorted tasks not covered under these categories. As a result of significant work volume, intern hours were expanded to a combined 16 hours a week in May 2018. The documented tasks may be slightly underestimated due to some brief gaps in data recording. In addition to the routine activities outlined previously, examples of some unique intern tasks include working with a pharmaceutical company to complete an adverse event report in response to a vaccine and clarifying dosing discrepancies on prescriptions with community pharmacies.

Table 1. Pharmacy intern completed tasks.

October 2017–October 2018	
Assigned Tasks	**Volume Completed**
PAs	1582
MAP applications	208
Appeals to PA rejections	21
Contraceptive device procurement	3
Inventory	4
Other tasks completed	252
Total tasks completed	2070

MAP = medication assistance program; PA = prior authorization.

3. Benefits of the Pharmacy Internship Program to Pharmacy Interns

The Fink Model of Significant Learning (FMSL) was applied in the development of the internship. In this model, Fink outlined six main categories of learning that create significant learning experiences for students. These six categories are: (1) foundational knowledge, (2) application, (3) integration, (4) human dimension, (5) caring, and (6) learning how to learn. Interns experienced each of these categories as a part of the internship program. The interns are utilizing their foundational knowledge of medication use from the didactic curriculum and integrating specific patient needs as part of the PA and MAP processes. Through their interaction with providers and patients, they are learning about the human dimension of patient care, as well as caring and advocating for others. Interns regularly inquire, or learn how to learn, to resolve drug-related problems and issues related to medication access [11].

Pharmacy interns participated in semi-structured interviews upon completion of their term. The pharmacy interns describe this position as rewarding for several reasons. Primarily, it offers an opportunity to work with vulnerable and underserved populations, a unique experience not always provided through traditional internships (FMSL categories: caring and human dimension). The diverse patient population requires multi-faceted approaches to obtaining medications that are often expensive. Interns regularly review pharmaceutical companies' MAPs, community pharmacy discount medication programs, discount medication cards, and websites (FMSL categories: Learning how to learn and application). Interns are also offered opportunities to shadow providers on their own unpaid time, if desired, to potentially gain a greater understanding of interprofessional relationships and comprehensive patient care that occurs in an ambulatory care setting. Additionally, interns participate in scholarly opportunities related to their work, resulting in two poster presentations and two manuscript preparation opportunities to date (FMSL categories: Learning how to learn, integration, and application). Finally, interns educate other student pharmacists who are completing curricular requirements, such as a rotation or service-learning activity about the intern responsibilities at the clinic (FMSL categories: Integration and human dimension).

Prescriber management of PAs is often unseen by student pharmacists. Both interns previously completed an introductory pharmacy practice experience (IPPE) in the community setting and observed the PA process in that setting. As processing PAs is the primary function of the intern position, it exposes interns to the challenges faced when working with a variety of insurance companies, while also ensuring patients receive their necessary prescribed medications. In processing PAs, interns critically review patient profiles and determine the patient-specific factors that are relevant in the selection of a medication (FMSL categories: foundational knowledge, application, and integration). Interns further advocate for patients with insurance companies by communicating the provider's rationale and decision-making process in prescribing the requested medication (FMSL categories: Caring, human dimension, and integration). Interns take part in an essential component of the prescribing process, leading to a better understanding of preferred medications, insurance formularies, and prior authorization approval criteria of prescription medications.

Additionally, the interns valued learning about the financial barriers experienced by some of the NCNC patient population (FMSL category: caring). Patients, especially those who are vulnerable or underserved, often see costs associated with their care as burdensome, and will periodically go without care, leading to poor health outcomes and increased healthcare costs [12]. Interns helped address these barriers by coordinating between providers and patients to complete MAP applications, resulting in increased medication access for patients and potentially improved patient outcomes (FMSL categories: Foundational knowledge, application, and integration). Interns identified barriers which slowed or complicated the MAP process, including the patient's motivation to provide and complete the required documentation, as well as provider understanding of application requirements. Solutions to these identified barriers were implemented as a result of intern observations, including provider education on the application processes, prefilled applications with provider information already completed, highlighted patient requirements on the applications, and increased availability of applications to providers and patients.

Skills learned by the interns in the pharmacy curriculum were applied and practiced through the internship program. Areas of emphasis include appropriate written communication and thorough documentation, interprofessional collaboration with providers to address insurance and/or patient barriers, and dissemination of key clinical information to insurance companies to justify a medication's necessity. Additionally, interns apply and integrate many of the tools and skills learned in the didactic portion of their pharmacy curriculum (i.e., foundational knowledge). Their role in the clinic allows them to practice skills prior to becoming pharmacists, when they will be expected to make clinical recommendations based on a variety of patient-specific factors.

4. Benefits of Pharmacy Internship Program to the FQHC Clinics

Pharmacist Fellows—Primarily, the pharmacy intern program allowed pharmacist fellows to explore and expand clinical pharmacy services, including an increase in direct patient care activities as a result of decreased time addressing PAs and MAPs. Subsequently, the fellows have implemented CPAs with the providers to manage multiple chronic disease states. The number of patients receiving anticoagulation management services has more than doubled, an event that has been aided by the transfer of administrative responsibilities. Providers are able to refer patients with diabetes to a pharmacist-directed telephone consult program designed to facilitate insulin management. Finally, in supervising the interns, the fellows gain additional management experience that will prove vital in their future careers as clinical faculty and preceptors.

Providers—The pharmacy interns provide on-site coverage for administrative paperwork four days a week, and are able to interact with providers, should the need arise. Interns facilitate MAP applications, obtain provider signatures for PAs, address any inventory issues, and communicate needed changes in a timely and efficient manner. Providers receive education on common prescribing issues with insurance formularies (e.g., prescribing omeprazole instead of Prilosec OTC®) and modify their prescribing habits to avoid these issues. Providers and their patients have also directly benefitted from the expansion of pharmacy services, including expanded direct patient care services, medication adjustment and monitoring through the CPAs, and clinical medication profile reviews for optimal chronic disease management.

Providers are regularly asked for feedback on the intern program and have not described any concerns with the transition of responsibilities from pharmacist to intern. Several providers have expressed appreciation for having the interns available on-site to answer insurance-related questions when the pharmacist is not at the clinic. Periodically, a patient will tell the provider during their office visit that they cannot afford the medication, or the insurance requires some action before approval. The interns have served as a valuable resource and are able to smoothly rectify the situation for the patient and the provider, deferring to the pharmacist when necessary.

Clinic—Implementation of the pharmacy internship program assisted in developing cost-effective pharmacy strategies for both the patient and the clinic. Prior to the fellowship program, other staff members (e.g., medical assistants, staff nurses, or support staff) would need to complete patient paperwork. A 2011 article estimated US physician and administrator costs related to time spent interacting with payers to be almost $83,000 annually [13]. The estimated cost of hiring the interns to manage these interactions with payers and other administrative responsibilities is approximately $10,800 annually, more than a seven-fold cost differential. Reduction in the burden of these administrative processes for providers, clinic staff and pharmacy fellows has increased efficiency in other areas and provides more time to deliver optimized patient-centered care.

Student pharmacist learners—Prior to the pharmacy internship program, APPE students at the clinics spent considerable time on PAs and MAP applications, resulting in few direct patient care activities. With the pharmacy internship program in place, APPE students engage in more hands-on patient interaction experiences, such as independently leading anticoagulation management visits, organizing medication and disease consult appointments, providing clinical recommendations to nurse practitioners through chart review, conducting in-service education to the interprofessional staff, and leading educational sessions with patients. APPE students also have the opportunity to participate in scholarly activities with the fellows and the institutions.

5. Challenges in Implementing the Pharmacy Internship Program

There were challenges in the implementation of the pharmacy internship program. First, there was an initial learning curve for the interns in identifying the best ways to contact insurance companies and communicating the information to successfully complete a PA or MAP application. This led to some trial and error in the beginning and resulted in some general delays with completing the daily assigned tasks. To reduce the transitional burden, one intern is recruited annually upon completion of their first professional year in the pharmacy program to fill the place of the intern advancing to the fourth year of the curriculum, while the other intern remains in place, providing stability and consistency during each period of transition. The "senior" intern serves as a resource and assists in orienting and training the "junior" intern. Further, semi-structured interviews occur at the end of each intern's time in the role to identify areas of improvement or difficulties that can be addressed by the fellows or the organization. Second, the position was originally approved for 12 h a week, which was often evenly split by the interns. This allowed for coverage three to four days a week, however, the clinics are open up to 12 h a day. As such, there was only a brief amount of time for the interns to complete paperwork for all four clinics, and the volume of patients cared for by the providers outpaced what the interns could provide. Requests would sometimes take several days to be processed, especially during holidays and weekends. The program expanded its hour limit to 16, which offset some of these delays and helped ensure timely processing of all responsibilities. Third, as part of their education, the pharmacy interns had academic requirements that periodically kept them from being able to work at the clinic, such as final exams or IPPEs. This challenge was managed by using a flexible schedule approach, requiring the interns to identify when their external responsibilities would be heaviest. The interns were able to adequately balance their academic and co-curricular needs through open communication with the pharmacist fellow, and no significant delays in service occurred.

6. Conclusions

This pharmacy internship program in an outpatient primary care organization is a unique learning and employment opportunity for student pharmacists. It provides them with a valuable experience while simultaneously benefitting the clinics, providers, and patients. From the intern perspective, working with the medically underserved was considered the most beneficial aspect of the program. Further, the interns utilized their acquired skills and experiences from the internship program during their APPEs. This experience also encouraged them to explore opportunities to work with underserved patient populations. The program demonstrates improvement in provider efficiency by spending less time on administrative paperwork and creates opportunities for the provision of direct patient care. Additional benefits are seen for the organization and student learners on required learning rotations. Primary care facilities may benefit from implementation and expansion of the pharmacy intern role to other basic clinical pharmacy needs.

Author Contributions: Conceptualization, N.E.F.III and K.S.P.; methodology, N.E.F.III and K.S.P.; investigation, N.E.F.III, N.R.G. and K.S.P.; writing—original draft preparation, N.E.F.III, N.R.G., G.J.S., S.L.C. and K.S.P.; writing—review and editing, N.E.F.III, N.R.G., G.J.S., S.L.C. and K.S.P.; visualization, N.E.F.III, N.R.G. and K.S.P.; supervision, N.E.F.III, N.R.G. and K.S.P.; project administration, N.E.F.III and N.R.G.

Funding: This research received no external funding.

Conflicts of Interest: The authors declare no conflict of interest.

References

1. Gillis, C.M.; Anger, K.E.; Cotugno, M.C. Enhanced responsibilities for pharmacy interns at a teaching hospital. *J. Am. Pharm. Assoc.* **2015**, *55*, 198–202. [CrossRef] [PubMed]
2. Schorr, S.G.; Eickhoff, C.; Feldt, S.; Hohmann, C.; Schulz, M. Exploring the potential impact of hospital ward-based pharmacy interns on drug safety. *Die Pharm. Int. J. Pharm. Sci.* **2014**, *69*, 316–320.
3. Nathan, J.P.; Schilit, S.; Zerilli, T.; Shah, B.; Plotkin, P.; Tykhonova, I. Functions performed by paid pharmacy interns in hospitals in New York. *Am. J. Health Syst. Pharm.* **2011**, *68*, 165–168. [CrossRef] [PubMed]
4. Pattin, A.J.; Kelling, S.E.; Szyskowski, J.; Izor, M.L.; Findley, S. The redesign of a community pharmacy internship program. *J. Pharm. Pract.* **2016**, *29*, 224–227. [CrossRef] [PubMed]
5. Gerdemann, A.; Griese, N.; Schulz, M. Pharmacy interns on the ward—A pilot study. *Pharm. World Sci.* **2007**, *29*, 34. [CrossRef] [PubMed]
6. Clark, J.S. Developing the future of pharmacy through health-system pharmacy internship programs. *Am. J. Health Syst. Pharm.* **2007**, *64*, 952–954. [CrossRef] [PubMed]
7. Derington, C.G.; Boom, G.D.; Choi, D.K.; Mader, K.; Johnson, J.D.; Trinkley, K.E. Pharmacy student involvement in the implementation of a student-run free clinic. *J. Basic Clin. Pharm.* **2017**, *8*, 3.
8. Mohammed, D.; Turner, K.; Funk, K. Pharmacy student involvement in student-run free clinics in the United States. *Curr. Pharm. Teach. Learn.* **2018**, *10*, 41–46. [CrossRef] [PubMed]
9. Moskowitz, D.; Glasco, J.; Johnson, B.; Wang, G. Students in the community: An interprofessional student-run free clinic. *J. Interprof. Care* **2006**, *20*, 254–259. [CrossRef] [PubMed]
10. Morello, C.M.; Singh, R.F.; Chen, K.J.; Best, B.M. Enhancing an introductory pharmacy practice experience at free medical clinics. *Int. J. Pharm. Pract.* **2010**, *18*, 51–57. [CrossRef] [PubMed]
11. Fink, L.D. *Creating Significant Learning Experiences: An Integrated Approach to Designing College Courses*; Jossey-Bass: San Francisco, CA, USA, 2003.
12. Lam, W.Y.; Fresco, P. Medication adherence measures: An overview. *BioMed Res. Int.* **2015**, *2015*, 217047. [CrossRef] [PubMed]
13. Morra, D.; Nicholson, S.; Levinson, W.; Gans, D.N.; Hammons, T.; Casalino, L.P. US physician practices versus Canadians: Spending nearly four times as much money interacting with payers. *Health Aff.* **2011**, *30*, 1443–1450. [CrossRef] [PubMed]

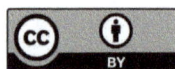

pharmacy

MDPI

Concept Paper

Training Community Pharmacy Staff How to Help Manage Urgent Mental Health Crises

Nathaniel Rickles [1,*], Albert Wertheimer [2] and Yifan Huang [1]

[1]   Department of Pharmacy Practice, University of Connecticut, Storrs, CT 06269, USA;
      yifan.huang@uconn.edu
[2]   Department of Sociobehavioral and Administrative Pharmacy, Nova Southeastern University,
      Fort Lauderdale-Davie, FL 33314, USA; awertheime@nova.edu
*   Correspondence: nathaniel.rickles@uconn.edu

Received: 9 July 2019; Accepted: 7 September 2019; Published: 16 September 2019

check for updates

Abstract: Nearly 44 million Americans are affected by mental illness every year. Many individuals, however, are not diagnosed and/or do not receive treatment. The present manuscript reviews the incidence of mental illness, the continuum from mental wellness to mental illness, and the role of the pharmacy staff in helping individuals manage different mental health needs. In particular, there is discussion of stigma of mental illness that those with mental health needs experience by those around them including health professionals such as pharmacy staff. One way to resolve such stigma is through training such as Mental Health First Aid (MHFA). The paper reviews key aspects of MHFA, the evidence supporting MHFA, and how MHFA relates specifically to pharmacy practice and services. A conceptual framework for MHFA and its relationship to individual factors, attitudes, behaviors, and outcomes. Lastly, a discussion is presented that briefly compares MHFA to other similar approaches to helping those in mental health crises, the limits of what is known about MHFA, and what future research might explore to better understand the outcomes of pharmacy staff providing mental health education, support, and referral to care.

Keywords: mental health care; pharmacy staff; mental health first aid; mental illness; pharmacist roles

1. Background

There are at least 43.8 million individuals in the US affected by mental illness every year [1]. There are several more millions of individuals, undertreated, who would be diagnosed and properly treated for mental illnesses who are not in the system [2]. In addition, there are numerous other individuals who do not meet the criteria for a diagnosis of mental illness or require treatment but experience episodes where they are unable to optimally cope or manage their temporary thoughts, feelings, and behaviors. For a variety of reasons, whether for those already diagnosed with mental illness, needing to be diagnosed and/or treated, or those with more transient/temporary mental health symptoms, these groups of individuals face significant challenges in obtaining resources to help them initiate and/or remain consistently engaged with a support system that can provide the needed support to help them resolve their temporary or long- term difficulties. Key reasons why these groups of individuals struggle to initially reach out for support or consistently engage in support include (1) the stigma experienced by all these groups that are afflicted with different levels of mental health challenges face, and (2) the lack of access to individuals trained to provide temporary supportive management of specific mental health crises and know when and what types of additional support is needed for such individuals [3].

The National Alliance on Mental Illness (NAMI) and many other mental health advocacy groups and organizations have promoted anti-stigma campaigns to target the first of these two reasons [4]. Clearly, there is still much work to do to make individuals with a variety of mental health symptoms feel more comfortable reaching out and having someone help them through their symptoms. There are many efforts that continue to focus on facilitating cultures at work places, health care environments, and other areas of the community that avoid judgement and distance away from the individual suffering from ongoing or temporary mental health symptoms [5]. One common example is using "person first" language that avoids labeling individuals by their illness such as "schizophrenics" and rather referring to these individuals as those with lived experience of schizophrenia or "individuals with schizophrenia." Rather, the focus of this anti-stigma work is to help bring the affected individual together with a community resource and together support the individual towards improved mental health management. As valued, trusted members of the community, pharmacists are at the frontlines of primary health care and thus regularly interact with individuals who may have mental illness and mental health crises. If pharmacists were equipped with tools that enhanced their engagement of individuals with mental health needs, it is possible pharmacists could help adults in need of mental health services seek mental health care. Mental illnesses are so prevalent throughout society, yet they are also some of the most severely undertreated. While 1 in 5 adults in the US is afflicted by mental health conditions in a given year, only 41% of those adults received mental health services [1]. Among adults with a serious mental illness, 62.9% received mental health services in the past [1]. Additionally, just over half (50.6%) of children with a mental health condition aged 8–15 received mental health services in the previous year [1]. Such disparities contribute to significant costs to the individuals with mental health symptoms and the healthcare system as a whole. Not only are individuals unable to optimally function that affects their quality of life, but they are actually also at greater risk for many comorbid conditions. On average, adults in the US living with mental illness die 25 years earlier than others, largely due to treatable medical conditions [1]. Suicide is also the 10th leading cause of death in the US, the 3rd leading cause of death for people aged 10–14, and the 2nd leading cause of death for people aged 15–24 [1]. Not only does mental illnesses severely impact individual lives, it has also contributed to $193.2 billion in economic losses per year [1].

Identifying mental health concerns and illness can be thought of on a continuum from what is considered mental wellness to mental illness (Table 1). The model presented in Table 1 is based on the definition and concepts in the Mental Health Continuum Model [6]. On the mental wellness end of the spectrum, we would expect healthy reactions including predictable mood fluctuations, general acceptance of challenges, sense of humor, high performance, average sleep patterns, moderate to high level of energy, and avoidance of excessive use of substances and engagement in addictive behaviors. Moving to the middle of continuum, an observer might start noticing the following: more unpredictable mood fluctuations, difficulty managing life challenges, diminishing sense of humor, reduced performance, poor sleep patterns, and moderate to low energy, more anxiousness about different activities, and gradual engagement in unhealthy behavior patterns. At the ill end of the spectrum, an individual will be observed to have: angry outbursts that are more significant and frequent, very labile moods with very low and/or low moods, significant anxiety, presence of unusual thoughts and behaviors, poor sleep, significant difficulties performing in daily activities and work, excessive substance use and risky and/or addictive behaviors, and thoughts of harming the self and others. Individuals presenting at different stages within this continuum are in need of different levels of support and professional help. Thus, awareness of the mental health continuum acts as a useful resource and context to clarify the severity of impairment of those suffering from mental health crises and illnesses, and what resources such individuals may need. Although Table 1 depicts a list of signs and symptoms under each aspect of the continuum from mental wellness to mental illness, this should not be interpreted that an individual needs to have all the signs and symptoms listed at one time to be considered mentally well or mentally ill. An individual may present with signs and symptoms from different parts of the continuum.

Table 1. Continuum of Mental Wellness and Illness.

Mental Wellness	Mild/Moderate Coping/Adjustment	Mental Illness Difficulties
Predictable mood fluctuations	Unpredictable mood fluctuations	Frequent & significant outbursts
General acceptance of challenges	Difficulty managing life challenges	Labile moods
Sense of humor	Diminishing sense of humor	Significant anger and/or anxiety
High performance	Reduced performance	Unusual thoughts and behaviors
Average sleep patterns	Irregular sleep patterns	Consistently poor sleep patterns
Moderate to high level of energy	Moderate to low energy	Significant dysfunction in daily activities and work
Avoidance of excessive use of substances	Anxiousness about activities	Excessive substance use &/or addictive behaviors
Avoidance of addictive behaviors	Gradual engagement in unhealthy behavior patterns	Thoughts of harm to self/others

While poor mental health can lead to poor physical health and mental illness, it is possible to have poor mental health temporarily and not lead to a diagnosed mental illness. For example, a person going through a hard life experience may have poor mental health during this time period without necessarily having a mental illness. Thus, feeling miserable or isolated may be red flags that your mental health requires attention and improvement. In these cases, it is important to utilize support from friends/families/other groups, focus on healthy lifestyle habits such as eating regularly and appropriate sleep hygiene, and even seeking support from a therapist can be beneficial. Poor mental health not leading to mental illness can be due to difficult life transitions, environmental challenges, and the lack of needed resources. It is also important to note that poor mental health may not lead to poor health and that an individual with mental illness may be in good physical health.

Diagnosed mental illnesses, however, are often associated with physiological alterations in the brain due to genetic predisposition, chemical changes, traumatic experiences, and/or major developmental challenges leading to significant changes in mood, thinking, and behavior that cannot be easily managed with self-help strategies or non-professional support systems. These individuals often require referrals to their primary care doctor, a psychologist, a psychiatrist, and occasionally a social worker for management of the various aspects of treatment. Some more severe cases may require hospitalization, or treatment programs with more intensive interventions and monitoring.

2. Role of the Pharmacy Staff

Pharmacists are considered the most accessible health care professionals, and see a large volume of patients in community pharmacies every day. The College of Psychiatric and Neurological Pharmacy (CPNP) and National Alliance on Mental Illness (NAMI) collaborated on a 2012 national survey and assessed the opinions of 1031 individuals with mental health concerns, or their caregivers, regarding their relationship with their pharmacist. Ninety-one percent felt very comfortable going to their community pharmacy, and 83% felt like the pharmacist respected them [7].

Pharmacists are involved in many services including: counseling, monitoring, and reducing side effects, assessing serum concentrations, identifying interactions, assisting in treatment plans, and developing ways to increase medication adherence. Pharmacists have also been repeatedly shown to enhance patients' knowledge, beliefs, and sense of treatment progress related to psychotropics such as antidepressants [8]. These findings illustrate the impact that pharmacists can have on the treatment, attitudes, and perceptions of their patients with mental illnesses. Such impact can help improve patient medication adherence. Pharmacy staff already have access to a large segment of this population. If pharmacy staff have the appropriate mental health skills, they can help to reshape the negative perceptions individuals with mental health needs and illness have about themselves and their illnesses. Such pharmacy support can remove a significant barrier to care, to be discussed in greater detail in next section [9]. In addition, pharmacy staff knowledgeable in the signs and symptoms of mental illnesses can also help identify individuals that may need to be referred to a clinician for follow-up and support. Pharmacy staff also can be excellent resources of information about mental health conditions and encourage various self-help and other strategies.

3. Barriers to Care: Presence of Stigma

A significant barrier to care for those individuals with mental illness is the stigmatization of their illness by others. Stigma has been developed and supported by a combination of media incorrectly portraying mental illness, and a lack of training/education regarding mental health awareness. With movies like *Friday the 13th—A New Beginning* (1985), *Psycho III* (1986), *Misery* (1990), and *Silence of the Lambs* (1991), many people have grown up with the misconceptions that mental illness disenables a person from logical thinking and makes them difficult to reason with, and even dangerous [10].

Stigma persists throughout all areas of the community, and healthcare is no exception [9,11]. In general, some healthcare professionals may view individuals with mental illness as incompetent, unpredictable, dangerous, difficult to communicate with, and require too much time to provide service. Even insurance companies have been shown to offer greater coverage for physical illness over mental illness [12]. Studies generally show that pharmacists have a positive view of people with mental illness, but are often uncomfortable with them [9,13–16]. Upon survey, pharmacists reported being more willing to counsel on a physical disorder (i.e., asthma) than a mental disorder [16].

In the 2012 national survey by CPNP and NAMI mentioned previously, a little over half of those sampled reported having a strong professional relationship with the pharmacist [7]. Approximately 40% of those in this latter sample actually reported no relationship with their pharmacist and 75% reported not receiving effectiveness and/or safety monitoring assistance from the pharmacist [7]. This illustrates a need for greater education focusing on how pharmacy staff can feel more comfortable in communicating with individuals with mental health needs and illnesses. Such greater comfort in communication will foster a stronger relationship between individuals with mental health needs, mental illnesses, and pharmacy staff. Through these stronger relationships, pharmacy staff can provide much needed education and motivational resource for individuals with mental health needs that may otherwise be overlooked by their system of care. Pharmacists need more training and skills to help improve their comfort in communication and build relationships with individuals with mental health needs. Such mental health training opportunities will be discussed in the next section.

4. Mental Health First Aid

Mental Health First Aid (MHFA) is a training program offered to the general public aiming to increase mental health literacy, and impart the participant with the skills required to provide an immediate response to a person experiencing an acute mental health crisis [17]. MHFA also helps train the participant to understand the signs and symptoms of different mental illnesses so they can help someone seek the appropriate support especially in the earlier stages of developing a mental health disorder or problem. The program originated in Australia in 2001 and was designed by Kitchener, a nurse specializing in health education, and Jorm, a mental health literacy professor. The program can be given as a one 8-hour day, two 4-hour days, or four 2-hour days. Programs delivered over the course of multiple days should not occur more than two weeks a part. During this time, participants obtain the skill set necessary to not only intervene in a mental health crisis, but to identify those at risk and/or having symptoms of mental illness, and direct them to the help they need. In both the participant and MHFA instructor manuals, MHFA is presented as being like first aid needed for cardiovascular support (American Red Cross' CPR program) but for mental health crises.

The program focuses on depression and other mood disorders, anxiety disorders, trauma, psychosis, and substance use disorders. Participants in the training learn the program's "Mental Health First Aid Action Plan," and are taught to apply the action plan to many different scenarios—specifically guiding interactions with others experiencing suicidal thoughts or behaviors, panic attacks, non-suicidal self-injury, overdose or withdrawal from substance use, and reaction to a traumatic event. The action plan consists of five steps:

1. Assess for risk of suicide or harm
2. Listen non-judgmentally

3. Give reassurance and information
4. Encourage appropriate professional help
5. Encourage self-help and other support strategies

The first letter of each step forms the acronym ALGEE. Throughout the training, instructors frequently refer to ALGEE and reinforce the ALGEE action plan.

There are no requirements for the training; it is available to the general public. The National Council for Behavioral Health (NCBH) that accredits the training programs strongly encourages professionals to participate who have frequent contact with those at risk or experiencing mental illness/crisis. Specific examples listed on the MHFA website include police officers, human resources workers, primary health care workers, schools, community faith organizations, and friends and family of someone experiencing mental illness or mental health crises. The Community Pharmacy Foundation supported a project by the National Community Pharmacist Association (NCPA) to develop and provide 8-hour of continuing education credits for pharmacists and technicians who participate in the 8-hour MHFA courses. This project also supported the creation of specific pharmacy-related cases that MHFA instructors can use when presenting topharmacists and pharmacy technicians. These cases are available to certified MHFA instructors who complete several days of NCBH training for certification. To use these NCPA cases, there is no additional training beyond needing to be certified to train others in MHFA.

There is a small but growing literature on MHFA in general and its application to pharmacy. A meta-analysis was performed estimating the effects of the MHFA program in participants of any occupation, both for adults and young people, based on results published up to March 2014 [18]. MHFA was found to be effective in increasing knowledge regarding mental health problems, and effectively decreasing negative attitudes toward individuals suffering from mental health problems. The program was also shown to increase help-providing behavior. Another publication reviewed three published trials, and found improved concordance with health professionals about treatments, improved helping behavior, greater confidence in providing help to others, and decreased social distance from people with mental disorders [19].

In Sweden, researchers conducted a randomized controlled trial involving a group of staff from various agencies who randomly received MHFA training and those who did not [20]. Results showed that the MHFA group had significantly greater knowledge and confidence in helping others with mental health disorders than the control group [20]. Such MHFA effects were shown to be maintained to a great extent after a two-year follow-up period [20]. The collective data reviewed in this section reinforces the central finding that taking a course in MHFA can significantly improve a participant's knowledge of mental health and mental health disorders, confidence in helping an individual manage a mental health crisis, decrease stigma, and sets the participant up for a more successful interaction when reaching out to those with mental illnesses.

In addition to the general literature regarding MHFA's impact on trainee outcomes, there is specific growing literature on MHFA's impact on pharmacists and pharmacy students. One study took place in eight rural Australian community pharmacies and entailed a survey assessing barriers to MHFA training and applications of the training to pharmacy [21]. Pharmacists identified and supported the need for MHFA, and had low confidence in their ability to handle an acute mental health crisis without the additional training [21]. The majority (72%) of pharmacists agreed they have a role to provide MHFA, but less than half (48%) were comfortable in providing this support. [21]. Most participants stated that they would be prepared to undertake this training. About a third of the sample thought the training should be administered during their intern year, 24% thought training should be administered during their pharmacist years, and the majority (76%) preferred administration of training as a one-day course with an online component [21]. The major barriers identified by pharmacists included time, geographic location, and resources [21]. These results show that pharmacists have both identified the need for and are willing to undertake MHFA training in order to improve access to mental health support in individuals at risk for or experiencing mental health crises and illnesses.

A controlled trial was conducted assessing 60 third year pharmacy students at the University of Sydney randomly chosen to complete one of two 12-hour sessions of MHFA and complete a follow up survey [22]. The survey (administered before and after the training) evaluated mental health literacy, the 7-item social distance scale, and 16 items related to self-reported behavior. Survey results showed that MHFA training reduced the pharmacy students' stigma towards individuals with mental illness, improved recognition of mental disorders and improved confidence in providing services to individuals with mental illnesses in a pharmacy setting [22].

Another randomized controlled study of 262 members of the Australian public demonstrated that students (pharmacy and other programs) who participated in an online MHFA course responded better to measures of stigma reduction compared to those that used a written manual [23]. This indicates that completing a training program such as the MHFA is more valuable than just offering educational materials to students. While pharmacy programs often provide clinical background on mental illnesses and evidence-based treatments to target these illnesses, they are typically less focused on helping students manage crises that might occur in their pharmacies. An additional study, taking place at University of Sydney, evaluated the differences in confidence and attitudes of their pharmacy students towards suicidal crisis in three groups of students: the first group simply completed MHFA training, the second group completed MHFA training and observed a simulation of a patient and pharmacist interaction with a person undergoing suicidal crisis, and the third completed the MHFA training and participated in the live simulated interaction [24]. Results displayed a statistically significant increase in confidence in all students who participated in the MHFA training. In particular, the greatest increases in confidence were among pharmacy students participating in the live interaction. Such data suggests that participating in a live simulation is critical to the MHFA training experience. This combined literature shows the clear value and impact of MHFA on learner attitudes and behaviors toward those at risk for mental health crises and/or experiencing mental illness.

These findings are likely supported by an underlying conceptual framework for how MHFA relates to individual factors, attitudes, behaviors, and outcomes. The authors depict this conceptual framework in Figure 1 as it specifically relates to MHFA by pharmacy staff and its effects on both the pharmacy staff and the outcomes of individuals experiencing mental health concerns and illnesses. Moving from left to right, the framework starts with the concept that background factors of both the individual with lived experience of mental health concerns and illness and the pharmacy staff affect the extent to which stigma of mental illness exists for both the individual and the pharmacy staff. From past extensive research on stigma of mental illness, it is well known that culture, education on mental illness, personal contact with individuals with mental health needs and illness, and demographics all impact the extent to which stigma towards mental illness develops [9,16,25,26]. In addition, there is a robust literature and framework development supporting the role of these background factors on pharmacy staff perceptions of counseling, relationships with patients, and the willingness to provide care and related counseling services to those with mental illnesses [16,27].

In the middle of Figure 1, MHFA can be seen as a variable with bi-directional impact on (1) stigma involving pharmacy staff and that of individuals with mental health needs, (2) attitudes of individuals with mental health needs and pharmacy staff towards each other, and (3) services provided by pharmacy staff to those with mental health needs. The research reviewed in this section supports MHFA's direct impact on these aspects of pharmacy practice [21,22]. Although not examined specifically, it is likely that the stigma changes and practice changes from MHFA would likely change the willingness to adopt and implement MHFA (reflected by the arrows going from stigma back to MHFA and practice-related perceptions and services back to MHFA).

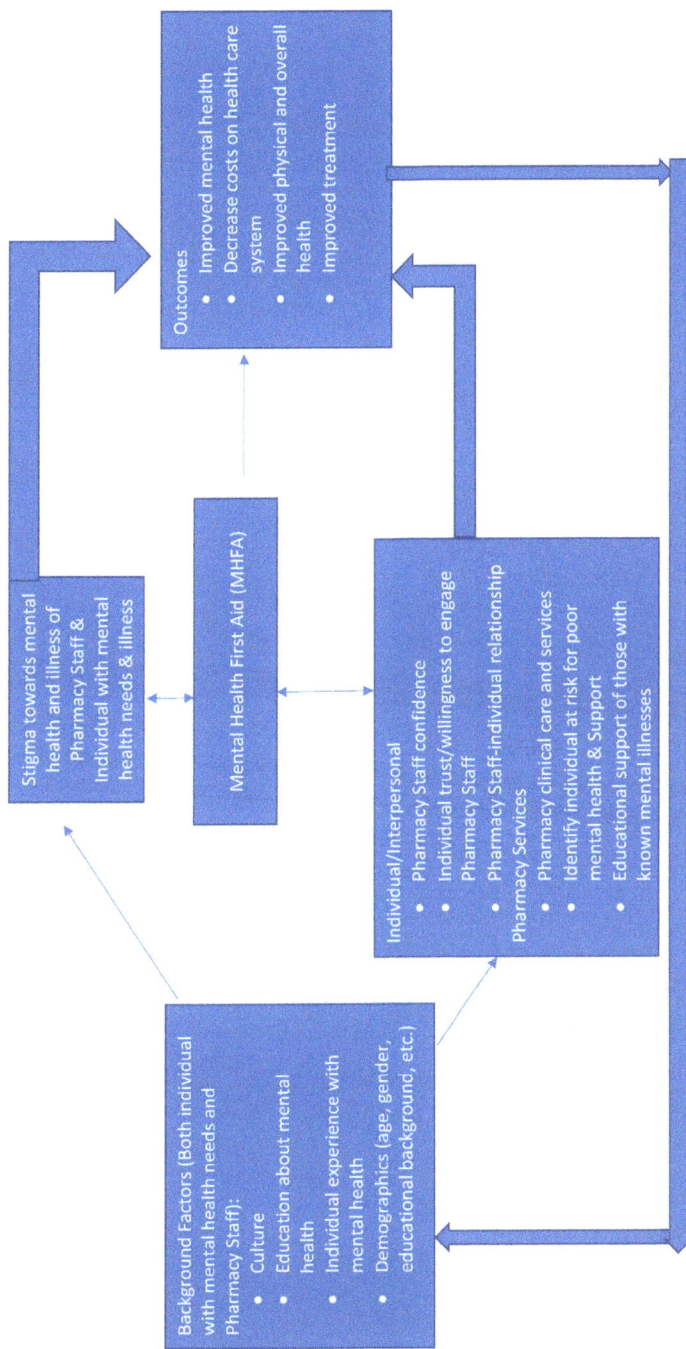

Figure 1. Conceptual framework of relationships between background factors, Mental Health First Aid (MHFA), and outcomes.

The arrows from pharmacy stigma, stigma of those with mental health needs, practice-related perceptions and services, and outcomes are all supported by decades of stigma and pharmacy practice research on these topics [25,27]. Many of the non-pharmacy literature reviewed also support how MHFA changes knowledge, willingness to help, negative attitudes toward those with mental health needs, and other process outcomes [18–20].

As for the right part of the Figure 1 linking MHFA to outcomes, there needs to be more research demonstrating the links between MHFA and various patient and health system outcomes such as mental and physical health of individuals helped by MHFA, cost of care and improved treatment [28]. Feedback models, such as Figure 1, often suggest that outcomes or outputs of the model will affect model inputs such as background characteristics. If MHFA improves mental and physical health, it is expected that one's background and experience would also change as well, and subsequently other relationships in the conceptual framework. One suggested research approach to testing the relationships in Figure 1 is through the secret shopper methodology whereby trained actors go into pharmacies showing signs of being in a mental health crisis and see how those trained in MHFA react differently from those not trained in MHFA and how the actor felt differently with a trained and untrained MHFA person. It would be useful to also conduct randomized controlled trials to see if practicing pharmacists trained in MHFA respond differently to individuals with mental health needs and illnesses than those not trained in MHFA.

5. Additional Considerations

MHFA is designed for administration to the general public. As noted by Chowdhary and colleagues, it may be prudent to give healthcare professionals a different program tailored to their education, training and experiences [28]. These programs should also highlight that pharmacists are not being trained in psychotherapy and other treatments. Rather, pharmacists being trained in MHFA need to remove their clinical intervention hats and focus on the ALGEE action plan to manage a mental health crisis.

MHFA is not the only program available to train participants on how to deal with mental health crisis and communicate effectively with those suffering. Other programs include options such as Psychological First Aid (PFA) and Emotional CPR (eCPR). PFA usually focuses more on protocol following a disaster. MHFA is more general than PFA by focusing on any mental health crisis [29]. eCPR, however, is another training geared toward the general public to assist a person experiencing an emotional crisis using three components [30].

1. C = Connecting with Compassion and Concern to Communicate
2. P = emPowerment to experience Passion, Purpose and Planning
3. R = Revitalize through Re-establishing Relationships, Routines and Rhythms in the community

eCPR is believed to involve consumers with lived experience of mental illness more actively in the trainings and, therefore, the voices of those with mental illnesses are heard first hand throughout the trainings. With no head to head studies comparing the different available training methods, it remains uncertain that MHFA is superior to these other programs in preparing the general public and pharmacy staff for these crisis-based interventions. MHFA, however, is gaining significant momentum throughout the country and recently Walgreens has announced its plan to train their pharmacists in MHFA [31]. Pharmacists are becoming certified train-the-trainers and offering MHFA sessions to pharmacy students and practicing pharmacists.

6. Conclusions

Although there is not yet enough evidence to support that MHFA improves patient outcomes, there is considerable support that it decreases existing stigma regarding mental illness (a leading barrier to individuals seeking care and pharmacy staff providing care). There is also evidence that MHFA increases pharmacist and pharmacy student confidence in identifying, approaching, interacting with an individual who is undergoing a mental health crisis, and helping them seek appropriate care. These are significant steps in improving access to needed help for individuals with mental illness or experiencing a mental health crisis. However, with no head to head studies comparing MHFA to other programs, it is still unclear which of the available programs are superior in creating sustainable changes in pharmacy staff confidence and engagement of individuals with mental health needs.

With the pharmacist being one of the most accessible and most frequently visited healthcare professionals, community pharmacists are well positioned to bridge the gap between those with a mental health crisis and/or illness and access to the treatment and support they need to begin the healing process. Community pharmacists clearly need to augment their knowledge regarding how to identify and respond to a mental health crisis. Training programs, like MHFA, are well designed to reduce stigma of mental illness, increase knowledge and confidence on how to manage mental health crises and support mental illnesses. By having more community pharmacists trained in MHFA or other similar programs, community pharmacists can meet a critical public health problem by being able to identify the urgent needs of someone in a mental health crisis, offer non- judgmental support, and provide critical information that allows the individual with mental health needs to quickly access the appropriate resources to help the individual achieve greater mental and physical wellness.

Funding: This research involved no external funding.

Conflicts of Interest: The authors declare no conflict of interest.

References

1. NIMH. Any Mental Illness (AMI) Among Adults. 2019. Available online: http://www.nimh.nih.gov/health/statistics/prevalence/any-mental-illness-ami-among-adults.shtml (accessed on 11 April 2019).
2. Bijl, R.V.; de Graaf, R.; Hiripi, E.; Kessler, R.C.; Kohn, R.; Offord, D.R.; Ustun, T.B.; Vicente, B.; Vollebergh, W.A.; Walters, E.E.; et al. The prevalence of treated and untreated mental disorders in five countries. *Health Aff.* **2003**, *22*, 121–133. [CrossRef] [PubMed]
3. Corrigan, P.W.; Druss, B.G.; Perlick, D.A. The Impact of Mental Illness Stigma on Seeking and Participating in Mental Health Care. *Psychol. Sci. Public Interest* **2014**, *15*, 37–70. [CrossRef] [PubMed]
4. Stigmafree. Available online: https://www.nami.org/stigmafree (accessed on 30 August 2019).
5. Framework to Help Eliminate Stigma. Available online: https://www.workplacestrategiesformentalhealth.com/psychological-health-and-safety/framework-to-help-eliminate-stigma (accessed on 30 August 2019).
6. Mental Health Continuum Model. Available online: https://bcfirstrespondersmentalhealth.com/wp-content/uploads/2017/06/MentalHealthContinuumModel.pdf (accessed on 31 August 2019).
7. Characterizing the Relationship between Individuals with Mental Health Conditions and Community Pharmacists-Results from a 2012 Survey. College of Psychiatric and Neurologic Pharmacists Foundation. Available online: https://cpnp.org/_docs/foundation/2012/nami-survey-report.pdf (accessed on 12 September 2019).
8. Rickles, N.M.; Svarstad BLStatz-Paynter, J.L.; Taylor, L.V.; Kobak, K.A. Pharmacist Telemonitoring of Antidepressant Use: Effects on Pharmacist–Patient Collaboration. *J. Am. Pharm. Assoc.* **2005**, *45*, 344–353. [CrossRef]
9. Calogero, S.; Caley, C.F. Supporting patients with mental illness: Deconstructing barriers to community pharmacist access. *J. Am. Pharm. Assoc.* **2017**, *57*, 248–255. [CrossRef] [PubMed]
10. Wahl, O.F. *Media Madness: Public Images of Mental Illness*; Rutgers University Press: New Brunswick, NJ, USA, 1995.
11. Chin, S.H.; Balon, R. Attitudes and perceptions toward depression and schizophrenia among residents in different medical specialities. *Acad. Psychiatry* **2006**, *30*, 262–263. [CrossRef] [PubMed]
12. Soumerai, S.B.; McLaughlin, T.J.; Ross-Degnan, S.; Casteris, C.S.; Bollini, P. Effects of limiting Medicaid drug-reimbursement benefits on the use of psychotropic agents and acute mental health services by patients with schizophrenia. *N. Engl. J. Med.* **1994**, *331*, 650–655. [CrossRef] [PubMed]
13. Cates, M.E.; Burton, A.R.; Wooley, T.W. Attitudes of pharmacists toward mental illness and providing pharmaceutical care to the mentally ill. *Ann. Pharm.* **2005**, *39*, 1450–1455.

14. Bells, J.S.; Johns, R.; Chen, T.F. Pharmacy students' and graduates' attitudes towards people with schizophrenia and severe depression. *Am. J. Pharm. Educ.* **2006**, *70*, 77. [CrossRef] [PubMed]

15. Bell, J.S.; Aaltonen, S.E.; Bronstein, E.; Desplenter, F.A.; Foulon, V.; Vitola, A.; Muceniece, R.; Gharat, M.S.; Volmer, D.; Airaksinen, M.S.; et al. Attitudes of pharmacy students toward people with mental disorders, a six country study. *Pharm. World Sci.* **2008**, *30*, 595–599. [CrossRef] [PubMed]

16. Rickles, N.M.; Dube, G.L.; McCarter, A.; Olshan, J.S. Relationship between attitudes toward mental illness and provision of pharmacy services. *J. Am. Pharm Assoc.* **2010**, *50*, 704–713. [CrossRef] [PubMed]

17. Mental Health First Aid USA. Available online: https://www.mentalhealthfirstaid.org/ (accessed on 5 July 2019).

18. Hadlaczky, G.; Hökby, S.; Mkrtchian, A.; Carli, V.; Wasserman, D. Mental Health First Aid is an effective public health intervention for improving knowledge, attitudes, and behaviour: A meta-analysis. *Int. Rev. Psychiatry* **2014**, *26*, 467–475. [CrossRef] [PubMed]

19. Kitchener, B.A.; Jorm, A.F. Mental Health First Aid training: Review of evaluation studies. *Aust. N. Z. J. Psychiatry* **2006**, *40*, 6–8. [CrossRef] [PubMed]

20. Svensson, B.; Hansson, L. Effectiveness of Mental Health First Aid Training in Sweden. A Randomized Controlled Trial with a Six-Month and Two-Year Follow-Up. *PLoS ONE* **2014**, *9*. [CrossRef] [PubMed]

21. Kirschbaum, M.; Peterson, G.; Bridgman, H. Mental health first aid training needs of Australian community pharmacists. *Curr. Pharm. Teach. Learn.* **2016**, *8*, 279–288. [CrossRef] [PubMed]

22. Oreilly, C.; Bell, J.S.; Kelly, P.; Chen, T.F. Impact of Mental Health First Aid training on pharmacy students' knowledge, attitudes and self-reported behaviour: A controlled trial. *Aust. N. Z. J. Psychiatry* **2011**, *45*, 549–557. [CrossRef] [PubMed]

23. Jorum, A.F.; Kitchener, B.A.; Fischer, J.A.; Cvetkovski, S. Mental health first aid training by e-learning: A randomized controlled trial. *Aust. N. Z. J. Psychiatry* **2010**, *44*, 1072–1081. [CrossRef] [PubMed]

24. Boukouvalas, E.A.; El-Den, S.; Chen, T.F.; Moles, R.; Saini, B.; Bell, A.; O'Reilly, C. Confidence and attitudes of pharmacy students towards suicidal crises: Patient simulation using people with a lived experience. *Soc. Psychiatry Psychiatr. Epidemiol.* **2018**. [CrossRef]

25. Link, B.G.; Phelan, J.C. Labeling and stigma. In *Handbook of Sociology of Mental Health*; Aneshensel, C.S., Phelan, J.C., Eds.; Kluwer Academic/Plenum: New York, NY, USA, 1999; pp. 481–494.

26. Jermain, D.M.; Crismon, M.L. Students' attitudes toward the mentally ill before and after clinical rotations. *Am. J. Pharm. Educ.* **1991**, *55*, 45–48.

27. Rickles, N.M.; Svarstad, B.L. The patient: Behavioral determinants. In *Remington: The Science and Practice of Pharmacy*, 22nd ed.; Allen, L., Ed.; Pharmaceutical Press: London, UK, 2012; pp. 1893–1902.

28. Chowdhary, A.; Zlotnikova, V.; Lucas, C.; Lonie, J.M. How do mental health first aid™ interventions influence patient help-seeking behaviours? A dilemma for pharmacist mental health first aid responders. *Res. Soc. Admin. Pharm.* **2019**, *15*, 106–108. [CrossRef]

29. Psychological First Aid: Guide for Field Workers. World Health Organization. Available online: http://www.who.int/mental_health/publications/guide_field_workers/en/ (accessed on 24 July 2018).

30. Emotional CPR (eCPR). Available online: https://www.emotional-cpr.org/ (accessed on 12 September 2019).

31. Johnson, S.R. Walgreens to Train Pharmacy Staff in Mental Health First Aid. Modern Healthcare. Available online: https://www.modernhealthcare.com/safety-quality/walgreens-train-pharmacy-staff-mental-health-first-aid (accessed on 5 July 2019).

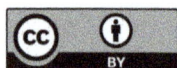

pharmacy

MDPI

Article

Uptake of Travel Health Services by Community Pharmacies and Patients Following Pharmacist Immunization Scope Expansion in Ontario, Canada

Sherilyn K. D. Houle [1,*], Kristina Kozlovsky [1], Heidi V. J. Fernandes [1] and Zahava Rosenberg-Yunger [2]

[1] School of Pharmacy, University of Waterloo, Waterloo, ON N2L 3G1, Canada; k.kozlovsky@hotmail.com (K.K); heidi.fernandes@uwaterloo.ca (H.V.J.F.)
[2] Ted Rogers School of Management, Ryerson University, Toronto, ON M5G 2C3, Canada; zahava.rosenberg@ryerson.ca
* Correspondence: sherilyn.houle@uwaterloo.ca; Tel.: +1-519-888-4567 (ext. 21378)

Received: 25 March 2019; Accepted: 11 April 2019; Published: 13 April 2019

check for updates

Abstract: In December 2016, pharmacists in Ontario, Canada with authorization to administer injections saw an expansion in their scope from a restriction to the influenza vaccination only to now including an additional 13 vaccine-preventable diseases, largely those related to travel. It was uncertain whether this change in scope would see sufficient uptake, or translate to a corresponding expansion in other travel health service offerings from community pharmacies. In October/November 2017 a survey was conducted of all licensed community pharmacists in Ontario, followed by semi-structured interviews with 6 survey respondents in June 2018. A web-based survey of members of the public from a single region of the province was also conducted in September 2018 to assess uptake of expanded vaccination services. Broad variability in uptake of these services was noted, ranging from the dispensing of travel-related medications and vaccinations only through to vaccine administration and prescribing under medical directive; however, uptake was generally at the lower end of this spectrum. This was evidenced by 94% of pharmacists reporting administering fewer than 10 travel vaccinations per month, fewer than 10% of patients reporting receiving a travel vaccine administered by a pharmacist, and a maximum of 30 pharmacies (of nearly 6000 in the province) designated to provide yellow fever vaccinations. Fewer than 1 in 3 pharmacists reported performing some form of pre-travel consultation in their practice, often limited to low-risk cases only. Barriers and facilitators reported were similar for these services as they were for other non-dispensing services, including insufficient time to integrate the service into their workload, perceived lack of knowledge and confidence in travel health, and low patient awareness of these new services available to them through community pharmacies.

Keywords: travel; immunization; vaccination; pharmacist; community pharmacy

---

1. Introduction

In 2012, pharmacists in Ontario, Canada, were authorized to administer the influenza vaccine to patients age 5 years and older following the successful completion of an immunization training program, and obtaining valid certification in cardiopulmonary resuscitation and first aid [1]. In December 2016, amendments were made to the Pharmacy Act to permit injection-trained pharmacists, pharmacy students, and interns to administer vaccines to patients for 13 travel and travel-related vaccine-preventable diseases [2], listed in Table 1. Of note, this legislation only authorizes the administration of each vaccine, with some still requiring a prescription as indicated in the table [3].

Pharmacists in Ontario currently do not have broad prescribing authorization for vaccines, although pharmacists can pursue medical directives from physicians or nurse practitioners to prescribe these vaccines under delegation [4]. Vaccines currently on Ontario's routine immunization schedule [5] can be obtained at no charge from a physician office or public health clinic; however, any of these vaccines received in a pharmacy must be paid for by the patient, as well as any administration fee that may be charged by the pharmacy. Some patients may be eligible for coverage through private insurance, although this varies by insurer and by vaccine.

Table 1. Vaccines that can currently be administered by authorized pharmacists in Ontario.

Vaccine	Prescription Required
Bacillus Calmette-Guérin	Yes
Haemophilus influenzae type B	No
Meningococcal	No
Pneumococcal	No
Typhoid	Yes
Typhoid / Hepatitis A Combination	Yes
Hepatitis A	Yes
Hepatitis B	Yes
Hepatitis A&B Combination	Yes
Herpes zoster	Yes
Human papillomavirus	No
Japanese encephalitis	Yes
Rabies	Yes
Varicella	Yes
Yellow Fever	Yes

This expansion in scope may have a positive impact on the health of travellers by offering additional points of access to vaccinations and other travel-related care. Indeed, the convenience of pharmacist-administered vaccinations has been cited as a key factor influencing patients' decisions to be vaccinated at a pharmacy [6]. One study reported that 30% of vaccinations administered by a U.S. pharmacy chain were administered outside of usual physician office hours, including weekday evenings, weekends, and national holidays [7]. However, vaccinations are only one component of travel-related risk reduction, with infectious diseases representing less than 2% of deaths among travelers [8]. However, seeking necessary vaccinations can be a driver for travelers to seek pre-travel healthcare advice. This creates the opportunity for clinicians to assess patient-, itinerary-, and destination-specific risks, as well as prophylactic drug therapy and education on non-drug health and safety measures [9].

There is evidence on the potential positive impact that pharmacists can have on patients' travel health care. With respect to vaccinations, previous studies have reported higher vaccination rates against seasonal influenza in jurisdictions that authorize pharmacists to administer vaccinations [10,11]. It is uncertain whether a similar trend is observed with travel vaccines. There is also evidence on the clinical outcomes achievable from pharmacist-performed travel consultations, including high acceptance rates of recommended vaccinations and medications, low incidence of illness while travelling, and patient confidence in their ability to self-manage illness abroad [12,13]. Finally, pharmacist-provided services were observed to lead to significant cost savings in one study as a result of lower use of unnecessary vaccinations and medicines when compared to consultations performed in a nurse-based travel service. This study also reported that pharmacists were able to identify and order missing vaccinations that were indicated for patients outside of just travel vaccinations (e.g., pneumococcal vaccine) [14]. Many of these studies were conducted among pharmacists with a specialized practice and additional training in travel health; moreover, other work has suggested that the general population of community pharmacists lack confidence in their ability to perform pre-travel consultations and assess the appropriateness of prescribed travel vaccines [15,16].

It is unknown whether an expansion in pharmacists' scope to include the administration of vaccines for travel-related purposes would translate to expanded offerings of multifaceted travel health services in community pharmacies, or if pharmacists would embrace this new scope in addition to their existing workload. The objective of this study is to examine data available to date on the landscape of travel health services in Ontario community pharmacies following this change in scope, pharmacists' perceptions of their ability to provide these services in practice, and patients' self-reported receipt of these additional vaccines by pharmacists, to determine the initial impact of this legislative change on pharmacy practice and patient care.

2. Materials and Methods

Triangulation of quantitative and qualitative data from four sources was performed:

2.1. Pharmacist Survey

Following a literature review, an online survey consisting of 38 questions was developed in consultation with a pharmacy practice researcher and an individual with expertise in health policy, and pilot tested for understandability and functionality among a sample of five third-year pharmacy students. The complete list of survey items is available in Appendix A. Questions sought basic demographic information about respondents, and explored the respondents' current travel health service offerings, changes around service offerings since the expansion in scope of December 2016, barriers and facilitators to service implementation, and further educational needs. Inclusion criteria for the survey were: (1) Current practice in a community pharmacy; and (2) Part A (active practice) licensure through the Ontario College of Pharmacists. The survey was administered using Qualtrics™ software (Qualtrics, Provo, UT, USA) and disseminated through the following methods: the Ontario Pharmacists Association's weekly email bulletins, social media, direct contact with known pharmacists, and through email to all Part A pharmacists in Ontario who provided permission to the Ontario College of Pharmacists to have their contact information utilized for research. Descriptive statistics were performed using IBM SPSS Statistics for Mac, Version 25 (Armonk, NY, USA). Ethics approval was received from the University of Waterloo Research Ethics Committee (ORE #22510) and Ryerson University's Research Ethics Board (REB 2018-282).

2.2. Pharmacist Interviews

At the conclusion of the pharmacist survey described above, respondents were asked to express interest in being contacted for a follow-up interview to gain deeper insight into reasons contributing to variable uptake across pharmacists and pharmacies, and to identify potential strategies to provide necessary support to pharmacists who wish to expand their patient care services in this area. Interested individuals were contacted and asked to participate in a telephone interview at a mutually agreeable time. A semi-structured interview guide was developed and is available in Appendix B. No compensation was provided for participants. Interviews were performed until data saturation was achieved, based on the perspective of the interviewer (JPS) and the principal investigator (SH). Interviews were audio-recorded and transcribed verbatim, with qualitative content analysis performed independently by two team members (ZRY and HF) for the first three transcripts to identify and summarize themes, and any disagreements resolved by consensus. The remaining transcripts were coded by one team member (HF). Analysis was performed using Microsoft Excel for Mac, version 15.33. Ethics approval was received from the University of Waterloo Research Ethics Committee (ORE #31442) and the Ryerson University Research Ethics Board (REB 2018–282).

2.3. Public Survey

Annually, the Survey Research Centre at the University of Waterloo conducts a Waterloo Regional Area Web Panel Survey. This omnibus survey allows researchers to pool resources for surveying the general public residing in the Waterloo region of Ontario, Canada. As such, the survey addresses a variety of topics of relevance to the general public. Members of the panel were identified through random digit dialing using both landline and cellular telephone numbers, followed by random selection of one member of the household for inclusion. Participants were then asked if they would be willing to be contacted by email to complete a web survey. Those who consent were invited by email to complete the survey, with two reminder emails at weekly intervals. Ethics approval for the survey was received from the University of Waterloo Research Ethics Committee (ORE #23309).

The 2018 survey included demographic questions such as employment status, household income, level of education, household size, and marital status, as well as a series of questions about receipt of pharmacist-administered vaccinations. Specifically, respondents were asked to indicate which (if any) vaccines they had ever received from a pharmacist. Each vaccine currently within the scope of practice for Ontario pharmacists was included. Web survey questions are provided in Appendix C.

Survey results were first analyzed descriptively using IBM SPSS Statistics for Mac, Version 25 (Armonk, NY, USA). Binary logistic regression was then performed to identify any associations between each demographic variable as independent variables and the receipt of any vaccine from a pharmacist, as well as each vaccine individually as the dependent variable. Statistical significance was defined a priori as $p < 0.05$.

2.4. Designated Yellow Fever Vaccination Centres

In Canada, the yellow fever vaccine is only distributed to healthcare facilities with current status as a Designated Yellow Fever Vaccination Centre through the Public Health Agency of Canada [17]. Pharmacies can obtain this designation, provided that they have either a pharmacist with authorization to prescribe the vaccine or have identified an individual with prescribing authority for the vaccine to serve as the site's nominated healthcare practitioner. This individual is responsible for overseeing operations to ensure compliance with designated site requirements. As yellow fever is not endemic in Canada [18], the use of its vaccine here is limited to international travellers. Additionally, given the complexity related to its use and other travel health risks associated with travel to yellow fever endemic countries, it can be assumed that only those sites providing pre-travel consultations and travel vaccinations on a regular basis would apply for designation. As such, the number of Designated Yellow Fever Vaccination Centers over time can serve as a proxy for the provision of travel health services.

All sites with this designation are publicly listed online, and searchable by province; however, the Public Health Agency of Canada does not retain historical records on the number and type of sites. To identify changes in the number of designated sites in Ontario over time, lists of all designated sites in the province of Ontario [19] were generated at 3-month intervals, beginning with March 2017. Pharmacies on this list were identified by cross-referencing pharmacy names and addresses with the list of licensed pharmacies maintained by the Ontario College of Pharmacists [20]. All other sites were coded as one of the following: travel clinic, medical clinic (includes interdisciplinary Family Health Teams and urgent care centers), public health unit, corporate or occupational health clinic, or other. Facilities whose categorization were uncertain based on their name alone were identified by performing an internet search to visit the website of the organization and determining the most applicable category. In the event that a facility was listed as a 'medical and travel clinic' it was coded as a travel clinic with the assumption that travel consultations performed here would be more representative of those performed at a specialized travel clinic than a general medicine practice.

As this analysis uses publicly available data, research ethics approval is not required. Descriptive statistics were performed using IBM SPSS Statistics for Mac, Version 25 (Armonk, NY, USA).

3. Results

3.1. Pharmacist Survey

Of the 222 respondents initiating the survey, 17 were excluded for failing to provide consent to participate (n = 5), not currently working in a community pharmacy (n = 11), or not currently holding Part A licensure (n = 1). The demographic characteristics of the 205 respondents completing the survey is provided in Table 2.

Table 2. Pharmacist survey respondent characteristics.

Characteristic	Frequency (%) N = 205
Type of community pharmacy	
Chain	78 (38.0%)
Independent	51 (24.9%)
Banner	50 (24.4%)
Mass merchandiser	15 (7.3%)
Grocery store	10 (4.9%)
Not specified	1 (0.5%)
Role in pharmacy	
Staff pharmacist	93 (45.4%)
Owner	47 (22.9%)
Manager	46 (22.6%)
Relief pharmacist	18 (8.8%)
Not specified	1 (0.5%)
Years in a community pharmacy practice	
Less than 1	3 (1.5%)
1–5	41 (20.0%)
6–10	46 (22.4%)
11–20	46 (22.4%)
21–30	35 (17.1%)
More than 30	32 (15.6%)
Not specified	2 (1.0%)
Average number of hours worked per week	
Less than 8	11 (5.4%)
8–16	12 (5.9%)
17–24	16 (7.8%)
25–32	25 (12.2%)
33–40	86 (42.0%)
More than 40	51 (24.9%)
Not specified	4 (2.0%)
Gender	
Male	97 (47.3%)
Female	102 (49.8%)
Gender variant / non-conforming	1 (0.5%)
Not specified	5 (2.4%)
Authorized to administer injections	
Yes	178 (86.8%)
No	21 (10.2%)
Not specified	6 (2.9%)

Most (n = 178, 87%) respondents had authorization to administer vaccines in Ontario; of these, 78% reported that they personally administer travel vaccines at their pharmacy (defined as any vaccines currently within their scope other than influenza). The most common way this service was offered was anytime by walk-in (69%), followed by appointment (24%) and during set days or hours such as a clinic day (6%); however, approximately half (54%) stated that appointment was their preferred method, with walk-in preferred by only 17% of respondents. Among the 137 individuals providing information on fees charged, 120 (88%) reported that their pharmacy charged patients a fee for this service, with CAD$20 per injection being most common (mean $18.32, SD $5.70, range $10–50). Uptake of this service appears to be low, as 94% of respondents reported administering fewer than 10 of these vaccines per month in total. Vaccines that respondents indicated they have personally administered since the expansion in scope are presented in Figure 1. Very few indicated administering any other vaccines under delegation, consisting of tetanus/diphtheria/pertussis (n = 3), measles/mumps/rubella (n = 2), and polio (n = 1).

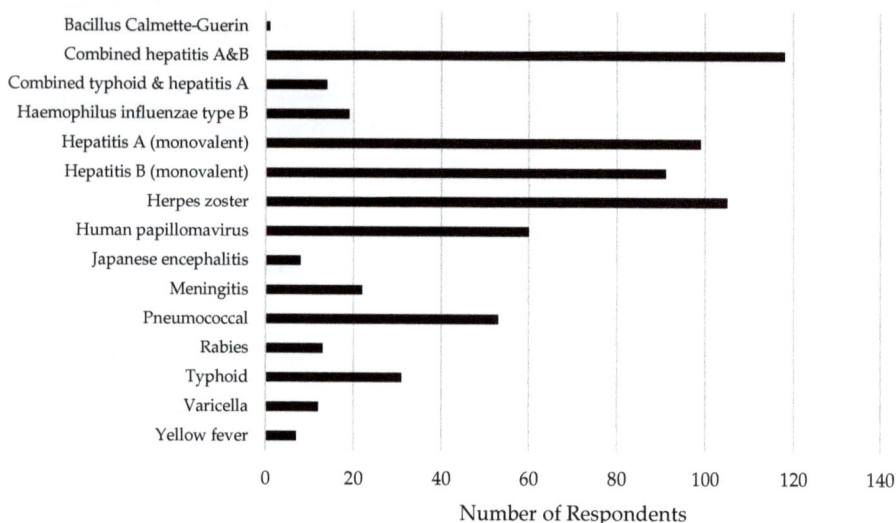

Figure 1. Pharmacist respondents' self-report of vaccinations they have personally administered to patients since December 2016.

Approximately 1 in 5 respondents (n = 56, 27%) reported that their pharmacy offers pre-travel consultation services, with walk-in being the most common model (55%) followed by an appointment basis (40%) and during clinic days (5%). By appointment is the preferred model by 62% of respondents, with only 16% preferring walk-in. Fees are charged by 35% of respondents offering this service, averaging CAD $34.17 (SD $12.81, range $20–50). As with vaccinations, pre-travel consultations are also infrequently performed, with 71% reporting performing fewer than 5 per month.

As illustrated in Figure 2, increases were noted in the number of respondents whose pharmacy offered a number of travel-related services following the expansion in scope, most notably an increase in pharmacies prescribing travel vaccines under delegation (relative increase of 50%) and offering pre-travel consultation services (relative increase of 33%). After vaccine administration, offering pre-travel consultations was the most frequent service, followed by the prescribing of oral medications under delegation and vaccine administration under delegation for vaccines currently outside of scope. In terms of future plans, 71% of respondents indicated an interest in receiving their Certificate in Travel Health designation from the International Society of Travel Medicine [19] within the next 5 years, and 77% expressed an interest in either implementing or further expanding their pharmacy's travel-related services. However, the stage of implementation was highly variable, with 38% stating they have a plan in place that they are working towards, while the remaining 62% have not established a plan.

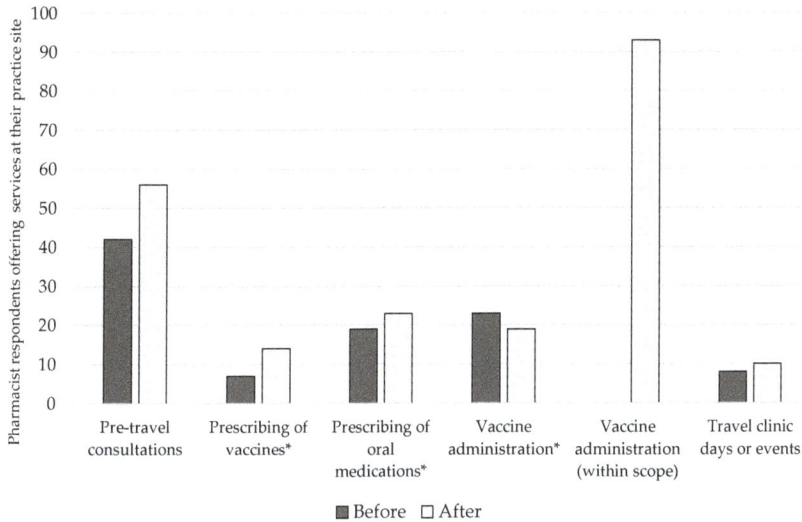

Figure 2. Travel-related services offered by respondents' practice site before and after scope expansion. Asterisk indicates activities requiring delegation or medical directive from a physician or other healthcare professional. Note: * indicates activities requiring a medical directive.

Respondents reported a number of barriers impacting uptake of these services by their pharmacy and by patients as indicated in Figure 3, and actual or potential facilitators as indicated in Figure 4. Taking both reported barriers and facilitators into account, education in travel health and the authorization to prescribe appear to be key priorities to better support this service in community pharmacy practice, followed by supports related to integrating these services into existing workflow. When asked if offering these services was revenue generating for the pharmacy, responses were split, with 50.6% feeling it was revenue generating and 49.4% feeling it was not. Revenue was primarily earned through service fees charged to patients (n = 69) followed by sale of non-prescription drugs for travel purposes (n = 43), the dispensing of prescriptions for travel purposes (n = 31), and new patient recruitment as a result of offering the service (n = 26).

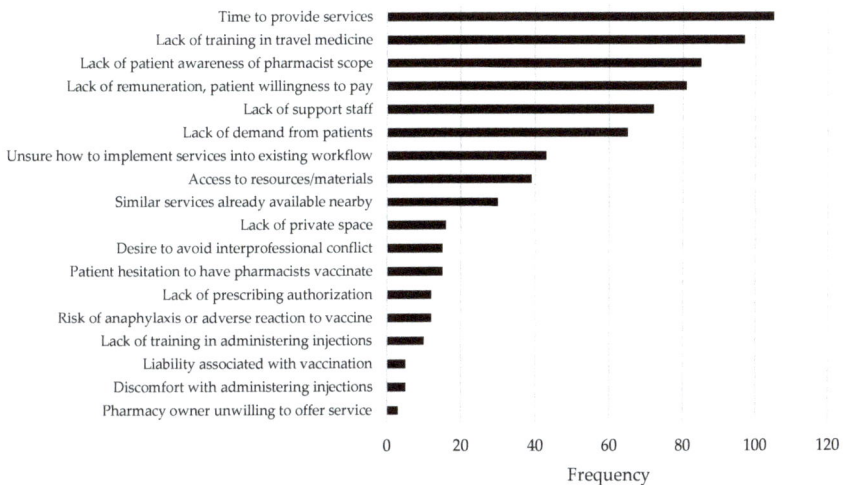

Figure 3. Barriers impacting ability to offer travel-related services.

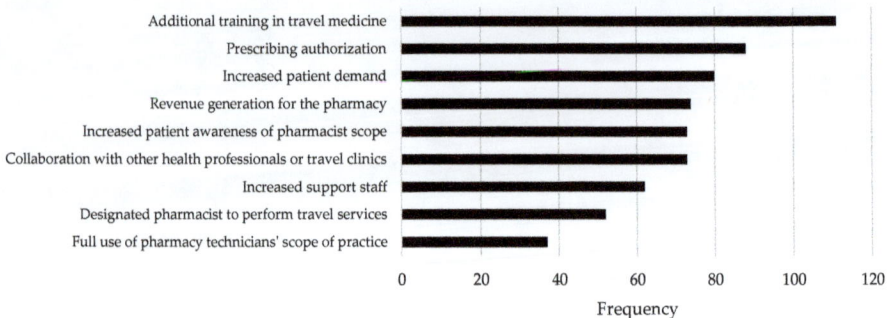

Figure 4. Facilitators (actual or potential) impacting ability to offer travel-related services.

3.2. Pharmacist Interviews

A total of six pharmacists (4 male, 2 female) from the above survey consented to participate in a semi-structured interview to further investigate pharmacy practice since the 2016 regulation change. Chain and independent practices were equally represented, as were staff pharmacists versus managers/owners. Years in practice ranged from 8–34, with one pharmacist reporting holding their Certificate in Travel Health from the International Society of Travel Medicine [21].

3.2.1. Confidence with New Scope

While all of the pharmacists were confident in administering influenza vaccinations, pharmacists experienced varying confidence levels and fewer number of patients accessing the pharmacy for administration of the other 13 vaccines within their scope. A number of factors appeared to influence the confidence level expressed:

- **Lower demand for non-influenza vaccinations.** The proportion of pharmacy patients who had an indication for influenza vaccine (the universal immunization program in Ontario advocates for all residents without contraindications to be vaccinated) versus the other vaccines means there are fewer opportunities to exercise the expanded scope.
- **Confidence is directly related to level of exposure.** Lower exposure to administration of the new vaccinations impacted pharmacists' confidence with both administering the vaccine and verifying its clinical appropriateness for a patient. One pharmacist practicing with a medical directive to administer non-influenza vaccinations since 2012 reported high confidence, while the others reported varying confidence based on the vaccine (e.g., more confident with herpes zoster than travel vaccines).
- **Duration of available scope.** Influenza vaccination by pharmacists in Ontario has been permitted since 2012, while additional vaccination authority was only initiated in December 2016. As such, there has been more time to gain experience with influenza vaccination, including administration and monitoring. For example, pharmacists are highly familiar with the volume, route, and adverse effects of influenza vaccination, but would need to look this information up for other vaccines. It was recognized that comfort and familiarity with the 13 new vaccines would likely increase with time as it did with influenza.

Pharmacists reported comfort with recognizing when a patient may need referral to another healthcare professional, such as last-minute travellers, those requiring yellow fever vaccination, and pediatric patients. For example, one respondent commented, "I may … refer them [the patient] to some place like … Travel Clinic because of their experience; they're going to know which things to get onboard right away, if there's alternative regimens that they might be able to use that I'm not comfortable suggesting" (Pharmacist 1).

Low-risk cases were considered to largely consist of healthy patients travelling to all-inclusive resorts in the Caribbean, and of those pharmacists that reported performing pre-travel consultations, most limited their practices to these low-risk cases.

3.2.2. Patient Identification and Interprofessional Collaboration

Patients requiring travel advice and other vaccinations were identified in one of three ways: (1) Patients self-identifying as needing advice; (2) Referral from other healthcare professionals; and (3) Pharmacist identification based on travel-related prescriptions presented for dispensing. Self-identified patients appeared motivated to present by an advertisement of the service or through an existing relationship with the pharmacist. Some pharmacists had collaborative relationships with other healthcare professionals who were aware of the regulation change and supported it. For example, one pharmacist described a relationship with a local nurse practitioner, saying "she has been sending a lot of her clients to us for the recommendation and then she provides a prescription" (Pharmacist 1). However, others reported pushback from other healthcare professionals who identified this expanded scope as overlapping or competing with their services. Pharmacist 2 found this differed with physician age, stating "Some of the newer physicians were keener to utilize the pharmacist whereas some of the ones that have been around for a bit longer were more reluctant." Pharmacist 3 similarly observed great variation, saying "Some doctors consider us as an equal and part of their practice. But some other doctors, they won't consider or they don't even take our recommendation."

3.2.3. Barriers and Facilitators

Barriers emerging from the interviews generally mirrored those of the broader survey, with the exception that inability to prescribe was a more frequently cited barrier among those interviewed than among survey respondents. As one respondent noted, "Right now our biggest barrier would be prescribing of course ... So we'll gather all the information and we'll first communicate directly with the patient, tell them what our recommendations are and whichever ones they approve or they agree with then we go through their primary care practitioner to try and get a prescription for those products" (Pharmacist 1).

1. **Awareness of Pharmacists Scope:** Depending on the pharmacy and its location (e.g., co-located with a medical clinic vs. standalone), lack of awareness of the regulatory change to pharmacists' scope was recognized among both patients and physicians, despite it being in effect for over a year at the time of the interviews. One pharmacist reported, "I don't think [regulation change] had a big change. I don't know if the patients are even aware about it or if it's advertised" (Pharmacist 3).

2. **Clinical Knowledge:** Travel health is a clinical area that is not routinely used daily in pharmacy practice, nor emphasized in university curricula. Pharmacists have to take it upon themselves to learn its extensive body of knowledge in order to become an expert in the field. In addition to the breadth and depth of clinical knowledge, it is also an ever-changing practice. Travel advisories, epidemics, and recommendations can change much quicker than other clinical areas (e.g., diabetes), which adds another difficulty for pharmacists to uptake travel health services. This distinction between travel health and other clinical areas was described by Pharmacist 1 as "[it's] kind of like you need to go above and beyond what is out there to make sure you have the background information ... .it's not like every day practice."

3. **Inability to Prescribe:** Pharmacists not being able to prescribe medications or vaccinations is a significant limitation to their provision of travel health services. Unlike receiving a consultation from a travel clinic, where a patient can receive their assessment, immunizations, education, and prescriptions in one appointment, patients that receive a consultation from a pharmacist must bear an additional wait time of a prescription being sent to the pharmacy from another health professional with prescribing ability. Many pharmacists expressed frustration at this limitation,

with Pharmacist 1 stating "I think our profession really needs to push towards having prescribing rights for those immunizations ... There is no harm in immunizing somebody, so I can't imagine what the barrier is to getting those prescribing rights."

4. **Remuneration:** The inability to prescribe also complicates remuneration for services, since pharmacists without medical directives to prescribe rely heavily on physicians to provide prescriptions for travelling patients. Some physicians may be hesitant to do so if they offer their own pre-travel consultations for a fee or could otherwise charge for a related office visit. It is perceived that they are contributing to the consultation but without receiving a fee like the pharmacist can, which may negatively impact collaboration. One pharmacist (Pharmacist 4) noted that this can also be confusing for patients, as "the doctors want to get paid for their service for writing a prescription, in which case [my consultation is] kind of redundant. Why is the patient paying [the pharmacist] as well?"

A strong facilitator of the service mentioned by all pharmacists was the added convenience that pharmacist-provided services offers for patients. Pharmacist 5 commented "We're open eight to eight Monday to Friday and we're open on weekends. We close three days a year, right, so finding a time to come in and get their vaccine or whatever is not an issue for them." While some patients were hesitant to pay an administration fee to receive the injection at a pharmacy versus at no charge from their physician's office, Pharmacist 1 explained the return on investment as: "You can wait and go to your doctor, if you like, go book an appointment, take another day off work .... Or you can get them right here, right now and maybe wait for five minutes or ten minutes for me."

3.3. Public Survey

Surveys were completed by 248 respondents (response rate 38.5%) with a mean age of 59.1 years (SD 14.0), of which 42.7%, 56.9%, and 0.4% identified as male, female, or transgendered, respectively. In total, 122 (49.2%) reported having never received a vaccine that was injected by a pharmacist. Vaccines received by a pharmacist, and the number and proportion of respondents reporting receiving each vaccine, are listed in Table 3. As influenza vaccination by pharmacists in Ontario has been in place since 2012, it is not surprising that it remains the most commonly-received vaccine by injection from a pharmacist. Interestingly, uptake of vaccines most commonly indicated for exposure related to travel were all administered by pharmacists to fewer than 5% of respondents, with the only exception being the hepatitis A&B combination vaccine at 5.6%.

Table 3. Vaccines reported by survey respondents as being received by injection from a pharmacist.

Vaccine	Frequency (%) (n = 248 Respondents)
Influenza	117 (47.2%)
Herpes zoster	16 (6.5%)
Pneumococcal	15 (6.0%)
Hepatitis A&B combination	14 (5.6%)
Bacillus Calmette-Guérin	8 (3.2%)
Meningococcal	8 (3.2%)
Varicella	7 (2.8%)
Typhoid	6 (2.4%)
Hepatitis B (monovalent)	6 (2.4%)
Hepatitis A (monovalent)	5 (2.0%)
Rabies	3 (1.2%)
Yellow fever	3 (1.2%)
Haemophilus influenzae type B	2 (0.8%)
Human papillomavirus	1 (0.4%)
Japanese encephalitis	1 (0.4%)

Binary logistic regression did not detect any statistically significant relationships between vaccination or non-vaccination by a pharmacist and the independent variables of age, employment status, household income, level of education, number of individuals in the household, and marital status, with the following exceptions:

- Negative relationship between increasing age and receipt of meningococcal (OR 0.847, p = 0.03), hepatitis B (OR 0.866, p = 0.004), and rabies (OR 0.839, p = 0.036) vaccines
- Positive association between increasing age and receipt of the herpes zoster vaccine (OR 1.05, p = 0.048)

3.4. Yellow Fever Vaccination Centres in Ontario

Prior to the expansion in pharmacist scope in December 2016, there were 220 Designated Yellow Fever Vaccination Centres in Ontario; unfortunately, data on the name of each site at this time could not be accessed; therefore, centres could not be categorized as of that date. At the first date of complete data availability, there were 227 designated centres with travel clinics and medical clinics comprising over 80% of all centres (Figure 5), followed in frequency by pharmacies and public health units, occupational health clinics, and a single nursing clinic. Small increasing trends in the number of designated sites were observed across travel clinics and general medical clinics over time, with pharmacies experiencing a near doubling between March 2017 and June 2018; however, this was immediately followed by a drop from 30 pharmacies to only 13 by September 2018 which remained consistent through December 2018. While reasons for this reduction in the number of pharmacies with designation are unavailable from the Public Health Agency of Canada, cross-referencing all pharmacies with discontinued designation against the register of licensed pharmacies in Ontario identified that all but two of these pharmacies remained licensed to operate, indicating that closure of the pharmacy was not the reason for discontinued designation status.

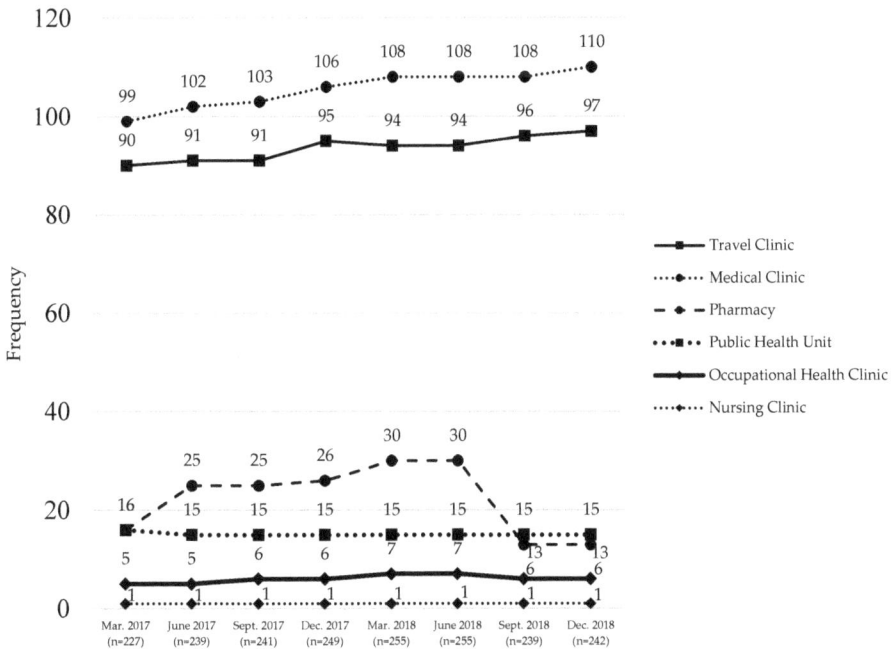

Figure 5. Designated Yellow Fever Vaccination Centres in Ontario, by category and date.

4. Discussion

Through the triangulation of multiple data sources, this study identified that the uptake of travel-related services by community pharmacies in Ontario has been generally slow, with some variation by activity and by pharmacist, since an expansion in scope to allow for the administration of travel-related vaccines in December 2016. Key challenges identified included lack of time to provide the service within existing workflow, knowledge needs related to making clinical recommendations and/or confirming the appropriateness of vaccines and prescribed drugs, and lack of prescribing authorization.

While triangulation of results from four different types of datasets was performed, limitations remain with these conclusions due to methodological design and data availability. With the pharmacist survey, the low response rate must be noted (n = 205, of over 16,000 pharmacists currently licensed in Ontario) [22], as well as under-representation of pharmacists practicing in independently-owned community pharmacies (24.9% of respondents, versus 52% of pharmacies in Ontario being independently owned), and over-representation of pharmacists with authorization to administer injections (86.8% of respondents vs. 46.8% of pharmacists in Ontario with injection administration authorization) [22,23]. Pharmacist interviews were also conducted with a small sample; however, it was felt that saturation was achieved with the responses obtained. Respondents from the public survey represented a 38.5% response rate among those contacted, but may not be representative of the overall population as the individuals invited to participate were those who had previously completed a telephone survey conducted by the Survey Research Centre at the University of Waterloo and opted-in to an online follow-up survey. Participants for the telephone survey were identified through random-digit dialing of both landline and cellular telephone numbers within the region, so individuals without access to a telephone, and individuals without internet access or comfort with internet technology, were likely excluded. Finally, as all facilities that administer the yellow fever vaccine must be registered as a Designated Yellow Fever Vaccination Centre, data on designated sites is complete; however, a worldwide shortage of yellow fever vaccine since November 2016 [24] may have negatively influenced the number of sites seeking this designation at this time.

The findings of this study are consistent with the literature on pharmacists' uptake of new services and pharmacists' perception of their ability to provide travel-related care. Slow uptake of new services by pharmacists in Canada was observed for activities including prescribing for medication renewals or adaptations and initial prescribing [25], prescribing for smoking cessation specifically [26], and medication reviews [27,28]. Similar trends have been observed internationally, even when remuneration is offered for the new service without having to request payment from patients [29]. Barriers and facilitators identified were consistent with those reported by pharmacists across other disease areas [30–33], in travel health specifically [14], and even by pharmacists in Ontario prior to the legislative change expanding their scope in December 2016 [16], including lack of confidence in their knowledge and skills, concerns with integrating new services into existing workflow, patient awareness of new services, and a desire for acceptance of (or enhanced collaboration with) physicians and other health professionals. We hypothesize that the clinical knowledge barrier may be more pronounced for travel health than other clinical areas due to minimal training received by many health professionals in travel health in their professional degree [34]; however, it was outside of the scope of this study to evaluate this assumption.

5. Conclusions

Similarities across barriers and facilitators with previous work in travel health and other services suggest that there are systemic changes that can be made to pharmacy practice to support non-dispensing services. A movement towards appointment-based patient care models when possible, pharmacy space layout modifications to provide adequate space and privacy for consultations, investment in continuing professional development and clinical software to aid with clinical decision-making and confidence with those decisions, and advocacy efforts targeting the public to increase awareness of pharmacists' expertise and scope will support all aspects of non-dispensing services performed in community pharmacies, with applicability to travel health and management of other clinical issues. Efforts to increase education in travel health in pharmacy curricula and the development of toolkits or standardized approaches to patient evaluation and risk management may also have a positive impact on reducing the broad variability observed related to pharmacist practice in travel health.

Author Contributions: Conceptualization, S.K.D.H.; Data curation, S.K.D.H., K.K., and Z.R.-Y.; Formal analysis, S.K.D.H., K.K., H.V.J.F., Z.R.-Y.; Funding acquisition, S.K.D.H. and Z.R.-Y.; Investigation, S.K.D.H.; Methodology, S.K.D.H., K.K., and Z.R.-Y.; Project administration, S.K.D.H.; Supervision, S.K.D.H.; Writing—original draft, S.K.D.H.; Writing—review and editing, S.K.D.H., K.K., H.V.J.F., Z.R.-Y.

Funding: Portions of this research were funded through an Applied Health Research Question submitted by the Ontario Pharmacists Association to the Ontario Pharmacy Evidence Network (OPEN). OPEN is funded by a grant from the Government of Ontario.

Acknowledgments: The authors wish to acknowledge the Ontario Pharmacy Evidence Network (www.open-pharmacy-research.ca) for their support allowing us to email Ontario pharmacists who consented to be contacted for research. We also wish to acknowledge the contribution of Jane Pearson-Sharpe for conducting the telephone interviews, and the Survey Research Centre at the University of Waterloo (https://uwaterloo.ca/survey-research-centre/) for conducting the Waterloo Regional Area Web Panel Survey.

Conflicts of Interest: Houle has received unrestricted research support from Valneva Canada, Inc. and unrestricted education grants from Merck and GSK. The remaining authors declare no conflict of interest. The funders had no role in the design of the study; in the collection, analyses, or interpretation of data; in the writing of the manuscript, or in the decision to publish the results.

Appendix A

Table A1. Pharmacist survey questions.

Question	Answer Options
Screening	
Do you currently work in a community pharmacy practice setting?	• Yes • No
Do you currently have an Ontario Part A license to practice pharmacy in the province?	• Yes • No
Demographics	
Which type of community pharmacy practice setting do you primarily work in?	• Independent community pharmacy • Community pharmacy associated with a chain • Community pharmacy associated with a banner • Community pharmacy associated with a grocery store • Community pharmacy associated with a mass merchandiser • Other (please specify)
What is your role in the community pharmacy practice setting you work in?	• Community pharmacy owner • Community pharmacy manager • Community pharmacy staff pharmacist • Community pharmacy relief pharmacist
Where is your community pharmacy practice setting located?	• Central East • Central South • Central West • East • North • South West • Toronto
How many years have you worked in a community pharmacy practice setting?	• Less than 1 • 1 to 5 • 6 to 10 • 11 to 20 • 21 to 30 • More than 30
On average, how many hours per week do you work in a community pharmacy practice setting?	• Less than 8 • 8 to 16 • 17 to 24 • 25 to 32 • 33 to 40 • More than 40

Table A1. *Cont.*

Question	Answer Options
Which gender do you most identify with?	• Male • Female • Gender Variant/Non-conforming
Are you authorized to administer injections in Ontario?	• Yes • No
Travel Vaccinations	
Do you currently administer travel or travel-related vaccinations at your pharmacy?	• Yes • No
When and how do you currently offer travel or travel-related vaccinations at your pharmacy? Select all that apply.	• Anytime by walk-in • During set days/hours by walk-in (e.g., clinic days) • By appointment
What would be your preferred method for offering travel or travel-related vaccinations at your pharmacy?	• Anytime by walk-in • During set days/hours by walk-in (e.g., clinic days) • By appointment • No preference
Does your pharmacy charge a fee to patients to administer travel or travel-related vaccinations?	• Yes (please specify the fee amount) • No
Which of the following travel or travel-related vaccines have you personally administered since the expansion of Ontario pharmacists' scope in December 2016? Select all that apply.	• Bacille Calmette-Guérin (BCG) (for tuberculosis) • Haemophilus influenza type b (Hib) • Hepatitis A • Hepatitis B • Combined hepatitis a and b • Herpes zoster (shingles) • Human papillomavirus (HPV) • Japanese encephalitis • Meningitis • Pneumococcus • Rabies • Typhoid • Combined typhoid and hepatitis A • Varicella zoster (chickenpox) • Yellow Fever • None of the above
Which other vaccines have you personally administered under delegation or a medical directive? Select all that apply.	• Diphtheria • IPV (poliomyelitis) • Measles, mumps, rubella (MMR) • Pertussis • Tetanus • Other (please specify) • None of the above
On average, how many travel or travel-related vaccinations do you administer in a month?	• Less than 5 • 5 to 10 • 11 to 15 • 16 to 20 • More than 20
Travel Consultations	
Do you currently perform travel consultations at your pharmacy?	• Yes • No
When and how do you currently offer travel consultations at your pharmacy? Select all that apply.	• Anytime by walk-in • During set days/hours by walk-in • By appointment
What would be your preferred method for offering travel consultations at your pharmacy?	• Anytime by walk-in • During set days/hours by walk-in • By appointment • No preference
Does your pharmacy charge a fee to patients to receive a travel consultation?	• Yes (please specify the fee amount) • No

Table A1. *Cont.*

Question	Answer Options
On average, how many travel consultations do you complete in a month?	• Less than 5 • 5 to 10 • 11 to 15 • 16 to 20 • More than 20
Practice Changes Related to Regulatory Expansion	
Which travel medicine services did you offer prior to the regulatory change? Select all that apply.	• Individual travel consultations • Prescribing of travel or travel-related vaccines under delegation • Prescribing of other drugs for travel purposes (e.g., travellers' diarrhea, altitude sickness, malaria) under delegation • Travel or travel-related vaccine administration under delegation • MedsCheck prior to travel • Travel medicine clinic days/events • Other (please specify) • Not applicable—I was not offering travel medicine services prior to the regulatory change
Which travel medicine services do you currently offer? Select all that apply.	• Individual travel consultations • Prescribing of travel or travel-related vaccines under delegation • Prescribing of other drugs for travel purposes (e.g., travellers' diarrhea, altitude sickness, malaria) under delegation • Travel or travel-related vaccine administration under expanded scope • Travel or travel-related vaccine administration under delegation • MedsCheck prior to travel • Travel medicine clinic days/events • Other (please specify) • Not applicable—I am not currently offering travel medicine services
Please choose one of the following statements that best describes how your pharmacy practice has changed since the regulatory expansion with respect to the number of travel medicine services you complete on a monthly basis. (Consider all travel medicine services you offer.)	• I am completing a higher number of services • I am completing a lower number of services • I am completing about the same number of services
How does your pharmacy promote your travel-related services (vaccinations, consultations, and other related services) to patients? Select all that apply.	• In-store posters • Signs outside of the pharmacy • Newspaper/radio ads • Bag stuffers • Website • Social media (e.g., Facebook, Twitter) • Word of mouth • Audio ads over pharmacy's intercom system • Audio ads while patients are on hold on the phone with the pharmacy • Other (please specify)
Practice Barriers and Facilitators	
What have been, or would you consider to be, the primary barrier(s) to implementing travel medicine services in your community pharmacy practice? Select all that apply.	• Lack of injection training • Lack of travel medicine training • Lack of knowledge of/access to resources/materials • Lack of time to dedicate to travel medicine services • Insufficient availability of support staff (e.g., pharmacy technicians, assistants) • Lack of demand from patients • Lack of patient awareness of pharmacists' expanded scope • Patients unwilling to have pharmacist vaccinate • Lack of remuneration • Unsure how to incorporate processes into daily work flow • Travel medicine services are already available near my place of practice • I am uncomfortable with administering injections

Table A1. *Cont.*

Question	Answer Options
Practice Barriers and Facilitators	
What have been, or would you consider to be, the primary barrier(s) to implementing travel medicine services in your community pharmacy practice? Select all that apply.	• Religious beliefs • I want to avoid conflict with other professionals who can vaccinate • I do not want to be professionally responsible for the act of vaccination • I do not feel prepared to handle allergic or adverse reactions in my pharmacy • Lack of private space • Other (please specify)
Of the options you selected in the previous question, please select the ONE that you consider to be the PRIMARY barrier to implementing travel medicine services in your community pharmacy practice.	• Lack of injection training • Lack of travel medicine training • Lack of knowledge of/access to resources/materials • Lack of time to dedicate to travel medicine services • Insufficient availability of support staff (e.g., pharmacy technicians, assistants) • Lack of demand from patients • Lack of patient awareness of pharmacists' expanded scope • Patients unwilling to have pharmacist vaccinate • Lack of remuneration • Unsure how to incorporate processes into daily work flow • Travel medicine services are already available near my place of practice • I am uncomfortable with administering injections • Religious beliefs • I want to avoid conflict with other professionals who can vaccinate • I do not want to be professionally responsible for the act of vaccination • I do not feel prepared to handle allergic or adverse reactions in my pharmacy • Lack of private space • Other (please specify)
What have been, or would you consider to be, the primary facilitator(s) for the implementation of travel medicine services in your community pharmacy practice? Select all that apply.	• Completion of additional training in immunization or travel medicine • Collaboration with other healthcare professionals or health clinics • Increased patient demand • Increased awareness of pharmacists' expanded scope • Increased support staff hours • Increased use of pharmacy technicians' scope of practice • Designated travel medicine services pharmacist • Pharmacists' ability to prescribe travel vaccines or travel-related medicine • Revenue generation • Other (please specify)
Of the options you selected in the previous question, please select the ONE that you consider to be the PRIMARY facilitator to implementing travel medicine services in your community pharmacy practice.	• Completion of additional training in immunization or travel medicine • Collaboration with other healthcare professionals or health clinics • Increased patient demand • Increased awareness of pharmacists' expanded scope • Increased support staff hours • Increased use of pharmacy technicians' scope of practice • Designated travel medicine services pharmacist • Pharmacists' ability to prescribe travel vaccines or travel-related medicine • Revenue generation • Other (please specify)
Do you find your pharmacy's travel medicine service(s) to be revenue generating?	• Yes • No

Table A1. *Cont.*

Question	Answer Options
What do you feel primarily contributes to the profitability of your service(s). Select all that apply.	• A fee-for-service is charged to patients • More people are becoming patients at my pharmacy because of the travel medicine services I/we offer • More travel-related OTC sales after counselling are occurring • More patients are bringing in their travel-related prescriptions because of the travel medicine service I/we offer • Efficiencies (through optimal use of staff, materials/resources used, implementation of processes, etc.) have been created as a result of implementing travel medicine services • Not applicable—a business evaluation of this service has not yet been conducted by our pharmacy • Other (please specify)
Education Needs and Preferences	
Which areas of additional travel medicine-related education would facilitate the implementation or improve the quality of pharmacist-led travel medicine services in your community pharmacy? Select all that apply.	• Processes for completing a pre-travel assessment • Pre-travel assessment knowledge based on geographical location(s) during travel • Pre-travel assessment knowledge based on activity/activities during travel • Pre-travel assessment knowledge based on patients' health status, comorbidities, and special patient populations • Travel-related diseases • Travel-related vaccines • Travel-related prescription medication use • Travel-related self-care and non-prescription drug measures • Other travel health risks • Other (please specify) • Not applicable—I feel confident in my travel medicine-related knowledge and training background
With respect to acquiring further travel medicine-related education, which forms of education would be most appealing to you? Select up to 5 options.	• Self-directed online continuing education course of <2 h duration • Self-directed online continuing education course of 2+ h duration • Webinar • In-person or live continuing education course (half day) • In-person or live continuing education course (full day) • Downloadable clinical practice guidelines on travel medicine topics • Downloadable or printable educational materials (e.g., booklets) • Mobile app or online resources • Self-assessment tools • Diploma/certificate level training in travel medicine • Other (please specify)
Would you be interested in pursuing a Certificate in Travel Health designation from the International Society of Travel Medicine in the next 5 years?	• Yes • No • Unsure
Future Plans and Advocacy	
Which of the following statements best describes your future plans with respect to offering travel medicine services in your pharmacy?	• Already implementing, and not currently working on a plan to further expand • Already implementing, and wanting/working on a plan to further expand • Intend to implement, and currently working on a plan • Interested in implementing, but not currently working on a plan • No intention to implement in the near future

Table A1. *Cont.*

Question	Answer Options
In addition to allowing additional vaccines to be administered, the regulatory changes under the *Pharmacy Act* also now allow for injection trained pharmacy students and interns to administer the same vaccines. Which of the following statements best describes how your pharmacy practice has changed since the regulatory change with respect to pharmacy students and interns administering vaccines?	• My pharmacy now has pharmacy students and/or interns administering vaccines • My pharmacy does not have pharmacy students or interns administering vaccines and does not intend to have them administering vaccines • My pharmacy does not have pharmacy students or interns administering vaccines but is considering having them administer vaccines in the future • Unsure • Not applicable—vaccines are not administered at my pharmacy
Would you want OPA to advocate for pharmacists' ability to prescribe travel and travel-related vaccines?	• Yes • No • Unsure
Would you want OPA to advocate for pharmacists' ability to prescribe travel-related drugs (e.g., travellers' diarrhea, malaria, altitude sickness, etc.)?	• Yes • No • Unsure

OPA, Ontario Pharmacists Association; OTC, over-the-counter.

Appendix B

Semi-structured interview guide for pharmacists.

Let's start with some questions about your current practice:

- Please describe your pharmacy's patient population *(Prompt if needed: for example, age, socioeconomic status, health conditions)*
- Please describe your relationships with other healthcare providers in your community and their perception of your role as a patient care provider.
- Is there a travel clinic or another health professional that currently provides travel health services in your community? Does this effect the types of services you offer?
- Can you explain your experience, if any, with administering influenza vaccines in your pharmacy? *(Prompt if needed: How long have you been doing this? How many patients have you administered to? What is your comfort level with this?)*
- Can you explain your experience, if any, with administering other vaccines that are generally **not** used for travel, such as pneumococcal, zoster, or HPV vaccine? *(Prompt if needed: How long have you been doing this? How many patients have you administered to? What is your comfort level with this?)*

Tell me about your experiences with travel health services in your practice? (Prompt if needed to discuss both administering travel vaccines and performing consultations. A consultation is an individualized assessment of a person's health risks while travelling, considering patient-specific, destination-specific, and activity-specific factors).

What impact, if any, has the regulatory change to expand the list of vaccinations that pharmacists can administer had on your services? Why?

IF they have experience with administering travel vaccines in their pharmacy:

Regarding administering travel vaccines, such as those for hepatitis A or B, typhoid, Japanese encephalitis, or yellow fever:

- Describe your process for administering these vaccines and how it fits within your workflow.
- How do you identify eligible patients?
- Are there any clinical or non-clinical circumstances where you would not administer travel vaccinations to a patient who requested it? *(Prompt if needed: What are these, and why?)*
- Describe your process for documentation. *(Prompt if needed: Do you inform the patient's primary care provider that you administered these vaccines?)*

- Do you provide patients with any written educational materials about these vaccines? If so, which resources do you provide? *(Prompt if needed: Information from website online, pamphlet provided by vaccine manufacturer, written information developed in-house)*
- Tell me about your rationale for either charging, or not charging, a fee for administering these vaccines. **IF a fee is charged:** How have your patients responded to being asked to pay for this service?

IF they have experience with performing travel consultations in their pharmacy:

Regarding providing travel consultations:

- Describe your process for providing this service and how it fits within your workflow.
- How do you identify eligible patients?
- Are there any clinical or non-clinical circumstances where you would refer a patient to another healthcare professional for a consultation? *(Prompt if needed: What are these, and why?)*
- Describe your process for documentation. *(Prompt if needed: Do you inform the patient's primary care provider that you performed this consultation?)*
- Do you provide patients with any written educational materials about travel health? If so, which resources do you provide? *(Prompt if needed: Information from website online, pamphlet provided by vaccine manufacturer, written information developed in-house)*
- Tell me about your rationale for either charging, or not charging, a fee for this consultation? **IF a fee is charged:** How have your patients responded to being asked to pay for this service?

For any pharmacists with experience with either or both of the activities above:

Let's talk about your overall experience as a travel health care provider:

- Tell me about facilitators and barriers you have experienced in delivering travel health services to your patients? What strategies have you tried to make it easier for you to provide this care in practice?
- Please describe for me your level of confidence with providing travel health services?
- What feedback, if any, have you received from your patients?
- What feedback, if any, have your received from other healthcare providers in your community?

For pharmacists that report NOT administering travel vaccines and NOT providing travel consultations:

- Under what clinical circumstances would you consider providing your patients with:

  - Travel vaccine administration?
  - Travel consultations and education?

- What are some reasons why you have not offered these services in your pharmacy? *(Prompt if needed: Some examples might be staffing, management support, need for more training or confidence, or do you feel this is outside of the scope of practice for pharmacists?)*
- What are some supports that would help you to offer these types of services?
- If your pharmacy were to start providing travel health services, would you charge a fee for administering vaccines or providing travel consultations? Why or why not?

Appendix C

Waterloo Region Area Survey questions.

Demographic Questions:

Please select your gender:

- Male
- Female
- Transgendered

What is your current employment status? **(SELECT ONE ONLY)**

- Full-time
- Part-time
- Retired
- Unemployed
- Student
- Homemaker
- Other (Please specify: _____)

What is your current household income before taxes? **(SELECT ONE ONLY)**

- Less than $20,000
- $20,000 to less than $50,000
- $50,000 to less than $80,000
- $80,000 to less than $100,000
- $100,000 or more

What is the highest level of formal education that you have completed? **(SELECT ONE ONLY)**

- Grade school
- High school
- College or trade apprenticeship
- University degree
- Other (Please specify: _____)

Not including yourself, how many people live in your household? Please include all adults, other than yourself, and any children that live with you all or most of the time.

At present, are you married, living with a partner, widowed, divorced, separated, or have you never been married? **(SELECT ONE ONLY)**

- Married
- Living with partner/common-law
- Widowed
- Divorced or separated
- Never married

Pharmacist-Administered Vaccines Question:

Please indicate which vaccines, if any, you have **ever** received **by injection** by a **pharmacist:** (Please select all that apply)

- Influenza (flu) vaccine
- Bacille Calmette-Guérin (tuberculosis) vaccine
- Haemophilus Influenzae type b (Hib) vaccine
- Meningococcal (meningitis) vaccine
- Pneumococcal (pneumonia) vaccine
- Typhoid vaccine

- Hepatitis A vaccine
- Hepatitis B vaccine
- Hepatitis A and B combined vaccines (e.g., Twinrix®)
- Herpes Zoster (shingles) vaccine
- Human Papillomavirus (HPV, cervical cancer) vaccine
- Japanese Encephalitis vaccine
- Rabies vaccine
- Varicella (chickenpox) vaccine
- Yellow Fever vaccine
- I have never received a vaccine that was injected by a pharmacist.

References

1. Leslie, K. Pharmacists in Ontario Can Give Flu Shots and Renew Non-Narcotic Prescriptions. *The Globe and Mail.* 9 October 2012. Available online: https://www.theglobeandmail.com/news/politics/pharmacists-in-ontario-can-give-flu-shots-and-renew-non-narcotic-prescriptions/article4598872/ (accessed on 2 January 2019).
2. Ontario College of Pharmacists. New Authority for Vaccinations (Effective Dec 15). Available online: http://www.ocpinfo.com/library/news/new-authority-vaccinations-effective-december-15/ (accessed on 2 January 2019).
3. National Association of Pharmacy Regulatory Authorities. Search National Drug Schedule. Available online: http://napra.ca/pages/Schedules/Search.aspx (accessed on 2 January 2019).
4. Ontario College of Pharmacists. Medical Directives and the Delegation of Controlled Acts. Available online: http://www.ocpinfo.com/regulations-standards/policies-guidelines/medical-directives/ (accessed on 2 January 2019).
5. Government of Ontario. Ontario's Routine Immunization Schedule. Available online: http://www.health.gov.on.ca/en/public/programs/immunization/static/immunization_tool.html (accessed on 6 April 2019).
6. Papastergiou, J.; Folkins, C.; Li, W.; Zervas, J. Community pharmacist-administered influenza immunization improves patient access to vaccination. *Can. Pharm. J.* **2014**, *147*, 359–365. [CrossRef] [PubMed]
7. Goad, J.A.; Taitel, M.S.; Fensterheim, L.E.; Cannon, A.E. Vaccinations administered during off-clinic hours at a national community pharmacy: Implications for increasing patient access and convenience. *Ann. Fam. Med.* **2013**, *11*, 429–436. [CrossRef] [PubMed]
8. Steffen, R.; Grieve, S. Chapter 2: Epidemiology: Morbidity and Mortality in Travelers. In *Travel Medicine*, 3rd ed.; Keystone, J.S., Freedman, D.O., Kozarsky, P.E., Connor, B.A., Nothdurft, H.D., Eds.; Saunders: Philadelphia, PA, USA, 2012.
9. Aw, B.; Boraston, S.; Botten, D.; Cherniwchan, D.; Fazal, H.; Kelton, T.; Libman, M.; Saldanha, C.; Scappatura, D.; Stowe, B. Travel medicine: What's involved? When to refer? *Can. Fam. Phys.* **2014**, *60*, 1091–1103.
10. Buchan, S.A.; Rosella, L.C.; Finkelstein, M.; Juurlink, D.; Isenor, J.; Marra, F.; Patel, A.; Russell, M.L.; Quach, S.; Waite, N.; et al. Impact of pharmacist administration of influenza vaccines on uptake in Canada. *Can. Med. Assoc. J.* **2017**, *189*, 146–152. [CrossRef] [PubMed]
11. Drozd, E.M.; Miller, L.; Johnsrud, M. Impact of pharmacist immunization authority on seasonal influenza immunization rates across states. *Clin. Ther.* **2017**, *39*, 1563–1580. [CrossRef] [PubMed]
12. Houle, S.K.D.; Bascom, C.S.; Rosenthal, M.M. Clinical outcomes and satisfaction with a pharmacist-managed travel clinic in Alberta, Canada. *Travel Med. Infect. Dis.* **2018**, *23*, 21–26. [CrossRef] [PubMed]
13. Tran, D.; Gatewood, S.; Moczygemba, L.R.; Stanley, D.D.; Goode, J.-V. Evaluating health outcomes following a pharmacist-provided comprehensive pretravel health clinic in a supermarket pharmacy. *J. Am. Pharm. Assoc.* **2015**, *55*, 143–152. [CrossRef] [PubMed]
14. Jackson, A.B.; Humphries, T.L.; Nelson, K.M.; Helling, D.K. Clinical pharmacy travel medicine services: A new frontier. *Ann. Pharmacother.* **2004**, *38*, 2160–2165. [CrossRef] [PubMed]

15. Bascom, C.S.; Rosenthal, M.A.; Houle, S.K.D. Are pharmacists ready for a greater role in travel health? An evaluation of the knowledge and confidence in providing travel health advice of pharmacists practicing in a community pharmacy chain in Alberta, Canada. *J. Travel Med.* **2015**, *22*, 99–104. [CrossRef] [PubMed]

16. Foong, E.A.; Edwards, D.; Houle, S.K.D.; Grindrod, K.A. Ready or not? Pharmacist perceptions of a changing scope of practice before it happens. *Can. Pharm. J.* **2017**, *150*, 387–396. [CrossRef] [PubMed]

17. Government of Canada. Procedures for Yellow Fever Vaccination Centres in Canada. Available online: https://www.canada.ca/en/public-health/services/travel-health/yellow-fever/procedures-yellow-fever-vaccination-centres-canada.html (accessed on 3 January 2019).

18. Centres for Disease Control and Prevention. Yellow Book, Chapter 3: Yellow Fever. Available online: https://wwwnc.cdc.gov/travel/yellowbook/2018/infectious-diseases-related-to-travel/yellow-fever (accessed on 3 January 2019).

19. Government of Canada. Yellow Fever Vaccination Centres in Ontario. Available online: https://www.canada.ca/en/public-health/services/travel-health/yellow-fever/vaccination-centres-canada-ontario.html (accessed on 3 January 2019).

20. Ontario College of Pharmacists. Find a Pharmacy. Available online: https://members.ocpinfo.com/search/ (accessed on 3 January 2019).

21. International Society of Travel Medicine. ISTM Certificate of Knowledge. Available online: http://www.istm.org/certificateofknowledge (accessed on 16 January 2019).

22. Ontario College of Pharmacists. Administering a Substance by Injection or Inhalation. Available online: http://www.ocpinfo.com/regulations-standards/policies-guidelines/administering_a_substance_injection/inhalation/ (accessed on 17 February 2019).

23. Ontario College of Pharmacists. 2017 Annual Report: Putting Patients First. Available online: http://www.ocpinfo.com/library/annual-reports/download/ocp_annual_report_2017.pdf (accessed on 6 March 2019).

24. Drug Shortages Canada. Drug Shortage Report for YF-VAX. Available online: https://www.drugshortagescanada.ca/shortage/1247 (accessed on 13 January 2019).

25. Guirguis, L.M.; Makowsky, M.J.; Hughes, C.A.; Sadowski, C.A.; Schindel, T.J.; Yuksel, N. How have pharmacists in different practice settings integrated prescribing privileges into practice in Alberta? A qualitative exploration. *J. Clin. Pharm. Ther.* **2014**, *39*, 390–398. [CrossRef] [PubMed]

26. Wong, L.; Burden, A.M.; Liu, Y.Y.; Tadrous, M.; Pojskic, N.; Dolovich, L.; Calzavara, A.; Cadarette, S.M. Initial uptake of the Ontario Pharmacy Smoking Cessation Program: Descriptive analysis over 2 years. *Can. Pharm. J.* **2015**, *148*, 29–40. [CrossRef] [PubMed]

27. MacCallum, L.; Consiglio, G.; MacKeigan, L.; Dolovich, L. Uptake of Community Pharmacist-Delivered MedsCheck Diabetes Medication Review Service in Ontario between 2010 and 2014. *Can. J. Diabetes* **2017**, *41*, 253–258. [CrossRef] [PubMed]

28. Dolovich, L.; Consiglio, G.; MacKeigan, L.; Abrahamyan, L.; Pechlivanoglou, P.; Rac, V.E.; Pojskic, N.; Bojarski, E.A.; Su, J.; Krahn, M.; et al. Uptake of the MedsCheck annual medication review service in Ontario community pharmacies between 2007 and 2013. *Can. Pharm. J.* **2016**, *149*, 293–302. [CrossRef] [PubMed]

29. Houle, S.K.D.; Grindrod, K.A.; Chatterley, T.; Tsuyuki, R.T. Paying pharmacists for patient care: A systematic review of remunerated pharmacy clinical care services. *Can. Pharm. J.* **2014**, *147*, 209–232. [CrossRef] [PubMed]

30. Berbatis, C.G.; Sunderland, V.B.; Joyce, A.; Bulsara, M.; Mills, C. Enhanced pharmacy services, barriers and facilitators in Australia's community pharmacies: Australia's National Pharmacy Database Project. *Int. J. Pharm. Pract.* **2007**, *15*, 185–191. [CrossRef]

31. Roberts, A.S.; Benrimoj, S.I.; Chen, T.F.; Willians, K.A.; Aslani, P. Practice change in community pharmacy: Quantification of facilitators. *Ann. Pharmacother.* **2008**, *42*, 861–868. [CrossRef] [PubMed]

32. Blake, K.B.; Madhavan, S.S.; Scott, V.; Elswick, B.L.M. Medication therapy management services in West Virginia: Pharmacists' perceptions of educational and training needs. *Res. Soc. Adm. Pharm.* **2009**, *5*, 182–188. [CrossRef] [PubMed]

33. Kritikos, V.S.; Reddel, H.K.; Bosnic-Anticevich, S.Z. Pharmacists' perceptions of their role in asthma management and barriers to the provision of asthma services. *Int. J. Pharm. Pract.* **2010**, *18*, 209–216. [PubMed]

34. Flaherty, G.; Thong, Z.Y.C.; Browne, R. The missing link; introducing travel medicine into the undergraduate medical curriculum. *J. Travel Med.* **2013**, *23*, 1–3. [CrossRef] [PubMed]

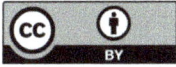

pharmacy

MDPI

Commentary

Pharmacist Services in the Opioid Crisis: Current Practices and Scope in the United States

Tanvee Thakur [1,*], Meredith Frey [2] and Betty Chewning [1]

[1] Social and Administrative Sciences Division, School of Pharmacy, University of Wisconsin-Madison, Madison, WI 53705, USA; betty.chewning@wisc.edu
[2] School of Pharmacy, University of Wisconsin-Madison, Madison, WI 53705, USA; mlfrey@wisc.edu
*   Correspondence: tmthakur@wisc.edu

Received: 23 April 2019; Accepted: 6 June 2019; Published: 13 June 2019

check for
updates

Abstract: Introduction: Pharmacist roles promoting safe opioid use are recognized in literature and practice. Pharmacists can offer services such as counseling on opioid risks, naloxone dispensing, education on opioid storage and disposal, prescription drug monitoring program (PDMP) utilization, opioid deprescribing, and providing resources for addiction treatment to help mitigate the opioid crisis. **Objective:** This commentary seeks to describe current and potential roles for pharmacists to combat the United States opioid crisis and identify key factors affecting service provision. **Methods:** The paper summarizes evidence-based studies describing current pharmacist roles and services, factors affecting service implementation, and strategies to further improve pharmacist roles and services related to promoting safe opioid use for patients. **Results:** Pharmacists recognize their roles and responsibilities to counsel patients on opioid risks, dispense naloxone, educate on opioid storage and disposal, utilize prescription drug monitoring programs (PDMPs), offer opioid deprescribing, and provide resources for addiction treatment. However, pharmacists express low confidence, time, and training as barriers to service provision. This suggests a need for structured training, resources, and organizational support for pharmacists to improve confidence and participation in such services. **Conclusions:** Although pharmacists are aware of roles and responsibilities to help reduce the opioid crisis, more training, education, organizational support and resources are needed to increase their ability to embody these roles.

Keywords: pharmacist services; opioid; communication; naloxone; misuse; disposal; safety; counseling

1. Introduction

Opioid medications have the potential to cause dependence characterized by a strong desire to take opioids, persistent opioid use despite harmful consequences, increased tolerance, a physical withdrawal reaction when opioids are discontinued, and potential fatal overdose [1]. In 2016, 34 million people globally reported using opioids consistently and about 19 million people used opioids at least once [2]. Deaths attributed to opioid overdose contribute up to half of all drug-related deaths globally [2]. There are effective treatments for opioid use disorders, and yet less than 10% of people who would benefit from treatment are receiving it [2].

In the United States (U.S.), prescription opioids specifically contribute largely to the current opioid crisis, with more than 40% of all opioid overdose deaths in 2016 involving a prescription opioid, and more than 46 people dying every day from overdoses involving prescription opioids [3]. From 1999–2016, more than 200,000 people died from overdose related to prescription opioids alone [4]. Approximately 1000 individuals are treated in emergency departments (ED) each day for prescription opioid misuse [5]. Deaths related to opioid overdose have increased exponentially and will likely continue to grow, making this an important national issue in the U.S. and the focus of this commentary.

Although many individuals and organizations are involved in combating the opioid crisis nationwide, healthcare professionals are primarily responsible for appropriate opioid prescribing and promoting safe opioid use [6]. Pharmacists are especially well-positioned to contribute to safe opioid use due to their role dispensing opioid prescriptions and accessibility to patients [7,8]. Pharmacists utilize prescription drug monitoring programs (PDMP) to help prevent diversion of opioids and detect inappropriate prescribing, and can monitor and recognize signs of opioid misuse [8]. PDMP is a state-based electronic database accessed by prescribers and pharmacists to track controlled substance prescribing and dispensing [9]. Specific information collected from the pharmacy includes what controlled substances were dispensed, how much, to whom, and by whom [9]. Pharmacists can extend patient counseling responsibilities by educating patients on risks associated with opioid use, proper storage and disposal of medication, and the consequences of sharing medications with another person [10]. Additionally, many pharmacists can distribute naloxone, an opioid antagonist effective in reversing respiratory depression from opioid use, enabling a family member, friend, or potential bystander to prevent death associated with opioid overdose [11]. Pharmacists are knowledgeable about addiction treatment options and can connect patients to resources within the community [8]. Although pharmacists are equipped to provide these services to help mitigate the opioid crises, current literature documents that pharmacists' breadth of opportunities for services is far from fully realized. Underlying factors need to be considered to help pharmacist meet their potential to provide services related to opioid use.

2. Objectives

This commentary seeks to describe current and potential roles for pharmacists to reduce the opioid crisis, identify key factors affecting service provision, and suggest strategies for improvement.

3. Methods

An exhaustive search of PubMed and Cinhal databases was conducted to identify evidence-based studies describing current pharmacist roles and services, factors affecting service implementation, and strategies to further pharmacist roles and services related to promoting safe opioid use for patients. The following search terms and combinations were used: opioids, pharmacy, pharmacist, safety, counseling, disposal, naloxone, PDMP, and deprescribing. Only studies conducted in the United States were included. The available evidence was summarized into six main categories based on pharmacist roles: counseling on opioid risks, naloxone dispensing, opioid storage and disposal, PDMP utilization, opioid deprescribing, and addiction treatment resources.

4. Results

4.1. Counseling on Opioid Risks and Safety

A nationally distributed case vignette survey of primary care physicians (PCPs), pain specialists, and pharmacists, along with nested chart reviews and surveys of patients with chronic pain revealed that prescribers and pharmacists often omit key messages during patient counseling regarding safe opioid use [12]. Among pharmacists, safety counseling is generally limited to informing patients of potential side effects [12]. The omission of information provided may be due to limited self-efficacy among pharmacists in communicating with patients regarding prescription drug abuse and misuse. Pharmacists cited common barriers to communication as lack of confidence, training, and time [13]. Barriers to discussing opioid therapy were similar to those cited for discussing drug abuse and pain with patients, including lack of confidence, training and inadequate access to health information [7]. These barriers are compounded by uncertainty among pharmacists and patients regarding pharmacists' roles in opioid safety. Patients and pharmacists perceived pharmacists to be responsible for medication safety, yet the majority of pharmacists were uncomfortable dispensing opioids and felt they were "policing" opioid prescriptions [14]. Overall, there is a paucity of literature describing current counseling practices pharmacists use to educate patients about opioid risks, such as dependence and overdose, or mechanisms to promote safe opioid use.

4.2. Naloxone Dispensing

Increased state and national legislative and regulatory initiatives are partly due to greater recognition and acceptance of naloxone use by the general public, people who use drugs (PWUD), and healthcare professionals such as pharmacists. About half of states have increased funding to expand patient access to naloxone, pharmacologic treatment options for PWUD, and guidelines for safe opioid prescribing [15]. Standing orders have been implemented on a national level, and allow for naloxone dispensing by pharmacists or other healthcare professionals without a patient-specific prescription [16]. Pharmacists have successfully utilized standing orders to increase patient access to and distribution of naloxone in many pharmacy settings [17]. State and national policies have facilitated the expansion of pharmacist roles, enabling pharmacist to be a key resource in opioid overdose prevention [18]. Pharmacists utilize these policies and standing orders to identify patients who are at risk of overdose and would benefit from naloxone given their medication regimens, medical history, and comorbidities [11,19,20].

In two surveys about pharmacist roles in naloxone dispensing and education, simultaneously administered to patients receiving treatment for substance use disorders and pharmacists in Ohio, patients expressed interest in naloxone-based interventions [21]. Meanwhile, many pharmacists were opposed to facilitating naloxone-based interventions [21]. Some of the same concerns were raised for naloxone consultations as had been identified for consultation with patients about opioid safety and risks. Pharmacists identified barriers to delivering these interventions or services as a lack of training to identify eligible patients, and challenges communicating with patients about the need for naloxone. Pharmacists also identified lack of time, reimbursement, and lack of support from management as barriers to implementing naloxone services [22,23]. Institution-specific guidelines and protocols addressing pharmacist roles, criteria for screening for eligibility, and flowcharts for education and dissemination of naloxone have facilitated identification of patients at risk of overdose, and serve as important resources for pharmacists and other healthcare professionals [24,25]. These resources along with structured programs regarding naloxone use have helped pharmacists successfully dispense naloxone to patients at risk of overdose [18,24,25].

4.3. Opioid Storage and Disposal

Pharmacists have a unique opportunity to educate patients on the importance of proper medication disposal and storage and disposal programs available in the community [8,26,27]. Student pharmacists can partner with community officials and businesses to provide safe and appropriate medication disposal [28]. While it is widely understood that medications such as opioids and other controlled substances contribute to environmental pollution when improperly disposed, it has proven hazardous to the population and community health as well [28]. Drug take-back programs have been popular across schools and pharmacies in the country and drug take-back days are helpful in facilitating these activities. Some community pharmacy chains, such as CVS, have installed drug take-back boxes in the pharmacies for patients to dispose of unused or expired prescription medications [29].

4.4. PDMP Utilization

Statewide prescription drug monitoring programs (PDMP) are a useful tool for healthcare professionals to track and monitor controlled substance prescriptions [9]. Specific legislative initiatives that support safe opioid prescribing and naloxone use include the 2016 21st Century Cures Act, which awarded funding to improve state PDMPs [30]. The PDMP can serve as a resource for pharmacists to identify patients that might be misusing opioids or those at risk of overdose. Additionally, the 2018

SUPPORT for Patients and Communities Act requires checking the PDMP for Medicare beneficiaries prior to controlled substance prescription. This may prompt further conversations with patients regarding opioid safety [31]. States have varying requirements for PDMP use among pharmacists and prescribers, ranging from voluntary to mandated use [9]. The majority of pharmacists have viewed the PDMP as an objective resource to support clinical decisions, make professional judgements, and prevent diversion and drug abuse [9,32–34]. Pharmacists also felt the PDMP helped support patient and prescriber communication regarding suspected drug abuse and helped provide patient education about opioid-specific risks and controlled substance abuse [9,32,35]. While the majority of pharmacists agreed that the PDMP was important in the prescribing and dispensing process, some pharmacists reported barriers to using the PDMP [36]. Pharmacists were less likely to use the PDMP if use was not mandated, if they were unfamiliar with it, didn't like the user interface, or if no training was provided on using the PDMP platform [9,36]. Some pharmacists also reported challenges in working with prescribers or patients in response to PDMP reports [9]. Factors that facilitated regular use of the PDMP included providing training and education on PDMP use. Integrating the PDMP interface into dispensing software and electronic health records was shown to be particularly powerful, along with mandating use for pharmacists and prescribers at the point of prescribing and dispensing, and the ability to contact the prescriber directly through the PDMP [9,32,36].

4.5. Opioid Deprescribing

Deprescribing is a necessary mechanism to reduce the use of inappropriate medications, including medications that cause patient harm or unnecessary adverse effects, medications not providing benefit, or medications with no indication [37]. Deprescribing programs initiated by pharmacists, or that included pharmacists in a multidisciplinary team, have measured successful outcomes such as decreased pill burden or decreased use of inappropriate medications [38–43]. However, few guidelines have been developed to guide healthcare professionals in a systematic process to deprescribe or taper inappropriate medications. Systematic processes for deprescribing or tapering inappropriate medications are limited to a few specific classes of medications, and no guidelines exist for opioid discontinuation or tapering [44–48]. Further barriers exist to deprescribing practices in general. Prescribers cite barriers related to lack of time, limited resources to support deprescribing, patient fear, patient withdrawal symptoms, or patient criticism among deprescribing programs involving pharmacists [49,50]. Pharmacists report barriers related to pressures to focus on productivity, rather than clinical interactions or decision-making with patients. Other barriers identified by pharmacists and prescribers include challenges working with patients and caregivers, lack of policies or guidelines specific to deprescribing, and difficulty partnering inter-professionally across health care settings due to lack of shared health information and patients visiting multiple pharmacies [50]. Factors cited by pharmacists and prescribers that would facilitate deprescribing include further involvement of patients and caregivers, staff education, financial incentives, and involvement in initiatives that expand evidence supporting deprescribing practices [50].

4.6. Providing Resources for Opioid Misuse and Addiction Treatment

Pharmacists play a key role in recognizing opioid toxicity and preventing diversion of opioids [26]. Compared to prescriber colleagues, pharmacists perceived a larger percentage of patients to be abusing opioids (17% prescribers and 41% pharmacists, respectively) [51]. Pharmacists understand the importance of providing appropriate counseling and resources to such patients but believed that engaging with patients potentially abusing opioids may cause loss of customers. Pharmacists identified regulatory agencies and patients' family or friends as most likely to influence their willingness to refer patients to resources for opioid misuse [20]. As with the earlier topics, pharmacists cited many of the same barriers to effectively communicating with patients such as lack of confidence, training, and time. Time required for counseling was found to be the most commonly cited control belief [51]. Pharmacists who had greater amounts of addiction-specific education had a higher likelihood of substance abuse counseling and felt more confident about counseling; however, the majority of pharmacists received no addiction education [52]. This suggests that the neurobiological basis for addiction, standards of care, and pain management guidelines are likely not understood by a subset of pharmacists.

5. Discussion

Pharmacists are considered gatekeepers for dispensing opioid medications by other health care professionals and in the literature [53]. They are well positioned to facilitate safe opioid use through counseling patients on opioid risks, educating about safe storage and disposal, providing naloxone, participating in deprescribing initiatives, utilizing the PDMP, and connecting patients to resources for addiction treatment [8]. Although these roles for pharmacist services exist, there are opportunities for broader implementation. Pharmacists are interested in providing these services and have identified mechanisms to support safe opioid use among patients as well as barriers to service implementation. Lack of confidence, training and resources, structured guidelines, and limited time were the most commonly cited barriers by pharmacists for providing all the services addressed in this commentary [7,9,14,22–25,32,50,51,54].

5.1. Counseling on Opioid Risks and Safety

Although pharmacists are expected by the Centers For Disease Control and Prevention (CDC) to communicate dependency, overdose, and other opioid risks during patient counseling, pharmacists reported barriers such as lack of confidence, training, and time [7,14,55] * (*The Centers for Disease Control and Prevention (CDC) is a federal agency that conducts and supports health promotion, prevention, and preparedness activities in the United States.). Pharmacists would benefit from additional training and resources in pharmacy school curricula and in practice to facilitate effective counseling for opioid medications. Due to the paucity of research and few initiatives focusing on pharmacist communication for opioid medications, additional research is needed to inform effective training strategies.

5.2. Naloxone Dispensing

Pharmacists are recognized as stewards of naloxone dispensing and often stock naloxone in the outpatient setting, but do not necessarily dispense naloxone regularly [22]. Pharmacists expressed a lack of training and confidence to detect patients who would benefit from naloxone and to provide education about the necessity and use of naloxone [22,56]. Targeted training and resources about naloxone dispensing and communication techniques will facilitate further pharmacist involvement in naloxone dispensing and education [18,24].

5.3. Education on Opioid Storage and Disposal

Pharmacists recognize their role in informing patients about safe storage and disposal of opioids, yet few initiatives have measured pharmacist improvement, facilitators and barriers to providing such services [27]. There is a need for more evidence-based intervention research about how to help pharmacists offer services to promote safe disposal of opioids [29].

5.4. Guidelines and Protocols for PDMP Use and Opioid Deprescribing

Most pharmacists agreed that PDMP was a useful tool, especially when linked to the electronic health record and utilized as a platform to contact prescribers. However, pharmacists also reported challenges when working with patients and prescribers about issues detected in PDMP reports [9,32,36]. Policies and procedures highlighting pharmacists' roles within the PDMP can help promote more frequent PDMP use and help involve pharmacists in the monitoring process. Beyond the monitoring of prescribed opioids, pharmacists also play an important role in eliminating unnecessary medication when it is inappropriate or no longer needed. Specific algorithms and guidelines would facilitate opioid deprescribing practices in a variety of pharmacy settings. Integrating these into electronic health records would strengthen the intervention even further.

5.5. Providing Resources for Addiction Treatment

Pharmacists recognized and valued their role in detecting and communicating with patients potentially misusing prescription opioids [51]. They also expressed lacking confidence and time when talking to patients about opioid abuse [13,51]. Training and resources about addiction treatment should be offered by schools of pharmacy and continuing education programs to facilitate better understanding and identification of resources available to patients in the community.

Overall, training, education, and guidelines for pharmacist roles specific to increasing their readiness to deliver services regarding prescription opioids is warranted for ensuring that pharmacists participate in services that promote safe opioid use among patients. This commentary summarizes services that pharmacists currently offer, assesses factors that affect pharmacists providing these services, suggests strategies for improvement, including areas that should be augmented with education or advocacy in order to ensure enhanced pharmacist services that promote safe opioid use. This commentary has limitations to acknowledge. The scope of this commentary focuses on the opioid crisis and pharmacist services within the U.S., reducing generalizability to other countries. The methodology does not follow a rigorous data extraction and data analysis procedure, but rather includes articles which the authors deemed most applicable and appropriate to include. This paper points to a lack of evidence demonstrating that pharmacist services are directly impacting patient outcomes. All of these services in theory have beneficial effects but it is difficult to find evidence of direct effect of pharmacist services in the literature. Thus, there is need for future research about the impact of pharmacist services in mitigating the opioid crisis.

6. Conclusions

This commentary paper is one of its kind to describe current practices and roles of pharmacists and factors that affect pharmacists' behaviors and attitudes dispensing these services. Pharmacists successfully recognize the importance of their involvement in services to promote safe opioid use. While pharmacists are expected to participate in service provision to mitigate the opioid crisis, it is evident that pharmacists need more targeted training, education, resources, and structured guidelines to increase confidence and self-efficacy in delivering such services.

Author Contributions: All authors (T.T., M.F., and B.C.) have contributed to this manuscript. Conceptualization, T.T. and M.F.; methodology, T.T. and M.F.; investigation, T.T. and M.F.; resources, T.T., M.F. and B.C.; writing—original draft preparation, T.T. and M.F.; writing—review and editing, B.C.; visualization, T.T. and M.F.; supervision, T.T.

Funding: This research received no external funding.

Conflicts of Interest: The authors declare no conflict of interest.

References

1. Center for Disease Control and Prevention. Opioid Overdose. Available online: https://www.cdc.gov/drugoverdose/opioids/prescribed.html (accessed on 28 March 2019).
2. World Health Organization. Management of Substance Abuse. Available online: https://www.who.int/substance_abuse/information-sheet/en/ (accessed on 23 May 2018).
3. National Institute of Health. Opioid Overdose Crisis. Available online: https://www.drugabuse.gov/drugs-abuse/opioids/opioid-overdose-crisis (accessed on 30 July 2018).
4. Center for Disease Control and Prevention. Opioid Overdose—Understanding the Epidemic. Available online: https://www.cdc.gov/drugoverdose/epidemic/index.html (accessed on 23 July 2018).
5. Seth, P.; Scholl, L.; Rudd, R.A.; Bacon, S. Increases and Geographic Variations in Overdose Deaths Involving Opioids, Cocaine, and Psychostimulants with Abuse Potential—United States, 2015–2016. *MMWR Morb. Mortal. Wkly. Rep.* **2018**. [CrossRef] [PubMed]

6. Woodard, D.; Van Demark, R.E., Jr. The Opioid Epidemic in 2017: Are We Making Progress? *S. D. Med.* **2017**, *70*, 467–471. [PubMed]
7. Marlowe, K.F.; Geiler, R. Pharmacist's role in dispensing opioids for acute and chronic pain. *J. Pharm. Pract.* **2012**, *25*, 497–502. [CrossRef] [PubMed]
8. Compton, W.M.; Jones, C.M.; Stein, J.B.; Wargo, E.M. Promising roles for pharmacists in addressing the U.S. opioid crisis. *Res. Soc. Adm. Pharm.* **2017**. [CrossRef]
9. Johnston, K.; Alley, L.; Novak, K.; Haverly, S.; Irwin, A.; Hartung, D. Pharmacists' attitudes, knowledge, utilization, and outcomes involving prescription drug monitoring programs: A brief scoping review. *J. Am. Pharm. Assoc. (2003)* **2018**, *58*, 568–576. [CrossRef] [PubMed]
10. Compton, W.M.; Boyle, M.; Wargo, E. Prescription opioid abuse: Problems and responses. *Prev. Med.* **2015**, *80*, 5–9. [CrossRef] [PubMed]
11. Adams, A.J.; Weaver, K.K. The Continuum of Pharmacist Prescriptive Authority. *Ann. Pharm.* **2016**, *50*, 778–784. [CrossRef]
12. Salinas, G.D.; Susalka, D.; Burton, B.S.; Roepke, N.; Evanyo, K.; Biondi, D.; Nicholson, S. Risk assessment and counseling behaviors of healthcare professionals managing patients with chronic pain: A national multifaceted assessment of physicians, pharmacists, and their patients. *J. Opioid Manag.* **2012**, *8*, 273–284. [CrossRef]
13. Hagemeier, N.E.; Murawski, M.M.; Lopez, N.C.; Alamian, A.; Pack, R.P. Theoretical exploration of Tennessee community pharmacists' perceptions regarding opioid pain reliever abuse communication. *Res. Soc. Adm. Pharm.* **2014**, *10*, 562–575. [CrossRef]
14. Hartung, D.M.; Hall, J.; Haverly, S.N.; Cameron, D.; Alley, L.; Hildebran, C.; O'Kane, N.; Cohen, D. Pharmacists' Role in Opioid Safety: A Focus Group Investigation. *Pain Med.* **2018**, *19*, 1799–1806. [CrossRef]
15. Wickramatilake, S.; Zur, J.; Mulvaney-Day, N.; Klimo, M.C.; Selmi, E.; Harwood, H. How States Are Tackling the Opioid Crisis. *Public Health Rep.* **2017**, *132*, 171–179. [CrossRef] [PubMed]
16. Naloxoneinfo.org. Case Studies. Available online: http://naloxoneinfo.org/case-studies/standing-orders (accessed on 23 July 2018).
17. The Network for Public Health Law. Using Law to Support Pharmacy Naloxone Distribution. Available online: networkforphl.org/_asset/qdkn97/Pharmacy-Naloxone-Distributions.pdf (accessed on 23 July 2018).
18. Penm, J.; MacKinnon, N.J.; Boone, J.M.; Ciaccia, A.; McNamee, C.; Winstanley, E.L. Strategies and policies to address the opioid epidemic: A case study of Ohio. *J. Am. Pharm. Assoc. (2003)* **2017**, *57*, S148–S153. [CrossRef] [PubMed]
19. Bailey, A.M.; Wermeling, D.P. Naloxone for opioid overdose prevention: pharmacists' role in community-based practice settings. *Ann. Pharm.* **2014**, *48*, 601–606. [CrossRef] [PubMed]
20. Cochran, G.; Hruschak, V.; DeFosse, B.; Hohmeier, K.C. Prescription opioid abuse: pharmacists' perspective and response. *Integr. Pharm. Res. Pract.* **2016**, *5*, 65–73. [CrossRef] [PubMed]
21. Riley, T.B.; Alemagno, S. Pharmacist utilization of prescription opioid misuse interventions: Acceptability among pharmacists and patients. *Res. Soc. Adm. Pharm.* **2019**. [CrossRef] [PubMed]
22. Nielsen, S.; Van Hout, M.C. What is known about community pharmacy supply of naloxone? A scoping review. *Int. J. Drug Policy* **2016**, *32*, 24–33. [CrossRef] [PubMed]
23. Green, T.C.; Case, P.; Fiske, H.; Baird, J.; Cabral, S.; Burstein, D.; Schwartz, V.; Potter, N.; Walley, A.Y.; Bratberg, J. Perpetuating stigma or reducing risk? Perspectives from naloxone consumers and pharmacists on pharmacy-based naloxone in 2 states. *J. Am. Pharm. Assoc. (2003)* **2017**, *57*, S19–S27.e14. [CrossRef] [PubMed]
24. Devries, J.; Rafie, S.; Polston, G. Implementing an overdose education and naloxone distribution program in a health system. *J. Am. Pharm. Assoc. (2003)* **2017**, *57*, S154–S160. [CrossRef]
25. Tewell, R.; Edgerton, L.; Kyle, E. Establishment of a pharmacist-led service for patients at high risk for opioid overdose. *Am. J. Health Syst. Pharm.* **2018**, *75*, 376–383. [CrossRef]
26. Cobaugh, D.J.; Gainor, C.; Gaston, C.L.; Kwong, T.C.; Magnani, B.; McPherson, M.L.; Painter, J.T.; Krenzelok, E.P. The opioid abuse and misuse epidemic: Implications for pharmacists in hospitals and health systems. *Am. J. Health Syst. Pharm.* **2014**, *71*, 1539–1554. [CrossRef]
27. Athern, K.M.; Linnebur, S.A.; Fabisiak, G. Proper Disposal of Unused Household Medications: The Role of the Pharmacist. *Consult. Pharm.* **2016**, *31*, 261–266. [CrossRef] [PubMed]

28. Gray-Winnett, M.D.; Davis, C.S.; Yokley, S.G.; Franks, A.S. From dispensing to disposal: The role of student pharmacists in medication disposal and the implementation of a take-back program. *J. Am. Pharm. Assoc. (2003)* **2010**, *50*, 613–618. [CrossRef] [PubMed]

29. CVS Health. Expanding Access to Safe and Convenient Drug Disposal. Available online: https://cvshealth.com/thought-leadership/expanding-access-to-safe-and-convenient-drug-disposal (accessed on 28 March 2019).

30. H.R.34—21st Century Cures Act. Available online: https://www.congress.gov/bill/114th-congress/house-bill/34 (accessed on 28 March 2018).

31. H.R.6—Support for Patients and Communities Act. Available online: https://www.congress.gov/bill/115th-congress/house-bill/6?q=%7B%22search%22%3A%5B%22hr6-2018%22%5D%7D&s=2&r=1 (accessed on 28 May 2018).

32. Norwood, C.W.; Wright, E.R. Integration of prescription drug monitoring programs (PDMP) in pharmacy practice: Improving clinical decision-making and supporting a pharmacist's professional judgment. *Res. Soc. Adm. Pharm.* **2016**, *12*, 257–266. [CrossRef] [PubMed]

33. Strand, M.A.; Eukel, H.; Burck, S. Moving opioid misuse prevention upstream: A pilot study of community pharmacists screening for opioid misuse risk. *Res. Soc. Adm. Pharm.* **2018**. [CrossRef] [PubMed]

34. Lal, A.; Bai, J.; Basri, D.; Yeager, K.A. Pharmacists' Perspectives on Practice, Availability, and Barriers Related to Opioids in Georgia. *Am. J. Hosp. Palliat. Care* **2018**. [CrossRef]

35. Fendrich, M.; Bryan, J.K.; Hooyer, K. Prescription Drug Monitoring Programs and Pharmacist Orientation Toward Dispensing Controlled Substances. *Subst. Use Misuse* **2018**, *53*, 1324–1330. [CrossRef]

36. Freeman, P.R.; Curran, G.M.; Drummond, K.L.; Martin, B.C.; Teeter, B.S.; Bradley, K.; Schoenberg, N.; Edlund, M.J. Utilization of prescription drug monitoring programs for prescribing and dispensing decisions: Results from a multi-site qualitative study. *Res. Soc. Adm. Pharm.* **2018**. [CrossRef]

37. Scott, I.A.; Hilmer, S.N.; Reeve, E.; Potter, K.; Le Couteur, D.; Rigby, D.; Gnjidic, D.; Del Mar, C.B.; Roughead, E.E.; Page, A.; et al. Reducing inappropriate polypharmacy: The process of deprescribing. *JAMA Intern. Med.* **2015**, *175*, 827–834. [CrossRef] [PubMed]

38. Potter, K.; Flicker, L.; Page, A.; Etherton-Beer, C. Deprescribing in Frail Older People: A Randomised Controlled Trial. *PLoS ONE* **2016**, *11*, e0149984. [CrossRef]

39. Kaur, S.; Mitchell, G.; Vitetta, L.; Roberts, M.S. Interventions that can reduce inappropriate prescribing in the elderly: A systematic review. *Drugs Aging* **2009**, *26*, 1013–1028. [CrossRef]

40. Spinewine, A.; Fialová, D.; Byrne, S. The role of the pharmacist in optimizing pharmacotherapy in older people. *Drugs Aging* **2012**, *29*, 495–510. [CrossRef] [PubMed]

41. Mudge, A.; Radnedge, K.; Kasper, K.; Mullins, R.; Adsett, J.; Rofail, S.; Lloyd, S.; Barras, M. Effects of a pilot multidisciplinary clinic for frequent attending elderly patients on deprescribing. *Aust. Health Rev.* **2016**, *40*, 86–91. [CrossRef] [PubMed]

42. Martin, P.; Tamblyn, R.; Benedetti, A.; Ahmed, S.; Tannenbaum, C. Effect of a Pharmacist-Led Educational Intervention on Inappropriate Medication Prescriptions in Older Adults: The D-PRESCRIBE Randomized Clinical Trial. *JAMA* **2018**, *320*, 1889–1898. [CrossRef] [PubMed]

43. Tannenbaum, C.; Martin, P.; Tamblyn, R.; Benedetti, A.; Ahmed, S. Reduction of inappropriate benzodiazepine prescriptions among older adults through direct patient education: The empower cluster randomized trial. *JAMA Intern. Med.* **2014**, *174*, 890–898. [CrossRef] [PubMed]

44. Farrell, B.; Black, C.; Thompson, W.; McCarthy, L.; Rojas-Fernandez, C.; Lochnan, H.; Shamji, S.; Upshur, R.; Bouchard, M.; Welch, V. Deprescribing antihyperglycemic agents in older persons: Evidence-based clinical practice guideline. *Can. Fam. Physician* **2017**, *63*, 832–843. [PubMed]

45. Farrell, B.; Pottie, K.; Thompson, W.; Boghossian, T.; Pizzola, L.; Rashid, F.J.; Rojas-Fernandez, C.; Walsh, K.; Welch, V.; Moayyedi, P. Deprescribing proton pump inhibitors: Evidence-based clinical practice guideline. *Can. Fam. Physician* **2017**, *63*, 354–364. [PubMed]

46. Bjerre, L.M.; Farrell, B.; Hogel, M.; Graham, L.; Lemay, G.; McCarthy, L.; Raman-Wilms, L.; Rojas-Fernandez, C.; Sinha, S.; Thompson, W.; et al. Deprescribing antipsychotics for behavioural and psychological symptoms of dementia and insomnia: Evidence-based clinical practice guideline. *Can. Fam. Physician* **2018**, *64*, 17–27.

47. Pottie, K.; Thompson, W.; Davies, S.; Grenier, J.; Sadowski, C.A.; Welch, V.; Holbrook, A.; Boyd, C.; Swenson, R.; Ma, A.; et al. Deprescribing benzodiazepine receptor agonists: Evidence-based clinical practice guideline. *Can. Fam. Physician* **2018**, *64*, 339–351. [PubMed]

48. Reeve, E.; Farrell, B.; Thompson, W.; Herrmann, N.; Sketris, I.; Magin, P.J.; Chenoweth, L.; Gorman, M.; Quirke, L.; Bethune, G.; et al. Deprescribing cholinesterase inhibitors and memantine in dementia: Guideline summary. *Med. J. Aust.* **2019**, *210*, 174–179. [CrossRef]

49. Anderson, K.; Stowasser, D.; Freeman, C.; Scott, I. Prescriber barriers and enablers to minimising potentially inappropriate medications in adults: A systematic review and thematic synthesis. *BMJ Open* **2014**, *4*, e006544. [CrossRef]

50. Conklin, J.; Farrell, B.; Suleman, S. Implementing deprescribing guidelines into frontline practice: Barriers and facilitators. *Res. Soc. Adm. Pharm.* **2018**. [CrossRef] [PubMed]

51. Hagemeier, N.E.; Gray, J.A.; Pack, R.P. Prescription drug abuse: A comparison of prescriber and pharmacist perspectives. *Subst. Use Misuse* **2013**, *48*, 761–768. [CrossRef] [PubMed]

52. Lafferty, L.; Hunter, T.S.; Marsh, W.A. Knowledge, attitudes and practices of pharmacists concerning prescription drug abuse. *J. Psychoact. Drugs* **2006**, *38*, 229–232. [CrossRef] [PubMed]

53. Shimane, T. The Pharmacist as Gatekeeper of Prescription Drug Abuse: Return to "Community Scientists". *Yakugaku Zasshi* **2016**, *136*, 79–87. [CrossRef]

54. Freeman, P.R.; Goodin, A.; Troske, S.; Strahl, A.; Fallin, A.; Green, T.C. Pharmacists' role in opioid overdose: Kentucky pharmacists' willingness to participate in naloxone dispensing. *J. Am. Pharm. Assoc. (2003)* **2017**, *57*, S28–S33. [CrossRef]

55. Opioid Overdose-Communicating with Patients. Available online: https://www.cdc.gov/drugoverdose/training/communicating/ (accessed on 10 September 2018).

56. Green, T.C.; Dauria, E.F.; Bratberg, J.; Davis, C.S.; Walley, A.Y. Orienting patients to greater opioid safety: Models of community pharmacy-based naloxone. *Harm. Reduct. J.* **2015**, *12*, 25. [CrossRef]

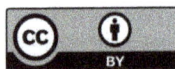

Article

Systematic Analysis of the Service Process and the Legislative and Regulatory Environment for a Pharmacist-Provided Naltrexone Injection Service in Wisconsin

James H. Ford II [ID]**, Aaron Gilson and David A. Mott ***

Sonderegger Research Center, University of Wisconsin School of Pharmacy, Madison, WI 53705, USA;
jhfordii@wisc.edu (J.H.F.II); aaron.gilson@wisc.edu (A.G.)
* Correspondence: david.mott@wisc.edu; Tel.: +1-608-265-9268

Received: 29 April 2019; Accepted: 6 June 2019; Published: 12 June 2019

Abstract: Community pharmacists are viewed by the public as convenient and trustworthy sources of healthcare and pharmacists likely can play a larger role in addressing the major public health issue of the opioid epidemic affecting Wisconsin residents. Approved medications, including long-acting injectable naltrexone, can transform the treatment of individuals with opioid use disorder (OUD). Due to shortages of behavioral health providers in the U.S., and pharmacists' knowledge about the safe use of medications, pharmacists can be a significant access point for treating OUD with naltrexone. Wisconsin's pharmacy practice laws authorize pharmacists to administer medications via injection, and a small number of pharmacists currently are using this authority to provide a naltrexone injection service. This exploratory study had two objectives: (1) describe the pharmacist injection service process and identify barriers and facilitators to that service and (2) analyze the legislative/regulatory environment to ascertain support for expanding naltrexone injection service. Semi-structured pharmacist interviews (n = 4), and an analysis of Wisconsin statutes/regulations governing public health and social services, were undertaken to explore the objectives. Findings suggest that the service process requires considerable coordination and communication with practitioners, patients, and pharmacy staff, but many opportunities exist to broaden and sustain the service throughout Wisconsin.

Keywords: naltrexone; opioid use disorder; implementation; service process; regulatory; community pharmacy

---

1. Introduction

The current opioid epidemic, including prescription opioid misuse or abuse and associated overdose deaths, represents a major public health issue in the United States [1–3]. The impact of opioid-related harms, including overdoses, is significant. Nationally, the opioid epidemic has resulted in an increase in inpatient stays and emergency department visits [4–9]. The rate of opioid related deaths also increased by 345% from 2001 to 2016 with the percent of deaths attributable to opioids increasing from 0.4% to 1.5%, a 292% increase over the same time period [10]. The increase in deaths has led to a decline in life expectancy for the third consecutive year due in part to opioid use disorder (OUD) [11]. An OUD represents a chronic relapsing condition similar to diabetes or hypertension, where individuals will experience patterns of treatment and abstinence from opioid use followed by a resumption of opioid use and relapse [12–14].

Wisconsin has not evaded this public health crisis. From 2006 to 2016, the number of Wisconsinites with an OUD tripled from 5828 to 20,590 [15]. During the same time, the number of inpatient hospital discharges per 100,000 residents associated with OUD increased 93% as compared to a 308% increase in OUD-related emergency department discharges [16]. Mortality associated with OUD for Wisconsinites is also increasing. Over a 15-year period (2001 to 2016), opioid-related deaths have increased by 529%, an increase primarily influenced by prescription opioids deaths [17]. The rate of change in opioid-related deaths experienced in Wisconsin from 2001 to 2016 is 53% higher than the national average [17].

1.1. Medication for Opioid Use Disorder

Potential access to FDA-approved medications is transforming how treatment is delivered to individuals with OUD. Medication for OUD (MOUD) includes methadone (an opioid agonist), buprenorphine (a partial opioid agonist) in all forms (sublingual, injectable or implantable), or oral naltrexone (tablet) or extended-release naltrexone (an injectable opioid antagonist, also known as Vivitrol®). The medications can be used to manage symptoms of opioid withdrawal or maintenance (methadone or buprenorphine) or abstinence from opioids (naltrexone) [14]. Managing OUD with medications has been shown to be more effective than treatment as usual [12,18,19]. For example, patients who receive oral naltrexone experienced reduced time in inpatient substance abuse and mental health treatment [20] or reduced opioid use [21]. More importantly, individuals who received six naltrexone injections experienced improvements in employment, mental health and psychosocial functioning, and reduced opioid craving and drug use [22]. Improving MOUD access is broadly considered a crucial public health strategy in confronting the opioid epidemic [23–26].

Despite demonstrated effectiveness as a treatment for OUD and federal agencies' calls for increased access, MOUD is underused in the United States [27,28]. Current delivery models for MOUD rely on patients accessing MOUD in primary care physician's offices or through a local addiction treatment provider. However, problems exist with current delivery models for MOUD, such as there not being enough practitioners who are registered (i.e., DATA-waived) with the Drug Enforcement Administration (DEA) to prescribe buprenorphine for office based opioid addiction treatment, negative practitioner attitudes about becoming DATA-waived, concerns about diversion of methadone and buprenorphine, insufficient infrastructure in practitioner offices/clinics to provide injections while maintaining patient anonymity, and lack of knowledge about naltrexone as a viable treatment modality for OUD [29–40]. This final issue is especially problematic, given that naltrexone is not a controlled substance. As a result, unlike both methadone and buprenorphine, any licensed physician can prescribe naltrexone without requiring an additional registration. Thus, new approaches are needed to improve access to and underutilization of MOUD.

1.2. Pharmacist Involvement in Patient Access to MOUD

Approaches to the treatment of individuals with OUD have largely eschewed pharmacists' involvement despite calls that specifically suggest that pharmacists be involved in such efforts [41–43]. Pharmacists can especially facilitate provision of MOUD because pharmacists commonly are one of the most accessible health care providers in communities [44,45], they provide a myriad of patient care services that contribute to public health [46,47], and patients are very accepting of the services provided by pharmacists [46–48]. In Wisconsin, an emerging pharmacist service is naltrexone injections for patients with OUD.

Pharmacists licensed in Wisconsin have legal authority to become an active partner in the care team for treating patients with OUD. The authority for pharmacists to provide patient care services, which can include naltrexone injections, is codified in Wisconsin law governing both medical and pharmacy practice (see Table 1), and represents a significant facilitating factor for pharmacists to be involved in OUD treatment. Beginning in March 2016 (2015 WI Act 290), pharmacists have had the legal authority to administer non-vaccine medications via injection provided they comply with training and reporting requirements. Additionally, Wisconsin's medical practice laws provide statutory authority for physicians to use a collaborative practice agreement to delegate patient care services to a pharmacist. Interpretation of the laws suggest that activities allowed under collaborative practice agreements between physicians and pharmacists would include the management of patients with OUD, including administering drugs via injection and/or administering oral drugs.

Table 1. Wisconsin State Statutes and Regulations Related to Pharmacist Authority to Provide Patient Care Services.

Wisconsin State Law Section	Intended Purpose of Cited Section of Wisconsin State Law
Wisconsin statute for Medical Practices [Section 448.03(2)]	Authorizes physicians to delegate patient care services to other health care providers through a collaborative practice agreement between physicians and pharmacists.
Wisconsin statute for Pharmacy Practice [(Section 450.033)]	Provides statutory authority for pharmacists to perform any patient care service delegated to a pharmacist by a physician
Wisconsin statute for Pharmacy Practice [(Section 450.035 (1r)]	Provides statutory authority for pharmacists to administer *non-vaccine drugs* via injection after completing specific training
Wisconsin statute for Pharmacy Practice [(Section 450.035 (1t))]	Provides statutory authority for pharmacist interns to administer *non-vaccine drugs* via injection after completing specific training
Wisconsin Pharmacy Examining Board (in Chap Phar 7 Section 7.10)	Establishes additional requirements for pharmacists and pharmacist interns who are administering *non-vaccine drugs* via injection

As Table 1 suggests, state legislatures, agencies, and regulatory boards play an important role in facilitating access to care for patients with OUD by creating and passing statutes and interpreting statutory language in regulations that have the potential to affect OUD treatment. As an employer, a provider of social services, and a payer of health care services, state government can influence greatly whether pharmacists can have an accepted role in the treatment process for patients with OUD, as well as the extent to which pharmacists are expected to be involved in such treatment. As such, the broad analysis of state statutes and regulations related to requirements for public health and human services can identify the potential demand for a pharmacist-provided naltrexone injection service. Understanding where and how pharmacists potentially can fit into the treatment processes for patients with OUD established by states is an important step in expanding the injection service across the state and/or the U.S.

Objectives

Pharmacists providing naltrexone injections to patients with OUD is a new service and a limited number of Wisconsin pharmacists currently are providing naltrexone injections to patients with OUD. The first objective of this exploratory study was to describe how pharmacists are currently providing the injection service, the processes used by pharmacists to provide the injection service, and barriers and facilitators for the injection service. Exploring the process and implementation barriers and facilitators will provide areas of future research and provide strategies to expand the service to other pharmacists.

The second objective of this exploratory study was to examine the legislative and regulatory environments in Wisconsin that can influence pharmacist involvement in treatment for patients with OUD. The review of both statutes and regulations governing a variety of healthcare practices and state social health or welfare agencies was meant to highlight a number of provisions that could potentially facilitate or impede the expansion of pharmacist-provided naltrexone treatment services for patients with OUD. Exploring provisions currently in state law will provide suggestions for ways to expand pharmacist service for naltrexone injections to treat OUD.

2. Materials and Methods

2.1. Objective 1—Service Process and Implementation

2.1.1. Interview Guide

Since the naltrexone injection service has been emerging in Wisconsin since 2016, qualitative research methods, including interviews, were used to collect and analyze data about the process and implementation strategies developed and used by pharmacists providing the service. We constructed a semi-structured interview guide for the interviews. The interview guide was developed to obtain descriptive information from pharmacists about how the service was being provided. The interview guide included questions about topics such as how patients were referred to the pharmacy, the process developed by the pharmacist to provide the service, costs to the pharmacy for itemized inputs needed for the service process, system, prescriber, patient, and pharmacy barriers and facilitators to accessing and implementing the service, and a question related to any miscellaneous items related to the development, implementation, and experience with providing the service. Question probes were included to obtain more details about various aspects of the service.

2.1.2. Sample

A snowball sampling technique was used to identify and sample pharmacists who were providing the injection service to interview. Initially, we obtained the names and contact information for two pharmacists providing the service from staff members at the Pharmacy Society of Wisconsin. When we contacted the initial pharmacists, we obtained the names of additional pharmacists providing the service by asking those pharmacists for names of other pharmacists that were providing naltrexone injections in their community.

2.1.3. Data Collection

We conducted four interviews with a purposeful sample of five pharmacists. Four of the five pharmacists were currently providing naltrexone injections in community pharmacy environments and the other pharmacist was planning the development of the service within a health system. All interviews took place between April and June 2018. Four pharmacists were practicing in urban areas and one pharmacist was practicing in a rural area of Wisconsin. One interview included two pharmacists providing the service and was conducted via telephone. The other three interviews were conducted in person, two were conducted in a private room at the University of Wisconsin School of Pharmacy and one was conducted at the pharmacy site. In the interviews with pharmacists, which were conducted conversationally, we asked about the naltrexone injection process at the community pharmacy with additional questions intended to seek clarification or learn more about specific process steps (e.g., interaction with behavioral health provider or actual injection process). The interviews were not recorded; however, each author took extensive notes during the interviews. Since this was neither conceptualized nor viewed by the IRB as research, a systematic data collection procedure was not necessary to meet the purpose of a quality improvement investigation.

2.1.4. Data Analysis

The notes from the interviews were reviewed to identify specific points and themes related to the naltrexone injection process at each community pharmacy. Authors analyzed the content of the interviews separately and then met to achieve consensus about their interpretation of identified content, and to discuss and negotiate the classification and naming of the processes and thematic domains related to the naltrexone injection process derived from the interview data.

2.2. Objective 2—Analysis of Wisconsin Statutes and Regulations

The purpose of the legislative and regulatory analyses was to identify requirements in state law that have the potential to either facilitate, allow, or impede pharmacist services to provide treatment to patients with OUD throughout Wisconsin. A synopsis of all identified policy requirements was created, as well as the implication of those requirements on pharmacists' roles in countering the current shortage of treatment services for patients with OUD in local communities.

2.2.1. Identification of Wisconsin Laws

All potentially relevant statutes and regulations were identified using Lexis® Academic, an electronic legal database available to all faculty, staff, and students at the University of Wisconsin—Madison. Identification of applicable language in all statutes and regulations involved two phases: (1) a keyword search of electronic text, and (2) manual review of potentially-relevant sections or subsections of laws. Relevant legislative statutes, as well as related regulations, which serve as the "sample" for this study objective, are listed in Table 2 and demonstrate the state agencies that are most central to the clinical issue of drug abuse treatment. For professional practice regulation and licensing laws, this search was confined to physicians, advanced practice nurses, and pharmacists, who are authorized to prescribe, dispense, or administer medications for chronic diseases or conditions. In addition to the specific laws in Table 2, an effort was made to determine applicable provisions that relate to the ability of practitioners to engage in telehealth (i.e., using electronic communication for exchanging health information to facilitate patient care) around OUD-related issues.

Table 2. Reviewed Statutes and Regulations that can Influence Pharmacist-Provided Medication-Assisted Treatment with Naltrexone.

Legislation	Regulations
Veterans Chapter 45	Department of Veterans Affairs
Social Services Chapter 46	
State Alcohol Drug Abuse, Developmental Disabilities, and Mental Health Act Chapter 51	
Chapter 150 Regulation of Health Services, Subchapter IV	Department of Health Services
Corrections Chapter 301	Department of Corrections
Regulation and Licensing Chapter 440 for prescribers Chapter 450 for pharmacists	Department of Regulation and Licensing
	Department of Children and Families

2.2.2. Policy Analysis

All content of the policies contained in Table 2 was collected, downloaded, and reviewed to select provisions that could be related to treatment with naltrexone. Regulation and Licensing laws, specifically pharmacy practice statutes and regulations, were examined first since they provide the legal authority for pharmacists' involvement in treatment of patients with OUD (see Table 1). The other areas of legislation and regulations identified in Table 2 were then analyzed to determine the other areas in law that likely impact pharmacists' roles in treatment of patients with OUD. Since state statutes provide the authority for state agencies to engage in certain activities, and regulations implement the statutory authority by defining the process for engaging in those activities, whenever possible related statutes and regulations (e.g., pharmacy practice act and pharmacy board regulations) were described together to reduce redundancy. All policy provisions identified for this analysis were current as of 30 September 2018.

3. Results

3.1. Objective 1—Service Process and Implementation

3.1.1. Pharmacy Infrastructure

Prior to offering naltrexone injections, the pharmacies had to create the service infrastructure. Infrastructure development comprised: (a) completing training on how to provide injectable medications in general; (b) working with Alkermes (manufacturer of injectable naltrexone) or other nurse educators to complete naltrexone injection training; (c) obtaining a Clinical Laboratory Improvement Amendment waiver to administer the rapid urine drug screen; and (d) establishing policies and procedures (e.g., urine drug screen testing, naltrexone procurement). Pharmacists also discussed setting aside a private consultation room or area to provide the injections that was located away from the prescription counter and other pharmacy and customer activities.

3.1.2. Summary of How Patients are Referred to the Pharmacist

All of the pharmacists providing the service reported that they had established collaborative practice agreements with a behavioral health practitioner or physician prescriber in accordance with Wisconsin statutes and regulations outlined in Table 1; although prescribing practitioners can refer patients to a pharmacy for naltrexone injections without a collaborative practice agreement, using such a document better assures coordination of care, especially for the provision of long-term care. One pharmacist said that 80% of their patients receiving the injections were from provider referrals, but that 20% of patients were walk-ins. These unscheduled patient walk-ins require immediate pharmacy staff attention creating a coordination burden for the pharmacist and patient, which may conflict with their ongoing counseling and dispensing responsibilities. The pharmacist planning the service said that a referral process from primary care providers whose clinics could not provide the injections would need to be established to bring patients with OUD to the pharmacy for the injections.

3.1.3. Development of a "Straw Model"

Results of the analysis of the data collected from the semi-structured pharmacist interviews were used to develop a "straw-model" (see Figure 1) of the pharmacist-provided naltrexone injection service. The term "straw-model" provides an initial representation of a process that is then utilized to generate discussion and revision [49,50]. The "straw-model" we developed for the naltrexone injection service starts with access and acceptability barriers that may prevent a patient with OUD from using, or their practitioner from referring the patient to, a pharmacist for the naltrexone injection service. The next three steps of the "straw-model" focus on the activities that occur prior to (e.g., scheduling), during (e.g., urine drug screen, injection) and after the actual service encounter (e.g., scheduling follow-up appointment) with the pharmacist.

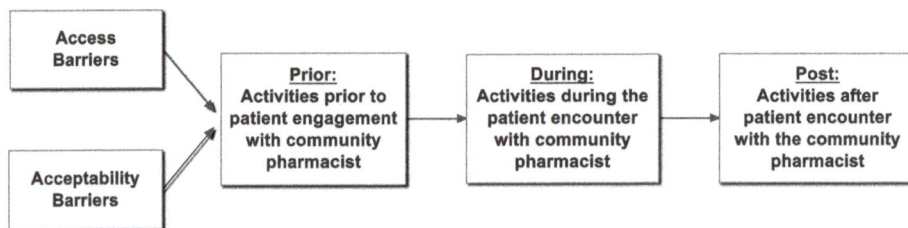

Figure 1. Community Pharmacy Medication Assisted Treatment with Naltrexone "Straw-Model".

Access and Acceptability Barriers. The interviews with pharmacists providing the naltrexone injection service identified perceived access and acceptability barriers (Table 3) from both the patient and the pharmacist perspectives. Pharmacists shared comments they heard from patients about barriers to medication and treatment for OUD in general and to naltrexone injections. Access barriers, broadly defined, related to the infrastructure and access issues. Acceptability barriers included issues related to prescribers' perceptions about treating OUD, and patients' perceptions about OUD. There was consensus that pharmacists thought patients feel less stigma receiving OUD treatment in the pharmacy since other customers remain unaware of the reasons for the patient presence in the pharmacy.

Table 3. Access and Acceptability Barriers to Pharmacist-provided Naltrexone Injection Service.

Access Barriers	Acceptability Barriers
Infrastructure	Prescriber Perceptions about Treating OUD
- Lack of clinic infrastructure to support providing injections - Prescriber unaware of naltrexone - Naltrexone covered as a Specialty Medication—limited pharmacy access	- Patients with OUD are difficult to manage - Prescriber concerns about the use and potential diversion of medications
Access	Patient perceptions
- Lack of transportation to prescriber and/or pharmacy (especially in rural areas) - Poor Access to prescribers (especially rural areas) - Access to naltrexone Injections	- Stigma associated with MAT - Patient knowledge and fear about medication

Injection Service Process Steps. During the interviews, pharmacists outlined the sequence of steps involved in the injection service and provided details about each step, in response to the interviewer's prompts. Prior to providing a naltrexone injection, the pharmacist must work with the prescriber and/or patient to schedule the appointment, and obtain the naltrexone injection after receiving the order from the prescriber. In some circumstances the drug can be ordered directly from the drug wholesaler. If the naltrexone injection is covered by a private prescription drug insurance plan that places the drug in a specialty drug tier, the pharmacist needs to make arrangements to obtain the drug from the specialty pharmacy.

Pharmacists described a general process involved in providing the injections for a patient that is seeing a psychiatry provider via tele-psychiatry at the pharmacy. Once the patient arrives at the pharmacy, to initiate the visit, the provider sends a code to the pharmacist to start the tele-psychiatry service session that includes just the patient and the provider using an i-pad in a private room in the pharmacy. At the end of the session, the psychiatry provider asks the patient if the injection can be provided to the patient today while the patient is in the pharmacy. If the patient responds affirmatively, the psychiatry provider asks the patient to go and get the pharmacist. Once the pharmacist is in the room, they engage in a three-way conversation between the pharmacist, provider and the patient to tailor the dose for the patient and also communicate with the provider/pharmacist about the dosing. After approval is given for the injection, the pharmacist collects relevant patient demographic information (e.g., age, gender) and conducts a rapid urine drug screen. The purpose of the drug screen is to ensure that a patient is opioid free. After preparing the naltrexone injection, the pharmacist administers the injection and monitors the patient (approximately 30 min) for any adverse reactions to the medication. Typically, the patient remains in the private area of the pharmacy until the monitoring is completed. During their visit to the pharmacy, the patient may receive behavioral health counseling from a counselor prior to receiving the injection or during the post-injection observation period via telemedicine.

After the appointment is completed, the pharmacist will schedule a follow-up appointment with the patient, bill for the service, and communicate the administration of the drug and monitoring feedback to the prescriber. Billing for services for Medicaid patients typically occurred under Healthcare

Common Procedure Coding System (HCPCS) code Q-3014 (Telehealth originating site facility fee). One pharmacist indicated that they could charge the patient an injection administration fee if the patient provided the naltrexone medication. Under this scenario, the patient picked up the medication from a specialty pharmacy as required by their private insurer and then transported the medication to the local pharmacy who administered the medication and the patient then paid the administration injection fee directly to the community pharmacy.

3.1.4. Perceived Facilitators and Barriers

Pharmacists identified facilitators as well as internal and external barriers to providing naltrexone injections in the community pharmacy (Table 4). Internal barriers were categorized as those barriers that related to aspects of the pharmacy or pharmacists that were providing the injection. External barriers were categorized as those that occurred outside of the pharmacy and related to patient, community, and health system factors. Since community pharmacies are more convenient for the patient and reduce patient perceptions about stigma, pharmacists in one pharmacy expressed a belief that physicians actually prefer that pharmacies provide the naltrexone injections because it facilitates access to care. However, these same pharmacists believe that insurance drives the locations where naltrexone can be administered, thus limiting patient access to the injections. Internal barriers reflect concerns expressed by the pharmacist about the viability of providing naltrexone injections (e.g., fixed cost investment, liability risks and inadequate reimbursement); and inexperience in providing naltrexone injections or process concerns (e.g., time to coordinate activities, lack of experience and training on how to schedule patients and manage no-shows).

Table 4. Naltrexone Administration: Preliminary Facilitators and Barriers in Community Pharmacies.

Facilitators	Internal Barriers	External Barriers
Motivated pharmacists and pharmacy ownership structure	Frontend fixed costs associated with staff, training, remodeling, on-site drug testing and billing.	Lack of adequate patient transportation and care coordination with prescriber, caseworker and other entities leads to poor adherence
Patient trust in the community pharmacist	Lack of a business case including insufficient reimbursement for drug administration and testing	Lack of supportive wraparound services (e.g., behavioral health)
Pharmacists' and behavioral health providers' knowledge of telemedicine and its role in proving health care.	Time to coordinate activities associated with administration including prior authorization, patient scheduling & managing appointment no-shows	Lack of awareness on ability to refer patients to pharmacies via collaborative practice agreement.
Flexible scheduling: community pharmacy vs. physician office to provide injections	Liability risks associated with providing MAT in the pharmacy	Misperceptions: pharmacists do not provide patient services/not treatment team member
Availability of training courses that allow pharmacist to meet regulations regarding injections	Pharmacists' lack of training and experience in MAT injections and induction.	Patient reluctance to pay drug co-pays or pharmacy injection fees
Willingness of pharmacists already engaged in practice to share knowledge with others		Pharmacy seen as a retail establishment versus clinic service provider

The external barriers generally differ from the access and acceptability barriers described previously in Table 4. Identified external barriers focus on issues such as the absence of resources in the community to support care coordination or to provide wrap-around services that are needed by the patient to adequately manage their chronic disease related to OUD. For example, one pharmacist mentioned a desire to connect patients with a recovery coach in the community to support the patient and improve the likelihood that the patient will return for subsequent naltrexone injections. The final set of external barriers focus on provider and patient misperceptions about their community pharmacy and the available services. For example, residents in the community may believe that the local community pharmacy primarily fills prescriptions in a retail capacity and does not offer clinical services, including naltrexone injections for persons with an OUD.

3.2. Objective 2—Analysis of Wisconsin Statutes and Regulations

The content of identified provisions and their implications, as well as the accompanying legal citations, are detailed in Table 5 for each state agency that has relevant activities involving drug abuse treatment and control.

Table 5. Statutory and Regulatory Provisions Relevant to Pharmacist Services for Naltrexone Injections.

Section of Law (Statutory Citation) (Regulatory Citation)	Description of Identified Provisions	Implication for Pharmacist Service
Children and Families (Statutes—none) (Regulations—Wisconsin Administrative Code; Department of Children and Families)	Applicants for work experience programs require substance abuse screening, testing, and referrals treatment (Wis. Adm. Code DCF 105.01), and a positive test requires treatment participation (Wis. Adm. Code DCF 105.06)	Requirements could increase demand for naltrexone injection service
Corrections (Statutes—Corrections) (Regulations—Wisconsin Administrative Code; Department of Corrections)	Prisoners are provided drug abuse assessment and treatment at each facility within the corrections system, while parolees or people on extended supervision also are to receive drug testing (Wis. Stat. § 301.03). For healthcare services, a prescription drug formulary is used (Wis. Stat. § 301.103), but covered medications are not specified	If naltrexone is included on the drug formulary, it conceivably could be offered through pharmacist service as a viable modality if positive assessments lead to treatment
	Substance abuse treatment also can seem to be a component of a variety of correctional programs and services, including: • for inmates selected for the challenge incarceration program (Wis. Stat. § 302.045; Wis. Adm. Code DOC 302.38(3)(e)) • for inmates transferred from state prisons (Wis. Stat. § 302.05) • those in an earned release program (Wis. Adm. Code DOC 302.39(3)(c)) • for those on-site or in hospitals using crisis intervention services (Wis. Stat. § 302.365) • when transferring a prisoner to a hospital or an approved treatment facility (Wis. Stat. § 302.38) • within residential, outpatient, and aftercare settings, as a means to reduce recidivism (Wis. Stat. § 301.068)	There are a variety of opportunities throughout the corrections system for identifying inmates as needing substance abuse treatment, and to potentially engage pharmacists to provide naltrexone injections either directly through the corrections facility or through their community pharmacies

Table 5. *Cont.*

Section of Law (Statutory Citation) (Regulatory Citation)	Description of Identified Provisions	Implication for Pharmacist Service
	• when in intensive sanctions program, as an alternative to incarceration (Wis. Adm. Code DOC 333.01(3) & (4)) • when transferring to the Wisconsin resource center (a specialized treatment program for inmates in need of mental health services) (Wis. Stat. § 302.055) • for those in jail using a prisoner classification system to provide services and programs based on medical/mental health needs (Wis. Stat. § 302.36; Wis. Adm. Code DOC 302.02) • for those in municipal lockup facilities and jails using a health screening form to identify drug abuse problems (Wis. Adm. Code DOC 349.03(9) & (17); Wis. Adm. Code DOC 350.03(12) and policies and procedures to provide drug abuse treatment services (Wis. Adm. Code DOC 349.16(1)(b); Wis. Adm. Code DOC 350.13(1) & (2))	
	Under certain circumstances, the DOC must notify local law enforcement before releasing a person into extended supervision (Wis. Stat. § 302.113) and can facilitate inmate release (Wis. Adm. Code DOC 302.34(5)(e) & (7)(g); Wis. Adm. Code DOC 302.35(3)(e)(2)) and can even expedite a risk reduction sentence (Wis. Adm. Code DOC 302.40(3)(e))	Such notification offers an opportunity to coordinate substance abuse treatment needs within the community, which could involve pharmacist naltrexone injection services if pharmacists are identified as a viable community resource
	Wisconsin counties must provide emergency mental health services (Wis. Adm. Code DHS 34.01), for conditions contained in the American Psychiatric Association's Diagnostic and Statistical Manual (Wis. Adm. Code DHS 34.02(14))	The American Psychiatric Association's Diagnostic and Statistical Manual includes an OUD diagnosis, providing a clear context for pharmacists' naltrexone injection service
	A number of specific health services programs and services permit SUD treatment, including: • outpatient mental health clinic services (Wis. Adm. Code DHS 35.17(1)(b)(4)) • comprehensive community services programs (Wis. Adm. Code DHS 36.02)	

Table 5. *Cont.*

Section of Law (Statutory Citation) (Regulatory Citation)	Description of Identified Provisions	Implication for Pharmacist Service
Health Services (Statute—none) (Regulation—Wisconsin Administrative Code; Department of Health Services)	• treatment alternative program (TAP) for people involved in the criminal justice system, as a means to avoid imprisonment (Wis. Adm. Code DHS 66.01(1)) • for applicants of certain employment and training programs (Wis. Adm. Code DHS 38.06(1) & (2)) • for people with an SUD diagnosis who have a functional impairment that interferes with major life activities (Wis. Adm. Code DHS 36.14(1) & (2)) • community support programs (Wis. Adm. Code DHS 63.08(1) • community substance abuse prevention and treatment services (Wis. Adm. Code DHS 75.01(1)) • prevention services and strategies to reduce the risk of substance abuse (Wis. Adm. Code DHS 75.04) • emergency outpatient service (Wis. Adm. Code DHS 75.05(1)) • medically-managed inpatient treatment service (Wis. Adm. Code DHS 75.10(1)) • individual and group counseling (Wis. Adm. Code DHS 75.10(6)(f)) • day treatment service (Wis. Adm. Code DHS 75.12(1)) • outpatient treatment service (Wis. Adm. Code DHS 75.13(1)) • transitional residential treatment service (Wis. Adm. Code DHS 75.14(1) & (6)(b))	There are a variety of opportunities throughout the Health Services system for identifying people as needing substance abuse treatment, all of which could be used to coordinate naltrexone treatment with community pharmacists
	• opioid treatment service for OUD providing methadone or other FDA-approved medications, as well as other medical or psychological services, counseling, or social services (Wis. Adm. Code DHS 75.15(1)) • intervention services that includes case management (Wis. Adm. Code DHS 75.16(1))	This provision provides a direct role for pharmacists and their authorization to provide naltrexone injections for the treatment of OUD

Table 5. *Cont.*

Section of Law (Statutory Citation) (Regulatory Citation)	Description of Identified Provisions	Implication for Pharmacist Service
Regulation and Licensing (Statutes—Regulation and Licensing; Chapter 448. Medical Practices/Chapter 450. Pharmacy Examining Board) (Regulations—Wisconsin Administrative Code; Medical Examining Board/Pharmacy Examining Board)	Healthcare examining boards can establish practice standards (Wis. Stat. § 450.02)	Practice standards could include pharmacist services in providing naltrexone injections
	Advisory committees can be convened to address behavioral health issues (Wis. Stat. § 440.043)	An advisory committee could be convened to address pharmacist services for OUD prevention and treatment
	Any licensed physician can use telemedicine as a patient engagement tool, after documenting a patient evaluation (Wis. Adm. Code Med 24.07)	Telemedicine authorization does not involve pharmacists, and it is unclear how this provision extends to pharmacists who are part of a collaborative agreement with a physician
Social Services (Statutes—Charitable, Curative, Reformatory and Penal Institutions and Agencies; Chapter 46. Social Services) (Regulations—none)	DHS has established a drug abuse program that creates the foundation for education, diagnosis, and treatment (Wis. Stat. § 46.973), and county-level DHS offices are developed to address, in part, drug abuse issues (Wis. Stat. § 46.23) Through a variety of funding mechanisms, community-based drug abuse prevention and treatment can focus on residential care, prisoner reintegration into communities, urban communities, and underserved populations (Wis. Stat. § 46.48), as well as to facilitate long-term care transitions (Wis. Stat. § 46.2803), for low-income Hispanics and Black Americans in urban areas, the Native American population, and women (Wis. Stat. § 46.975), and for inmates in the criminal justice system as an alternative to imprisonment (Wis. Stat. § 46.65)	Implementation of community-based program funding could increase demand for naltrexone injection service, especially when DHS efforts acknowledge the role of and establish relationships with community pharmacists that provide those services
State Alcohol, Drug Abuse, Developmental Disabilities and Mental Health Act (Statutes—Charitable, Curative, Reformatory and Penal Institutions and Agencies; Chapter 51. State Alcohol, Drug Abuse, Developmental Disabilities and Mental Health Act) (Regulations—none)	This statute addresses a broad range of AODA prevention and treatment services and is designed to assure continuity of care for such treatment (Wis. Stat. § 51.001), which reinforces DHS's authority to establish a comprehensive and coordinated drug abuse program for education, diagnosis, and treatment (Wis. Stat. § 51.45)	Pharmacist-provided drug abuse treatment services could be a regular component of DHS coordinated care efforts
	Methadone treatment programs include the provision of methadone, buprenorphine, and naltrexone (Wis. Stat. § 51.4223)	The provisions for methadone treatment programs could allow pharmacist services for naltrexone injections

Table 5. *Cont.*

Section of Law (Statutory Citation) (Regulatory Citation)	Description of Identified Provisions	Implication for Pharmacist Service
Veteran's Affairs (Cultural and Memorial Institutions; Veteran's Affairs; Chapter 45. Veterans) (Wisconsin Administrative Code; Department of Veteran's Affairs)	Healthcare assistance from a variety of health care providers is available to all needy veterans (Wis. Stat. § 45.40)	Under this section, the definition of "health care provider" does not include pharmacists
	Substance abuse treatment programs approved by the U.S. Department of Veteran's Affairs (USDVA) or Wisconsin-certified AODA programs are available for needy veterans (Wis. Adm. Code VA 2.01), and treatment in such programs can facilitate subsistence aid when veterans lose income due to drug abuse (Wis. Adm. Code VA 2.01(3)(b))	Given the description of AODA-related programs in Wisconsin's Health Services and Social Services regulations, as well as in the State Alcohol, Drug Abuse, Developmental Disabilities and Mental Health Act, it is likely that such treatment could involve injection naltrexone
	Federal grant to counties can be issued to improve services to veterans (Wis. Stat. § 45.82), and the Tribal veterans' service office can apply for American Indian grants (Wis. Adm. Code VA 15.02(1))	Veteran-related funding may potentially be applied to drug abuse issues, but pharmacist involvement in providing such services may be limited due to their not being a recognized "health care provider"

A systematic analysis of Wisconsin statutes and regulations identified a variety of provisions that could facilitate a pharmacist service for providing naltrexone injections to treat patients with OUD. Requirements contained in Correction laws and in Health Services regulations provide ample chances, under a variety of situations, for pharmacists to be a member of the patient care team for OUD. This role is further strengthened by DHS's authority to maintain treatment coordination for people with drug abuse problems (Wis. Stat. § 51.45). Treatment continuity would be especially important for people transitioning within the corrections, health services, and social services systems, or for inmates who are released into the community. Despite these opportunities, there are instances of legal language that could impede pharmacists providing the injection service. For example, healthcare assistance to needy veterans does not seem to involve pharmacists, even though drug abuse issues can be a problem with which needy veterans are struggling. In addition, telemedicine authorization is not contained in pharmacy practice laws, although it is permitted for physicians. As a result, it is ambiguous whether a pharmacist could be involved in distance consultations with a physician even as a function of a collaborative practice agreement between the two healthcare professionals.

4. Discussion

The results of this study suggest that a pharmacist-provided naltrexone injection service can be an access point for the treatment of patients with OUD. Additionally, the legislative and regulatory analysis documented numerous opportunities for the service to be incorporated into the current infrastructure for public health and social services in Wisconsin. Given the shortage of behavioral health providers in Wisconsin, and that pharmacies are more accessible to patients, a pharmacist-provided naltrexone injection service can broaden patients' treatment options. A pharmacist-provided naltrexone injection service has the potential to be a "game changer" for OUD treatment [51]. The study identified five key factors that explain why MOUD from pharmacists is not widely available: transportation; awareness and acceptance; inter-organizational coordination of care; reimbursement and funding; and service infrastructure including telemedicine.

Transportation to and from the pharmacy for patients needing MOUD is a critical issue that needs to be addressed. Community pharmacists have a long history of offering delivery service to patients to facilitate prescription drug access. Perhaps pharmacists can use their experience with delivery service to develop a cost-effective method to convey patients to and from the pharmacy for naltrexone injections. Another model that could be considered is pharmacists making monthly trips to treatment facilities and providing the injections to groups of patients. Further research is required to understand the needs of patients with OUD to access the injection service and to study the costs and effectiveness of different methods to access the service.

Similar to other pharmacist services, increasing awareness about the service and promoting acceptability are important for the spread of the service. According to the interview results, pharmacists said that patients were universally accepting of the service since it reduced the stigma of treating OUD. However, additional research needs to determine the generalizability of these interview findings, and more broadly assess the perceptions and attitudes of patients with OUD about receiving naltrexone injections from a pharmacist. Learning which aspects of the service—before, during, and after the injection—are most beneficial to patients could help pharmacists to better promote the service and generate better adherence outcomes.

Increasing prescriber acceptance of the service is integral to more widespread adoption and sustainability of the service. A strategy to promote practitioners' acceptance of the service is informed by the process illustrated by the interviewed pharmacists to provide the naltrexone injections, as well as described in a previous study [52]: (1) establishing and following a protocol that is used in clinics when treating patients with OUD and (2) meeting quality benchmarks to show that the process and service is of high quality. Approaches to promote the acceptability of the service to prescribers could focus on advantages of naltrexone (i.e., it is not a controlled substance, and prescribers do not have to be DATA-waived) and how pharmacists can facilitate access to naltrexone and can provide the injection and post-injection monitoring. As also suggested by our analysis of legislative and regulatory language, public health and social services administrators and affiliated prescribing practitioners need to be accepting of the service as well. Importantly, understanding practitioners' attitudes and perceptions about pharmacists' involvement in OUD treatment, including providing naltrexone injections, would be a useful gauge for the viability of the service. Attitudes and perceptions could be used to develop approaches and messaging to increase acceptability of the service. Additionally, researchers and pharmacists are encouraged to propose comparative effectiveness trials of pharmacist-provided naltrexone injections to study the relative advantages of the service. Dissemination of the results could be used to promote acceptance of the service.

One implication of the injection service process is that it requires extensive engagement, communication, and coordination to get the patient into the pharmacy for the first injection, as well as additional coordination to assure their return for follow-up. The finding that coordination and communication is a key component of successful OUD treatment is consistent with research about OUD treatment in clinics [53]. The pharmacists we interviewed had spent significant time working with the behavioral health provider to be part of the patient care team, including mechanisms for communication. Although telemedicine with a behavioral health provider was a component of the injection service described by the interviewed pharmacists, OUD treatment with naltrexone can be initiated by local primary care providers. Pharmacists interested in starting a naltrexone injection service should be aware of OUD treatment providers and access issues in their immediate and surrounding communities. Such efforts should focus on the connection with community resources to promote awareness and acceptance of community pharmacy provided naltrexone injections by non-prescribers.

Interviewed pharmacists reported that reimbursement for costs associated with the administration of the naltrexone injection is not widely available. One pharmacist even provided an itemized list of naltrexone administration costs, and it was estimated that each administered injection resulted in approximately $102 of unreimbursed cost. It should not be surprising that the non-remunerated cost of providing the service can be a substantial barrier impacting the initial decision to provide the service and for the sustainability of the service in a community. Although the analysis of state laws did not involve reimbursement laws due to their complexity, it did identify conceivable opportunities for payment for the injection administration service through separate funding from the public health and social services areas.

As mentioned, there are many additional sources of state-level funding that possibly could help expand pharmacists' role in OUD treatment across the state, and pharmacists may put themselves in a beneficial position by learning whether possibilities for payment for the injection administration, or other mechanisms for payment, are available through these sources. In fact, an entire statute (Charitable, Curative, Reformatory and Penal Institutions and Agencies, Chapter 46) is devoted to preventing substance abuse, and providing community-based services for people experiencing difficulties with substance abuse issues, primarily through the establishment of program funding opportunities. Table 5 also identifies additional funding opportunities available through DHS-distributed grants, specific drug abuse treatment funds, and veterans' service grants. Each of these potential funding sources presumably creates the prospect of expanding MOUD around the state. As pharmacist-provided naltrexone injections become increasingly normalized as a convenient and reliable avenue for OUD treatment within the community, it is likely that such funding would broaden the availability of that essential service.

In addition to legally-sanctioned funding opportunities, it is clear from the analysis of statutes and regulations that Wisconsin law provides broad legal capacity, through a variety of government agencies, for the treatment of people with an OUD—even though demand often outstrips available resources. Infrastructures for OUD treatment seem especially robust for the areas of corrections, health service, and social services, as well as through the State Alcohol, Drug Abuse, Developmental Disabilities and Mental Health Act. Although considerable systems exist by law for people needing AODA treatment, the role of pharmacists and their ability to administer injectable naltrexone is currently either undefined or underutilized. The extensive legal foundation for comprehensive AODA assessment and treatment in Wisconsin is still advantageous, because, as this pharmacy service develops and spreads, statutes and regulations could more clearly define the role of pharmacists and facilitate demand for the service.

While Wisconsin law permits pharmacists to give naltrexone injections either pursuant to or without a collaborative practice agreement with a physician, little additional guidance is provided to pharmacists about engaging in such treatment. However, it would be possible for the pharmacy board to develop practice standards for pharmacist-involved OUD treatment, including with injectable naltrexone. Such a standard, potentially coupled with an appointed committee's advisory statement about OUD-related behavioral health issues, would offer important clarification about the extent of pharmacists' potential contributions to treatment with naltrexone. In addition, the State Alcohol, Drug Abuse, Developmental Disabilities and Mental Health Act identifies "methadone maintenance programs" as including the use of naltrexone; although there are no legislative notes to provide information about the contributions that pharmacy service can make to these programs, agency policies and procedures could be modified to specifically describe the role of pharmacists providing treatment in methadone maintenance programs. As such results suggest, clarifying these standards could contribute to promoting awareness of the pharmacist service, as well as better assure that health and social services administrators and practitioners are more accepting of the service.

In relation to general healthcare practice, physicians can engage in telemedicine to facilitate distance treatment. When pharmacists and physicians collaborate to conduct a visit via telemedicine, as done by the pharmacists we interviewed, it offers a new location (i.e., community pharmacy) for the provider-patient visit. The process then facilitates the pharmacist providing the naltrexone injection. The lack of a parallel telemedicine provision in pharmacy practice laws, absent clarifying authoritative statements, creates uncertainty about the legality of pharmacists' involvement in physician or patient interactions through telemedicine consults. To establish well-defined authority for pharmacists to engage in telehealth, the pharmacy examining board could modify its regulations to permit such practice. Such regulatory change, coupled with a communications strategy to its licensees about the change, has the potential to facilitate pharmacist service around naltrexone treatment for patients with OUD and expand access to MOUD treatment.

Limitations

A few limitations characterize this initial analysis of state laws. First, it is possible that relevant provisions were contained in either statutes or regulations but were overlooked or inappropriately disregarded during the review. Second, due to the complexity of reimbursement-related laws (at the Federal, state, and local levels, and either public or private sector), description of state insurance laws were excluded for this project. Since the applicability of state insurance laws does not function in isolation of other types of reimbursement laws, a more detailed discussion of these policies is necessary for providing an accurate account of the coverage of pharmacy-provided naltrexone treatment, as well as providing telemedicine services, which was outside the scope of this article. However, further research is indeed necessary to examine the potential influence of the variety of reimbursement-related laws affecting the use of injection naltrexone for OUD treatment.

Our understanding of the process of community pharmacists providing naltrexone injections was based on a purposeful sample, and thus has a few limitations. First, it is possible that there are other community pharmacists in Wisconsin who provide naltrexone injections and use service processes that vary from the initial straw model we developed. Research to further describe the service process is needed. Second, the perceived prescriber and patient acceptability barriers, as well as the identified facilitators and barriers, may be understated, which in turn could impact the willingness to utilize community pharmacists as a provider of naltrexone injections. Further research is needed to conduct a broad environmental scan of community pharmacists, including if they are currently providing (or would be willing to provide) naltrexone injections and identifying other perceived facilitators and barriers to offering the service. Also, additional information is needed about the existing infrastructure in community pharmacies offering naltrexone injections. The information could be used to develop a toolkit for other community pharmacists and the toolkit's effectiveness could be examined in a comprehensive dissemination and implementation research study design.

5. Conclusions

The nascent growth of the partnership between community pharmacists, individuals with an OUD and prescribers in Wisconsin to offer naltrexone injections highlights the potential for community pharmacists to be active partners in addressing issues related to the growing opioid crisis. However, barriers associated with transportation, service infrastructure, reimbursement, awareness and acceptance by practitioners including communication and service coordination need to be studied to facilitate implementation and sustainability of this service in community pharmacies. In addition, the design, implementation and effectiveness of current naltrexone injection service delivery approaches by community pharmacists are not well understood. Operating in a supportive legislative and regulatory environment, community pharmacists, as an already trusted and acceptable provider of service within their community, could provide individuals a significant access point for OUD treatment with naltrexone injections.

Author Contributions: Conceptualization, A.G., D.A.M. and J.H.F.II; methodology, A.G., D.A.M. and J.H.F.II; validation, A.G., D.A.M. and J.H.F.II; formal analysis, A.G., D.A.M. and J.H.F.II; investigation, A.G., D.A.M. and J.H.F.II; resources, A.G., D.A.M. and J.H.F.II; data curation, A.G., D.A.M. and J.H.F.II; writing—original draft preparation, A.G., D.A.M. and J.H.F.II; writing—review and editing, A.G., D.A.M. and J.H.F.II; visualization, A.G., and J.H.F.II; supervision, D.A.M.; project administration, D.A.M.

Funding: This research received no external funding.

Acknowledgments: Marty Skemp Brown, Gina Bryan and Martha Maurer for helping to facilitate and assist in data collection. Community pharmacist who participated in the interviews sharing their insights about naltrexone injections in their pharmacy.

Conflicts of Interest: The authors declare no conflict of interest.

References

1. Abraham, A.J.; Andrews, C.M.; Yingling, M.E.; Shannon, J. Geographic disparities in availability of opioid use disorder treatment for Medicaid enrollees. *Health Serv. Res.* **2018**, *53*, 389–404. [CrossRef] [PubMed]

2. Skolnick, P. The opioid epidemic: Crisis and solutions. *Annu. Rev. Pharmacol. Toxicol.* **2018**, *58*, 143–159. [CrossRef] [PubMed]

3. U.S. Department of Health and Human Services (HHS), Office of the Surgeon General. *Facing Addiction in America: The Surgeon General's Report on Alcohol, Drugs, and Health*; HHS: Washington, DC, USA, November 2016.

4. Compton, W.M.; Jones, C.M.; Baldwin, G.T. Relationship between nonmedical prescription-opioid use and heroin use. *N. Engl. J. Med.* **2016**, *374*, 154–163. [CrossRef] [PubMed]

5. Weiss, A.; Elixhauser, A.; Barrett, M.; Steiner, C.; Bailey, M.; O'Malley, L. *Opioid-Related Inpatient Stays and Emergency Department Visits by State, 2009–2014*; Healthcare Cost and Utilization Project, Statistical Brief# 219; Agency for Healthcare Research and Quality: Rockville, MD, USA, 2017.

6. Wurcel, A.G.; Anderson, J.E.; Chui, K.K.H.; Skinner, S.; Knox, T.A.; Snydman, D.R.; Stopka, T.J. Increasing Infectious Endocarditis Admissions Among Young People Who Inject Drugs. *Open Forum Infect. Dis.* **2016**, *3*, ofw157. [CrossRef] [PubMed]

7. Peterson, C.; Xu, L.; Mikosz, C.A.; Florence, C.; Mack, K.A. US hospital discharges documenting patient opioid use disorder without opioid overdose or treatment services, 2011–2015. *J. Subst. Abus. Treat.* **2018**, *92*, 35–39. [CrossRef]

8. Centers for Disease Control Prevention. *Annual Surveillance Report of Drug-Related Risks and Outcomes—United States, 2017*; Surveillance Special Report 1; CDC: Atlanta, GA, USA, 2017.

9. Vivolo-Kantor, A.M.; Seth, P.; Gladden, R.M.; Mattson, C.L.; Baldwin, G.T.; Kite-Powell, A.; Coletta, M.A. Vital signs: Trends in emergency department visits for suspected opioid overdoses—United States, July 2016–September 2017. *Morb. Mortal. Wkly. Rep.* **2018**, *67*, 279. [CrossRef]

10. Gomes, T.; Tadrous, M.; Mamdani, M.M.; Paterson, J.M.; Juurlink, D.N. The Burden of Opioid-Related Mortality in the United States. *JAMA Netw. Open* **2018**, *1*, e180217. [CrossRef]

11. Madras, B.K.; Connery, H. Psychiatry and the opioid overdose crisis. *Focus J. Am. Psychiatr. Assoc.* **2019**, *17*, 128–133. [CrossRef]

12. Lee, J.D.; Friedmann, P.D.; Kinlock, T.W.; Nunes, E.V.; Boney, T.Y.; Hoskinson, R.A., Jr.; Wilson, D.; McDonald, R.; Rotrosen, J.; Gourevitch, M.N. Extended-Release Naltrexone to Prevent Opioid Relapse in Criminal Justice Offenders. *N. Engl. J. Med.* **2016**, *374*, 1232–1242. [CrossRef]

13. Palis, H.; Marchand, K.; Guh, D.; Brissette, S.; Lock, K.; MacDonald, S.; Harrison, S.; Anis, A.H.; Krausz, M.; Marsh, D.C. Men's and women's response to treatment and perceptions of outcomes in a randomized controlled trial of injectable opioid assisted treatment for severe opioid use disorder. *Subst. Abus. Treat. Prev. Policy* **2017**, *12*, 25. [CrossRef]

14. Schuckit, M.A. Treatment of Opioid-Use Disorders. *N. Engl. J. Med.* **2016**, *375*, 357–368. [CrossRef]

15. WIDHS. Opioids: Data, Reports, Studies. Available online: https://www.dhs.wisconsin.gov/opioids/data-reports-studies.htm (accessed on 22 July 2018).

16. WIDHS. Wisconsin Interactive Statistics on Health (WISH) Query System: Opioid-Related Hospital Encounters. Available online: https://www.dhs.wisconsin.gov/wish/opioid/hospital-encounters.htm (accessed on 22 July 2018).

17. WIDHS. Wisconsin Interactive Statistics on Health (WISH) Query System: Drug Overdose Deaths. Available online: https://www.dhs.wisconsin.gov/wish/opioid/mortality.htm (accessed on 22 July 2018).

18. Krupitsky, E.; Nunes, E.V.; Ling, W.; Illeperuma, A.; Gastfriend, D.R.; Silverman, B.L. Injectable extended-release naltrexone for opioid dependence: A double-blind, placebo-controlled, multicentre randomised trial. *Lancet* **2011**, *377*, 1506–1513. [CrossRef]

19. Krupitsky, E.; Zvartau, E.; Blokhina, E.; Verbitskaya, E.; Wahlgren, V.; Tsoy-Podosenin, M.; Bushara, N.; Burakov, A.; Masalov, D.; Romanova, T.; et al. Randomized trial of long-acting sustained-release naltrexone implant vs oral naltrexone or placebo for preventing relapse to opioid dependence. *Arch. Gen. Psychiatry* **2012**, *69*, 973–981. [CrossRef] [PubMed]

20. Robertson, A.G.; Easter, M.M.; Lin, H.-J.; Frisman, L.K.; Swanson, J.W.; Swartz, M.S. Associations between pharmacotherapy for opioid dependence and clinical and criminal justice outcomes among adults with co-occurring serious mental illness. *J. Subst. Abus. Treat.* **2018**, *86*, 17–25. [CrossRef]

21. Jarvis, B.P.; Holtyn, A.F.; Subramaniam, S.; Tompkins, D.A.; Oga, E.A.; Bigelow, G.E.; Silverman, K. Extended-release injectable naltrexone for opioid use disorder: A systematic review. *Addiction* **2018**, *113*, 1188–1209. [CrossRef]

22. Saxon, A.J.; Akerman, S.C.; Liu, C.C.; Sullivan, M.A.; Silverman, B.L.; Vocci, F.J. Extended-release naltrexone (XR-NTX) for opioid use disorder in clinical practice: Vivitrol's Cost and Treatment Outcomes Registry. *Addiction* **2018**, *113*, 1477–1487. [CrossRef] [PubMed]

23. Crowley, R.; Kirschner, N.; Dunn, A.S.; Bornstein, S.S. Health and public policy to facilitate effective prevention and treatment of substance use disorders involving illicit and prescription drugs: An American College of Physicians position paper. *Ann. Intern. Med.* **2017**, *166*, 733–736. [CrossRef] [PubMed]

24. Kolodny, A.; Courtwright, D.T.; Hwang, C.S.; Kreiner, P.; Eadie, J.L.; Clark, T.W.; Alexander, G.C. The prescription opioid and heroin crisis: A public health approach to an epidemic of addiction. *Annu. Rev. Public Health* **2015**, *36*, 559–574. [CrossRef]

25. Murthy, V.H. Ending the opioid epidemic—A call to action. *N. Engl. J. Med.* **2016**, *375*, 2413–2415. [CrossRef]

26. Volkow, N.D.; Frieden, T.R.; Hyde, P.S.; Cha, S.S. Medication-Assisted Therapies—Tackling the Opioid-Overdose Epidemic. *N. Engl. J. Med.* **2014**, *370*, 2063–2066. [CrossRef]

27. Larochelle, M.R.; Bernson, D.; Land, T.; Stopka, T.J.; Wang, N.; Xuan, Z.; Bagley, S.M.; Liebschutz, J.M.; Walley, A.Y. Medication for Opioid Use Disorder After Nonfatal Opioid Overdose and Association With Mortality: A Cohort Study. *Ann. Intern. Med.* **2018**, *169*, 137–145. [CrossRef] [PubMed]

28. Volkow, N.D.; Wargo, E.M. Overdose Prevention Through Medical Treatment of Opioid Use Disorders. *Ann. Intern. Med.* **2018**, *169*, 190–192. [CrossRef] [PubMed]

29. Abraham, A.J.; Knudsen, H.K.; Rieckmann, T.; Roman, P.M. Disparities in access to physicians and medications for the treatment of substance use disorders between publicly and privately funded treatment programs in the United States. *J. Stud. Alcohol Drugs* **2013**, *74*, 258–265. [CrossRef] [PubMed]

30. Andrilla, C.H.A.; Moore, T.E.; Patterson, D.G.; Larson, E.H. Geographic Distribution of Providers With a DEA Waiver to Prescribe Buprenorphine for the Treatment of Opioid Use Disorder: A 5-Year Update. *J. Rural Health* **2019**, *35*, 108–112. [CrossRef] [PubMed]

31. Morgan, J.R.; Schackman, B.R.; Leff, J.A.; Linas, B.P.; Walley, A.Y. Injectable naltrexone, oral naltrexone, and buprenorphine utilization and discontinuation among individuals treated for opioid use disorder in a United States commercially insured population. *J. Subst. Abus. Treat.* **2018**, *85*, 90–96. [CrossRef] [PubMed]

32. Rosenblatt, R.A.; Andrilla, C.H.A.; Catlin, M.; Larson, E.H. Geographic and Specialty Distribution of US Physicians Trained to Treat Opioid Use Disorder. *Ann. Fam. Med.* **2015**, *13*, 23–26. [CrossRef]

33. Substance Abuse and Mental Health Services Administration. *National Survey of Substance Abuse Treatment Services (N-SSATs): 2016. Data on Substance Abuse Treatment Facilities*; TBHSIS Series S-93, HHS Publication No. (SMA) 17-5039; Substance Abuse and Mental Health Services Administration: Rockville, MD, USA, 2017.

34. Andraka-Christou, B.; Capone, M.J. A qualitative study comparing physician-reported barriers to treating addiction using buprenorphine and extended-release naltrexone in U.S. office-based practices. *Int. J. Drug Policy* **2018**, *54*, 9–17. [CrossRef]

35. Andrilla, C.H.A.; Coulthard, C.; Patterson, D.G. Prescribing practices of rural physicians waivered to prescribe buprenorphine. *Am. J. Prev. Med.* **2018**, *54*, S208–S214. [CrossRef]

36. Johnson, Q.; Mund, B.; Joudrey, P.J. Improving Rural Access to Opioid Treatment Programs. *J. Law Med. Ethics* **2018**, *46*, 437–439. [CrossRef]

37. Alanis-Hirsch, K.; Croff, R.; Ford, J.H.; Johnson, K.; Chalk, M.; Schmidt, L.; McCarty, D. Extended-release naltrexone: A qualitative analysis of barriers to routine use. *J. Subst. Abus. Treat.* **2016**, *62*, 68–73. [CrossRef]

38. Aletraris, L.; Edmond, M.B.; Roman, P.M. Adoption of injectable naltrexone in US substance use disorder treatment programs. *J. Stud. Alcohol Drugs* **2015**, *76*, 143–151. [CrossRef] [PubMed]

39. Jones, C.M.; Campopiano, M.; Baldwin, G.; McCance-Katz, E. National and State Treatment Need and Capacity for Opioid Agonist Medication-Assisted Treatment. *Am. J. Public Health* **2015**, *105*, e55–e63. [CrossRef] [PubMed]

40. Molfenter, T.; Sherbeck, C.; Zehner, M.; Quanbeck, A.; McCarty, D.; Kim, J.-S.; Starr, S. Implementing buprenorphine in addiction treatment: Payer and provider perspectives in Ohio. Subst. *Abus. Treat. Prev. Policy* **2015**, *10*, 13. [CrossRef] [PubMed]

41. Cobaugh, D.J.; Gainor, C.; Gaston, C.L.; Kwong, T.C.; Magnani, B.; McPherson, M.L.; Painter, J.T.; Krenzelok, E.P. The opioid abuse and misuse epidemic: Implications for pharmacists in hospitals and health systems. *Am. J. Health-Syst. Pharm.* **2014**, *71*, 1539–1554. [CrossRef] [PubMed]

42. Compton, W.M.; Jones, C.M.; Stein, J.B.; Wargo, E.M. Promising roles for pharmacists in addressing the US opioid crisis. *Res. Soc. Adm. Pharm.* **2017**. [CrossRef]

43. Reynolds, V.; Causey, H.; McKee, J.; Reinstein, V.; Muzyk, A. The Role of Pharmacists in the Opioid Epidemic An Examination of Pharmacist-Focused Initiatives Across the United States and North Carolina. *N. C. Med. J.* **2017**, *78*, 202–205.

44. Ullrich, F.; Salako, A.; Mueller, K. Issues Confronting Rural Pharmacies after a Decade of Medicare Part D. *Rural Policy Brief* **2017**, *3*, 1–5.

45. *National Association of Chain Drug Stores 2011–2012 Chain Pharmacy Industry Profile*; National Association of Chain Drug Stores: Alexandria, VA, USA, 2011.

46. Scott, D.M.; Strand, M.; Undem, T.; Anderson, G.; Clarens, A.; Liu, X. Assessment of pharmacists' delivery of public health services in rural and urban areas in Iowa and North Dakota. *Pharm. Pract. (Granada)* **2016**, *14*. [CrossRef]

47. Strand, M.A.; Tellers, J.; Patterson, A.; Ross, A.; Palombi, L. The achievement of public health services in pharmacy practice: A literature review. *Res. Soc. Adm. Pharm.* **2016**, *12*, 247–256. [CrossRef]

48. Drozd, E.M.; Miller, L.; Johnsrud, M. Impact of pharmacist immunization authority on seasonal influenza immunization rates across states. *Clin. Ther.* **2017**, *39*, 1563–1580.e1517. [CrossRef]

49. Folsom, W.D. *Understanding American Business Jargon: A Dictionary*; Greenwood Publishing Group: Westport, CT, USA, 2005; p. 293.

50. Gustafson, D.H.; Sainfort, F.; Eichler, M.; Adams, L.; Bisognano, M.; Steudel, H. Developing and testing a model to predict outcomes of organizational change. *HSR Health Serv. Res.* **2003**, *38*, 739–764. [CrossRef]

51. Boesl, S.; (Sauk County Human Services Department, Baraboo, WI, USA). Personal communication, 2018.

52. Hebbard, A.M.; Colvard, M.J.; Book, S.W.; VandenBerg, A.M. Development of a collaborative drug therapy management protocol for extended-release intramuscular naltrexone. *Ment. Health Clin.* **2013**, *3*, 292–294. [CrossRef]

53. Korthuis, P.T.; McCarty, D.; Weimer, M.; Bougatsos, C.; Blazina, I.; Zakher, B.; Grusing, S.; Devine, B.; Chou, R. Primary care–based models for the treatment of opioid use disorder: A scoping review. *Ann. Intern. Med.* **2017**, *166*, 268–278. [CrossRef] [PubMed]

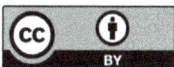

Article

Impact of the 2016 Policy Change on the Delivery of MedsCheck Services in Ontario: An Interrupted Time-Series Analysis

Ahmad Shakeri [1], Lisa Dolovich [1,2,3], Lori MacCallum [1,4], John-Michael Gamble [2], Limei Zhou [5] and Suzanne M. Cadarette [1,5,6,7,*]

1   Leslie Dan Faculty of Pharmacy, University of Toronto, Toronto, ON M5S 3M2, Canada
2   School of Pharmacy, University of Waterloo, Kitchener, ON N2L 3G1, Canada
3   Department of Family Medicine, McMaster University, Hamilton, ON L8P 1H6, Canada
4   Banting & Best Diabetes Centre, Faculty of Medicine, University of Toronto, Toronto, ON M5G 2C4, Canada
5   ICES, Toronto, ON M5T 3M6, Canada
6   Dalla Lana School of Public Health, University of Toronto, Toronto, ON M5T 3M7, Canada
7   Eshelman School of Pharmacy, University of North Carolina, Chapel Hill, NC 27599-7355, USA
*   Correspondence: s.cadarette@utoronto.ca; Tel.: +1-416-978-2993

Received: 1 June 2019; Accepted: 6 August 2019; Published: 12 August 2019

check for updates

Abstract: MedsCheck (MC) is an annual medication review service delivered by community pharmacists and funded by the government of Ontario since 2007 for residents taking three or more medications for chronic conditions. In 2010, MC was expanded to include patients with diabetes (MCD), home-bound patients (MCH), and residents of long-term care homes (MCLTC). The Ontario government introduced an abrupt policy change effective 1 October 2016 that added several components to all MC services, especially those completed in the community. We used an interrupted time series design to examine the impact of the policy change (24 months pre- and post-intervention) on the monthly number of MedsCheck services delivered. Immediate declines in all services were identified, especially in the community (47%–64% drop MC, 71%–83% drop MCD, 55% drop MCH, and 9%–14% drop MCLTC). Gradual increases were seen over 24 months post-policy change, yet remained 21%–76% lower than predicted for MedsCheck services delivered in the community, especially for MCD. In contrast, MCLTC services were similar or exceeded predicted values by September 2018 (from 5.1% decrease to 3.5% increase). A more effective implementation of health policy changes is needed to ensure the feasibility and sustainability of professional community pharmacy services.

Keywords: community pharmacy services; health policy; interrupted time series analysis; medication reconciliation

1. Introduction

Chronic medications are often critical to an individual's ability to maintain and improve their health [1]. However, drug therapy problems, such as unnecessary therapy, ineffective dosage, and adverse drug reactions are common [2,3]. Effective strategies to identify and decrease drug therapy problems are important to reduce the potential harms from medication [4]. Community pharmacists are widely accessible and commonly maintain a comprehensive record of an individual's prescription medications [5]. Community pharmacists are thus well positioned to effectively identify drug therapy problems and prevent adverse drug events [6,7]. Community-pharmacist medication review programs are well-established and publicly funded in Australia, Denmark and the United Kingdom [8–10]. Canada has universal Medicare that covers all medically necessary physician services, and at minimum, partial coverage of medications listed on provincial formularies for seniors and specialized vulnerable groups [11]. In April 2007, the government of Ontario launched the MedsCheck program as the first publicly funded community-pharmacy delivered professional service outside of drug dispensation. When it was originally introduced, the MedsCheck (MC) service was a one-on-one annual consultation service in a community pharmacy that provided education and assessed adherence to therapy. The program targeted Ontario residents taking three or more medications for chronic conditions, and pharmacy reimbursement was limited to once every 12 months [12]. The opportunity for pharmacies to be reimbursed for unlimited follow-up services was added in November 2007. In September 2010, the MedsCheck program was expanded to include people with diabetes (MCD), people unable to physically attend a medication review service in a pharmacy due to physical or mental incapability (MedsCheck at Home [MCH]), and residents in long-term care (MCLTC) [13,14]. In addition, unlimited follow-up services within the year were included for MCD and quarterly services were included for MCLTC. MC and MCD annuals and their respective follow-ups are completed in community pharmacies, whereas MCH and MCLTC occur in a person's place of residence. Pharmacies are reimbursed for these services by submitting a claim to the Ontario Drug Benefit program. Of interest is the fact that all long-term care (LTC) homes are required by legislation to ensure pharmacist participation in quarterly and annual medication reviews with each patient [13].

The Ontario government announced changes to MedsCheck service delivery in July 2016 that were implemented on 1 October 2016. The mandatory changes added several components to each service, including follow-up services, such as requiring written patient consent, structured pharmacist documentation, and the provision of summary information and recommendations to physicians (Table 1) [15]. MCD included an extra set of assessment parameters related to diabetes education and goal-setting, and new requirements that pharmacists have either a certified diabetes educator designation or have gained adequate diabetes management knowledge through a professional continuing education program approved by the Canadian Council on Continuing Education in Pharmacy [13,16]. However, MCD follow-up services were less rigorous, intended for education and did not require a complete medication review. The objective of this study was to estimate the change in the monthly number of MedsCheck services delivered following the 2016 policy change.

We hypothesized that the increased workload accompanying the policy change and added documentation and training requirements for MCD delivery would impact the feasibility of community services, and thus, an immediate decline in the number of services would be identified. However, given that regular medication reviews are required in LTC, we hypothesized that pharmacies would leverage the MCLTC program to meet medication review requirements and thus, changes to the program would have minimal impact on the frequency of MCLTC services.

2. Materials and Methods

2.1. Study Design

We used an interrupted time-series segmented regression design to study trends in the monthly services delivered [17–19]. Interrupted time series is a robust, quasi-experimental approach for evaluating the effects of policy and public health interventions [17,20]. This method models changes in the level (immediate impact) and trend (slope) after a policy change; in our case, we examined the change in monthly MedsCheck services following the 1 October 2016 policy change.

Table 1. MedsCheck documentation requirement pre- and post-October 2016 policy change.

Before October 2016	Since October 2016 Policy Change
Patient Assessment Summary with Pharmacist's Signature and Date	1. *MedsCheck Patient Acknowledgement of Professional Pharmacy Service* *
	• Completed annually for all community MedsCheck services (not required for MCLTC)
	2. *Pharmacists Worksheet* * for professional notes, 4 pages
	3. *Personal Medication Record*, 1 or more pages (not required for MCLTC)
	• Signed and dated by the pharmacist indicating the date of the consultation
	• Documentation with assurance that the record is an accurate assessment of the patient's prescription, non-prescription and natural health product usage
	• Table format for: what, why, how and comments for each product
	• Includes evidence that drug therapy problems have been followed-up or have a plan for resolution
Specific to MCH	• Records if the optional patient take-home summary was provided
Medicine Cabinet Review:	4. *Healthcare Provider Notification of MedsCheck Services* *, 1 page
Review of the medicine storage areas Expired or unused medications itemized removed from the home with signed consent for removal	• Mandatory summary provided to the primary prescriber that includes the *Personal Medication Record* and lists follow-up issues identified for resolution (not required for MCLTC)
	5. *MedsCheck Patient Take-Home Summary* *, 1 or more pages (optional)
Specific to MCLTC	• Summary of discussion, patient goals, suggestions for how to achieve goals, lists of resources, contacts and referrals
Name of designate of long term care team with whom results reviewed	Specific to MedsCheck Diabetes annual services
	6. *Diabetes Education Checklist* *, 4 pages
	7. *Diabetes Education Patient Take-Home Summary* *, 1 or more pages
	• Summary of discussion, patient goals, suggestions for how to achieve goals, lists of resources, contacts and referrals
	• Unlike other community MedsCheck services, the take-home summary is required for patients receiving MedsCheck Diabetes services

* Standardized forms, available at http://www.forms.ssb.gov.on.ca/, accessed on 2 May 2019 [15]; MCH: MedsCheck at Home, MCLTC: MedsCheck Long-Term Care.

2.2. Data Sources

We identified all MedsCheck services from October 2014 to September 2018 based on the product identification number submitted to the Ontario Drug Benefit program (Table 2). Age and sex were identified from the Registered Persons Database. These data were linked using unique encoded identifiers and analyzed at ICES. Records with errors (death date prior to first service date, age <0, missing age or missing sex) were excluded, and duplicate claims in the same month were deleted. The total number of claims over the study period and the proportion of women and mean age of people receiving each service were summarized by MedsCheck type (MC, MCD, MCH or MCLTC) based on their first service date of each type.

Table 2. MedsCheck service administrative codes and reimbursement fees as of October 2016.

Service	PIN	Fee
MedsCheck (MC) [1]		
MC annual	93899979	$60 [1]
MC follow-up		
• Hospital discharge ≤ 2 weeks	93899981	
• Pharmacist decision	93899982	$25
• Physician or nurse practitioner referral	93899983	
• Planned hospital admission	93899984	
MedsCheck Diabetes (MCD) [2]		
MCD annual	93899988	$75
MCD follow-up	93899989	$25
MedsCheck at Home (MCH) [3]		
MCH annual	93899987	$150
MedsCheck Long Term Care (MCLTC) [4]		
MCLTC annual	93899985	$90
MCLTC quarterly	93899986	$50

[1] $50 before October 2016, eligible for residents with valid Ontario health card taking 3 or more chronic medications. [2] eligible for residents with diabetes and a valid Ontario health card. [3] eligible for residents with a valid Ontario health card and with diabetes or taking 3 or more chronic medications and unable to attend community pharmacy to have a MedsCheck service. [4] eligible for residents of licensed long-term care (LTC) homes with valid Ontario health card and taking 3 or more chronic medications. Pharmacist participation in annual and quarterly medication review services in LTC are required by legislation [13]. PIN: Product Identification Number.

2.3. Analytical Approach

The primary outcome was the monthly number of MedsCheck claims by MedsCheck service type (MC annual or follow-up, MCD annual or follow-up, MCH, MCLTC annual or quarterly). We used segmented regression to study trends in monthly service delivery, accounting for autocorrelation, non-stationarity and seasonality. Autocorrelation was examined in the data using the Durbin-Watson test [21] and autocorrelation plots, and stationarity was tested using the Dickey–Fuller test [22]. We specified our model to estimate level and trend changes in MedsCheck services in the 24-months pre-implementation and 24-months post-implementation periods, while accounting for seasonality, non-stationarity, and autocorrelation.

$$y = \beta_0 + \beta_1 \times time + \beta_2 \times implementation + \beta_3 \times time\ after + e \qquad (1)$$

Equation (1) Generalized equation (autoregressive and moving average terms not included).

Equation (1) includes the generalized equation, where y was the number of MedsCheck services delivered, β_0 the number of MedsCheck services delivered in October 2014, β1 the monthly trend in MedsCheck service delivery pre-implementation (October 2014–September 2016), β2 the immediate (level) change in monthly MedsCheck services after implementation (October 2016), β3 monthly trend in MedsCheck service delivery post-implementation (October 2016–September 2018), and *e* the random error. The pre-intervention level and linear trends were plotted using model coefficients, and the level and trend predicted values absent of the policy change were calculated for comparisons [23]. Analyses were completed using R 3.5.2 (Vienna, Austria) leveraging the Companion to Applied Regression (car) and Linear and Nonlinear Mixed Effects Models (nlme) packages [24].

3. Results

We identified 2,952,434 MC annual or follow-up services, 848,911 MCD annual or follow-up services, 103,591 MCH services, and 1,084,410 MCLTC annual or quarterly services over the 48-month study period, Table 3. The mean age at the first Medscheck service was lowest for MC (mean = 58.3,

SD = 17.3) and highest for MCLTC (mean = 82.6, SD = 10.5). Besides MCD, a higher proportion of MedsCheck service recipients were women.

Table 3. Demographic information of recipients and total number of Medscheck claims, by service type *.

Service Type	MedsCheck (Annual or Follow-Up)	MedsCheck Diabetes (Annual or Follow-Up)	MedsCheck at Home	MedsCheck Long Term Care (Annual or Quarterly)
Number of recipients	647,740	209,060	57,583	95,191
Number of Service claims	2,952,434	848,911	103,591	1,084,410
Age, mean (SD)	58.3 (17.3)	60.6 (14.2)	74.4 (16.4)	82.6 (10.5)
Women, %	52.4	45.2	62.1	64.0

* Age and sex for each service type based on first service date for that service type. SD = Standard Deviation.

In the two years pre-intervention, there was a significant monthly increase for MCD annual and MCH; yet, we observed a slight significant monthly decline for MCLTC annual (Table 4). A significant immediate and large drop in the monthly number of MedsCheck community services was seen after policy implementation (October 2016), ranging from 47% to 64% for MC (Figure 1), 71% to 83% for MCD (Figure 2), and was 55% for MCH (Figure 3). In contrast, a considerable smaller decline was seen for MCLTC, ranging from 9% to 14% (Figure 4). Gradual increases were seen over 24 months post-intervention period, yet remained 21% to 76% lower than predicted for MedsCheck services delivered in the community, particularly for MCD. In contrast, MCLTC services were similar to or exceeded predicted values by September 2018 (from a 5.1% decrease to a 3.5% increase).

Table 4. Results of interrupted time-series segmented regression models, October 2014–September 2018, with intervention (policy change) 1 October 2016.

Parameter	MedsCheck		MedsCheck Diabetes		MedsCheck at Home	MedsCheck Long Term Care	
	Annual	Follow-Up	Annual	Follow-Up		Annual	Quarterly
Total Claims	2,356,615	595,819	664,483	184,428	103,591	285,403	799,007
Monthly Claims							
• Minimum number	22,973	5768	4314	896	1151	4493	14,000
• Maximum number	70,554	21,353	23,443	8304	3482	7074	18,687
Results of Segmented Regression Models							
Baseline (October 2014), number (95% CI)	63,223 (60,452, 65,994)	16,698 (15,826, 17,771)	18,984 (18,069, 19,899)	6704 (6157, 7251)	2575 (2454, 2697)	6274 (6199, 6349)	16,848 (16,355, 17,341)
Pre-intervention slope, mean monthly claims (95%CI)	−173 (−373, 27)	67 (−1, 135)	81 (14, 149)	−19 (−57, 19)	15 (6, 24)	−6 (−11, −0.3)	18 (−17, 52)
Level Change at Intervention (October 2016)							
• Number of claims (95% CI)	−28,167 (−32,034, −24,302)	−11,854 (−13,205, −10,503)	−14,876 (−16,244, −13,508)	−5214 (−5942, −4487)	−1635 (−1828, −1442)	−929 (−1034, −825)	−1656 (−2348, −965)
• Relative percent change (95% CI)	−46.7 (−52.9, −40.4)	−64.3 (−71.1, −57.3)	−70.5 (−76.7, −64.3)	−83.2 (−94.3, −72.1)	−55.0 (−61.2, −48.8)	−14.4 (−16.0, −12.8)	−9.4 (−13.2, −5.6)
Post-intervention slope, mean monthly claims (95% CI)	521 (42, 1002)	52 (−110, 215)	139 (−17, 296)	16 (−77, 108)	22 (4, 40)	42 (30, 54)	50 (−33, 132)
Relative difference to forecast (September 2018), proportion (95% CI)	−21.0 (−27.7, −14.3)	−61.0 (−67.3, −54.5)	−58.9 (−64.6, −53.2)	−75.8 (−87.7, −63.8)	−44.9 (−50.4, −39.3)	3.5 (1.8, 5.1)	−5.1 (−8.8, −1.3)

CI: Confidence Interval.

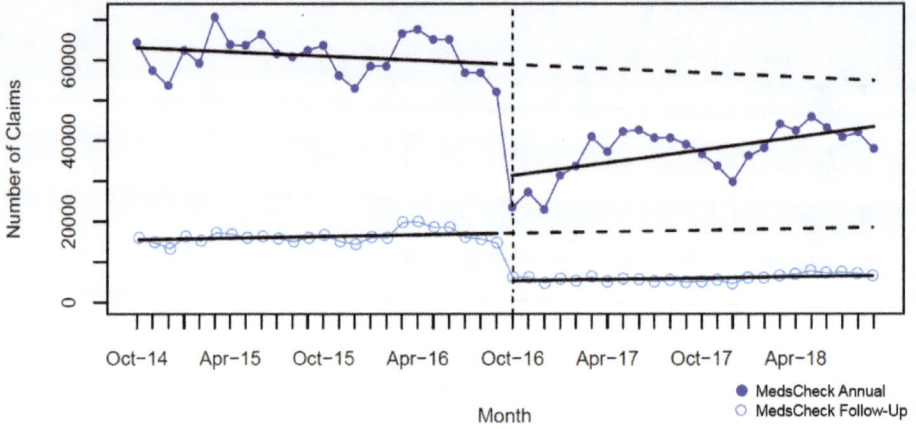

Figure 1. Monthly number of MedsCheck claims relative to the implementation of the October 2016 policy change (vertical dashed line = intervention date). The solid lines show fitted values from the interrupted time series model and the dashed lines show the predicted trend absent the policy change.

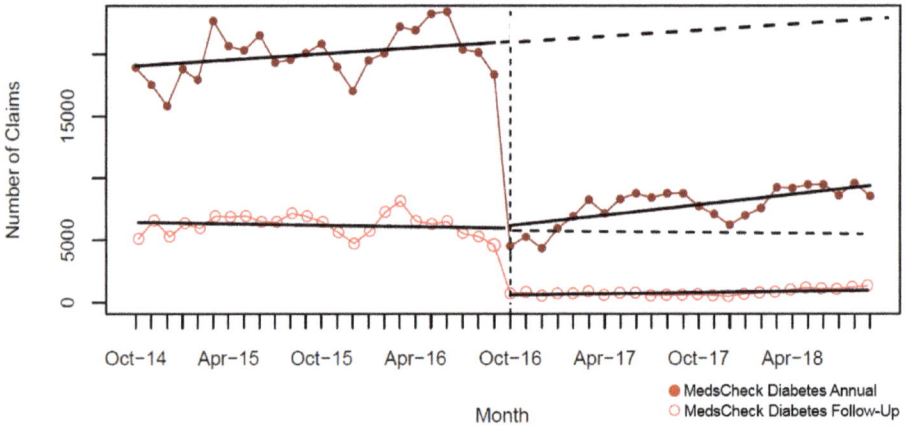

Figure 2. Monthly number of MedsCheck Diabetes claims relative to the implementation of the October 2016 policy change (vertical dashed line = intervention date). Solid lines show fitted values from the interrupted time series model, and dashed lines show the predicted trend absent the policy change.

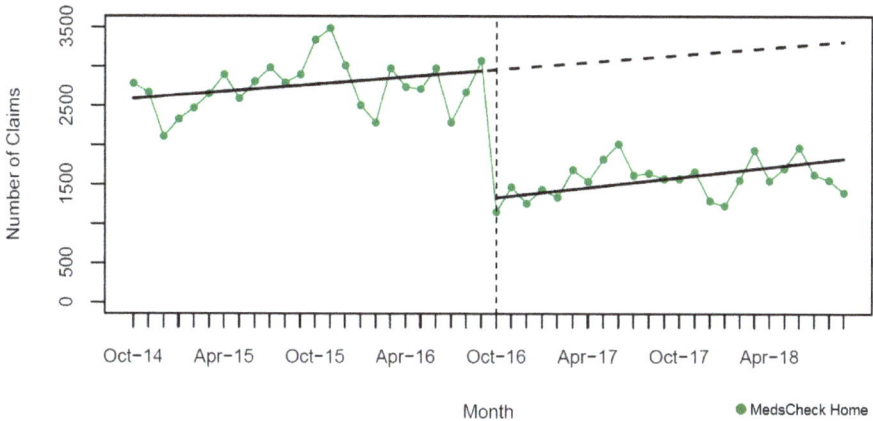

Figure 3. Monthly number of MedsCheck at Home claims relative to the implementation of the October 2016 policy change (vertical dashed line = intervention date). The solid lines show fitted values from the interrupted time series model and the dashed lines show the predicted trend absent the policy change.

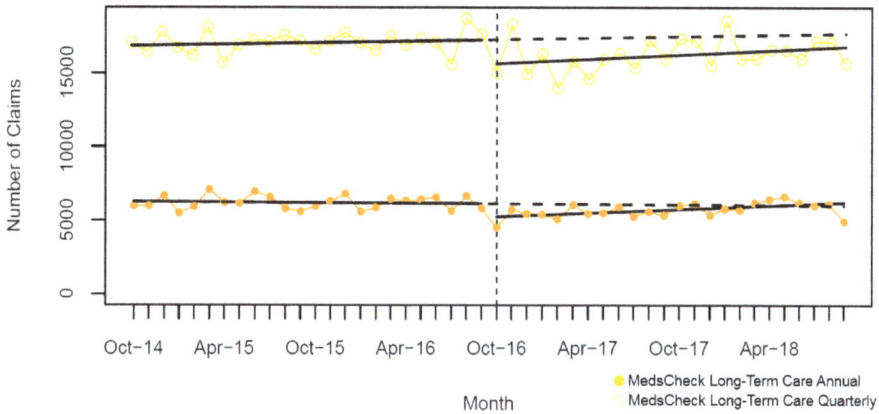

Figure 4. Monthly number of MedsCheck Long Term Care claims relative to the implementation of the October 2016 policy change (vertical dashed line = intervention date). The solid lines show fitted values from the interrupted time series model and the dashed lines show the predicted trend absent the policy change.

4. Discussion

MedsCheck was introduced in 2007 as a publicly funded medication review service for patients in the community taking multiple medications, and expanded in 2010 to target other high-risk groups (people with diabetes, home bound and residents of LTC homes) [12,13]. Despite the rapid uptake of these services [14,25], some concerns were raised about quality resulting from the lack of standard documentation or interprofessional coordination [26,27]. In response, the Ontario government consulted the Pharmacy Council—a body that includes representation from the Ontario Pharmacists Association and other stakeholders to provide advice and recommendations related to the pharmacy profession on the development of standardized documentation for the suite of MedsCheck services [28–30]. The added service components resulted in an immediate decline in the number of MedsCheck services delivered in the community. The decreases were generally sustained over the subsequent 2 years. However, there was minimal impact on the number of MedsCheck services delivered in LTC. Conceivably, the new requirements may have improved service quality. Future mixed method studies that consider the relative quantity and quality of MedsCheck services pre- and post-policy change are of high interest.

We found that MedsCheck follow-up services remained 61% (MC follow-up) to 76% (MCD follow-up) below predicted 24 months after the policy change. This may partially be attributed to pharmacies being ill-equipped to integrate routine follow-up services into their day-to-day workflow. Reminder systems to identify patients that may benefit from follow-up services are not routine. In addition, the use of part-time staffing and recent pharmacy funding cuts [31–34] may make it difficult for pharmacists to step away from their dispensing duties and reach out to patients to conduct a follow-up service [35]. Appointment-based pharmacy models are becoming more common in the United States and research demonstrates that appointment-based models improve the number of prescription fills, reduce the number of trips to the pharmacy, improve vaccination rates, and increase the proportion of patients adherent to therapy [36]. The significant impact of the policy change on the number of follow-up services in our study is concerning since monitoring and follow-up with patients on a consistent basis allows for the evaluation of drug therapy effectiveness and adherence, as well as identifying new drug therapy problems [37,38].

The impact on MCH is unexpected given the higher reimbursement ($150 MCH vs. $60 MC annual and $75 MCD annual). However, increased documentation and reporting on top of travel time and expense (i.e., fuel and parking) to visit a patient's home, medicine cabinet reviews and the removal of unused drugs for proper disposal at the pharmacy [39], may have made the service less feasible. MCH serves an important role in the community as it provides medication review to homebound individuals, typically frail and elderly or living in isolated settings. These patients are often more vulnerable to medication related errors [32]. Managing medications in the home setting is a unique challenge and MCH has the potential to educate patients and their families about medication therapy, and thus ultimately contribute to improved health and quality of life.

Of interest is the fact that the number of monthly MCLTC services changed minimally after the policy change and by 24 months after the policy change, services were above or close to the predicted values. The legislative requirement for annual and quarterly medication reviews together with existing infrastructure logically made MCLTC more feasible, i.e., much of the labour required in the community was already automated in LTC. MCLTC serves an important role since seniors make up about 12% of the Canadian population and 2.6% of all Canadian seniors reside in LTC [40].

Our study had a major strength by leveraging complete population-based level data submitted for reimbursement. However, we were limited in the ability to adjust monthly claims by the number of people eligible to receive MedsCheck services. Drug dispensation for chronic medication is increasing in Ontario [33], therefore, we expect the number of eligible patients for MC and MCH services to be increasing over time [41–43]. Similarly, the dispensation of diabetes medications is increasing, indicating an increase in the number of patients eligible to receive MCD services. Finally, the number of LTC beds increased by 2.5%, from 76,982 in 2016 to 78,872 in 2018 [40,44], thus, it is not surprising that we found a 3.5% higher than projected number of MCLTC annual services by September 2018. Despite our inability to adjust claims based on the number of eligible claimants, our results are population-based and compelling given the negligible to slow increase in the number of MedsCheck services over time.

Overall, the 2016 policy change that added several documentation and reporting requirements for MedsCheck services was well-intended to help standardize service delivery yet was followed by a substantive decline in the use of MedsCheck services. Although better standardization in program delivery is desirable, better understanding and pilot testing for feasibility before rolling-out new policies is encouraged. Indeed, leveraging a framework to optimize the design and implementation of new programs has the potential to improve success, value and impact [45,46]. On 25 April 2019, the Ontario Government announced a proposal to "modernize" the MedsCheck program with a sole focus on transitions in care and LTC [47]. The proposed change will lead to the discontinuation of all community MedsCheck services outside of transitions in care. The details have yet to be announced, yet we speculate that the termination of community-based MedsCheck programs relates to the keen interest by the new government to reduce the deficit, coupled with the decline in service delivery and lack of evidence of clinical benefit [48]. For example, the provincial budget notes that "Changing the way pharmacy fees are paid, including a tiered framework for drug mark-up fees; fees paid for filling prescriptions for long-term care home residents, and focusing the MedsCheck program on patients transitioning between health care settings, [will result] in annual savings of over \$140 million by 2021–22" [49]. The decision to continue supporting MedsCheck services around transitions in care may relate to evidence that supports the benefit of pharmacy-led medication review in reducing readmission rates among patients discharged from hospital [6,49–51].

The impact of the cuts to MedsCheck services on the quality of the Ontario healthcare system is in question, particularly related to the identification and resolution of drug therapy problems. A better understanding of the impact of changes in service delivery on different subgroups of patients is important. At minimum, we identified that patients with diabetes were possibly more impacted by the policy-change with proportionally fewer MCD completed post-policy changes compared to MCH or MC annual. However, it is also possible that pharmacies strategically switched from billing for MCD annual to billing for MC annual among patients with diabetes taking three or more medications to reduce some of the added paperwork specific to MCD. Further exploration of the use of MedsCheck services among patients with diabetes is of interest. Community pharmacists are increasingly involved in patient care through the conduct of regular medication review [52]. In particular, studies from Australia, Canada, the United Kingdom, and the United States show that diabetes education and support delivered through community pharmacies improves care and outcomes [53–55]. However, direct clinical evidence of the various types of medication review programs is scarce. There is a need for well-designed, rigorous studies with more sensitive and specific outcomes that consider the effect of community pharmacists' contributions to reviewing medications on improving health [52,56,57]. Our results provide compelling evidence of the immediate and sustained effects of policy decisions on the level of publicly reimbursed professional community pharmacy-delivered services. In the future, policy makers are encouraged to work closely with healthcare providers and fund research to provide evidence of the best mechanisms for the implementation of new pharmacy services [45,46]. Funding research to consider the benefits and harms of programs is also important instead of abruptly cancelling programs without considering how to better focus program delivery efforts.

Our research was limited in its ability to understand why the policy change had such a dramatic impact on the number of services delivered, or if the changes impacted the quality of service delivery. Future mixed-methods research is encouraged. Focus groups with community pharmacists will provide a deeper understanding of the experience of delivering MedsCheck services pre- and post-2016 policy change, and thus help uncover the reasoning behind reduced levels of service delivery. Survey research of MedsCheck program recipients may help to clarify the impact of changes on the quality of service delivery, as well as patient satisfaction and possible concerns about the decision by the Ontario government to cancel community services outside transitions in care. Finally, semi-structured interviews with policy decision makers and Pharmacy Council may help clarify the rationale behind the 2016 policy changes, as well as more recent changes to pharmacy practice in Ontario.

5. Conclusions

The Ontario government instituted a policy change October 2016 that abruptly changed reporting and documentation requirements that was followed by a sharp and sustained decline in community pharmacy MedsCheck services. Our findings highlight the importance of a well-executed implementation strategy for health policy changes to ensure the feasibility and sustainability of professional community pharmacy services. Despite consulting with pharmacy stakeholders through a formal Pharmacy Council to develop a more standardized service, the comprehensive documentation and interprofessional communication processes put in place were associated with a substantial

Pharmacy 2019, 7, 115

reduction in the number of professional services delivered. The immediate and profound reduction in service delivery speak to the importance and benefits of pilot studies that consider program feasibility in a real-world setting. Better understanding of the impacts of the 2016 policy change on the quality of MedsCheck services and outcomes, as well as potential harms from cancelling many of these services, are needed to inform future policy-decision making.

Author Contributions: Conceptualization, S.M.C.; data curation, L.Z. and S.M.C.; formal analysis, A.S.; funding acquisition, S.M.C. and L.D.; writing-original draft preparation, A.S. and S.M.C.; methodology, A.S., J.-M.G., L.D., S.M.C.; writing-review and editing, J.-M.G., L.D., L.M.C., L.Z. and S.M.C.; supervision, S.M.C.; project administration, S.M.C.

Funding: This research was funded by the Ontario Pharmacy Evidence Network (OPEN) grant from the Government of Ontario to S.M.C. A.S. is supported in part by the Leslie Dan Faculty of Pharmacy Dean's Fund. This study was supported by ICES, which is funded by an annual grant from the Ontario Ministry of Health and Long-Term Care (MOHLTC). The opinions, results and conclusions reported in this paper are those of the authors and are independent from the funding sources. No endorsement by ICES or the Ontario MOHLTC is intended or should be inferred. All analyses were completed at the ICES University of Toronto site, supported by the Leslie Dan Faculty of Pharmacy.

Acknowledgments: The authors thank Avery Loi and Qihang (Abby) Gan who completed undergraduate research project related to the MedsCheck long-term care (Avery) and MedsCheck at Home (Abby). In addition, Avery Loi assisted with summarizing documentation changes and provided details related to long-term care homes in Ontario. Authors also thank Maha Chaudhry, Nancy He and Natalia Konstantelos for assistance during manuscript revisions.

Conflicts of Interest: The authors declare no conflict of interest.

References

1. Ministry of Health and Long-Term Care. *Preventing and Managing Chronic Disease: Ontario's Framework*; Queen's Printer for Ontario: Toronto, ON, Canada, 2007.

2. Institute of Medicine Committee on Identifying and Preventing Medication Errors. *Preventing Medication Errors*; National Academies Press: Washington, DC, USA, 2007.

3. Sichieri, K.; Rodrigues, A.R.B.; Takahashi, J.A.; Secoli, S.R.; Nobre, M.R.C.; Mónica, M.A.; Julio, F.G. Mortality associated with the use of inappropriate drugs according Beers criteria: A systematic review. *Adv. Pharmacol. Pharm.* **2013**, *1*, 74–84.

4. Dormann, H.; Criegee-Rieck, M.; Neubert, A.; Egger, T.; Geise, A.; Krebs, S.; Schneider, T.; Levy, M.; Hahn, E.; Brune, K. Lack of awareness of community-acquired adverse drug reactions upon hospital admission: Dimensions and consequences of a dilemma. *Drug Saf.* **2003**, *26*, 353–362. [CrossRef]

5. Tsuyuki, R.T.; Beahm, N.P.; Okada, H.; Al Hamarneh, Y.N. Pharmacists as accessible primary health care providers: Review of the evidence. *Can. Pharm. J.* **2018**, *151*, 4–5. [CrossRef] [PubMed]

6. Schnipper, J.L.; Kirwin, J.L.; Cotugno, M.C.; Wahlstrom, S.A.; Brown, B.A.; Tarvin, E.; Kachalia, A.; Horng, M.; Roy, C.L.; McKean, S.C.; et al. Role of pharmacist counseling in preventing adverse drug events after hospitalization. *Arch. Intern. Med.* **2006**, *166*, 565. [CrossRef] [PubMed]

7. Knudsen, P.; Herborg, H.; Mortensen, A.R.; Knudsen, M.; Hellebek, A. Preventing medication errors in community pharmacy: Frequency and seriousness of medication errors. *Qual. Saf. Health Care* **2007**, *16*, 291–296. [CrossRef] [PubMed]

8. Roberts, A.S.; Benrimoj, S.I.; Chen, T.F.; Williams, K.A.; Hopp, T.R.; Aslani, P. Understanding practice change in community pharmacy: A qualitative study in Australia. *Res. Soc. Adm. Pharm.* **2005**, *1*, 546–564. [CrossRef] [PubMed]

9. Houle, S.K.D.; Carter, C.A.; Tsuyuki, R.T.; Grindrod, K.A. Remunerated patient care services and injections by pharmacists: An international update. *Can. Pharm. J.* **2019**, *152*, 92–108. [CrossRef] [PubMed]

10. Latif, A.; Pollock, K.; Boardman, H.F. Medicines use reviews: A potential resource or lost opportunity for general practice? *BMC Fam. Pract.* **2013**, *14*, 57. [CrossRef] [PubMed]

11. Martin, D.; Miller, A.P.; Quesnel-Vallée, A.; Caron, N.R.; Vissandjée, B.; Marchildon, G.P. Canada's universal health-care system: Achieving its potential. *Lancet* **2018**, *391*, 1718–1735. [CrossRef]

12. Ontario Ministry of Health and Long-Term Care. *The MedsCheck Program Guidebook*, 2nd ed.; Queen's Printer for Ontario: Toronto, ON, Canada, 2008.

13. Ontario Ministry of Health and Long-Term Care. *Professional Pharmacy Services Guidebook*, 3rd ed.; Queen's Printer for Ontario: Toronto, ON, Cananda, 2016.

14. MacCallum, L.; Consiglio, G.; MacKeigan, L.; Dolovich, L.; MacCallum, L. Uptake of community pharmacist-delivered MedsCheck diabetes medication review service in Ontario between 2010 and 2014. *Can. J. Diabetes* **2017**, *41*, 253–258. [CrossRef]

15. Government of Ontario. Central Forms Repository. Available online: http://www.forms.ssb.gov.on.ca/mbs/ssb/forms/ssbforms.nsf?opendatabase&ENV=WWE (accessed on 7 August 2019).

16. Canadian Council on Continuing Education in Pharmacy MedsCheck (Diabetes) Ontario. Available online: https://www.cccep.ca/pages/meds_check_diabetes_ontario.html (accessed on 17 May 2019).

17. Jandoc, R.; Burden, A.M.; Mamdani, M.; Lévesque, L.E.; Cadarette, S.M. Interrupted time series analysis in drug utilization research is increasing: Systematic review and recommendations. *J. Clin. Epidemiol.* **2015**, *68*, 950–956. [CrossRef] [PubMed]

18. Wagner, A.K.; Soumerai, S.B.; Zhang, F.; Ross-Degnan, D. Segmented regression analysis of interrupted time series studies in medication use research. *J. Clin. Pharm. Ther.* **2002**, *27*, 299–309. [CrossRef] [PubMed]

19. Bernal, J.L.; Cummins, S.; Gasparrini, A. Interrupted time series regression for the evaluation of public health interventions: A tutorial. *Int. J. Epidemiol.* **2016**, *46*, 348–355.

20. Lagarde, M. How to do (or not to do)... Assessing the impact of a policy change with routine longitudinal data. *Health Policy Plan.* **2012**, *27*, 76–83. [CrossRef] [PubMed]

21. Durbin, J.; Watson, G.S. Testing for serial correlation in least squares regression: I. *Biometrika* **1950**, *37*, 409–428. [PubMed]

22. Dickey, D.A.; Fuller, W.A. Distribution of the estimators for autoregressive time series with a unit root. *J. Am. Stat. Assoc.* **1979**, *74*, 427–431.

23. Zhang, F.; Wagner, A.K.; Soumerai, S.B.; Ross-Degnan, D. Methods for estimating confidence intervals in interrupted time series analyses of health interventions. *J. Clin. Epidemiol.* **2009**, *62*, 143–148. [CrossRef] [PubMed]

24. R Core Team. *R: A Language and Environment for Statistical Computing*; R Foundation for Statistical Computing: Vienna, Austria, 2013.

25. Dolovich, L.; Consiglio, G.; MacKeigan, L.; Abrahamyan, L.; Pechlivanoglou, P.; Rac, V.E.; Pojskic, N.; Bojarski, E.A.; Su, J.; Krahn, M.; et al. Uptake of the MedsCheck annual medication review service in Ontario community pharmacies between 2007 and 2013. *Can. Pharm. J.* **2016**, *149*, 293–302. [CrossRef]

26. Tracy, C.S.; Upshur, R.E.G. MedsCheck: An opportunity missed. *CMAJ* **2008**, *178*, 440. [CrossRef]

27. Pechlivanoglou, P.; Abrahamyan, L.; Mackeigan, L.; Consiglio, G.P.; Dolovich, L.; Li, P.; Cadarette, S.M.; Rac, V.E.; Shin, J.; Krahn, M. Factors affecting the delivery of community pharmacist-led medication reviews: Evidence from the MedsCheck annual service in Ontario. *BMC Health Serv. Res.* **2016**, *16*, 666. [CrossRef]

28. Ontario Public Drug Programs, Ministry of Health and Long-Term Care. Notice from the Executive Officer: MedsCheck Program Enhancements Standardization. Available online: http://www.health.gov.on.ca/en/pro/programs/drugs/opdp_eo/notices/exec_office_20160704.pdf (accessed on 20 May 2019).

29. Ontario Pharmacists Association. MedsCheck Program. Available online: https://www.opatoday.com/professional/resources/for-pharmacists/programs/medscheck (accessed on 2 July 2019).

30. Ontario Ministry of Health and Long-Term Care. MedsCheck Resources for Pharmacists—Health Care Professionals. Available online: http://www.health.gov.on.ca/en/pro/programs/drugs/medscheck/resources.aspx (accessed on 2 July 2019).

31. Ontario Ministry of Heath and Long-Term Care. Reforming Ontario's Drug System. Available online: https://news.ontario.ca/mohltc/en/2010/04/reforming-ontarios-drug-system.html (accessed on 29 May 2019).

32. Canadian Institute for Health Information; Canadian Patient Safety Institute; Institute for Safe Medication Practices Canada. *Medication Reconciliation in Canada: Raising the Bar*; Accreditiation Canada: Ottawa, ON, Canada, 2012.

33. Canadian Institute for Health Information. *Prescribed Drug Spending in Canada, 2018: A Focus on Public Drug Programs*; Accreditiation Canada: Ottawa, ON, Canada, 2018.

34. Strauss, M.; Howlett, K. Pharmacies Take Hit as Ontario Cuts Generic Drug Payments Again. Available online: https://www.theglobeandmail.com/globe-investor/pharmacies-take-hit-as-ontario-cuts-generic-drug-payments-again/article4170794/ (accessed on 29 May 2019).

35. Ministry of Finance; Ministry of Heath and Long-Term Care. Stronger, Healthier Ontario Act (Budget Measures). 2017. Available online: https://news.ontario.ca/mof/en/2017/05/stronger-healthier-ontario-act-budget-measures-2017.html (accessed on 29 May 2019).

36. Barnes, B.; Hincapie, A.L.; Luder, H.; Kirby, J.; Frede, S.; Heaton, P.C. Appointment-based models: A comparison of three model designs in a large chain community pharmacy setting. *J. Am. Pharm. Assoc.* **2018**, *58*, 156–162. [CrossRef] [PubMed]

37. MacCallum, L.; Dolovich, L. Follow-up in community pharmacy should be routine, not extraordinary. *Can. Pharm. J.* **2018**, *151*, 79–81. [CrossRef] [PubMed]

38. Cipolle, R.J.; Strand, L.M.; Morley, P.C. *Pharmaceutical Care Practice: The Patient-Centered Approach to Medication Management Services*, 3rd ed.; McGraw-Hill Education: New York, NY, USA, 2012.

39. Ontario Ministry of Health and Long Term Care. MedsCheck at Home. Available online: http://www.health.gov.on.ca/en/pro/programs/drugs/medscheck/medscheck_home.aspx (accessed on 23 May 2019).

40. Ontario Long Term Care Association. *This Is Long-Term Care 2018*; Ontario Long Term Care Association: Toronto, ON, Canada, 2018.

41. Lipscombe, L.L.; Hux, J.E. Trends in diabetes prevalence, incidence, and mortality in Ontario, Canada 1995–2005: A population-based study. *Lancet* **2007**, *369*, 750–756. [CrossRef]

42. Statistics Canada Diabetes, by Age Group and Sex (Number of Persons). Available online: http://www.statcan.gc.ca/tables-tableaux/sum-som/l01/cst01/health53a-eng.htm (accessed on 22 May 2018).

43. Ontario Ministry of Health and Long-Term Care. Diabetes: Strategies for Prevention. Available online: http://www.health.gov.on.ca/en/common/ministry/publications/reports/diabetes/diabetes.aspx (accessed on 22 May 2019).

44. Ontario Long Term Care Association. *This Is Long-Term Care 2016*; Ontario Long Term Care Association: Toronto, ON, Canada, 2016.

45. Craig, P.; Dieppe, P.; Macintyre, S.; Michie, S.; Nazareth, I.; Petticrew, M.; Medical Research Council guidance. Developing and evaluating complex interventions: The new Medical Research Council guidance. *BMJ* **2008**, *337*. [CrossRef] [PubMed]

46. Bleijenberg, N.; de Man-van Ginkel, J.M.; Trappenburg, J.C.A.; Ettema, R.G.A.; Sino, C.G.; Heim, N.; Hafsteindóttir, T.B.; Richards, D.A.; Schuurmans, M.J. Increasing value and reducing waste by optimizing the development of complex interventions: Enriching the development phase of the Medical Research Council (MRC) Framework. *Int. J. Nurs. Stud.* **2018**, *79*, 86–93. [CrossRef] [PubMed]

47. Drugs and Devices Division: Ministry of Health and Long-Term Care. Proposals to Establish More Efficient Pharmacy Reimbursement Policies. Available online: http://www.health.gov.on.ca/en/pro/programs/drugs/opdp_eo/notices/exec_office_20190426.pdf (accessed on 2 July 2019).

48. Office of the Auditor General of Ontario. *Chapter 3: Reports on Value-for-Money, 3.09: Ontario Public Drug Programs. 2017 Annual Report Volume 2*; Queen's Printer for Ontario: Toronto, ON, Canada, 2017.

49. Ministry of Finance. 2019 Ontario Budget|Chapter 3: Ontario's Fiscal Plan and Outlook. Available online: http://budget.ontario.ca/2019/chapter-3.html (accessed on 2 July 2019).

50. Al-Rashed, S.A.; Wright, D.J.; Roebuck, N.; Sunter, W.; Chrystyn, H. The value of inpatient pharmaceutical counselling to elderly patients prior to discharge. *Br. J. Clin. Pharmacol.* **2002**, *54*, 657–664. [CrossRef] [PubMed]

51. Jack, B.W.; Chetty, V.K.; Anthony, D.; Greenwald, J.L.; Sanchez, G.M.; Johnson, A.E.; Forsythe, S.R.; O'Donnell, J.K.; Paasche-Orlow, M.K.; Manasseh, C.; et al. A reengineered hospital discharge program to decrease rehospitalization: A randomized trial. *Ann. Intern. Med.* **2009**, *150*, 178–187. [CrossRef] [PubMed]

52. Nazar, H.; Nazar, Z.; Portlock, J.; Todd, A.; Slight, S.P. A systematic review of the role of community pharmacies in improving the transition from secondary to primary care. *Br. J. Clin. Pharmacol.* **2015**, *80*, 936–948. [CrossRef] [PubMed]

53. Ali, M.; Schifano, F.; Robinson, P.; Phillips, G.; Doherty, L.; Melnick, P.; Laming, L.; Sinclair, A.; Dhillon, S. Impact of community pharmacy diabetes monitoring and education programme on diabetes management: A randomized controlled study. *Diabet. Med.* **2012**, *29*, e326–e333. [CrossRef] [PubMed]

54. Krass, I.; Armour, C.L.; Mitchell, B.; Brillant, M.; Dienaar, R.; Hughes, J.; Lau, P.; Peterson, G.; Stewart, K.; Taylor, S.; et al. The Pharmacy diabetes care program: Assessment of a community pharmacy diabetes service model in Australia. *Diabet. Med.* **2007**, *24*, 677–683. [CrossRef]

55. Al Hamarneh, Y.N.; Charrois, T.; Lewanczuk, R.; Tsuyuki, R.T. Pharmacist intervention for glycaemic control in the community (the RxING study). *BMJ Open* **2013**, *3*, e003154. [CrossRef]

56. Kallio, S.E.; Kiiski, A.; Airaksinen, M.S.A.; Mäntylä, A.T.; Kumpusalo-Vauhkonen, A.E.J.; Järvensivu, T.P.; Pohjanoksa-Mäntylä, M.K. Community pharmacists' contribution to medication reviews for older adults: A systematic review. *J. Am. Geriatr. Soc.* **2018**, *66*, 1613–1620. [CrossRef]

57. Jokanovic, N.; Tan, E.C.; Sudhakaran, S.; Kirkpatrick, C.M.; Dooley, M.J.; Ryan-Atwood, T.E.; Bell, J.S. Pharmacist-led medication review in community settings: An overview of systematic reviews. *Res. Soc. Adm. Pharm.* **2017**, *13*, 661–685. [CrossRef]

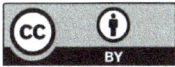

![pharmacy logo] *pharmacy*

MDPI

Article

Dispensing of Prescribed Medicines in Swiss Community Pharmacies-Observed Counselling Activities

Karen A. Maes [1], Jasmine A. Ruppanner [1], Tamara L. Imfeld-Isenegger [1], Kurt E. Hersberger [1]🔾,
Markus L. Lampert [1,2] and Fabienne Boeni [1,2,*]

[1] Pharmaceutical Care Research Group, University of Basel, 4056 Basel, Switzerland;
karen.a.maes@gmail.com (K.A.M.); j.ruppanner@gmail.com (J.A.R.); tamara.isenegger@unibas.ch (T.L.I.-I.);
kurt.hersberger@unibas.ch (K.E.H.); markus.lampert@unibas.ch (M.L.L.)
[2] Institute of Hospital Pharmacy, Solothurner Spitäler, 4600 Olten, Switzerland
* Correspondence: fabienne.boeni@unibas.ch; Tel.: +41-61-207-1426

Received: 22 November 2018; Accepted: 15 December 2018; Published: 21 December 2018

✓ check for updates

Abstract: Background: Patient counselling and addressing drug-related problems are the pharmacist's key activities to ensure the safe and effective use of medicines. This study aimed to describe the dispensing practice of prescribed medicines in daily community pharmacy practice and to identify factors influencing counselling provision; **Methods:** An observational study was conducted in community pharmacies in Basel, Switzerland. One master student in pharmacy performed non-participatory observations for one day at each of the participating community pharmacies. Patient characteristics, counselling content, additional activities, and pharmaceutical interventions were documented on a structured checklist; **Results:** 556 prescription encounters (PE) in 18 participating community pharmacies were observed (269 first prescriptions; 287 refill prescriptions). Patients were regular customers (n = 523, 94.1%) and 53.8 ± 23.4 years old. Counselling was provided to 367 (66.0%) customers on 2.9 ± 3.1 themes per PE. Factors influencing counselling were dispensing by the pharmacist, new customer, customer who did not refuse counselling, customer with a first prescription, with a prescription resulting in a pharmaceutical intervention, and a prescription filled by carers. During 144 PEs, 203 interventions were documented. Pharmacists proposed few additional activities and performed no cognitive pharmaceutical service; **Conclusions:** Our study quantified counselling and additional services at the dispensing of prescribed medicines and identified influencing factors on counselling provision at the patient, prescription, and pharmacy level.

Keywords: community pharmacy practice; dispensing; counselling; pharmaceutical intervention; pharmaceutical care; observation

---

1. Introduction

The Pharmaceutical Care Network Europe defined "Pharmaceutical Care" as "the pharmacist's contribution to the care of individuals in order to optimize medicines use and improve health outcomes provided" [1]. As part of pharmaceutical care, patient counselling and addressing drug-related problems (DRPs) are the pharmacist's key activities to ensure the safe and effective use of medicines [2,3]. Dispensing includes all activities between the reception of the patient with a prescription and the distribution of medicines to the patient with the provision of counselling [2]. During dispensing, community pharmacists help the patient to make the best use of prescribed medicines by providing written and oral information, responding to the patients' needs [4]. Patients have the opportunity to receive counselling and education about their health problems and medicines in several care situations, especially in community pharmacies at the time of dispensing prescribed medicines [5]. Patient counselling about their medicines (e.g., administration, risks and benefits) has been shown to be effective in improving medicine adherence [6,7], and in identifying DRPs [8]. In contrast, insufficient information about medicines can lead to patient non-adherence to drug therapy, and negative health outcomes [5].

The joint International Pharmaceutical Federation and World Health Organization (FIP/WHO) guidelines on Good Pharmacy Practice (GPP) describes the pharmacist's function of dispensing medicines concerning counselling as "providing advice to ensure that the patient receives and understands sufficient written and oral information to derive maximum benefit for the treatment" [3]. Prescription dispensing at the community pharmacy is an important contact point for patient counselling [8]. Patients regularly pick up their prescribed medicines in community pharmacies [9], hence pharmacy staff are usually one of the last healthcare providers who interact with patients prior to medication intake that has the possibility to counsel them [10,11]. The joint FIP/WHO GPP also suggests minimum national standards that should be established for this function.

In Switzerland, the Swiss Association of Pharmacists published standards for pharmaceutical counselling [12]. A service–based remuneration system for community pharmacies has been established since 2001 [13] and some cognitive pharmaceutical services are reimbursed by the health insurance [14,15]. The counselling provided during dispensing of prescribed medicines is remunerated by the 'drug check' (fixed fee for checking each dispensed item for dosage, interactions, risk factors, contraindications, misuse and for patient counselling, choice of optimal package size, etc.) and 'delivery check' (fixed fee for managing a patient record and checking medication history) [14]. In Switzerland, prescribers can issue refill prescriptions for up to 12 months for patients with ongoing long-term therapies, leaving responsibility for counselling and follow-up of therapy to the pharmacist.

The literature on counselling in community pharmacies described the communication between patient and provider about the medicines use [16,17] and compared counselling practice to guidelines [9,18]. A Swiss study described community staff-patient interactions with a focus on adherence [19]. This study showed that only 6.7% of all patient interactions comprised adherence counselling, and recommended an in-depth analysis of pharmacist-patient interaction. To the authors' knowledge, the full pattern of the daily community pharmacy practice, with all activities and interventions a prescription triggers at the time of dispensing in a setting with remuneration for prescription validation and counselling, have not been described yet.

For this reason, the aim of the study was to describe the observed dispensing practice of prescribed medicines at the counter in daily community pharmacy practice, focusing on counselling, pharmaceutical interventions and further activities, and to define factors influencing counselling provision.

2. Materials and Methods

A non-participatory observational study was conducted in community pharmacies in Basel, Switzerland to illustrate the observed dispensing practice of prescribed medicines. The Ethics Committee of Northwest and Central Switzerland approved the study on 25.01.2016 (EKNZ BASEC UBE-req. 16/00011).

2.1. Data Collection

Community pharmacies in Basel, Switzerland, were randomly invited for study participation, according to a prior study [19]. One master student in pharmacy observed pharmacy staff-customer interactions for one day at each participating community pharmacy in a non-participatory way during March and April 2016. The observation method was based on ad-hoc manual recording of exchanged information during a pharmacy staff-customer interaction and subsequent transcribing into quantitative information. After a quick briefing about the study, the pharmacy staff were neither actively involved in data collection, nor disturbed in their usual practice. At the dispensing of prescribed medicines, counselling content (information exchanged over the counter between customer and pharmacy staff), patient characteristics (e.g., age), pharmaceutical interventions (e.g., dose adjustment) and additional activities (offered and/or performed further activity/service) were documented on a structured checklist for each prescription encounter (PE). The non-participatory observer stood next to a pharmacy staff member and recorded a PE from the greeting of a customer (patient or carer) filling a prescription in the community pharmacy to closing salutations; where after, the next customer was observed. Customers were not informed about the study to avoid any influence on the counselling activities. Only communication in German was assessed.

The checklist was modified from a previous study [20] and enabled ad hoc coding of nine categories and 61 predefined themes: Patient characteristics (n = 4 themes), provider (pharmacy staff involved, n = 1), prescription (n = 7), counselling (n = 34), intervention (n = 2), physician contact (n = 2), situation (n = 6), and additional activities (n = 5). The category counselling, including 34 counselling themes that were considered as best practice, was derived from the 'drug check' of the Swiss service–based remuneration system [13], the literature [9,21,22], the requirement of the Omnibus Budget Reconciliation Act (OBRA, 1990) [23], the recommendations for internal audits of the Swiss Pharmacists' Association [24], and on expert discussions with five community pharmacists. Each theme was defined in a data dictionary to standardize the observer judgement. The checklist enabled to distinguish between the active and passive (e.g., asking and answering questions, respectively) involvement of the pharmacy staff and the customer during the PEs. After piloting, the checklist was refined and cases were discussed between the observer and two experienced community pharmacists to ensure data quality. An anonymized copy of the prescription and list of medicines from refill prescriptions of every observed patient were additionally collected and used to test the documentation of the observed PEs on consistency and plausibility. Observation time and characteristics of the pharmacies and their staff were recorded separately.

The systematic documentation of the pharmaceutical interventions, performed by pharmacists, were accomplished with aid of the Pharmacists' Documentation of Intervention in Seamless Care (PharmDISC) system. This classified the pharmaceutical interventions in different categories (problem, type of problem, cause, intervention, person involved, and the outcome of the intervention) [25].

At the end of the observation day, a semi-structured interview focusing the pharmacists' opinion on the counselling, triggers, facilitators, and barriers was conducted with one pharmacist per pharmacy. The results of the interviews are reported separately [26].

The main outcome measures were the number and type of themes covered in counselling, the factors influencing counselling provision, and number, frequency, and type of pharmaceutical interventions and additional activities.

2.2. Data Analysis

All coded data were quantified and analyzed descriptively using IBM SPSS Statistics for Windows, Version 24 (IBM Corp., Armonk, NY, USA). For the determination of factors influencing counselling provision, counselling theme ratios (sum of each counselling theme counselled divided by the number of medicines dispensed on one prescription) were expressed in percentage. A mean counselling theme ratio of 100% represented the maximum of all 34 possible counselling themes counselled for each dispensed medicine. A single factor variance–analysis, Chi-Square, Spearman, and Mann-Whitney U tests were used to compare variables. A p-value < 0.05 was considered statistically significant.

3. Results

Forty-nine community pharmacies were invited and 18 (37%) took part in the study. Reasons for participation refusal were no interest (n = 7), lack of staff resources (n = 4) or time (n = 4), holidays (n = 2), or unknown (n = 14). All pharmacies were located in the urban area of Basel. Thirteen were independent pharmacies (72.2%), while five belonged to a pharmacy chain (27.8%). They were on average open for 10.25 ± 1.5 h per day, and were observed during 8 ± 0.6 h (covering 78.0% of opening hours) per day, per pharmacy. The mean number of working staff per pharmacy at the observation day was 5.8 ± 2.6 (1.7 ± 0.9 pharmacists, 2.8 ± 1.7 pharmacy technicians, 1.0 ± 0.3 apprentices, and 0.2 ± 0.7 pharmacists in training).

During the total observation time of 145.5 h (18 observation days), 571 PEs (mean 31.2 ± 6.4 per pharmacy, range 22–45) were documented. Fifteen PEs had to be excluded because no medicines were dispensed (n = 9, e.g., drug not in stock), spoken language was foreign (n = 3), ordered medicines were picked-up (n = 1), physician-ordered medication (n = 1), or no documentation about the dispensed medicines was available (n = 1). A total of 556 PEs (269 first PEs and 287 refill PEs) constituted the sample for statistical analysis (each PE involved one customer).

Table 1 illustrates the characteristics of the patient, prescription, and provider. The number of medicines on a prescription varied from 1 to 25 (mean 3.2 ± 3.2).

Table 1. Patient, prescription, and provider characteristics.

Prescription Encounter	All	First	Refill
	(n = 556)	(n = 269)	(n = 287)
Patient			
Female n (%)	337 (60.6)	162 (60.2)	175 (61.0)
Mean age (years) ± SD	53.8 ± 23.4	45.6 ± 23.9	61.4 ± 20.2
Regular customer n (%)	523 (94.1)	242 (90.0)	281 (97.9)
Carer filled a prescription for a patient n (%)	105 (18.9)	62 (23.0)	43 (15.0)
Prescription			
Ambulatory n (%)	468 (84.2)	212 (78.8)	256 (89.2)
Hospital discharge n (%)	88 (15.8)	57 (21.2)	31 (10.8)
Provider of counselling *			
Pharmacist n (%)	149 (26.8)	70 (26.0)	79 (27.5)
Pharmacy technician n (%)	267 (48.0)	124 (46.1)	143 (49.8)
Apprentice n (%)	86 (15.5)	45 (16.7)	41 (14.3)
Pharmacist in training n (%)	13 (2.3)	8 (3.0)	5 (1.7)
Druggist n (%)	8 (1.4)	1 (0.4)	7 (2.4)
Combination of pharmacy staff n (%)	33 (5.9)	21 (7.8)	12 (4.2)

* Definition of the different counselling providers in Switzerland: Apprentice is a pharmacy technician in their 3-year training; pharmacist in training is a student in her/his last year of the master in pharmacy curriculum; druggist accomplished a 4-year apprenticeship.

3.1. Counselling

The PEs lasted on average 4.5 ± 3.0 min (first 5.2 ± 3.1; refill 3.9 ± 2.7, $p < 0.001$), ranging from 1.0 to 23.0 min. In 106 PEs (19.1%), pharmacy staff offered counselling by asking if the patient already knew about their medicines, or if they had any questions regarding the use of medicines (general closed questions that were intended to verify patient need for counselling). During the 556 PEs, counselling was provided to 367 (66.0%) customers, to 249 with first prescriptions and to 118 with refill prescriptions ($p < 0.001$). Of the 367 customers, 68 (12.2%) received counselling on one theme (out of the 34 counselling themes), 52 (9.4%) on two themes, 132 (36.0%) on three to five themes, and 115 (20.7%) on five to thirteen themes (Figure 1). Pharmacy staff did not provide any counselling in 169 refill PEs and in 20 first PEs. On average, customers were counselled on 2.9 ± 3.1 themes per PE (first PEs 4.9 ± 3.0; refill PEs 1.0 ± 1.7, $p < 0.001$). Customers who refused counselling (148 PEs [26.6%]; 51 first PEs vs. 97 refill PEs, $p < 0.001$) were significantly more often approached for counselling at first PEs than refill PEs (3.7 ± 2.9 theme vs. 1.7 ± 1.9, $p < 0.001$).

Table 2 presents the number of the counselling themes and their initiator. Pharmacy staff mainly counselled on administration (at first PEs 465 times and at refill PEs 73 times), dose (188; 46), and use (152; 36) and provided a label (189; 55). Of the 34 counselling themes, 8 were never addressed.

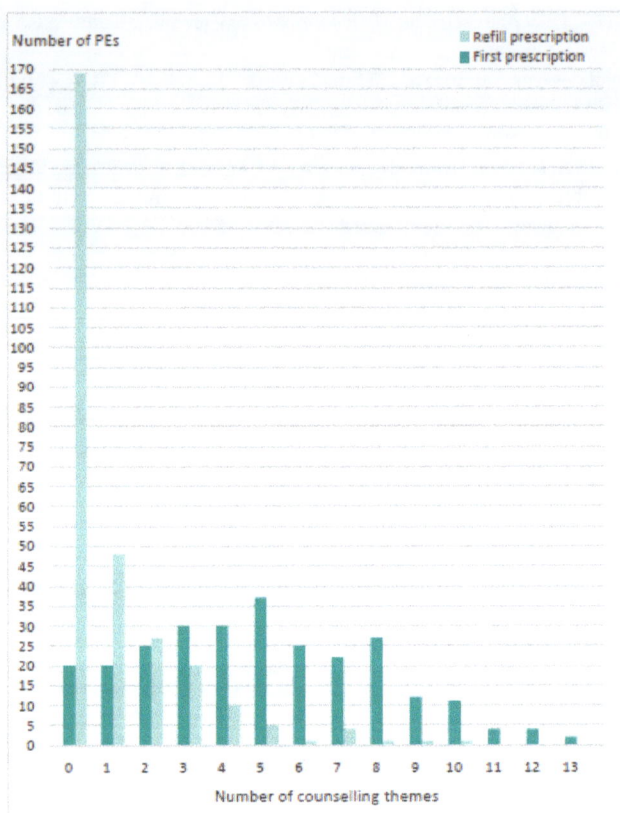

Figure 1. Number of themes counselled by the pharmacy staff per prescription encounter (PE) during first (n = 269) and refill PEs (n = 287).

3.1.1. Patient Involvement

The customer was actively involved in 193 (34.7%) of PEs by providing information (n = 149 PEs, 77.2%), asking questions (n = 25, 13.0%), or a combination of both (n = 19, 9.8%). During the first PEs, the customer was more often actively involved than during refill PEs (48.7% vs. 21.6%, $p < 0.001$).

3.1.2. Factors Influencing Counselling Provision

Table 3 presents factors influencing counselling provision at the patient, prescription and provider level. At patient level, new compared to regular customer received more counselling from the pharmacy staff (11.9% vs. 5.0%, $p < 0.001$) (Table 3). The type of prescription also influenced the rate of counselling. Significantly more counselling was provided with a first compared to a refill prescription (mean theme counselling ratio 9.6% vs. 1.5%, $p < 0.001$), and with prescriptions requiring a pharmaceutical intervention vs. no intervention (7.9% vs. 4.6%, $p < 0.001$). At the provider level, pharmacists provided counselling on significantly more themes per PE than pharmacy technicians (3.5 vs. 2.6 themes, $p < 0.05$), druggists (3.5 vs. 1.9, $p < 0.05$), and apprentices (3.5 vs. 2.3, $p < 0.05$). However, no significant difference between pharmacists and pharmacists in training (3.5 vs. 3.2, $p = 0.849$) or between pharmacists and a combination of a pharmacist and another staff member (3.5 vs. 4.2, $p = 0.194$) was seen.

The detection of factors influencing counselling provision allowed the illustration of counselling patterns (Figure 2).

Table 2. Number of counselling themes and their initiators. Bold p-values are considered as statistically significant ($p < 0.05$).

Counselling Themes (n = 34)	First Prescription Encounters (n = 269)					Refill Prescription Encounters (n = 287)					p-Value (First vs. Refill Prescription Encounters of Themes Counselled by Pharmacy Staff)
	Theme Counselled (Pharmacy Staff)	Theme Discussed (Pharmacy or Customer)	Pharmacy Staff as Initiator	Customer as Initiator	Initiator Not Known	Theme Counselled (Pharmacy Staff)	Theme Discussed (any Person)	Pharmacy Staff as Initiator	Customer as Initiator	Initiator Not Known	
	n (%)	n (%)	n (%)	n (%)	n (%)	n (%)	n (%)	n (%)	n (%)	n (%)	
Anamnesis (total)	100 (37.2)	101 (37.5)	99 (98.0)	1 (1.0)	1 (1.0)	8 (2.8)	9 (3.1)	8 (88.9)	1 (11.1)	0 (0)	**<0.001**
1. Medicines	34 (12.6)	35 (13.0)	33 (94.3)	1 (2.9)	1 (2.9)	3 (1.0)	4 (1.4)	3 (75.0)	1 (25.0)	0 (0)	**<0.001**
2. Diseases	9 (3.3)	9 (3.3)	9 (100)	0 (0)	0 (0)	0 (0)	0 (0)	0 (0)	0 (0)	0 (0)	**0.001**
3. Allergy	34 (12.6)	34 (12.6)	34 (100)	0 (0)	0 (0)	3 (1.0)	3 (1.0)	3 (100)	0 (0)	0 (0)	**<0.001**
4. Pregnancy/lactation	8 (3.0)	8 (3.0)	8 (100)	0 (0)	0 (0)	0 (0)	0 (0)	0 (0)	0 (0)	0 (0)	**0.003**
5. Family anamnesis	0 (0)	0 (0)	0 (0)	0 (0)	0 (0)	0 (0)	0 (0)	0 (0)	0 (0)	0 (0)	-
6. Lifestyle	0 (0)	0 (0)	0 (0)	0 (0)	0 (0)	0 (0)	0 (0)	0 (0)	0 (0)	0 (0)	-
7. Clinical parameter	15 (5.6)	15 (5.6)	15 (100)	0 (0)	0 (0)	2 (0.7)	2 (0.7)	2 (100)	0 (0)	0 (0)	**0.001**
8. Dose	188 (69.9)	191 (71.0)	180 (94.2)	8 (4.2)	3 (1.6)	46 (16.0)	50 (17.4)	46 (92.0)	4 (8.0)	0 (0)	**<0.001**
Drug use (total)	152 (56.5)	153 (56.9)	143 (93.5)	9 (5.9)	1 (0.6)	36 (12.5)	38 (13.2)	36 (94.7)	2 (5.7)	0 (0)	**<0.001**
9. Use	129 (48.0)	130 (48.3)	121 (93.1)	8 (6.2)	1 (0.8)	34 (11.8)	36 (12.5)	34 (94.4)	2 (5.6)	0 (0)	**<0.001**
10. Duration of use (single application)	14 (5.2)	14 (5.2)	13 (92.9)	1 (7.1)	0 (0)	1 (0.3)	1 (0.3)	1 (100)	0 (0)	0 (0)	**<0.001**
11. Instruction/training of use	9 (3.3)	9 (3.3)	9 (100)	0 (0)	0 (0)	1 (0.3)	1 (0.3)	1 (100)	0 (0)	0 (0)	**0.009**
Drug administration (total)	465 (172.9)	475 (176.6)	437 (92.0)	26 (5.5)	13 (2.7)	73 (25.4)	80 (27.9)	69 (86.3)	8 (10.0)	3 (3.7)	**<0.001**
12. Frequency of administration	159 (59.1)	163 (60.6)	154 (94.5)	6 (3.7)	3 (1.8)	34 (11.8)	37 (12.9)	33 (89.2)	3 (8.1)	1 (2.7)	**<0.001**
13. Therapy duration	90 (33.5)	91 (33.8)	85 (93.4)	4 (4.4)	2 (2.2)	13 (4.5)	13 (4.5)	11 (84.6)	1 (7.7)	1 (7.7)	**<0.001**
14. Timing of administration	120 (44.6)	125 (46.5)	111 (88.8)	6 (4.8)	8 (6.4)	20 (7.0)	24 (8.4)	19 (79.2)	4 (16.7)	1 (4.2)	**<0.001**
15. Modality of administration	96 (35.7)	97 (36.1)	87 (89.7)	10 (10.3)	0 (0)	6 (2.1)	6 (2.1)	6 (100)	0 (0)	0 (0)	**<0.001**
Written information											
16. Label	189 (70.3)	189 (70.3)	188 (99.5)	1 (0.5)	0 (0)	55 (19.2)	55 (19.2)	55 (100)	0 (0)	0 (0)	**<0.001**
17. Flyer	8 (3.0)	8 (3.0)	8 (100)	0 (0)	0 (0)	0 (0)	0 (0)	0 (0)	0 (0)	0 (0)	**0.003**
18. Schedule	0 (0)	0 (0)	0 (0)	0 (0)	0 (0)	0 (0)	0 (0)	0 (0)	0 (0)	0 (0)	-
19. Document	0 (0)	0 (0)	0 (0)	0 (0)	0 (0)	0 (0)	0 (0)	0 (0)	0 (0)	0 (0)	-
20. Indication	108 (40.1)	111 (41.3)	98 (88.3)	11 (9.9)	2 (1.8)	21 (7.3)	25 (8.7)	20 (80)	5 (20)	0 (0)	**<0.001**
21. Effect	51 (19.0)	52 (19.3)	49 (94.2)	3 (5.8)	0 (0)	7 (2.4)	7 (2.4)	6 (85.7)	1 (14.3)	0 (0)	**<0.001**
22. Mechanism of action	1 (0.4)	1 (0.4)	1 (100)	0 (0)	0 (0)	0 (0)	0 (0)	0 (0)	0 (0)	0 (0)	0.48
23. Benefit/purpose of therapy	3 (1.1)	4 (1.5)	3 (75)	1 (25.0)	0 (0)	8 (2.8)	9 (3.1)	7 (77.8)	2 (22.2)	0 (0)	0.226
24. Adverse effect	18 (6.7)	18 (6.7)	16 (88.9)	1 (5.6)	1 (5.6)	6 (2.1)	7 (2.4)	6 (85.7)	1 (14.3)	0 (0)	**0.011**
25. Red flag	3 (1.1)	3 (1.1)	3 (100)	0 (0)	0 (0)	0 (0)	0 (0)	0 (0)	0 (0)	0 (0)	0.11
26. Drug-drug interaction	17 (6.3)	18 (6.7)	13 (72.2)	5 (27.8)	0 (0)	4 (1.4)	4 (1.4)	4 (100)	0 (0)	0 (0)	**0.003**
27. Contraindication	1 (0.4)	1 (0.4)	1 (100)	0 (0)	0 (0)	0 (0)	0 (0)	0 (0)	0 (0)	0 (0)	0.48
Appropriate action in case of:											
28. Missed dose	0 (0)	0 (0)	0 (0)	0 (0)	0 (0)	0 (0)	0 (0)	0 (0)	0 (0)	0 (0)	-
29. Underdose	0 (0)	0 (0)	0 (0)	0 (0)	0 (0)	0 (0)	0 (0)	0 (0)	0 (0)	0 (0)	-
30. Overdose	0 (0)	0 (0)	0 (0)	0 (0)	0 (0)	0 (0)	0 (0)	0 (0)	0 (0)	0 (0)	-
31. Storage	5 (1.9)	5 (1.9)	5 (100)	0 (0)	0 (0)	0 (0)	0 (0)	0 (0)	0 (0)	0 (0)	**0.025**
32. Information transfer	0 (0)	0 (0)	0 (0)	0 (0)	0 (0)	0 (0)	0 (0)	0 (0)	0 (0)	0 (0)	-
33. Adherence	12 (4.5)	12 (4.5)	12 (100)	0 (0)	0 (0)	23 (8.0)	23 (8.0)	22 (95.7)	1 (4.3)	0 (0)	0.116
34. Self-/monitoring	0 (0)	0 (0)	0 (0)	0 (0)	0 (0)	1 (0.3)	1 (0.3)	1 (100)	0 (0)	0 (0)	-

Table 3. Factors influencing counselling provision. Bold *p*-values are statistically significant (*p* < 0.05).

Variable 1	Mean Ratio of PEs with at Least One Counselling Theme [%] Average ± SD	Variable 2	Mean Counselling Theme Ratio [%] Average ± SD	*p*-value
Patient				
Regular customer [n = 523]	5.0 ± 6.1	New customer [n = 33]	11.9 ± 6.3	**<0.001**
Female patient [n = 337]	5.2 ± 6.1	Male patient [n = 219]	5.8 ± 6.5	0.436
Counselling not refused [n = 408]	6.2 ± 6.7	Counselling refused [n = 148]	3.5 ± 4.6	**0.001**
Prescription filled by the patient [n = 451]	5.1 ± 6.2	Prescription filled by the carer [n = 105]	6.7 ± 6.7	**0.026**
Prescription				
First prescription [n = 269]	9.6 ± 6.2	Refill prescription [n = 287]	1.5 ± 3.1	**<0.001**
Ambulatory prescription [n = 468]	5.3 ± 6.2	Discharge prescription [n = 83]	6.7 ± 6.7	0.088
Prescription with interventions [n = 144]	7.9 ± 6.6	No intervention [n = 412]	4.6 ± 6.0	**<0.001**
Hand written prescription [n = 247]	7.5 ± 6.7	Printed prescription [n = 117]	7.0 ± 6.3	0.599
All medicines directly dispensed [n = 495]	5.7 ± 6.4	Some medicines picked up later [n = 61]	3.2 ± 4.6	**0.004**
>1 medicine dispensed [n = 290]	5.7 ± 5.9	1 medicine dispensed [n = 266]	5.2 ± 6.7	**0.027**
>1 medicine on prescription [n = 353]	5.0 ± 5.8	1 medicine on prescription [n = 182]	6.5 ± 7.2	0.129
Provider of counselling				
Pharmacist [n = 149]	6.3 ± 6.6	Pharmacy technician [n = 267]	5.0 ± 6.1	**0.018**
		Druggist [n = 8]	2.4 ± 6.8	**0.019**
		Apprentice [n = 86]	4.6 ± 5.4	**0.045**
		Combination of a pharmacist and a other staff member [n = 33]	7.6 ± 7.8	0.476
		Pharmacist in training [n = 13]	6.7 ± 5.7	0.651
Situation				
Stress factor by waiting customers [n = 89]	6.5 ± 6.6	No waiting customer [n = 467]	5.3 ± 6.2	0.059
Silent environment [n = 500]	5.4 ± 6.4	Loud environment [n = 56]	5.6 ± 5.9	0.582
No disruption during counselling [n = 550]	5.5 ± 6.3	Disruption during counselling [n = 6]	3.9 ± 4.8	0.610
No communication problem [n = 548]	5.4 ± 6.3	Communication problem [n = 8]	6.9 ± 6.5	0.525

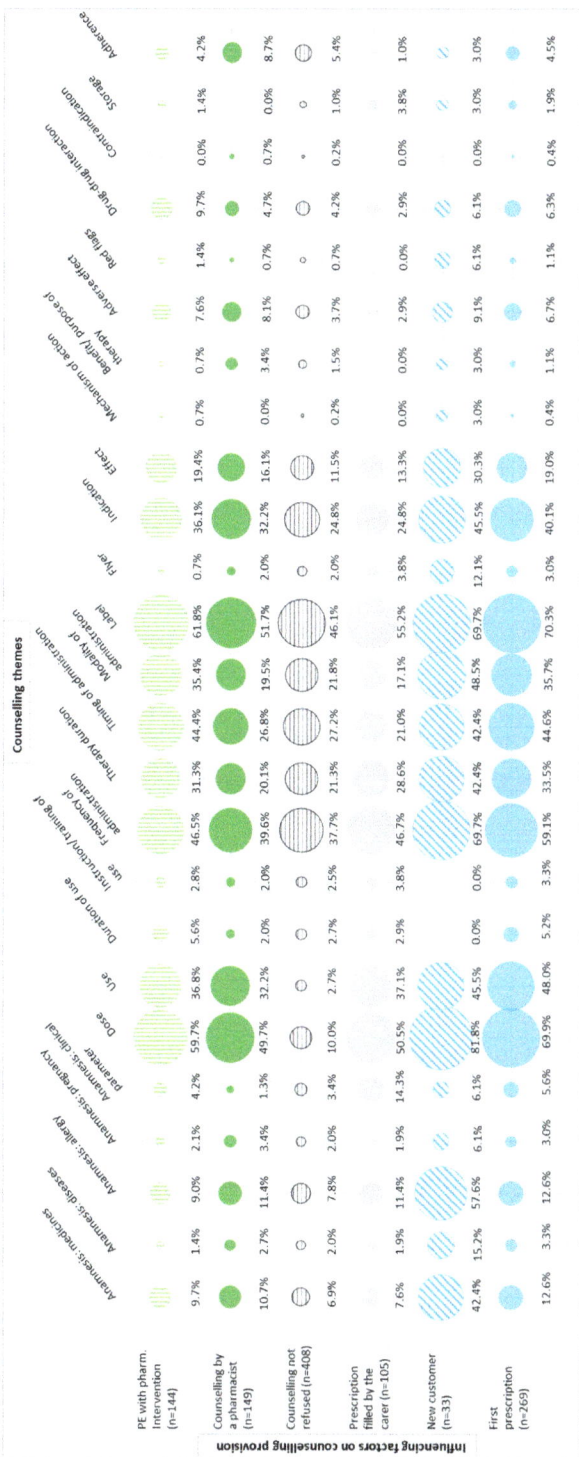

Figure 2. Patterns of counselling: Frequency of counselling themes as a function of the factors influencing counselling provision. These factors were selected in terms of significance. The size of the circle represents its frequency with respect to the factors influencing counselling provision. The color and the pattern of the circle help to distinguish the different factors.

3.2. Pharmaceutical Interventions

During all 18 observation days, 203 pharmaceutical interventions were documented at 144 PEs (intervention rate 25.9%). Interventions occurred significantly more at first PEs (n = 103) vs. refill PEs (n = 41; $p < 0.001$), with an average per prescription of 1.4 ± 0.7 (range 1–4). Pharmacists' intervention mainly included drug substitution (n = 89, 43.8%), clarification of information (n = 64, 31.5%), and adjustment of the package size/quantity (n = 39, 19.2%). Table 4 represents the most frequent pharmaceutical interventions. The cause was technical for 180 pharmaceutical interventions (88.7%) and clinical for 23 pharmaceutical interventions (11.3%). Active interaction with the prescriber was necessary in 11 (5.4%) pharmaceutical interventions, whereas the involvement of the patient was observed in 127 (62.6%) pharmaceutical interventions and neither the prescriber nor the patient was involved in 65 (32.0%) pharmaceutical interventions.

Table 4. The most frequently observed pharmaceutical interventions, their cause and type of problem (documented with the PharmDISC system).

Intervention	Cause of Intervention	Type of Problem	n (%)
Total interventions			203 (100.0)
	Technical		180 (88.7)
Clarification/addition of information	Incomplete/unclear prescription	Manifest, reactive	55 (27.1)
Substitution (generic)	Financial burden	Manifest, reactive	49 (24.1)
Substitution	Prescribed drug not available	Manifest, reactive	31 (15.3)
Adjustment of package size/quantity	Financial burden	Manifest, reactive	18 (8.9)
Adjustment of package size/quantity	Financial burden	Manifest, reactive	9 (4.4)
	Clinical		23 (11.3)
Adjustment of package size/quantity	Concerns about the treatment	Manifest, reactive	3 (1.5)
Substitution	No concordance with guidelines, only suboptimal therapy possible	Potential, preventive	2 (1)
Substitution	Concerns about the treatment	Manifest, reactive	2 (1)
Therapy stopped/no delivery	Drug-drug interaction	Potential, preventive	2 (1)
In-depth counselling of patient	Drug-drug interaction	Potential, preventive	2 (1)

The number of pharmaceutical interventions per PE increased with the frequency of counselled themes per PE (correlation r = 0.270, $p < 0.001$) and with the frequency of dispensed medicines per PE (r = 0.236, $p < 0.001$). The number of pharmaceutical interventions per PE did not increase with the age of the patients (r = -0.018, $p = 0.687$) or the work experience of the pharmacy staff (r = 0.032, $p = 0.470$).

3.3. Additional Activities

Of all PEs, 10 PEs resulted in a phone call with the physician, five in a referral to the physician, one PE in a consultation in a separate room, and one PE in a refusal of dispensing. The pharmacists reconstituted seven suspensions, and offered three follow-ups. Non-pharmacological counselling (e.g., balanced nutrition) was provided at 11 PEs (11 first, 0 refill, $p < 0.001$).

4. Discussion

This observation study allowed depicting the dispensing practice of prescribed medicines at the counter of Swiss community pharmacies and analysing factors influencing counselling provision.

4.1. Counselling

Counselling was provided to 66.0% of the customers receiving prescribed medicines, which is slightly more than in a previous observation study (57.3%) performed in Switzerland in 2010 [19]. A review of worldwide counselling practices on prescribed medicines reported counselling rates from 12% to 100%, when observational methods were used [17]. In this study, the customers were counselled on up to 13 out of the 34 predefined counselling themes per PE. However, in real daily practice, 34 different themes cannot be counselled at one PE, as this would overload the patient. Staff members have to decide on priorities during the interaction with the patient. With refill prescriptions, additional themes can be counselled at following visits. Written information in the form of an individualized label to reinforce verbal communication was provided in 43% of the PEs.

A quarter of customers refused counselling and one-third of the customers did not receive any counselling. The study design did not take into account the long-term relationship between the pharmacy staff and the patient as a regular customer, with pre-existing counselling provided at a prior PE, which could lead to PEs without observed counselling. This is in line with what was observed previously: New customers received more counselling than regular customers. Nevertheless, this study depicted how the patient received the counselling at the counter. The findings revealed that pharmacists were involved in direct patient contact at the counter in only a quarter of all PEs. Pharmacists' activities, such as drug interaction-check and investigating medication history, have often been done in the back office, and are neither visible, nor communicated to the customer. If pharmacy staff were more transparent and better communicated their activities to the customer during dispensing, this could improve trust and collaboration.

The themes of counselling were more product-centered (e.g., dose, administration) than patient-centered (e.g., adherence, therapy benefit), similar to the findings of other studies [17,19,27]. Indeed, the counselling patterns of Figure 2 illustrate the gaps in patient-centered counselling. Especially for patients refilling prescribed medicines, low counselling ratios were observed. Not addressing the patient-centered counselling themes at refill might be interpreted as a missed opportunity to improve patients' adherence to their drug therapy. It is known that patients often stop taking their newly prescribed medicines in the first months of therapy (medication non-persistence), because of concerns (e.g., adverse effect) and lack of perceived need (e.g., poor understanding of medicines/disease) [28,29]. To address adherence issues, remunerated cognitive pharmaceutical services (e.g., 'Polymedication check', 'Adherence fee') were introduced in Switzerland since 2010 [14], but during the observation, none of these services were performed.

Pharmacy staff–customer interactions have been observed before and the findings have been similar internationally. Although countries and guidelines adopted pharmaceutical care as one of the key roles for community pharmacist, they are reported to be delivered only in a limited way [21,30–33]. Counselling rates are usually rather low, and the content is mostly about the medication (product-centered) [16,17,19]. Patient-centered issues are seldom discussed in a pharmacy staff-customer interaction and pharmaceutical care services are not provided to their full potential [32]. Our study confirms these results although in Switzerland, counselling about prescribed medicines and certain pharmaceutical care services are remunerated by the health insurance. To our knowledge, this is the first study observing the daily practice of dispensing prescribed medicines at the community pharmacy under these conditions. Another possible barrier is the non-conformity of roles and expectations between pharmacy staff and customers [34]. Educational interventions have shown success in improving counselling by pharmacists [35].

4.1.1. Patient Involvement

This observational study showed that the pharmacy staff were the main initiators of discussion, confirming the findings of another observational Dutch study, which videotaped their encounters [9]. A systematic review revealed a mainly passive role of the patient in conversations with healthcare providers [36], even though guidelines encourage interactive communication [5]. This is in line with this observational study; customers asked only a few questions, although these questions might give the pharmacy staff the opportunity to tailor information on patients' needs [4]. Lack of privacy at the counter [37], lack of interest in pharmacy counselling [38–40], and patients' underestimation of pharmacists' role in healthcare are possible reasons for patients' barriers in asking questions [27,34,41]. Nevertheless, the patients' initiative would be important, knowing that the outcome of a dialogue depends on the person who initiates the discussion [42]. Indeed, in patient-centered care, the patient always comes first, and their needs should drive the PE [43]. Therefore, the patient should be encouraged in PEs to be more active in the discussion. Furthermore, the findings revealed that pharmacy staff sometimes offered counselling only by asking general closed questions (e.g., do you know this medicine already?), limiting the counselling provision and the patient involvement, and consequently not taking into account the patients' needs. It has been shown that the counselling provided to the patients does not fulfil their information needs [44]. A study exploring advice-giving behavior in British community pharmacies reported that the counselling was mostly based on product use, and that the customers wished information about the drug's effectiveness, while the pharmacists provided information on drug safety. The authors proposed a protocol to guide pharmacy staff, including the customers' perspective [27]. To meet patient needs, the pharmacists should better listen to the patients' problems and provide individualized counselling [45].

4.1.2. Factors Influencing Counselling Provision

Counselling was not equally provided, suggesting that pharmacy staff use different levels of counselling at PEs. If extended counselling at each first and refill PE is not possible in daily practice, pharmacy staff should target counselling for specific situations. However, it is important to notice that each PE offers to the pharmacist an opportunity to interact with the patient and hence to detect DRPs and patients' concerns. The study findings highlight some factors influencing counselling provision at the patient, prescription and provider level. These indicators could help in prioritizing prescriptions needing in-depth counselling.

Patient level

- New customers were more likely to receive counselling from the pharmacy staff than regular customers. The counselling patterns revealed that the pharmacy staff performed more likely an anamnesis (medicine, diseases, and allergy) with the new customers, while the counselling patterns of the other factors influencing counselling provision were comparable (Figure 2). Similarly, to a review [17], the pharmacy staff mainly counselled on administration, dose and use.
- Customers who did not refuse counselling received more counselling. Refusing counselling did not mean that the patient did not receive any counselling, but such refusal is known to be an important barrier for the provision of counselling [19]. Lack of patient interest is a common phenomenon during counselling in community pharmacy [38,39], up to 41–63% patients decline a counselling offer [33,40], leading to low counselling ratios [40].
- Carers who filled a prescription for a patient received more information on the prescribed medicines than the patients themselves. Possibly, the carer was not present at the consultation with the prescriber and did not receive information on the patient's drug therapy.

Prescription level

- Customers with a first prescription received more counselling than customers with a refill prescription. In a first PE, it is important to ensure that the patient receives the knowledge for using their medicines correctly [19]. Appropriate drug use is ensured by counselling on therapy duration, dosage, and optimal timing of drug intake [46]. At refill PE, pharmacists could suppose that patients with chronic medication were already informed about their use [47]. They could also be regular customers needing less clarification. Previous studies showed that pharmacy staff classified the communication with patients to be more difficult during refill PE than during the first PE [48,49]. It has been shown that patients' expectations towards counselling are different in first and refill PEs. More interest by patients during a first PE may facilitate more extensive counselling [40]. This is in line with the study findings: During the first PEs, patients showed more interest in counselling than during refill PEs, as two thirds of the counselling refusals were observed during refill PEs.
- Prescriptions that resulted in a pharmaceutical intervention required more counselling than prescriptions without any intervention, because interventions imply to inform the patient about

the DRP, and to involve him/her in solving it. Additionally, these prescriptions must involve the pharmacist, who is known to give more counselling than other pharmacy staff member.

Provider level

- Pharmacists provided more counselling to customers than other pharmacy staff members. Other studies reported this factor as well [19,47,50]. A reason could be that pharmacists have a larger knowledge about drug therapy. Counselling should be driven by the patient and the prescription, not by the randomly allocated pharmacy staff member.

Counselling quality can be improved by developing counselling skills through education (e.g., role-play with standardized patients [51]), patient-centered communication (concordance of provided care with patients' preferences and needs) [52,53], the implementation of established guidelines on Good Pharmacy Practice [3], and continuing evaluation with feedback (e.g., mystery shopper).

4.2. Pharmaceutical Interventions

The study findings confirm that the community pharmacists were effective in detecting, preventing, and solving DRPs [4,54]. By intervening during dispensing, pharmacists contributed to the safe, appropriate, and cost-effective use of drugs. Individual judgement and professional knowledge of the pharmacists and collaboration with the patient, carer, or prescriber was needed to respond satisfactorily to the patient needs. The rate of pharmaceutical interventions (25.9%) was comparable to a German study describing DRPs at time of dispensing prescribed medicines, which reported an intervention rate of 18.0% [54].

4.3. Additional Activities

Pharmacy staff proposed only a few additional activities during PE, missing the opportunity to offer additional care and ensure continuity of care and optimize patient therapy and health outcomes. Notably, each refill prescription is an opportunity for the pharmacists to offer follow-up and further cognitive pharmaceutical services. Although such services are remunerated in Switzerland [14], none of the pharmacists proposed a medication review (e.g., 'polymedication check') or an adherence aid (e.g., 'adherence fee') to the customer during the observation time of 18 days. However, they often performed 'generic substitution' for newly prescribed medicines. This limited practice of pharmaceutical care in community pharmacies confirms the results of previous findings [33,50,55] and indicates that the implementation of these cognitive pharmaceutical services is still challenging.

4.4. Strengths and Limitations

The approach of the study to describe the dispensing practice of prescribed medicines at the counter was a non-participant observation, which is a useful way to study the quality of services and consistency of care [56]. The full pattern of the real-life situation, with all of the activities and interventions triggered by a prescription at the time of dispensing could be described, which forms a basis to improve these processes. In general, observations allow the description of customers' behavior and practice in real daily life [57], avoiding consequently the biases of self-report methods [46]. The observation method used in this study was based on ad-hoc note-taking of exchanged information and subsequent transcribing into quantitative information. This demonstrated that observation is a feasible method to provide valuable insight into pharmacies' activities. The documentation of the observed PEs has been tested for consistency and plausibility. The data was collected in 18 randomly selected pharmacies; however, the study was restricted to one region in Switzerland. The principal limitation was the presence of an observer, which could positively influence the counselling performance of the pharmacy staff by triggering them to be more aware of their way of approaching customers (the Hawthorne effect) [58]. To minimize this effect, the observer became accustomed to the pharmacy staff prior data collection to make them feel comfortable. Moreover, the observation lasted a whole working day, which allowed observation of normal practice over time. Simulated client methods, such as mystery shopping, could minimize observation bias, but present limitations of their own. The extracted information corresponds to a small part (snapshot) of healthcare practice only, and is therefore hard to generalize to other healthcare situations [59]. The observations were not recorded and not reviewed by a second investigator, which might have limited the reliability of the results.

5. Conclusions

The observation of the dispensing practice of prescribed medicines at community pharmacies resulted in a picture about processes and activities triggered by a customer with a prescription in an everyday practice setting. We identified factors influencing counselling provision at the patient, prescription and provider level: Dispensing by the pharmacist, the customer with a first prescription, customer with a prescription requiring a pharmaceutical intervention, carer filling the prescription for a patient, new customer, and customer not refusing counselling. Counselling was not evenly provided, indicating that pharmacy staff counsel different customers to different degrees. The themes of counselling were more product-centered than patient-centered. With a more transparent practice and patient-centered counselling, pharmacy staff could improve to address the patients' needs on medicines information. Pharmacists intervened frequently, however, only a few additional activities and no further services (e.g., adherence support) were offered. Education of pharmacy staff should focus more on patient-centered counselling and the customers should be informed about the role of the pharmacist. Further research will analyze the pharmacists' opinions gathered within this project. Interventional studies could be used to investigate factors for enhancing pharmacy staff-customer interactions overcoming known barriers.

Author Contributions: Conceptualization, K.A.M., J.A.R., T.L.I.-I., K.E.H., M.L.L., and F.B.; methodology, K.A.M., T.L.I.-I., K.E.H., and F.B.; validation, J.A.R. and K.A.M.; formal analysis, J.A.R. and K.A.M.; investigation, J.A.R.; resources, J.A.R. and K.A.M.; data curation, J.A.R. and K.A.M.; writing—original draft preparation K.A.M.; writing—review and editing, T.L.I.-I., K.E.H., M.L.L., and F.B.; visualization, K.A.M.; supervision, K.E.H., M.L.L., and F.B.

Funding: This research received no external funding.

Acknowledgments: The authors gratefully thank the participating pharmacies from Basel to allow us to observe their practices and William Caddy for proofreading.

Conflicts of Interest: The authors declare no conflict of interest.

References

1. Allemann, S.S.; van Mil, J.W.; Botermann, L.; Berger, K.; Griese, N.; Hersberger, K.E. Pharmaceutical care: The PCNE definition 2013. *Int. J. Clin. Pharm.* **2014**, *36*, 544–555. [CrossRef] [PubMed]
2. Spivey, P. Ensuring good dispensing practices. In *MDS-3: Managing Access to Medicines and Health Technologies*; Management Sciences for Health: Arlington, VA, USA, 2012.
3. *Joint FIP/WHO Guidelines on Good Pharmacy Practice: Standards for Quality of Pharmacy Services*; World Health Organization, Ed.; WHO Technical Report Series; World Health Organization: Geneva, Switzerland, 2011. Available online: https://www.fip.org/www/uploads/database_file.php?id=331&table_id= (accessed on 27 August 2018).
4. Blom, L.; Krass, I. Introduction: The role of pharmacy in patient education and counselling. *Patient Educ. Couns.* **2011**, *83*, 285–287. [CrossRef] [PubMed]
5. American Society of Health-System Pharmacists. ASHP guidelines on pharmacist-conducted patient education and counselling. *Am. J. Health-Syst. Pharm.* **1997**, *54*, 431–434.
6. Ngoh, L.N. Health literacy: A barrier to pharmacist-patient communication and medication adherence. *J. Am. Pharm. Assoc.* **2009**, *49*, e132–e146. [CrossRef] [PubMed]
7. Osterberg, L.; Blaschke, T. Adherence to medication. *N. Engl. J. Med.* **2005**, *353*, 487–497. [CrossRef] [PubMed]

8. Patel, M.; Campbell, M.; Moslem, M.; Spriggel, P.; Warholak, T. Identifying drug therapy problems through patient consultation at community pharmacies: A quality improvement project. *J. Patient Saf.* **2015**. [CrossRef]

9. van Dijk, M.; Blom, L.; Koopman, L.; Philbert, D.; Koster, E.; Bouvy, M.; van Dijk, L. Patient–provider communication about medication use at the community pharmacy counter. *Int. J. Pharm. Pract.* **2016**, *24*, 13–21. [CrossRef]

10. Blom, L.; Wolters, M.; Ten Hoor–Suykerbuyk, M.; van Paassen, J.; van Oyen, A. Pharmaceutical education in patient counselling: 20h spread over 6 years? *Patent Educ. Couns.* **2011**, *83*, 465–471. [CrossRef]

11. Alkhawajah, A.M.; Eferakeya, A.E. The role of pharmacists in patients' education on medication. *Public Health* **1992**, *106*, 231–237. [CrossRef]

12. Benedetti, C.; Berger, J.; Bugnon, O.; Burnier, M.; Dommer-Schwaller, J.; Hugentobler-Hampaï, D.; Mesnil, M. Pharmazeutische Beratung: Notwendige Fragen. In *pharManuel*; PharmaSuisse, Schweizerischer Apothekerverband: Bern, Switzerland, 2016.

13. Tarifvertrag (LOA IV) Zwischen dem Schweizerischen Apothekerverband (pharmaSuisse) und Santésuisse—Die Schweizer Krankenversicherer (Santésuisse). Available online: http://www.pharmasuisse. org/data/Oeffentlich/de/Themen/Tarifvertrag_LOA-IV_def_d_09-03-6.pdf (accessed on 26 January 2016).

14. Hersberger, K.E.; Messerli, M. Development of Clinical Pharmacy in Switzerland: Involvement of Community Pharmacists in Care for Older Patients. *Drugs Aging* **2016**, *33*, 205–211. [CrossRef]

15. Guignard, E.; Bugnon, O. Pharmaceutical care in community pharmacies: Practice and research in Switzerland. *Ann. Pharmacother.* **2006**, *40*, 512–517. [CrossRef] [PubMed]

16. Murad, M.S.; Chatterley, T.; Guirguis, L.M. A meta-narrative review of recorded patient-pharmacist interactions: Exploring biomedical or patient-centered communication? *Res. Soc. Adm. Pharm.* **2014**, *10*, 1–20. [CrossRef] [PubMed]

17. Puspitasari, H.P.; Aslani, P.; Krass, I. A review of counselling practices on prescription medicines in community pharmacies. *Res. Soc. Adm. Pharm.* **2009**, *5*, 197–210. [CrossRef] [PubMed]

18. Koster, E.S.; van Meeteren, M.M.; van Dijk, M.; van de Bemt, B.J.; Ensing, H.T.; Bouvy, M.L.; Blom, L.; van Dijk, L. Patient-provider interaction during medication encounters: A study in outpatient pharmacies in the Netherlands. *Patient Educ. Couns.* **2015**, *98*, 843–848. [CrossRef] [PubMed]

19. Boeni, F.; Arnet, I.; Hersberger, K.E. Adherence counselling during patient contacts in swiss community pharmacies. *Patient Prefer. Adher.* **2015**, *9*, 597–605. [CrossRef] [PubMed]

20. Rüfenacht, I. BABS 2010 Basler Apothekenbeobachtungsstudie–7: The Frequency of the Four Clients' Demands Concerning Analgesics and the State of Compliance Support in Community Pharmacies. Master's Thesis, University of Basel, Basel, Switzerland, 2010.

21. Chong, W.W.; Aslani, P.; Chen, T.F. Pharmacist–patient communication on use of antidepressants: A simulated patient study in community pharmacy. *Res. Soc. Adm. Pharm.* **2014**, *10*, 419–437. [CrossRef] [PubMed]

22. Schommer, J.C.; Wiederholt, J.B. A field investigation of participant and environment effects on pharmacist–patient communication in community pharmacies. *Med. Care* **1995**, *33*, 567–584. [CrossRef]

23. Omnibus Budget Reconciliation Act of 1990 (OBRA'90). *Public Law* **1990**, *4206*, 101–508.

24. PharmaSuisse. Schweizer QUALITÄTSMANAGEMENTSYSTEM für Apotheken—Auditbericht. Available online: http://www.pharmasuisse.org/data/Oeffentlich/de/Themen/QMS/Musterbericht_QMS.pdf (accessed on 5 August 2016).

25. Maes, K.A.; Bruch, S.; Hersberger, K.E.; Lampert, M.L. Documentation of pharmaceutical care: Development of an intervention oriented classification system. *Int. J. Clin. Pharm.* **2017**, *39*, 354–363. [CrossRef]

26. Boeni, F. Dispensing of prescribed medicines in community pharmacies—Part B: Observations deviate from pharmacists' opinions. 45th ESCP-NSF international symposium on clinical pharmacy: Clinical pharmacy tackling inequalities and access to health care, Oslo, Norway, 5–7 October 2016. *Int. J. Clin. Pharm.* **2017**, *39*, 208–341. [CrossRef]

27. Hassell, K.; Noyce, P.; Rogers, A.; Harris, J.; Wilkinson, J. Advice provided in British community pharmacies: What people want and what they get. *J. Health Serv. Res. Policy* **1998**, *3*, 219–225. [CrossRef]

28. Gadkari, A.S.; McHorney, C.A. Medication nonfulfillment rates and reasons: Narrative systematic review. *Curr. Med. Res. Opin.* **2010**, *26*, 683–705. [CrossRef]

29. Kreps, G.L.; Villagran, M.M.; Zhao, X.; McHorney, C.A.; Ledford, C.; Weathers, M.; Keefe, B. Development and validation of motivational messages to improve prescription medication adherence for patients with chronic health problems. *Patient Educ. Couns.* **2011**, *83*, 375–381. [CrossRef] [PubMed]

30. Olsson, E.; Ingman, P.; Ahmed, B.; Kälvemark Sporrong, S. Pharmacist-patient communication in Swedish community pharmacies. *Res. Soc. Adm. Pharm.* **2014**, *10*, 149–155. [CrossRef] [PubMed]

31. Berger, K.; Eickhoff, C.; Schulz, M. Counselling quality in community pharmacies: Implementation of the pseudo customer methodology in Germany. *J. Clin. Pharm. Ther.* **2005**, *30*, 45–57. [CrossRef] [PubMed]

32. Melton, B.L.; Lai, Z. Review of community pharmacy services: What is being performed, and where are the opportunities for improvement? *Integr. Pharm. Res. Pract.* **2017**, *6*, 79–89. [CrossRef] [PubMed]

33. Kaae, S.; Mygind, A.; Saleem, S. A characterization of the current communication patterns in Danish community pharmacies—An observational study. *Res. Soc. Adm. Pharm.* **2013**, *9*, 958–964. [CrossRef]

34. Worley, M.M.; Schommer, J.C.; Brown, L.M.; Hadsall, R.S.; Ranelli, P.L.; Stratton, T.P.; Uden, D.L. Pharmacists' and patients' roles in the pharmacist–patient relationship: Are pharmacists and patients reading from the same relationship script? *Res. Soc. Adm. Pharm.* **2007**, *3*, 47–69. [CrossRef]

35. Liekens, S.; Vandael, E.; Roter, D.; Larson, S.; Smits, T.; Laekeman, G.; Foulon, V. Impact of training on pharmacists' counselling of patients starting antidepressant therapy. *Patient Educ. Couns.* **2014**, *94*, 110–115. [CrossRef]

36. Stevenson, F.A.; Cox, K.; Britten, N.; Dundar, Y. A systematic review of the research on communication between patients and health care professionals about medicines: The consequences for concordance. *Health Expect* **2004**, *7*, 235–245. [CrossRef]

37. Pronk, M.C.M.; Blom, A.T.G.; Jonkers, R.; Bakker, A. Evaluation of patient opinions in a pharmacy-level intervention study. *Int. J. Pharm. Pract.* **2003**, *11*, 143–151. [CrossRef]

38. Barner, J.C.; Bennett, R.W. Pharmaceutical care certificate program: Assessment of pharmacists' implementation into practice. *J. Am. Pharm. Assoc.* **1999**, *39*, 362–367. [CrossRef]

39. Barnes, J.M.; Riedlinger, J.E.; McCloskey, W.W.; Montagne, M. Barriers to compliance with OBRA'90 regulations in community pharmacies. *Ann. Pharmacother.* **1996**, *30*, 1101–1105. [CrossRef] [PubMed]

40. Puspitasari, H.P.; Aslani, P.; Krass, I. Pharmacists' and consumers' viewpoints on counselling on prescription medicines in Australian community pharmacies. *Int. J. Pharm. Pract.* **2010**, *18*, 202–208. [CrossRef] [PubMed]

41. Assa-Eley, M.; Kimberlin, C.L. Using interpersonal perception to characterize pharmacists' and patients' perceptions of the benefits of pharmaceutical care. *Health Commun.* **2005**, *17*, 41–56. [CrossRef] [PubMed]

42. Kaae, S.; Traulsen, J.M.; Norgaard, L.S. Challenges to counselling customers at the pharmacy counter—Why do they exist? *Res. Soc. Adm. Pharm.* **2012**, *8*, 253–257. [CrossRef] [PubMed]

43. Cipolle, R.J.; Strand, L.M.; Morley, P.C. *Pharmaceutical Care Practice: The Patient-Centered Approach to Medication Management Services*, 3rd ed.; McGraw-Hill Companies: New York, NY, USA, 2012.

44. van Hulten, R.; Blom, L.; Mattheusens, J.; Wolters, M.; Bouvy, M. Communication with patients who are dispensed a first prescription of chronic medication in the community pharmacy. *Patient Educ. Couns.* **2011**, *83*, 417–422. [CrossRef] [PubMed]

45. Clifford, S.; Barber, N.; Elliott, R.; Hartley, E.; Horne, R. Patient-centred advice is effective in improving adherenceto medicines. *Pharm. World Sci.* **2006**, *28*, 165–170. [CrossRef] [PubMed]

46. Westerlund, T.; Gelin, U.; Pettersson, E.; Skarlund, F.; Wagstrom, K.; Ringbom, C. A retrospective analysis of drug–related problems documented in a national database. *Int. J. Clin. Pharm.* **2013**, *35*, 202–209. [CrossRef] [PubMed]

47. Aslanpour, Z.; Smith, F.J. Oral counselling on dispensed medication: A survey of its extent and associated factors in a random sample of community pharmacies. *Int. J. Pharm. Pract.* **1997**, *5*, 57–63. [CrossRef]

48. Schommer, J.C.; Wiederholt, J.B. Pharmacists' views of patient counselling. *Am. Pharm.* **1994**, *34*, 46–53.

49. Schommer, J.C.; Wiederholt, J.B. The association of prescription status, patient age, patient gender, and patient question asking behavior with the content of pharmacist–patient communication. *Pharm. Res.* **1997**, *14*, 145–151. [CrossRef] [PubMed]

50. Kimberlin, C.L.; Jamison, A.N.; Linden, S.; Winterstein, A.G. Patient counselling practices in U.S. pharmacies: Effects of having pharmacists hand the medication to the patient and state regulations on pharmacist counselling. *J. Am. Pharm. Assoc.* **2011**, *51*, 527–534. [CrossRef] [PubMed]

51. Martin, B.A.; Chewning, B.A. Evaluating pharmacists' ability to counsel on tobacco cessation using two standardized patient scenarios. *Patient Educ. Couns.* **2011**, *83*, 319–324. [CrossRef] [PubMed]

52. Sepucha, K.; Ozanne, E.M. How to define and measure concordance between patients' preferences and medical treatments: A systematic review of approaches and recommendations for standardization. *Patient Educ. Couns.* **2010**, *78*, 12–23. [CrossRef] [PubMed]

53. Epstein, R.M.; Franks, P.; Fiscella, K.; Shields, C.G.; Meldrum, S.C.; Kravitz, R.L.; Duberstein, P.R. Measuring patient-centered communication in patient-physician consultations: Theoretical and practical issues. *Soc. Sci. Med. (1982)* **2005**, *61*, 1516–1528. [CrossRef] [PubMed]

54. Nicolas, A.; Eickhoff, C.; Griese, N.; Schulz, M. Drug-related problems in prescribed medicines in Germany at the time of dispensing. *Int. J. Clin. Pharm.* **2013**, *35*, 476–482. [CrossRef] [PubMed]

55. Hughes, C.M.; Hawwa, A.F.; Scullin, C.; Anderson, C.; Bernsten, C.B.; Bjornsdottir, I.; Cordina, M.A.; da Costa, F.A.; De Wulf, I.; Eichenberger, P.; et al. Provision of pharmaceutical care by community pharmacists: A comparison across Europe. *Pharm. World Sci.* **2010**, *32*, 472–487. [CrossRef] [PubMed]

56. Green, J.A.; Norris, P. Quantitative Methods in Pharmacy Practice Research. In *Pharmacy Practice Research Methods*; Babar, Z.-U.-D., Ed.; Springer: Cham, Switzerland, 2015.

57. Kaae, S.; Traulsen, J.M. Qualitative methods in pharmacy practice research. In *Pharmacy Practice Research Methods*; Babar, Z.-U.-D., Ed.; Springer: Cham, Switzerland, 2015.

58. Wickstrom, G.; Bendix, T. The "Hawthorne effect"–What did the original Hawthorne studies actually show? *Scand. J. Work Environ. Health* **2000**, *26*, 363–367.

59. Madden, J.M.; Quick, J.D.; Ross-Degnan, D.; Kafle, K.K. Undercover careseekers: Simulated clients in the study of health provider behavior in developing countries. *Soc. Sci. Med.* **1997**, *45*, 1465–1482. [CrossRef]

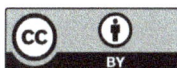

pharmacy

MDPI

Article

Patients', Pharmacy Staff Members', and Pharmacy Researchers' Perceptions of Central Elements in Prescription Encounters at the Pharmacy Counter

Susanne Kaae [1,*][iD]**, Lotte Stig Nørgaard** [1][iD]**, Sofia Kälvemark Sporrong** [1][iD]**,**
Anna Birna Almarsdottir [1]**, Mette Kofoed** [2]**, Rami Faris Daysh** [1] **and Nima Jowkar** [1][iD]

[1]   Social and Clinical Pharmacy, Department of Pharmacy, Faculty of Health and Medical Sciences, University of Denmark, 2100 København Ø, Denmark

[2]   Department of Public Health, University of Southern Denmark, 5000 Odense C, Denmark

*   Correspondence: susanne.kaae@sund.ku.dk

Received: 7 May 2019; Accepted: 2 July 2019; Published: 4 July 2019

check for
updates

Abstract: Background: Studies suggest that the way pharmacy counselling takes place does not fully support patients in obtaining optimal medicine use. To understand the basis of current challenges in pharmacy counselling, we investigated which selected related cues, i.e., objects, sounds, or circumstances in prescription encounters, patients, and pharmacy staff notice, and how they interpret these cues. Pharmacy practice researchers' cue orientation was also investigated to explore possible differences to those of staff and patients. **Methods**: Twelve focus group interviews representing 5 community pharmacies (staff and patients) and 2 universities (researchers) were conducted during 2017–2018 in Denmark. A total of 20 patients, 22 pharmacy staff, and 6 pharmacy researchers participated. A theoretical analysis based on cue orientation and social appraisal was conducted. **Results:** Pharmacy staff, patients and researchers noticed different selected related cues in prescription encounters. Staff particularly noticed 'types of patients'. Patients were more divided and grouped into three overall categories: 'types of staff', medical content, and the situation around the encounter. Pharmacy researchers noticed multiple cues. Different emotions were integrated in the construction of the cues. **Conclusion:** Differences in the cue orientation between all three groups were identified. The identified types of cues and emotions can explain an underlying dissatisfaction with the encounters. Patients lack, in particular, more personal contact. Staff need to consider these aspects to provide relevant counselling.

Keywords: pharmacy communication; cue orientation; focus group interviews; Denmark

1. Introduction

Communication between pharmacy staff and patients at the pharmacy counter is important for community pharmacies to fulfil their societal obligations of offering professional counselling to patients. Medication counselling is a challenging process that should take the wishes and needs of the patient into consideration, while at the same time performing quality dispensing and keeping waiting times to a minimum.

Several aspects of medication counselling have been investigated, especially those regarding how often staff provide information, what the information concerns, the duration of the encounters, the quality of the counselling, and staff and patient characteristics with an influence on the communication [1–8]. Studies suggest that the way pharmacy counselling takes place today does not fully support patients in obtaining optimal medicine use. Identified problems include patient reliance on doctors rather than pharmacy staff to provide relevant information [9], that staff do not activate patients in the encounters [10–13], and that patients do not always find information from the pharmacy relevant [14]. However, the underlying reasons for the identified challenges remain unknown.

One important aspect in improving pharmacy counselling is to understand how counselling is perceived by pharmacy staff and patients since the ways they approach and react to the encounters are shaped by these perceptions. In any face-to-face encounter, there are, according to classic communication theory, potentially many elements/cues i.e., objects, sounds, or circumstances to be taken into consideration by participants in order for them to interpret what is taking place [15]. Cues in a pharmacy could be the architecture, characteristics of the person at the counter, etc. Which cues are selected for interpretation and how they are interpreted differ from preconceptions based on cultural learning and personal experiences [15]. Hence, examining what cues pharmacy staff and patients notice in pharmacy encounters, and which meanings and values they ascribe to them, will help us understand their basic understanding of pharmacy encounters. The underlying perceptions of pharmacy encounters could give valuable insight into why counselling challenges exist, especially in the case of discrepancies between patients and staff.

One might assume that pharmacy practice researchers also develop certain perceptions of pharmacy encounters that influence their research, both in terms of perspectives and interpretations. It is important to find out what these are, especially since they may differ from those of both community pharmacy staff and patients.

The aim of this study was, therefore, to investigate what cues in community pharmacy encounters patients, staff and pharmacy practice researchers notice, and how they interpret these cues.

Due to identified differences in pharmacy patients' interest in receiving over-the-counter versus prescription counselling [14,16], the study was restricted to prescription encounters. This choice was also made because prescription encounters, especially those involving refill prescriptions, appear to be particularly challenging in terms of counselling [14,16].

2. Materials and Methods

To investigate pharmacy patients', staff members' and researchers' cue orientation in prescription encounters, focus group interviews were conducted. This method is ideal for stimulating discussion, gaining insights and generating ideas of social issues under investigation [17].

2.1. Theoretical Framework

Only a small fraction of data from our surroundings is ever consciously perceived in any way by an individual. Of this fraction, only a selected portion (cues) is in some sense chosen by the individual. We further simplify the waves of incoming data by recording their contents into meaningful '*summary codes*'. The overall meaning we make of selected and usually related cues is influenced by our 'expectancy set', which is described as: "One's cultural belief system learned through socialization, the sum of one's experiences, and one's currently salient roles" [15]. With regard to the selection of incoming data, individuals tend to focus on cues that reinforce past or emerging interpretations [18].

In this study, the articulated focus of incoming data is defined as 'selected related cues' i.e., of all the possible impressions in a pharmacy prescription encounter, what types of cues do the different actors overall notice? The summary and interpretation of the 'selected related cues' i.e., which elements do participants include in their description of 'selected related cues', are defined as 'summary codes'. Patients, pharmacy staff and researchers have individual knowledge and experiences but are expected to share some cultural belief systems (in particular staff and researchers through education and workplace socialization), which might create different patterns of cue orientation and summary codes between the groups.

2.2. Design

To investigate selected related cues and summary codes, an exploratory study design was chosen to cover participants' untainted perceptions of and experiences with prescription encounters. The interview guide was thus kept short and open and consisted of only two major questions. The first question was presented in three ways to stimulate as many reflections as possible:

- What types of encounters have you experienced at the pharmacy counter?
- What types of meetings have you experienced at the pharmacy counter?
- Which types of different (human) interactions have you experienced at the pharmacy counter?

The second question concerned participants' opinions about the role of community pharmacies in society, this was to explore if and how these views might influence the way participants react in the pharmacy encounters.

To identify participants' original cue orientation, they were first asked to write their immediate thoughts about the first question for 5–10 minutes, and each participant was then asked to tell the other participants about their notes. Participants then commented on each other's remarks to generate more reflections. By this design, both the individuals' untainted cue orientation was identified along with the benefit of the focus group participants discussing the cues with each other. By the end of the interview, the second question was presented. Data collectors used probing questions when necessary. The three types of interviewees were interviewed in separate focus groups to explore their perceptions in depth. The interviews were recorded and transcribed verbatim.

2.3. Recruitment

Five community pharmacies in Denmark were approached for purposeful yet convenient sampling ensuring heterogeneity between the pharmacies according to location (provincial/urban) and overall socio-demographic background of inhabitants in the area. All agreed to participate. The pharmacies were asked to recruit 4–6 staff members (both pharmacy technicians and pharmacists) and 4–6 patients from the pharmacy for the interviews. Inclusion criteria for patients were adulthood, recipient of prescription medicine and a variation in gender and age. Two groups of researchers from the University of Copenhagen and from the University of Southern Denmark both engaged in pharmacy practice research represented the views of pharmacy researchers.

The interviews took place at the five pharmacies and at the two universities. Four of the authors (first, fifth, sixth and last author) conducted the interviews.

2.4. Analysis

Transcripts were read, and relevant citations were extracted and coded in NVivo12. Codes were divided into whether the findings were from staff, patients or researchers. The codes and extracts were theoretically interpreted according to the type of *selected related cues* (what items were mentioned when participants were speaking of pharmacy encounters) and *summary code* (what different elements were described by participants in relation to the selected related cues) [19]. All authors, individually, carried out the initial stage of the analysis for three pharmacies (patient and staff focus groups). Selected related cues and summary codes identified were then compared in consensus discussions. Based on these discussions the first author undertook the analysis of the pharmacy researchers. This was as three of the authors participated as interviewees in one university interview, and hence were not suited for this.

Interviews at pharmacies (pharmacy staff and patients) were conducted in two more pharmacies (by sixth and last author). Data saturation was then observed. The analysis indicated that emotions were an integrated part of cue orientation and the development of summary codes, why (social) appraisal theory was integrated into the analyses. Appraisal theory highlights how cognition and emotions are interdependent in peoples' appraisal and reactions to the events in which they take part [20,21]. Hence, the same pharmacy meeting might arouse different feelings in staff and patients and between different staff and patients based on their evaluation of what is going on in the situation. Therefore, apart from registering selected related cues and summary codes as pure cognitive processes, the analysis allowed the identification of emotional responses linked to the selected related cues and summary codes. Besides, it was registered whether an appraisal of a pharmacy meeting leading to an emotional response appeared to be on an individual level or as a member of a social group, i.e., pharmacy staff [21]. Two authors (first and third) carried out this supplementary analysis.

2.5. Ethics

Written information about the study was provided to patients and pharmacy staff at the time of recruitment. Oral informed consent from all interviewees was further obtained at the beginning of the interviews. The study was approved by the Danish Data Protection Agency (ref.no. 514-0310/19-3000). The collected data were stored according to the EU rules of GDPR.

3. Results

Twelve focus group interviews were conducted during 2017 and 2018. Forty-eight persons participated in the focus groups, including 20 patients, 22 pharmacy staff members and 6 pharmacy researchers. Between 3 and 5 participants were included in each interview. Patient gender was equally represented, but the majority of patients were over 50 years, whereas approximately 2/3 of the staff participants were women and the majority were under 50 years of age. The majority of researchers were women over 50 years of age. The interviews lasted between 55–95 minutes.

Quotes illustrating central elements of the identified '*selected related cues*' and related '*summary codes*' are presented in Tables 1–3 for the three different groups.

3.1. Pharmacy Staff

3.1.1. Selected Related Cues

The predominant selected related cue noticed by staff was the (type of) patient. Types of meetings were mentioned by participants in especially one focus group. Further, many communication elements were described, such as language barriers and power balance (please see Table 1).

Table 1. Examples of elements (transcript data) built into the summary codes of the selected related cues noticed by pharmacy staff.

Selected Related Cues	Elements in Summary Code
Type of patient	'I have counseled those [ed. patients] who are open, that like to know more and who seek insight into their own disease. That's a good dialogue, I would say.' (Pharmacy 1)
	'And then I have written a regular customer who is used to coming here and they are used to us helping them and it is at our place that they look for advice and confirmation—and we have to help them with all kind of things related to their treatment.' (Pharmacy 1)
	'And then there are some who are a bit defiant who don't want to listen because the doctor knows best and we should not interfere … In those cases, I always try to plant a seed, so perhaps they can think about it and then come back.' (Pharmacy 2)
	'I experience that there is a bit of difference between customers, sometimes we have new customers who are not well informed, who should have some counseling, in contrast to people who have had it [ed. the medicine] for 20 years. There is a difference if they really want to listen.' (Pharmacy 4)
	'There is a big difference if you are speaking to a man or a woman because women like to share and men don't.' (Pharmacy 4)

Table 1. *Cont.*

Selected Related Cues	Elements in Summary Code
Types of meetings	'I think we have a lot of what I have called 'the intimate meeting', where the customer opens up, where we get to talk about it, where we are allowed to get under their skin and become intimate in our talk.' (Pharmacy 3)
	'I have divided into a professional academic meeting where you are allowed to bring some information to the customer which the customer was not aware of.' (Pharmacy 3)
	'I have divided them into quick encounters without information. The customers knows everything or they had the medicines for many years and think they know everything about it … And then we have the in-depth encounters where you take into consideration that the customer is a new user of the medicine and where the customer is interested in receiving information.' (Pharmacy 5)
Communication elements	'Cultures, high/low status, habits of informing, those who know better, the busy ones, it all have an influence on us in the interaction. It can be noise, a printer which is noisy, a telephone that rings, somebody who wants you to answer the phone or who wants to ask you something: 'where can I find this product?' There are so many things that influence the encounter which makes it different for the customer.' (Pharmacy 1)
	'And I have written the interactions in which the customer comes in with certain expectations and then meets something else – and that can go both ways: 'Thank you so much' or 'Can't we finish so I can get out of here?'' (Pharmacy 2)
	'I agree that if you have a bad start of the encounter then it can influence the rest of the meeting with this customer.' (Pharmacy 3)
	'Person 2: Language barriers, I think we experience that with every second customer Person 4: And it gives, as you said, impatient customers because if we have the language barriers then it takes time.' (Pharmacy 4)

3.1.2. Summary Codes

Various types of patients were described by staff, including positive patients with a general interest in counselling and an interest in their own health, indifferent patients, busy patients, sensitive patients needing discretion, insecure patients with many questions, and patients who sought information prior to entering the pharmacy. The different types of patients were mainly perceived according to their interest in receiving counselling from staff. This was often described as a personal trait of the patient and, in fewer cases, as a consequence of other demographics, such as age, education, and language.

Pharmacy staff perceived that the type of patient impacted how the encounter developed. If the patient was interested in a dialogue about medicines, the encounter often developed to address the needs of the patient, whereas a meeting with a patient without interest would be rather short. However, some participants in one pharmacy (pharmacy 2) described how they tried to develop the patients' interest in counselling by 'planting seeds'.

A few staff participants, particularly in pharmacy 3, described different types of meetings that differed according to the degree of empathy between the individuals, if the content was technical and if staff managed to interest the patient in counselling. Short meetings (with no communication about medicines) were mentioned in all pharmacies.

Several communication elements that were perceived to influence the meetings were described: expectations, language barriers, a similar notion by both parties of what should take place, the power balance, the importance of getting a good start to the encounter and staff feeling disturbed by phones. A few staff members described how they themselves influenced the encounters. In these cases, the way staff phrased their questions and their body language was perceived to influence the meetings, but a few also added that it depended on whether they had a good day, whether they felt the topic to be embarrassing and whether they were able to read the patient correctly. Variations were seen between the focus groups in the different pharmacies in how many communication issues were discussed, including if pharmacy staff's own performance was perceived to influence the development of the encounters.

The emotions of staff linked to the described cues and summary codes were in many cases related to the fact that staff felt dependant on the interest of the customer regarding whether or not they could fulfil their perceived social role as medicine counsellors. Hence, different types of patients to a large extent evoked the same types of feelings in staff. For example, those patients being interested in counselling provoked positive emotions in staff whereas those patients refusing counselling evoked negative emotions in terms of disappointment.

3.2. Patients

3.2.1. Selected Related Cues

Patients were more varied than staff with regard to predominant selected related cues. Approximately one-third of the patients noticed the type of staff they met at the pharmacy. Another third noticed the content of the meeting. Finally, some patients emphasized the situation 'around' the meetings, i.e., if it was a busy pharmacy day and if the requested medicine was in stock. Some patients also described communication elements (please see Table 2).

Table 2. Examples of elements (transcript data) built into the summary codes of different selected related cues noticed by patients.

Selected Related Cues	Elements in Summary Code
Type of staff	'Yes, then you get one of the staff with whom you have special interaction.' (Pharmacy 1) 'I don't mind [ed. getting information] but when I say: "Yes I've taken it for 25 years" they say: "Yes, but you have to be aware of … "—"But try to listen to what I'm telling you. I know it. I discuss it with my doctor" and then they say: "Yes, yes but … " and they keep on.' (Pharmacy 1) 'I just want more personal contact, something more personal than a conversation only about the medicine or how expensive it is.' (Pharmacy 5)
Content of meeting	'They ask whether you have any questions regarding the medicine, if the medicine is new to you or if you have any side effects, you would like to discuss.' (Pharmacy 2) 'I have experienced very professional encounters … It's: "Do you know how to take it?" and the dosage they focus on.' (Pharmacy 4) 'With regard to the counseling, I often feel that they advise you on how many tablets to take and how often.' (Pharmacy 5)
Situation around the meeting	'I think it's quite nice to come to Copenhagen because they always have the products I need.' (Pharmacy 3) 'You could observe that there is some kind of stress from their (ed. the staff) side. I think some times that if there is a long queue waiting then they perceive that it should be a bit quicker.' (Pharmacy 4) 'When they are very busy then they try to make it very short and concise – and then it's out with this guy and in with the next.' (Pharmacy 5)
Communication elements	'I have lived in many different places and been a customer in many pharmacies. You sense if there is a good spirit in the pharmacy. I haven't yet sensed the spirit of the new owner down here.' (Pharmacy 1) 'Interviewer: have you ever experienced to be positively surprised?K3: Oh yes. It concerns all aspects of life—also down here. Oh no not him and then it turns out well. And then it's a good experienceK2: basically it's because your first judgment is wrong.' (Pharmacy 1) 'And it might be that there is another tone here in the counseling area after the new owner has started … You feel it when you enter … .It has a positive influence on the staff.' (Pharmacy 2) 'I feel the quality can be different from pharmacy to pharmacy. It can be very different … depending if you are in a big pharmacy or in a small branch and who is behind the counter.' (Pharmacy 4)

3.2.2. Summary Codes

Patients who noticed staff discussed whether there was good personal chemistry between them and staff and if they felt pharmacy staff listened to them. Some emphasized that having a personal interaction with staff was important. A few patients said they liked meetings where the two parties had a laugh and did not necessarily talk about the medicine. A central element in the interpretation of staff was whether staff members were explaining too much and/or asking too many questions about the medicine. This element was important because staff were perceived as sometimes overlooking that the patient was not interested in the counselling, and staff thereby displayed a basic lack of interest in the patient. A few patients defended the routine of (over-) informing the patient since this was perceived to be in the best interest of the patient and that staff were only fulfilling their healthcare role.

Other patients focused on the content of the encounter and how it proceeded. Examples of content included how to take the medicine, correct dosage, possible adverse drug events, and drug-drug interactions, and who initiated the discussion about the medicine.

Some communication elements influencing the meetings were also described; however, fewer than by staff. The aspects mentioned were differences between pharmacies including how the pharmacy owner influenced the atmosphere of the pharmacy also with regard to counselling. Patients who had experienced management responsibilities themselves in their professional career seemed to notice this aspect. A few patients described how they themselves influenced the meeting, for example, by being too quick to judge (negatively) the staff.

Patient ascribed different emotions to pharmacy meetings with some being in general highly content whereas others were more dissatisfied thereby clearly illustrating that patients bear different meanings and emotional responses to the same type of events. There seemed to be a certain pattern between emotions evoked by pharmacy encounters in relation to the cue orientation. Hence, patients who were satisfied with the encounters appeared to focus on the content in their cue orientation, whereas patients who were not always satisfied focused more on the staff ability to create a personal meeting (or the situation around the encounter).

3.3. Pharmacy Researchers

3.3.1. Selected Related Cues

The pharmacy researchers described multiple selected related cues, i.e., more and different types of cues than staff and patients. The selected related cues included content of the meetings, the situation around the meeting, the length and outcome of meetings, the type of patient, and various communication elements, for example, how the two parties were influencing each other (please see Table 3).

Table 3. Examples of elements (transcript data) built into the summary codes of different selected related cues noticed by pharmacy researchers.

Selected Related Cues	Elements in Summary Code
Content	'I have myself experienced what could be defined as generic substitution where we discuss the price, the package, the looks, the drug and I have a lot of different experiences with that.' (University 1)
Situation around meeting (influencing content)	'And then there are the problems when the doctor hasn't sent the prescription and you [ed. being the staff] talk a lot about that, problems with the doctor sending the wrong medicine.' (University 1)
	'And the problems can be related to the people or due to IT-problems, it can be the prescription-server, it can be something with the IT that doesn't work, it can be drug-shortages ... ' (Pharmacy 1)
	'And then there are very practical matters such as the customer complains because there has been a mistake, or the customer can't get the medicine due to drug shortages, the customers finds the medicine expensive, the customer doesn't speak Danish. So there are a lot of meetings being event-dependent.' (University 2)
Type of patient	'And then I thought about some of the customers who are very worried about something or that you received some new medicine or that you received a new diagnosis.' (University 1)
	'There are many different kinds of meetings depending on what type of customer you have, and that's the way it should be.' (University 2)
	' ... the customer is in a hurry, the customer doesn't want to talk about something because it's a taboo, that the customer is emotionally affected ... ' (University 2)

Table 3. *Cont.*

Selected Related Cues	Elements in Summary Code
Communication elements (including interaction and emotions)	'And then we have customers with misuse problems and the pharmacist knows this, and then the customer thinks that the staff member looks at him in a strange way and perhaps the pharmacist does, but even so, the pharmacist doesn't, you feel awkward as the customer. But also, where the pharmacist doesn't dare or care to make the effort because it's unpleasant.' (Pharmacy 1)
	'I think in most cases that it is the customer who is a bit aggressive. They have been waiting in the queue for a long time, they are aggressive, then you [ed. being the staff] turn a bit aggressive because the other party, whoever that is, is influenced by it.' (University 1)
	' … where the pharmacist or the pharmacy technician invites you for a talk about the treatment or the drug counseling. Where the patient accepts – and other scenarios where the pharmacist or the pharmacy technician invites for talk about drug advice where the patient declines.' (University 2)
	'There can be different parameters which have an influence such as age, language – is there a language barrier which you often experience in the pharmacies and how it influences the meeting.' (Pharmacy 2)

3.3.2. Summary Codes

The content of a meeting that was influenced by a specific situation was specifically described by the researchers. Examples included an encounter about the medicine being out of stock or discussions about high prices, errors in the prescription, IT problems (electronic prescription not available), etc.

Hence, researchers, in contrast to staff and patients, gave specific examples of non-medical content in the encounters. The researchers specifically made a distinction between whether the content was about medicine or not, and noted if the staff took the initiative during the meetings to discuss the medicine, and how the patients responded. Further, they described elements such as the length and occurrence of a problem, for example, whether the problem was solved and the satisfaction with the encounter of the involved parties.

Different types of patients were also described by the researchers; for example, some patients were perceived as asking many questions, but patients were also perceived as emotional, complaining, affected by a psychological disease, and getting the medicine for the first time – aspects that in some way influenced the encounters. Researchers also stressed the challenges around obtaining fruitful meetings and gave examples of how the two parties influenced each other, for example, on an emotional level. One example of this was how an unpleasant situation might arise because the two parties repeatedly reacted towards the other person's stress. The staff skills to cope with such situations were discussed. Otherwise, the researchers did not distinguish between types of staff as much as between types of patients. In general, as part of the construction of summary codes, the researchers explicitly described emotional aspects as an integral part of prescription encounters as compared to staff and patients who were influenced by emotions but did not describe this specifically.

Researchers were in general reluctant to describe what they perceived to be the optimal pharmacy encounter hence were hesitant to display their own emotions towards pharmacy meetings. However, some criticism or dissatisfaction of pharmacy staff was shown with regard to them not always being able to assess adequately the needs of the patient. Researchers appeared aligned in their deliberate lack of emotional response to pharmacy encounters perhaps thinking that displaying emotions is not an acceptable social role of a pharmacy researcher or that they are looking at the encounters from a distance and are hence not personally involved.

4. Discussion

Many and different types of selected related cues in prescription encounters were described by pharmacy staff, patients and researchers. The three groups noticed different cues. Staff particularly noticed patients whereas patients were more divided and grouped into three overall cues, including staff, medical content, and the situation around the encounter. Pharmacy researchers noticed multiple cues. Different elements including emotions were included in the construction of the cues. For example, patients' interest in talking about the medicine or not was a central element in staff's perception of 'types of patients' and influenced their emotional response towards the encounters, whereas staff skills to create a personal meeting were included in patients' descriptions of and satisfaction with 'types of staff'. Pharmacy staff and pharmacy researchers' emotional responses involved in their perception of pharmacy encounters were more univocal than those of patients.

4.1. Differences in Cue Orientation between Patients and Staff

Considerable difference as described above was found in the selected related cues noticed by staff and patients and the meaning (summary codes) they ascribe to them. To our knowledge, this is the first study to focus on cue and cue differentiation between community pharmacy staff and patients; however, other researchers have previously identified differences between staff and patients, for example, with regard to preferences of the roles of the community pharmacist [22,23]. In these studies, staff more than patients was shown to think that they should be involved in detecting and solving patients' drug-related problems. Such results were partly observed in our study, in particular, in relation to some patients feeling content by having a casual talk rather than a talk about medicines; in contrast to staff who focused on whether a patient was interested in a dialogue about medicine or not. Hence, staff and (some) patients do not agree on the items they appreciate being discussed in prescription encounters. Yet patients in this study appeared to differ in this view as we also identified a group of patients who were satisfied with staff asking questions about their use of medicines.

That staff primarily focused on types of patients and how they influenced the encounter, which might be explained by staff aiming at fulfilling their perceived social role as medical counsellors. Hence, pharmacists in many countries base their counselling on the individual patients, and trying to 'read' the patient is perceived as an integral part of good communication skills [24].

A reason for the identified differences in cue orientation between patients and staff could be that when relationships do not work optimally the involved parties focus more on the underlying relationship than the content [15]. In fact, the predominant type of cue of the majority of staff and some patients pertained to the relationship i.e., a focus on the opposite person and how this person influenced the meeting. In supplement, the patients who appeared satisfied with the counter meetings focused primarily on the content. This result thus indicates that both patients and staff are dissatisfied with prescription counselling today, yet for different reasons. Hence, the dissatisfaction is shown by the aspects/cues they notice around pharmacy encounters and the meaning built into them. Assa-Eley at al. (2005) noted the fact that disagreement between patients and staff of what ought to take place during the encounters often goes unrecognized [23], which might explain why unsatisfactory practices are being repeated.

4.2. Differences in Cue Orientation between Patients

We observed two overall types of patients: those who focused on the type of staff and those who focused on content of the dialogue. A few patients noticed the situation around the encounter.

Renberg et al. (2011) investigated how patients differed according to their ideal prescription pharmacy encounter and found two overall groups: those who focused on the 'drug product' and those who focused on 'personal support' from staff [25]. Each overall group consisted of sub-groups/factors. For example, 'personal support' included both the sub-group IV emphasizing a competent pharmacist who should offer individual advice since the patient usually does not like to make health decisions alone, as well as sub-group V emphasizing privacy and personal contact as some patients are not fond of a traditional professional-client relationship [25].

When comparing our results to those of Renberg, the two predominant patient groups in this study both pertain to the 'personal support' group but in different ways representing both sub-group IV and V. Hence, in contrast to the study of Renberg, only a few of the patients in this study described the pharmacy as a place that is only relevant for them in order to pick up medicine. However, this type of patient was described by staff in our study, which might have to do with how patients were recruited and the willingness of patients to participate. The study by Renberg was conducted using Q-methodology with a more overall perspective on pharmacy practice. Also, the study was conducted in 2008 (in Sweden), which might explain some of the differences. Further, community pharmacies worldwide have, for the last decade, attempted to embrace an expanded role in patient-centred counselling, which some patients may now have started noticing and appreciating.

4.3. Practice Implications

Researchers described many types of selected related cues compared to pharmacy patients and staff, which might be considered both appropriate and explainable considering the complexity of the field [26]. Hence, researchers in the field of pharmacy communication seem to be open to studying many different elements related to pharmacy encounters. However, for future pharmacy practice research aiming to improve counselling, researchers and educators should consider paying special attention to the issues of importance to staff and patients.

Another important aspect relates to the staff's focus on the types of patients, i.e., the majority of staff seem to perceive that the way the encounter develops is influenced by the type of patient and not by themselves. This perception affected staff emotionally. Rather than trying to change the situation many staff members appeared to accept it. Appraisal theory points to the phenomenon of applying relevant adaptive emotions, i.e., a situation where emotions are selected based on the individual's evaluation of the situation comparing the capabilities and resources of the individual with the requirements of the situation [20]. Hence, on one side disappointment as the emotional response to lack of patient interest in pharmacy counselling is relevant in the sense that it conserves resources in a situation that cannot be changed. However, this emotional response is at the same time unfortunate since staff then prevents themselves from trying to develop the encounters further. Hence, being aware of emotional responses in relation to pharmacy encounters might be one way of furthering communication at the counter for pharmacy staff.

An indication of lack of satisfaction with prescription encounters of both patients and staff was identified. Patients, through their descriptions of prescription encounters, displayed the aspects they appreciate and often lack in the encounters, in particular, more personal contact. As most staff participants didn't describe this aspect, a particular attention by staff in this area is warranted to improve counselling.

4.4. Limitations

The results of this study might be influenced by selection bias. Contact persons in the five pharmacies responsible for recruiting staff and patients might have (subconsciously) selected certain kinds of participants, for example, those who are more in favour of pharmacy counselling. Social desirability might also have played a role as the interviews with patients and staff took place in the pharmacy. However, a group of patients who were not overly satisfied with pharmacy encounters was also included in the sample.

Some of the discrepancies between staff and patients with regard to cue orientation might be explained by the fact that the majority of patients were older than 50 years, whereas the majority of staff were younger than 50 years. As cues and summary codes are influenced by both individual and collective experiences, age is expected to play a role in forming expectations.

The enrolled researchers reflected on different kinds of experiences when contemplating pharmacy encounters. Some of the researchers reflected on experiences as former community pharmacists, and others reflected on their experiences as patients or insights gained through their research. These different approaches might explain why researchers were particularly varied in their cue orientation. That researchers noticed more selected related cues than staff and patients also illustrates how selective the last two groups are in their cue orientation and, thus, how the theoretical approach of cue orientation

Pharmacy **2019**, *7*, 84

is useful in investigating differences in cognitive (and emotional) elements constituted in underlying perceptions of pharmacy encounters.

The perceptions and views of pharmacy encounters described by interviewees do not necessarily reflect how the pharmacy counter meetings take place. To verify how meetings actually occur, observational studies are needed. However, identified cues and summary codes are important tools when trying to understand why pharmacy encounters today are not perceived as satisfactory by all involved parties. This knowledge might be used as a basis for community pharmacy staff to further develop their communication skills.

5. Conclusions

Cue orientation, summary codes, and related emotions in pharmacy prescription encounters differ considerably between community pharmacy staff, patients, and pharmacy practice researchers. These differences could constitute some of the identified challenges in pharmacy counselling today. For example, some patients noticed aspects around a personal encounter whereas staff appeared more oriented towards discussing the patient's medicine. A group of patients, however, was content with the current counselling practices of staff.

Author Contributions: Conceptualization: S.K. and L.S.N. and S.K.S. and A.B.A.; Methodology: S.K. and M.K.; Formal Analysis: S.K. and L.S.N. and S.K.S. and A.B.A. and M.K. and R.F.D. and N.J; Investigation: S.K. and M.K. and R.F.D. and N.J.; Data Curation: S.K.; Writing—Original Draft Preparation: S.K.; Writing—Review & Editing: L.S.N. and S.K.S. and A.B.A. and M.K. and R.F.D. and N.J.; Supervision: S.K. and L.S.N.; Project Administration: S.K.

Funding: This research received no external funding.

Acknowledgments: We like to thank the pharmacy patients and staff members who participated in the study.

Conflicts of Interest: The authors declare no conflict of interest.

References

1. Paluck, E.; Green, L.; Frankish, C.; Fielding, D.; Havercamp, B. Assessment of communication barriers in community pharmacies. *Eval. Health Prof.* **2003**, *26*, 380–403. [CrossRef] [PubMed]
2. Schommer, J.; Wiederholt, J. The association of prescription status, patient age, patient gender, and patient question asking behavior with the content of pharmacist-patient relationship. *Pharm. Res.* **1997**, *14*, 145–151. [CrossRef] [PubMed]
3. Shah, B.; Chewning, B. Conceptualizing and measuring pharmacist-patient communication: A review of published studies. *Res. Soc. Adm. Pharm.* **2006**, *2*, 153–185. [CrossRef] [PubMed]
4. Puspitasari, H.; Aslani, P.; Krass, I. A review of counseling practices on prescription medicines in community pharmacies. *Res. Soc. Adm. Pharm.* **2009**, *5*, 197–210. [CrossRef] [PubMed]
5. Sabater-Galindo, M.; Fernandez-Llimos, F.; Sabater-Hernandez, D.; Martinez-Martinez, F.; Benrimoj, S. Healthcare professional-patient relationships: Systematic review of theoretical models from a community pharmacy perspective. *Pat. Educ. Couns.* **2016**, *99*, 339–347. [CrossRef] [PubMed]
6. Nusair, M.B.; Guirguis, L.M. Thoroughness of community pharmacists' assessment and communication using the patient care process. *Res. Soc. Adm. Pharm.* **2018**, *14*, 564–571. [CrossRef] [PubMed]
7. Chong, W.W.; Aslani, P.; Chen, T.F. Pharmacist-patient communication on use of antidepressants: A simulated patient study in community pharmacy. *Res. Soc. Adm. Pharm.* **2014**, *10*, 419–437. [CrossRef] [PubMed]
8. Olsson, E.; Ingman, P.; Ahmed, B.; Kalvemark Sporrong, S. Pharmacist-patient communication in Swedish community pharmacies. *Res. Soc. Adm. Pharm.* **2014**, *10*, 149–155. [CrossRef] [PubMed]
9. Schommer, J.; Gaither, G. A segmentation analysis for pharmacists' and patients' views of pharmacists' roles. *Res. Soc. Adm. Pharm.* **2014**, *10*, 508–528. [CrossRef] [PubMed]
10. Dijk, M.V.; Blom, L.; Koopman, L.; Philbert, D.; Koster, E.; Bouvy, M.; Dijk, L.V. Patient–provider communication about medication use at the community pharmacy counter. *Int. J. Pharm. Pract.* **2016**, *24*, 13–21. [CrossRef]

11. Garner, M.; Watson, M. Using linguistic analysis to explore medicine counter assistants' communication during consultations for nonprescription medicines. *Patient Educ. Couns.* **2007**, *65*, 51–57. [CrossRef] [PubMed]

12. Koster, E.; Meeteren, M.V.; Dijk, M.V.; Bemt, B.V.D.; Ensing, H.; Bouvy, M.; Blom, L.; Dijk, L.V. Patient–provider interaction during medication encounters: A study in outpatient pharmacies in the Netherlands. *Patient Educ. Couns.* **2015**, *98*, 843–848. [CrossRef] [PubMed]

13. Nusair, M.B.; Guirguis, L.M. How pharmacists check the appropriateness of drug therapy? Observations in community pharmacy. *Res. Soc. Adm. Pharm.* **2017**, *13*, 349–357. [CrossRef] [PubMed]

14. Kaae, S.; Mygind, A.; Saleem, S. A characterization of the current communication patterns in Danish community pharmacies—An observational study. *Res. Soc. Adm. Pharm.* **2013**, *9*, 958–964. [CrossRef] [PubMed]

15. Simmons, G.; McCall, J. Social perception and appraisal. In *Communication Theory*; Mortensen, C., Ed.; Transaction Publishers: New Brunswick, NJ, USA, 2009; Volume 2, pp. 58–73.

16. Kaae, S.; Traulsen, J.; Nørgaard, L. Customer interest in and experience with various types of pharmacy counselling—A qualitative study. *Health Expect.* **2012**, *17*, 852–862. [CrossRef] [PubMed]

17. Bowling, A. Unstructured interviewing and focus groups. In *Research Methods in Health. Investigating Health and Health Services*; Bowling, A., Ed.; Open University Press: Berkshire, UK, 2006; Volume 2, pp. 377–401.

18. Barnlund, D. A transactional model of communication. In *Communication Theory*; Mortensen, C., Ed.; Transaction Publishers: New Brunswick, NJ, USA, 2009; Volume 2, pp. 47–57.

19. Kvale, S. *Interviews: An Introduction to Qualitative Research Interviewing*; Kvale, S., Ed.; Sage Publications: London, UK, 1996.

20. Roseman, I.; Smith, C.A. Appraisal theory: Overview, assumptions, varieties, controversies. In *Appraisal Processes in Emotion: The Theory, Methods, Research*; Scherer, K.R., Johnstone, T., Eds.; Oxford University Press: New York, NY, USA, 2001; pp. 3–19.

21. Tran, V.; Garcia-Prieto, P.; Schneider, S.C. The role of social identity, appraisal, and emotion in determining responses to diversity management. *Hum. Relat.* **2001**, *64*, 161–176. [CrossRef]

22. Worley, M.M.; Schommer, J.C.; Brown, L.M.; Hadsall, R.S.; Ranelli, P.L.; Stratton, T.P.; Uden, D.L. Pharmacists' and patients' roles in the pharmacist-patient relationship: Are pharmacists and patients reading from the same relationship script? *Res. Soc. Adm. Pharm.* **2007**, *3*, 47–69. [CrossRef] [PubMed]

23. Assa-Eley, M.; Kimberlin, C.L. Using interpersonal perception to characterize pharmacists' and patients' perceptions of the benefits of pharmaceutical care. *Health Commun.* **2005**, *17*, 41–56. [CrossRef]

24. McDonough, R.P.; Bennett, M.S. Improving communication skills of pharmacy students through effective precepting. *Am. J. Pharm. Educ.* **2006**, *70*, 58. [CrossRef] [PubMed]

25. Renberg, T.; Wichman Tornqvist, K.; Kalvemark Sporrong, S.; Kettis Lindblad, A.; Tully, M.P. Pharmacy users' expectations of pharmacy encounters: A Q-methodological study. *Health Expect. Int. J. Public Particip. Health Care Health Policy* **2011**, *14*, 361–373. [CrossRef] [PubMed]

26. Sporrong, S.; Kaae, S. Trends in Pharmacy Practice Communication Research. *Pharmacy* **2018**, *6*, 127. [CrossRef] [PubMed]

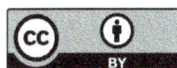

pharmacy

MDPI

Article

Administration, Billing, and Payment for Pharmacy Student-Based Immunizations to Medicare Beneficiaries at Mobile Medicare Clinics

Joseph A. Woelfel, Edward L. Rogan *[ID], Rajul A. Patel, Winnie Ho, Hong Van Nguyen, Emily Highsmith, Claire Chang, Nhat-Thanh Nguyen, Morgan Sato and Daniel Nguyen

Department of Pharmacy Practice, Thomas J. Long School of Pharmacy, University of the Pacific, Stockton, CA 95211, USA; jwoelfel@pacific.edu (J.A.W.); rpatel@pacific.edu (R.A.P.); w_ho1@u.pacific.edu (W.H.); h_nguyen40@u.pacific.edu (H.V.N.); e_highsmith@u.pacific.edu (E.H.); c_chang15@u.pacific.edu (C.C.); n_nguyen68@u.pacific.edu (N.-T.N.); m_sato4@u.pacific.edu (M.S.); d_nguyen36@u.pacific.edu (D.N.)
* Correspondence: erogan@pacific.edu

Received: 30 January 2019; Accepted: 21 February 2019; Published: 25 February 2019

check for
updates

Abstract: Training student pharmacists to administer vaccinations requires a substantial investment in vaccines, supplies, and time. Few schools of pharmacy seek out or receive any reimbursement for the provision of vaccines, despite the fact it is a covered service. This study sought to implement, deliver, and demonstrate an innovative, financially sustainable curriculum-based immunization program by trained pharmacy students as part of their experiential learning. Thirty-nine community health clinics targeting Medicare beneficiaries were conducted throughout Northern/Central California during Medicare's fall open enrollment periods between 2014–2016. American Pharmacists Association (APhA)-trained student pharmacists (under licensed pharmacist supervision) administered 1777 vaccinations. Vaccines were billed via a secure Health Insurance Portability and Accountability Act of 1996 (HIPAA)-compliant web-based portal. The total net income was $11,905 and $8032 for 2015 and 2016, respectively. Return on investment was greatest for the influenza vaccine > Tdap > pneumococcal. Pharmacy students are already being trained to provide immunizations and can utilize their skills to deliver financially viable public health programs.

Keywords: immunization programs; mobile health units; experiential learning; billing; healthy people 2020

1. Introduction

Vaccinations are a well-known, cost-effective, way to reduce morbidity and mortality. For each group of individuals born in the same year (birth cohort) that is properly vaccinated, the following could be prevented; 14 million cases of disease, 33,000 deaths, and almost $10 billion in direct health care costs. However, approximately 42,000 adults in the United States still die from vaccine-preventable diseases each year [1].

The Department of Health and Human Services initiated the Healthy People 2020 program with the intent to promote the health of Americans by encouraging collaboration across communities, empowering individuals, and measuring the impact of these interventions [1]. One notable goal is the improvement of vaccination rates. Healthy People 2020 seeks a goal of at least 90% of adults 65 years of age and older to be vaccinated against both influenza and pneumococcal disease [1]. In 2014, data released by the Centers for Disease Control and Prevention (CDC) showed that approximately 70% of seniors 65 years old and over were vaccinated against influenza and approximately 61% against pneumococcal [2].

Inadequate vaccination rates could be a result of multiple factors, including a lack of perceived value, insufficient information and education, fear or opposition to vaccines, cost, accessibility, and operational or systemic barriers [3]. Despite the fact that Medicare is the primary insurance for most seniors, 36% to 71% of general internists and family physicians reported a lack of knowledge of Medicare vaccine coverage [4].

Lower adult vaccination rates may also be due to the lack of immunization programs that support and promote adult vaccinations. Vaccines for Children (VFC), a federally funded program through the CDC, provides discounted vaccines to agencies that then distribute them to doctors' offices and public health clinics. The VFC program has proven successful in improving childhood vaccination rates. Further contributing to the disparity in vaccination rates between children and seniors is the fact that many older patients may be unaware of the importance of indicated vaccines, a pattern first observed during adulthood [3]. The lack of proper education on immunizations remains an issue. Studies that examined attitudes toward the influenza vaccine found that the main concern among those eschewing the vaccine was the belief they would get influenza from the vaccination or experience adverse effects [5]. Barriers to vaccination uptake among patients 65 years and older include a lack of awareness of the need to get vaccinated and the perceived belief that they were unlikely to catch "the flu" [5]. Interestingly, greater than half of unvaccinated patients studied did not know that the entire cost of the influenza vaccine was a covered Medicare benefit [5]. Increased understanding of this benefit should encourage greater uptake of the influenza vaccine by older patients. The study also found that patients who were recommended immunizations by a healthcare professional were more likely to be vaccinated. Immunization rates can be increased due to pharmacists' easy accessibility and their ability to dispel vaccine safety concerns and explain the risks of being unvaccinated. [5].

Expanding the provision of vaccines into non-traditional settings, such as worksites and pharmacies, has been proven to be a cost-effective way to improve adult vaccination rates. Prosser reported that the mean cost of providing vaccines was 40%–60% lower in non-traditional settings when compared to traditional settings, such as physician offices [6]. Moreover, it was found that the cost of preventing an episode of influenza was $90 in a pharmacy setting (e.g., when a pharmacist provides the vaccine), $210 in a mass vaccination setting, and $870 in traditional settings. Providing vaccines in non-traditional settings helps increase patient convenience, improves vaccination coverage rates, and is cost-effective [6].

Since pharmacists can play a major part in increasing community vaccination rates, student pharmacist training is crucial to preparing tomorrow's pharmacists to take up this vital public health role. As of June 2017, 67/135 schools of pharmacy throughout the United States are certified to provide the American Pharmacists Association's (APhA's) Pharmacy-Based Immunization Delivery program to their students [7]. The APhA's Pharmacy-Based Immunization Delivery Program is a national training certificate program employed to educate pharmacists on how to become vaccination providers [7]. After completion of this training, and subject to their state's scope of practice laws, student pharmacists are able to provide vaccinations to patients. Previous research by Turner and colleagues has shown that the provision of vaccines by student pharmacists during introductory pharmacy practice experiences can enhance students' vaccine knowledge and increase students' self-confidence in the administration of vaccines [8]. Chou and colleagues showed that student pharmacist consultation can improve patient perceptions and attitudes towards receiving vaccinations, further increasing adult vaccination uptake and changing the public's view of the pharmacist's role in preventive health [9]. The provision of vaccines by student pharmacists also helps schools of pharmacy satisfy accreditation standards for disease prevention promotion set by the Center for the Advancement of Pharmacy Education [10].

While the majority of pharmacy schools across the county have pharmacy students provide vaccinations to the community, few provide vaccines other than influenza, and even fewer bill for provided vaccines. A previous study at The University of Oklahoma College of Pharmacy described the integration of introductory and advanced pharmacy practice experiences within campus-based influenza clinics to provide vaccinations to faculty, staff, and their families [11]. They reported that billing through their on-campus retail pharmacy generated a net income for their clinics [11].

Even though students from schools of pharmacy have been providing vaccinations for some time now, little literature exists on the provision of any other vaccines besides influenza being provided by student pharmacists. This may be due to the fact that the influenza vaccine is considerably less expensive to provide than all other available vaccines, and thus more financially feasible given limited school budgets.

This study details the creation and application of a curriculum-based, financially self-sustaining pharmacy school program designed to increase vaccination rates in ambulatory Medicare beneficiaries while providing an experiential learning environment.

2. Materials and Methods

During the fall Medicare open enrollment periods from 2014–2016, the University of the Pacific School of Pharmacy & Health Sciences held thirty-nine Mobile Medicare Clinics in 10 different cities throughout Northern/Central California. Beneficiaries at each clinic site were able to take advantage of multiple health services/screenings, including: Medicare Part D plan reviews, Medication Therapy Management (MTM), health screenings, and immunizations.

The following vaccines were available at each clinic location: influenza (TIV and/or QIV); Pneumovax 23 (PPSV 23); Prevnar 13 (PCV13); and the tetanus, diphtheria, and pertussis vaccine (Tdap). The influenza vaccine was both purchased by the School and also donated by multiple different county public health departments. All other vaccines and supplies were purchased by the School. During each MTM session, assisted beneficiaries were asked a series of questions so as to ascertain their vaccination history. State vaccination registries and immunization providers were contacted when patients were unsure of their vaccination history. To improve convenience, patients were able to receive vaccinations at one of two locations at each clinic site: (1) a designated vaccination station or (2) the table at which they were receiving the MTM intervention. Walk in patients not receiving MTM services could also receive vaccinations.

Beneficiaries expressing interest in receiving any of the available vaccines provided personal information (including their Medicare ID number) and were asked a series of standard APhA vaccine screening questions, such as those relating to allergies, previous reactions to vaccines, pregnant or could be pregnant, etc. All answers were reviewed by a licensed, immunization-certified pharmacist and vaccine appropriateness was determined. School faculty and/or staff would verify beneficiary eligibility and financial responsibility for Part B (influenza or pneumococcal vaccine) or Part D (Tdap) vaccines using TransactRx, an internet-based billing and integrated claims processing platform. TransactRx provides real-time patient eligibility and on-line billing and payment for all covered Medicare Part B and D vaccines.

If the beneficiary was eligible for Part B billing of the influenza or pneumococcal vaccines, there was no co-pay sharing. However, if the beneficiary was eligible for Part D billing of the Tdap vaccine, the co-pay amount would be communicated to the patient and collected if they were interested in receiving the vaccine. Co-pays were collected via cash, personal check, or credit card using a University-approved PCI-compliant electronic payment system (CashNet). Vaccine doses that could be successfully billed were drawn from the School's purchased supply. The Public Health influenza vaccine was used whenever an uninsured or unqualified beneficiary needed vaccination. 'Vouchered vaccines' were non-billable (e.g., Public Health donated vaccine, vaccines subsidized through grant funds, or vaccines given away to the community) administered vaccines. Once vaccine billing was initiated and an individual dose prepared, a certified student pharmacist administered the vaccine under the supervision of a pharmacist preceptor and provided the beneficiary with necessary paperwork (Vaccine Information Sheet (VIS) and proof of vaccination).

The number and type of vaccines provided at each mobile clinic were recorded. Return on investment (ROI) was calculated as follows: ROI = [(Total revenue − Total Cost)/(Total Cost)] × 100.

Along with ROI, net income was computed each season from TransactRx billing software reports. Descriptive statistics (e.g., absolute frequency for types of vaccinations administered/billed and average ROI for each vaccination type provided) were calculated and reported for these items.

Students received introductory pharmacy practice experiences (IPPE) credit as part of a required health care outreach class that contributed approximately 8% of their total required hours. Vaccinations were coordinated by a student group, Operation Immunization, and were responsible for bringing supplies, set up, and other logistics necessary for a mobile health clinic. Additional students enrolled in the outreach class signed up to participate in the vaccination or one of the other health screenings being provided at the clinic. Students were not required to spend a specific amount of time per each station, but were required to stay at the same station for which they signed up for the duration of that event. Each event, on average, had two students from Operation Immunization and four to eight students administering vaccines. Students participated in multiple health care outreach events to acquire the required number of hours.

This study was approved by the University of the Pacific's Institutional Review Board.

3. Results

A total of 4083 beneficiaries were served at our Mobile Medicare Clinics from 2014–2016. Senior immunizations were a major part of the services provided. Overall, 1777 vaccines were administered during the study time period. Table 1 identifies the type and number of vaccines administered and billed at clinic sites from 2014–2016. As shown in Table 1, about two out of three of the vaccines provided during the study period were for influenza. Of the 1777 administered vaccines, 1345 (75.7%) were billed through TransactRx (Table 1); 832 (68.2%) influenza, 449 (99.6%) pneumococcal, and 64 (60.4%) Tdap. As shown in Table 1, 629 vaccines in 2014 were billed through an independent partnering pharmacy as a proof of concept. In 2015 and 2016, 411 and 305 vaccines, respectively, were billed directly using the TransactRx platform. A total of 432 vouchered vaccines were provided during the study period; 388 (89.8%) of which were for influenza. Figure 1 highlights the ROI for each provided vaccine in 2015 and 2016. The ROI was greatest for the influenza vaccine > Tdap > pneumococcal. The total net income was $11,905 and $8032 for 2015 and 2016, respectively (data not shown).

Table 1. Number and Types of Vaccines Administered and Billed at Clinic Sites from 2014–2016.

Vaccination Type	Number of Vaccinations Administered and Billed by Year (Billing System)			
	2014 (Partnering Pharmacy)	2015 (TransactRx)	2016 (TransactRx)	Total
Influenza				
administered	436	397	387	1220
billed	436	214	182	832
Pneumococcal				
administered	138	191	122	451
billed	138	191	120	449
Tdap				
administered	55	35	16	106
billed	55	6	3	64
Total				
administered	629	623	525	1777
billed	629	411	305	1345

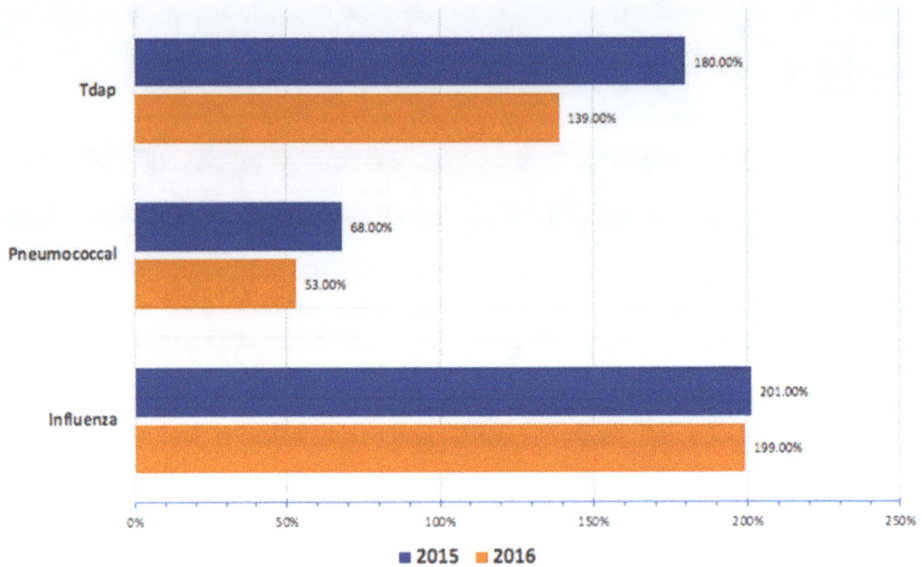

Figure 1. Return on Investment for Each Vaccine from 2015–2016.

4. Discussion

The present study describes a new, fiscally self-sustainable vaccination program in which trained student pharmacists provided vaccinations to Medicare beneficiaries in community settings as part of their IPPE. Our study describes a program that utilizes a live-claim processing platform (e.g., TransactRx) for vaccines at community-based health clinics that can: (1) provide students with practical experience of immunization administration, coverage, and billing; (2) help increase vaccination rates of older adults and other Medicare beneficiaries; and (3) generate income for the provision of such services by a school of pharmacy. The above criteria set up a true "win-win-win" proposition for the target population, pharmacy students, and the school of pharmacy.

During the fall of 2015 and 2016, successful Medicare vaccine billing generated a total net income of $19,937 for our School of Pharmacy. The generation of this net income was the first step in building an effective community outreach program in which students delivered essential and needed services in a budget-neutral way for our School. Profits from the program are used to purchase vaccines and supplies for the next season. The vaccine billing model discussed here can be duplicated at other schools of pharmacy throughout the country, with the ability to increase the types and numbers of vaccines that students can provide to their communities.

While the majority of pharmacy schools across the county have pharmacy students providing vaccinations to the community, few provide vaccines other than influenza, and even fewer bill for provided vaccines. Our study adds to the current literature in that it describes the structure, implementation, billing, and benefit of vaccination services in a mobile, community-based setting. Utilization of a web-based claims processing platform (e.g., TransactRx) allows vaccine administration and billing in areas outside of a traditional school/university's campus or clinic. Using an on-line claims billing service also allows patient eligibility to be checked and billed in real-time, virtually eliminating billing denials and potential loss of revenue. Furthermore, implementation of such a system can be used by any school of pharmacy across the country, regardless of whether they have an on-site medical center or pharmacy.

Program models such as ours present schools of pharmacy a means to help fulfill the various requirements of accrediting bodies and national objectives for improving public health. In 2011, the American Association of Colleges of Pharmacy, encouraged by the Healthy People 2020 curriculum task force, instituted a new requirement in which core public health concepts were to be integrated into every pharmacy school curricula (objective ECBP-17) [12]. Additionally, our program model also helps to satisfy the Healthy People 2020's Immunization and Infectious Diseases objective of increasing the vaccination rates of adults 65 years of age and older (Objectives IID-12.7 and IID-13.1) [13].

The return on investment for the three vaccines we provided varied according to the type of vaccine administered. The influenza vaccine was the highest, with about a 200% ROI. Of the three, the influenza vaccine was the most inexpensive and had the highest margin. The influenza vaccine is indicated to be administered annually and can be a continuous source of revenue for a school-based immunization clinic. The other vaccines, pneumococcal and Tdap, had a lower ROI and are only administered as a one-time dose or as a booster. The number of these vaccines declined notably after the initial year because many of our clinics are held at the same locations and draw many of the same patients every year. These vaccines did not function as a major source of revenue, but their availability was essential to providing comprehensive vaccination services to an ambulatory Medicare population with a vaccination rate below the goals of Healthy People 2020.

Some limitations of our study were that students at the time were not specifically trained to counter vaccine hesitancy from patients and that cost/coverage was a main factor impacting patients' acceptance of vaccination. Preparing students to better address vaccine myths and misinformation could further improve vaccination rates and acceptance. Learning modules on vaccine hesitancy have been developed and incorporated into didactic classes and vaccine clinics and are currently being evaluated for their effectiveness. Another limitation is that the implementation of our program by other schools will require a contract with Medicare to bill for Medicare covered services. The associated application paperwork and administrative constraints can be lengthy, cumbersome, and require considerable time for approval.

5. Conclusions

Vaccination billing through a web-based transaction platform provides schools of pharmacy with a net income to boost the availability and variety of vaccinations administered by student pharmacists. This incentivized and replicable vaccine billing model can be implemented by any school of pharmacy, creating an economically sustainable, community-based vaccination program that provides students with experiential training and addresses suboptimal vaccination rates of older adults and other Medicare beneficiaries.

Author Contributions: Conceptualization, J.A.W., R.A.P. and E.L.R.; Methodology, J.A.W., R.A.P. and E.L.R.; Software, R.A.P.; Validation, J.A.W., R.A.P. and E.L.R.; Formal Analysis, R.A.P., J.A.W. and E.L.R.; Investigation, J.A.W., R.A.P., E.L.R., W.H., H.V.N., E.H., C.C., N.-T.N., M.S. and D.N.; Writing-Original Draft Preparation, J.A.W., R.A.P., E.L.R., W.H., H.V.N., E.H., C.C., N.-T.N., M.S. and D.N.; Writing-Review & Editing, J.A.W., R.A.P., E.L.R., W.H., H.V.N., E.H., C.C., N.-T.N., M.S. and D.N.

Funding: This research received no external funding.

Conflicts of Interest: The authors declare no conflict of interest.

References

1. U.S Department of Health and Human Services. Healthy People 2020: Immunization and Infectious Disease. Healthy People 2020 Web Site. Updated 2017. Available online: https://www.healthypeople.gov/2020/topics-objectives/topic/immunization-and-infectious-diseases (accessed on 8 May 2017).
2. *Health, United States, 2015: With Special Feature on Racial and Ethnic Health Disparities*; National Center for Health Statistics (US): Hyattsville, MD, USA, 2016.
3. Ventola, C.L. Immunization in the United States: Recommendations, Barriers, and Measures to Improve Compliance: Part 2: Adult Vaccinations. *Pharm. Ther.* **2016**, *41*, 492–506.

4. Hurley, L.P.; Lindley, M.C.; Allison, M.A.; Crane, L.A.; Brtnikova, M.; Beaty, B.L.; Snow, M.; Bridges, C.B.; Kempe, A. Primary care physicians' perspective on financial issues and adult immunization in the era of the affordable care act. *Vaccine* **2017**, *35*, 647–654. [CrossRef] [PubMed]

5. Zimmerman, R.K.; Santibanez, T.A.; Janosky, J.E.; Fine, M.J. What affects influenza vaccination rates among older patients? An analysis from inner-city, suburban, rural, and veterans affairs practices. *Am. J. Med.* **2003**, *114*, 31–38. [CrossRef]

6. Prosser, L.A.; O'Brien, M.A.; Molinari, N.M. Non-traditional settings for influenza vaccination of adults. *Pharmacoeconomics* **2008**, *26*, 163–178. [CrossRef] [PubMed]

7. Pharmacy-Based Immunization Delivery. American Pharmacists Association Web. Available online: http://www.pharmacist.com/pharmacy-based-immunization-delivery (accessed on 9 August 2017).

8. Turner, C.J.; Ellis, S.; Giles, J.; Altiere, R.; Sintek, C.; Ulrich, H.; Valdez, C.; Zadvorny, E. An introductory pharmacy practice experience emphasizing student-administered vaccinations. *Am. J. Pharm. Educ.* **2007**, *71*, 3. [CrossRef] [PubMed]

9. Tony, I.; Chou, F.; Lash, D.B.; Malcolm, B.; Yousify, L.; Quach, J.Y.; Dong, S.; Yu, J. Effects of a student pharmacist consultation on patient knowledge and attitudes about vaccines. *J. Am. Pharm. Assoc.* **2014**, *54*, 130–137.

10. CAPE Educational Outcomes. AACP. Available online: https://www.aacp.org/resource/cape-educational-outcomes (accessed on 12 February 2019).

11. Conway, S.E.; Johnson, E.J.; Hagemann, T.M. Introductory and Advanced Pharmacy Practice Experiences Within Campus-based Influenza Clinics. *Am. J. Pharm. Educ.* **2013**, *77*, 61. [CrossRef] [PubMed]

12. Healthy People 2020. American Association of Colleges of Pharmacy. Available online: http://www.aacp.org/resources/research/institutionalresearch/Pages/HealthyPeople2020.aspx (accessed on 7 August 2017).

13. Immunization and Infectious Diseases. Immunization and Infectious Diseases | Healthy People 2020. Available online: https://www.healthypeople.gov/2020/topics-objectives/topic/immunization-and-infectious-diseases/objectives (accessed on 7 August 2017).

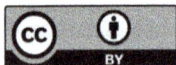

pharmacy

MDPI

Article

Feasibility of a Coordinated Human Papillomavirus (HPV) Vaccination Program between a Medical Clinic and a Community Pharmacy

William R. Doucette [1],*, Kelly Kent [2], Laura Seegmiller [1], Randal P. McDonough [2] and William Evans [1]

[1] Department of Pharmacy Practice & Science, University of Iowa, Iowa City, IA 52242, USA
[2] Towncrest Pharmacy, Iowa City, IA 52240, USA
*   Correspondence: william-doucette@uiowa.edu; Tel.: +01-1-319-335-8786

Received: 28 April 2019; Accepted: 8 July 2019; Published: 14 July 2019

check for updates

Abstract: Human papillomavirus (HPV) vaccination coverage could be enhanced by community pharmacies working with medical clinics to coordinate completion of the HPV vaccination series. The objective for this study was to assess the feasibility of a coordinated model of HPV vaccine delivery in which a clinic gives the first dose and refers patients to a partnering community pharmacy to receive subsequent doses. A medical clinic-community pharmacy team was established in a Midwestern state to develop and operate a coordinated care model for HPV vaccinations. Under the coordinated model, the clinic identified patients needing HPV vaccination(s), administered the first dose and described the option to complete the vaccination series at the pharmacy. Interested patients then had an information sheet faxed and electronic prescriptions sent to the pharmacy. The pharmacy contacted the patients to schedule administration of 2nd and 3rd doses of the HPV vaccine. Over a 12-month period, 51 patients were referred to the pharmacy by the clinic. Of these, 23 patients received a total of 25 vaccinations. Clinic and pharmacy personnel mostly rated the coordinated program favorably. An initial study of a coordinated HPV vaccination program between a medical clinic and a community pharmacy supported patients getting HPV vaccinations.

Keywords: human papilloma virus; HPV vaccination; pharmacy; coordinated care

1. Introduction

Human papillomavirus (HPV) is the most common sexually transmitted infection, with 14 million infections occurring in women and men in the United States (U.S.) annually [1]. HPV is responsible for approximately 33,700 cases of cancer each year, including virtually all cases of cervical cancer [2]. The infection is most common among young adults in their early teens through late twenties, in which it is transmitted sexually through contact with an infected person. The FDA approved the first vaccine for HPV in 2006. The HPV vaccine is recommended for adolescents beginning at 11 years of age, and consists of two doses administered over a course of six to twelve months, or three doses for those ages 15 and over [3]. In the four years following the recommendation, HPV infections in teenage girls decreased by 56% [4]. Despite the efficacy and safety of the vaccine, HPV vaccination rates have been substandard. In 2017, only 48.6% of teens reported HPV vaccination series completed, showing HPV vaccination rates are well below the *Healthy People 2020* national goal of 80% [5].

Innovative strategies should be considered in order to improve the vaccination rates among at-risk populations. In some countries, school-based approaches to delivering HPV vaccinations have been successful [6,7]. However, due to limited availability and concerns about payment, such school-based solutions are a challenge in the U.S. Pharmacists are healthcare professionals in a unique position to improve vaccine access and provide convenient administration of vaccines to patients, including the HPV vaccine. The National Vaccine Advisory Committee recommended using pharmacies to raise patient access to HPV vaccines [8]. Pharmacist involvement in vaccinations varies globally, with some countries allowing pharmacists to administer vaccines. These countries include Argentina, Australia, Philippines, South Africa, the UK and USA. These countries most commonly allow pharmacists to administer influenza vaccines, though other vaccines are allowed. In the US, pharmacists typically can administer influenza vaccines and other adult vaccines (e.g., for pneumococcus, or shingles) and travel vaccines. Much less common is ability of pharmacists to administer the "childhood vaccines" [9]. Pharmacists have historically offered several immunizations (e.g., influenza and pneumococcal) in the community setting and continually demonstrate their contribution to improved vaccination rates. A recent study assessed a 10 year span and compared vaccination rates between states that permitted pharmacy vaccination services and those that did not. The investigators found a significant increase in influenza vaccination rates among the states permitting pharmacist vaccinations [10]. Community pharmacies have collaborated with clinics to increase influenza vaccination rates [11]. Though such a coordinated model could be effective for raising HPV vaccination rates, no descriptions of this approach have been reported. It could be helpful to tap the potential of community pharmacists working in coordination with a clinic to address HPV vaccine series completion rates. The objective for this study was to assess the feasibility of a coordinated model of HPV vaccine delivery in which a clinic gives the first dose and refers patients to a partnering community pharmacy to receive subsequent doses.

2. Materials and Methods

This study recruited one primary care medical clinic and one community pharmacy to develop and evaluate a coordinated HPV vaccination program. To recruit a clinic-community pharmacy team, based on an author's experience (W.R.D.) several progressive community pharmacies were approached, and interested pharmacists provided contact information for a clinician or clinic with which they wished to partner with for HPV vaccine delivery. An independent pharmacy located in a micropolitan area (population at least 10,000 but not more than 50,000) agreed to participate, along with a primary care medical clinic. The pharmacy provided traditional dispensing services, immunizations, adherence packaging services, medication management, and compounding services. The pharmacy employed a total of five pharmacist full-time equivalents (FTEs), a community pharmacy resident, and five technician FTEs. The two partners were located about two miles apart. The clinic is affiliated with a university health system, and employs about 20 providers. Once a clinic-pharmacy team was identified, the investigators contacted both providers and scheduled a 60 min face-to-face team building session for the pharmacy-clinic team members, including providers, the clinic manager, other clinic staff and pharmacy personnel. The team building session was facilitated by the research team, and consisted of an explanation of the project objectives with team discussion of roles and responsibilities in a coordinated HPV vaccination program.

In the USA, the credentialing of pharmacists to administer vaccinations varies by state. That is, each state's governing/licensing body for pharmacists sets the requirements for pharmacists to be able to administer vaccines in that state. All 50 states have authorized pharmacists to administer vaccines at some level. Three states did not allow pharmacists to administer HPV vaccines (in 2015). In Iowa, the Board of Pharmacy allows pharmacists to administer HPV vaccines pursuant to a prescription order. It requires that a licensed pharmacist must complete an approved program on vaccine administration and complete training on basic life support for healthcare providers which includes hands-on training. There are not specific requirements for pharmacies other than providing proper storage for vaccines. Vaccinations typically are paid for by private insurance or through government program coverage, such as Vaccines for Children or Medicare for older patients. The preferred workflow of the coordinated program was determined by the clinic and pharmacy team members, including how patients would be identified, communication with the patients and between providers, reporting of immunizations in the state registry, and payment for the vaccinations. After the program was planned, practice changes and tools were made during a 4 month period, and then the coordinated program operated for a planned 12 month period. A brief online survey was used to collect feedback about the program from clinic and pharmacy staff. The survey asked about overall performance of the coordinated approach using a five-point scale (poor, fair, good, very good, excellent), challenges and benefits of the model using checklists, and an open-ended question about suggested improvements to the coordinated model. The Human Subjects Office at the University of Iowa approved this study.

The coordinated HPV vaccination program worked as follows. The clinic identified patients in need of HPV vaccination during its established patient care processes for preventive care for young patients. The first dose of the HPV series was administered within the participating clinic. To incorporate the coordinated program, all patients then were offered a choice of receiving the remainder of the HPV series vaccinations at the clinic or the pharmacy. For the patients who selected the pharmacy, the clinic then used electronic order sets developed with their IT personnel for second and third HPV vaccine doses and sent them to the participating pharmacy along with a patient information sheet, which contained demographic and contact information. The pharmacy was then responsible for working with the patient to schedule the remaining HPV vaccinations. During the administration visit at the pharmacy, patients were offered educational materials available in English and Spanish languages. The clinic and pharmacy served patients who spoke Spanish as their primary language. The pharmacist recorded the vaccinations in the Iowa Immunization Registry Information System (IRIS) and sent a clinical note in SOAP (Subjective, Objective, Assessment, Plan) format to the clinic partner. The pharmacy submitted billing to private insurers or to the Vaccines for Children (VFC) program for the doses administered there.

Prior to this study, the pharmacy had experience in administering vaccinations, including for influenza, pneumococcus, herpes zoster, and others. The pharmacy staff participated in a provider training session on the HPV vaccine provided by Merck. The patient education materials in English and Spanish were obtained from the CDC and other sources. During the study period, the pharmacy utilized a contact log to track communications with the patients, and used a texting service to remind patients of scheduled vaccinations.

The primary outcome variable for the coordinated HPV vaccination program was the number of HPV vaccinations delivered at the pharmacy. In addition, data were collected on the number of patients referred to the pharmacy by the clinic and the number of patients receiving an HPV vaccination at the pharmacy. Finally, changes in practice and tools developed for the program were collected from clinic and pharmacy staff.

3. Results

Both practices made changes in their operations to be able to work together within the coordinated HPV program. The clinic added electronic prescription order sets to be able to e-prescribe the second and third doses of the HPV vaccine to the pharmacy. In addition, the clinic developed a patient information sheet to fax to the pharmacy whenever they referred a patient for an HPV vaccine. This information included patient name, date of birth, address, insurance coverage and numbers, parent or guardian identification, and contact information. Finally, the clinic incorporated into their workflow a discussion with eligible patients about the option of completing the HPV vaccination series at the pharmacy. All providers participating at the clinic were physicians.

The pharmacy developed materials for patient communication, including a flyer about the HPV vaccination service in English and in Spanish, as well as a script for pharmacists to use when calling patients and/or their families about the HPV vaccination at the pharmacy. They also used "Oh Don't Forget" texting to send patients a reminder before a scheduled vaccination. The pharmacy already routinely recorded vaccinations in Iowa's Immunization Registry Information System (IRIS), and did so with the HPV vaccinations. For communicating with the clinic, the pharmacy utilized a clinical note template they already had in use that followed a SOAP format to inform the providers about each HPV vaccination administered. They also sent to the clinic a quarterly summary of the patients receiving an HPV vaccination. This report listed the patients receiving an HPV vaccination during that period, as well as the date of administration and the number of vaccine in the HPV series (e.g., 2nd or 3rd). Other practice changes made by the pharmacy included establishing themselves as a provider for the Vaccines for Children (VFC) program in Iowa, and developing a vaccination log to track communications with patients. The Vaccines for Children is a federal program that pays for vaccines for low income children.

During the 12 month study period, 51 patients were referred to the pharmacy by the clinic. Of these, 23 patients received a total of 25 vaccinations. All 23 patients completed their HPV series. Eighteen (78.3%) of the patients were female, while the mean age was 13.4 years (SD = 1.4). The insurance payments to the pharmacy were 13 (56.5%) commercial payers and 10 (43.5%) VFC. The other 28 patients either could not be reached by the pharmacy or declined to come to the pharmacy after being contacted. Surveys were received from five people at the clinic (four physicians and the clinic manager) and one from the pharmacy (pharmacist). Of the five respondents who rated the program's performance, two rated it as excellent, and one each as very good, fair and poor. Reported difficulties in collaborating included having few interested patients, challenges with workflow, lack of staff time and some language barriers with the patients. Reported benefits to the coordinated program were that it made it easier for patients to complete the HPV vaccination series, increased opportunity for pharmacists and improved communication between the providers and pharmacists. When asked about changes to support such a team approach, having community pharmacist access to an electronic health record was the most common suggestion.

4. Discussion

The coordinated delivery of the HPV vaccine using clinic-pharmacy partnerships is a promising model for the improvement of HPV immunization rates through the use of alternative settings. As reported by the participating providers, some patients appreciated the convenience of getting an HPV vaccination at a pharmacy, which was open more hours than most clinics. This coordinated model improved patient access to HPV vaccinations, similar to the enhanced access provided for other vaccines, especially influenza. Previous work has shown that provider referrals are vital for pharmacies seeking to administer vaccines [12]. The coordinated model builds in provider referrals from the participating clinic. This study shows community pharmacies as a viable location for administration of HPV vaccinations. Future research should be conducted to investigate how a coordinated model could be implemented on a broader scale, perhaps involving a whole community instead of a single clinic-pharmacy team.

Positive provider recommendations to patients are key in getting them to agree to receive vaccinations, especially an HPV vaccine [13]. A strength of the coordinated program was that two voices were used to inform and encourage parents and patients to complete the HPV vaccination series. In addition to clinic personnel explaining the need for the HPV vaccine, a community pharmacist also discussed the HPV vaccination series with the patients and parents/caretakers. Pharmacists have been recognized as a trusted provider of medication and health information by patients [14], and can serve in a public health role. In addition, most pharmacists have completed training in providing immunizations, which supports their role in discussing HPV vaccinations with patients and/or their parents [15]. Together, primary care providers and pharmacists can help overcome parental hesitancy for HPV vaccinations [16]. This complementary communication can readily derive from a coordinated care approach being followed by a clinic-pharmacy partnership.

Another facilitator of this coordinated HPV program was that the clinic and the pharmacy exchanged patient information in a timely and usable manner. The patient information sheet sent by the clinic to the pharmacy allowed the pharmacy to receive necessary patient information, and provided successful patient hand-off communication [17]. The pharmacist was then able to contact the patient's caretaker to discuss and schedule the next dose of the HPV vaccine. Similarly, the clinical note sent by the pharmacy to the clinic after vaccine administration let the clinic providers know that the patient had received another HPV vaccination. Another facilitator was the presence of HPV vaccination champions in both the clinic and the pharmacy. These people, a registered nurse and a pharmacist, helped assure that their respective organizations implemented the program and remained committed to it during the 12 month follow-up period.

As reported by the FIP in 2016, four countries allowed pharmacists to administer HPV vaccinations: Canada (some provinces), Portugal, the UK and USA [9]. It is hoped that the number of countries giving pharmacists authority to administer HPV vaccines will increase as more experience is gained with such services. A number of other countries allow pharmacists to administer influenza vaccines. As flu shots become more expected at pharmacies, it could be that other vaccines will be added to those that can be given by a pharmacist. Such changes likely would improve patient access to vaccines.

This study has several limitations. First is that only one clinic-community pharmacy team was studied. This limits the variability in the practice characteristics involved with the coordinated care model, including staff commitment, patient characteristics and community context. Having multiple clinics and multiple pharmacies using a coordinated care model likely would uncover more obstacles to be addressed in making the model work. This study showed that the coordinated care model involving a clinic and community pharmacy can be successful. However, future research with multiple clinic-pharmacy teams in a more rigorous design can address the limitation of just one team being studied. Another limitation is that no patient feedback was collected about their experiences with the coordinated care model. We do not know how satisfied they were with the vaccinations delivered at the pharmacy. As community pharmacists deliver more HPV vaccinations, patient feedback could be collected about their experiences with them.

5. Conclusions

An initial study of a coordinated HPV vaccination program between a medical clinic and a community pharmacy supported patients getting HPV vaccinations. More research is needed to extend and further test the effectiveness of this model.

Author Contributions: The authors contributed to this work as follows: Conceptualization, W.R.D., L.S. and R.P.M.; methodology, W.R.D., K.K., L.S. and R.P.M.; formal analysis, W.R.D.; investigation, W.R.D., L.S. and W.E.; writing—original draft preparation, W.R.D., L.S. and W.E.; writing—review and editing, W.R.D., K.K., L.S., R.P.M. and W.E.; project administration, W.R.D. and L.S.; funding acquisition, W.R.D. and L.S.

Funding: This research was funded by the American Cancer Society and the Centers for Disease Control and Prevention's Cancer Prevention and Control Research network.

Conflicts of Interest: The authors declare no conflict of interest. The funders had no role in the design of the study; in the collection, analyses, or interpretation of data; in the writing of the manuscript, or in the decision to publish the results.

References

1. Centers for Disease Control and Prevention. Genital HPV Infection—Fact Sheet. Available online: http://www.cdc.gov/std/HPV/STDFact-HPV.htm#a7 (accessed on 18 October 2018).
2. Centers for Disease Control and Prevention. HPV and Cancer. Available online: http://www.cdc.gov/hpv/parents/cancer.html (accessed on 18 October 2018).
3. Centers for Disease Control and Prevention. HPV Vaccine Recommendations. Available online: https://www.cdc.gov/hpv/parents/Vaccine-for-hpv.html (accessed on 18 October 2018).
4. Centers for Disease Control and Prevention. HPV Vaccine Safety and Effectiveness. Available online: https://www.cdc.gov/vaccines/vpd/hpv/hcp/safety-effectiveness.html (accessed on 18 October 2018).
5. Walker, T.Y.; Elam-Evans, L.D.; Singleton, J.A.; Yankey, D.; Markowitz, L.E.; Fredua, B.; Williams, C.L.; Meyer, S.A.; Stokley, S. National, regional, state and selected local area vaccination coverage among adolescents aged 13–17 years—United States, 2017. *MMWR Morb. Mortal. Wkly. Rep.* **2018**, *67*, 909–917. [CrossRef] [PubMed]

6. Kempe, A.; Allison, M.A.; Daley, M.F. Can school-located vaccination have a major impact on human papillomavirus vaccination rates in the United States? *Acad. Pediatr.* **2018**, *18*, S101–S105. [CrossRef] [PubMed]

7. Vandelaer, J.; Olaniran, M. Using a school-based approach to deliver immunization-global update. *Vaccine* **2015**, *33*, 719–725. [CrossRef] [PubMed]

8. Committee, National Vaccine Advisory. Recommendations to address low HPV vaccination coverage rates in the United States. *June* **2015**, *9*, 2015.

9. International Pharmaceutical Federation (FIP). *An Overview of Current Pharmacy Impact on Immunization—A Global Report 2016*; International Pharmaceutical Federation: The Hague, Netherlands, 2016.

10. Drozd, E.M.; Miller, L.; Johnsrud, M. Impact of pharmacist immunization authority on seasonal influenza immunization rates across states. *Clin. Ther.* **2017**, *39*, 1563–1580.e17. [CrossRef] [PubMed]

11. Luder, H.R.; Shannon, P.; Kirby, J.; Frede, S.M. Community pharmacist collaboration with a patient-centered medical home: Establishment of a patient-centered medical neighborhood and payment model. *J. Am. Pharm. Assoc.* **2018**, *58*, 44–50. [CrossRef] [PubMed]

12. Weitzel, K.W.; Goode, J.V. Implementation of a pharmacy-based immunization program in a supermarket chain. *J. Am. Pharm. Assoc.* **2000**, *40*, 252–256. [CrossRef]

13. Brewer, N.T.; Fazekas, K.I. Predictors of HPV vaccine acceptability: A theory-informed, systematic review. *Prev. Med.* **2007**, *45*, 107–114. [CrossRef] [PubMed]

14. Frazier, K.R.; McKeirnan, K.C.; Kherghehpoush, S.; Woodard, L.J. Rural patient perceptions of pharmacist-provided chronic condition management in a state with provider status. *J. Am. Pharm. Assoc.* **2019**, *59*, 210–216. [CrossRef] [PubMed]

15. Sommers Hanson, J. Pharmacists Engaging Adults to be Vaccinated. March 2017 Immunization Supplement. Pharmacy Times. 2017. Available online: https://www.pharmacytimes.com/publications/supplementals/2017/immunizationsupplementmarch2017/pharmacists-engaging-adults-to-be-vaccinated/ (accessed on 24 April 2019).

16. Shay, L.A.; Baldwin, A.S.; Betts, A.C.; Marks, E.G.; Higashi, R.T.; Street, R.L.; Persaud, D.; Tiro, J. Parent-provider communication of HPV vaccine hesitancy. *Pediatrics* **2018**, *141*, e20172312. [CrossRef] [PubMed]

17. Sentinel Event Alert: Inadequate Hand-off Communication. Joint Commission. 2017, 58, SEP 12. Available online: https://www.jointcommission.org/assets/1/18/SEA_58_Hand_off_Comms_9_6_17_FINAL_(1).pdf (accessed on 24 April 2019).

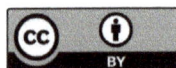

pharmacy

MDPI

Article

A Study to Identify Medication-Related Problems and Associated Cost Avoidance by Community Pharmacists during a Comprehensive Medication Review in Patients One Week Post Hospitalization

Roxane L. Took [1], Yifei Liu [2,*] and Peggy G. Kuehl [2]

[1]   Division of Pharmacy Practice, St. Louis College of Pharmacy, St. Louis, MO 63110, USA;
     roxane.took@stlcop.edu
[2]   Division of Pharmacy Practice and Administration, School of Pharmacy, University of Missouri-Kansas City,
     Kansas City, MO 64108, USA; kuehlp@umkc.edu
*   Correspondence: liuyif@umkc.edu

Received: 29 April 2019; Accepted: 22 May 2019; Published: 29 May 2019

check for updates

Abstract: Objectives: To determine the numbers of medication discrepancies and medication-related problems (MRPs) identified and resolved when providing a transitions of care comprehensive medication review (CMR) after hospital discharge within a community pharmacy; and to estimate the cost-avoidance value of this service. **Methods:** Community pharmacists provided CMRs to covered employees and dependents of a self-insured regional grocery store chain who were discharged from the hospital. Data was collected prospectively over 4 months. Discrepancies were identified among patients' medication regimens by comparing the hospital discharge record, the pharmacy profile, and what the patient reported taking. MRPs were categorized into ten categories, as defined by the OutcomesMTM® Encounter Worksheet. Interventions were categorized using the severity scale developed by OutcomesMTM®, a Cardinal Health company. Data were analyzed using descriptive statistics and bivariate correlations. **Results:** Nineteen patients were enrolled in the program. Pharmacists identified 34 MRPs and 81 medication discrepancies, 1.8 and 4.3 per patient, respectively. The most common type of MRP was underuse of medication (70.6%). Significant positive correlations were found between the number of scheduled prescription medications and the number of medications with discrepancies ($p \leq 0.01$; $r = 0.825$) and number of scheduled prescription medications and the number of MRPs ($p \leq 0.01$; $r = 0.697$). Most commonly, the severity levels associated with the MRPs involved the prevention of physician office visits or addition of new prescription medications ($n = 10$ each); however, four emergency room visits and three hospitalizations were also avoided. The total estimated cost avoidance was $92,143, or $4850 per patient. Extrapolated annual cost savings related to this service would be $276,428. **Conclusions:** This transitions of care service was successful in identifying and addressing MRPs and discrepancies for this patient population. By providing this service, community pharmacists were able to prevent outcomes of various severities and to avoid patient care costs.

Keywords: community pharmacy; medication therapy management; medication-related problems; medication discrepancies; continuity of patient care; cost avoidance

1. Introduction

Medication errors resulted in an estimated 251,454 hospital deaths in 2013 [1]. It is estimated that $17 to $29 billion is spent on preventable adverse events annually. In addition, up to 80% of serious medical errors involve miscommunication among medical providers [2]. Given the high prevalence, morbidity, and cost of such errors, much attention has been drawn to discrepancies and medication-related problems (MRPs) that occur during transitions of care, a time when patient care is handed off among inpatient and outpatient providers.

Previous research has shown the value of pharmacist involvement in transitions of care. Inclusion of a pharmacist has lowered rates of re-hospitalizations and emergency department visits, improved patient satisfaction with care, and increased medication adherence [3,4]. Many hospitals and pharmacy directors have also recognized the importance of involving pharmacists in transitions of care activities for hospitalized patients [5].

Community pharmacists have aided in the transition process by calling patients within 2 to 7 days after discharge to reinforce the discharge plan, provide patient education, address any medication-related issues, and review medications [6–9]. The extent to which pharmacists have been involved has varied from a brief phone call to an extensive face-to-face visit with a pharmacist and 2-week follow-up [6–10]. For instance, in the study of TransitionRx, community pharmacists performed face-to-face visits with patients admitted for congestive heart failure, chronic obstructive pulmonary disease, and pneumonia [10]. These visits consisted of medication reconciliation, comprehensive medication review (CMR), disease state education, patient counseling on new medications, and self-management education. Patients were provided with a personal medication list (PML), medication action plan (MAP), self-monitoring logs, and educational materials. Physicians were provided with a summary of this face-to-face visit and any MRPs or discrepancies were resolved. There was a readmission rate of 7% for patients who met with a pharmacist vs. 20% in the usual care group.

Kelling et al. described the implementation of medication therapy management (MTM)-based transitions of care with a Medicaid population in a grocery store setting [11]. In the study, 17 Medicaid patients met face-to-face with a pharmacist in either a supermarket chain pharmacy or a local federally qualified health center. Patients were asked to bring all prescription and non-prescription medications along with discharge paperwork. Pharmacists completed a medication reconciliation using the discharge paperwork and resolved any MRPs or side effects via phone or fax. Patients were mailed a PML and MAP. Reimbursement was provided through Medicaid, and additional payments for each MRP were identified, resolved, and entered into the OutcomesMTM® Connect™ Platform. For these 17 patients, 50 pharmacologic recommendations and 36 behavior modification recommendations were advised.

While these studies demonstrated that pharmacists could identify and resolve MRPs during transitions of care, none provided an estimate of the cost avoidance of these interactions or examined the severity of MRPs involved. Therefore, the objectives of this study were to determine the numbers of medication discrepancies and MRPs identified and resolved when community pharmacists performed a CMR for employees and dependents of a self-insured regional grocery store/pharmacy chain following hospital discharge; and to associate each MRP with cost-avoidance to quantify the value of this service.

2. Service Description

Balls Food Stores (BFS) is a self-insured regional grocery store and pharmacy chain with approximately 2600 covered lives under their health insurance plan. The company provides many BFS pharmacist-led employee health programs and patient services, including one-on-one disease state management visits for employees and dependents with uncontrolled hypertension, dyslipidemia, diabetes mellitus, and history of myocardial infarction or stroke; tobacco cessation classes for employees and dependents; immunizations including travel vaccine clinics; MTM services; and health screenings are also conducted. BFS implemented a transitions of care service in the fall of 2013 to provide transitions of care for covered employees and dependents. Three clinical pharmacists, employed by BFS, performed this service.

Using information provided by BFS' insurance plan administrator, pharmacists were able to identify covered employees and dependents discharged from a hospital or long-term care facility. Patients were eligible for this service if they were ≥18 years old, insured by BFS, and hospitalized for at least two consecutive days. Patients were not eligible for this service if hospitalized for childbirth, suicidal attempts, or psychiatric conditions. Eligible patients were assigned to one of three pharmacist providers who contacted these patients within 7 days of discharge to schedule a one-on-one CMR. These providers were clinical pharmacists who had residency-training or were undergoing residency training. Visits were completed as soon as the patient and pharmacist were available and performed either in-person or via telephone. Pharmacists asked patients to provide discharge papers, all prescription medications, over-the-counter products, herbal products, and supplements for the CMR visit. If the patient did not have their discharge paperwork, the pharmacist requested a copy from the medical records department of the discharging hospital. These visits were 30 to 60 min long and were documented using a modified CMR worksheet and the OutcomesMTM® Encounter Worksheet (see Supplementary Materials). Pharmacists compared the patient's current medications to the discharge orders and the active medications in the pharmacy dispensing profile. Pharmacists were able to determine the number of MRPs detected and categorize them using the "drug therapy problem detected" section of the OutcomesMTM® Encounter Worksheet. When an MRP was identified, pharmacists took action to resolve it either directly with the patient or by communicating with the patient's health care provider.

Within 7 days of CMR completion, patients were mailed a PML, MAP, and cover letter with the pharmacist's hours of availability and contact information. Pharmacists completed documentation for each MRP identified and followed up with each patient 1 week after mailing/delivering the medication list to ensure that the patient received the letter and understood the action items required to resolve the MRP.

3. Methods

For this research, data for all patients seen by this service from 1 December 2013 to 31 March 2014 were included for analysis. All MRPs and medication discrepancies were transcribed from the patient care chart and recorded onto a master data collection sheet. Discrepancies were identified by comparing the pharmacy dispensing profile, discharge paperwork, and patient interview. MRPs were categorized into 10 categories, as defined by the OutcomesMTM® Encounter Worksheet and discrepancies were assigned to one of three categories: Discrepancy between discharge instructions and pharmacy medication profile, discrepancy between discharge instructions and patient self-report, and discrepancy between pharmacy medication profile and patient self-report.

After completion of a premium subscription agreement and data use agreement with OutcomesMTM®, encounters were entered into the OutcomesMTM® Connect™ Platform [12], and severity levels were reviewed and validated by OutcomesMTM® staff. OutcomesMTM® is an MTM administrative service company that allows pharmacists to bill for MTM services through their electronic platform. This platform has been used primarily by community pharmacies to document CMRs and targeted interventions (TIPs). OutcomesMTM® can also be used to identify cost savings associated with pharmacist's interventions to resolve therapy and adherence problems.

Each MRP was assigned a severity level and cost avoidance was assigned to each intervention using the OutcomesMTM Actuarial Investment Model® [13]. All data were stored in accordance with applicable federal privacy regulations. The methodology of OutcomesMTM® was used to document severity level and cost savings associated with resolution of MRPs. MRPs included: Needs additional drug therapy, unnecessary drug therapy, suboptimal drug, dose too low, adverse drug reaction, drug interaction, dose too high, overuse of medication, underuse of medication, and inappropriate administration or technique. Variables collected included patient demographics, types of discrepancies, types of MRPs, severity levels, number of physicians per patient, and number of prescriptions. Data were analyzed using descriptive statistics and bivariate correlations. A *p* value ≤ 0.05 was regarded as statistically significant. This study was approved by the University of Missouri—Kansas City Adult Health Sciences Institutional Review Board.

4. Results

For the 4 months during which the transitions of care service was studied, 63 patients were discharged from a hospital or intermediate care facility, and 40 met the inclusion criteria. Figure 1 represents the patients included and excluded from the service. Because of initial issues with reporting from the insurance administrator, seven patients were not identified as eligible for this service until after 7 days post-discharge. These patients were not contacted for this service. Pharmacists attempted to reach 13 patients three or more times regarding this service with no response; therefore, these patients could not be included in the service. One eligible patient declined to participate. All 19 participating patients received a CMR and either a complete or incomplete medication reconciliation. Sixteen patients completed all aspects of the service (CMR, provision of discharge paper work, and medication reconciliation). For three patients, pharmacists were unable to obtain discharge paperwork from the hospital or the patient and thus had an incomplete medication reconciliation. For the 19 participating patients, the majority were male (68%), and the mean age was 60 (range 46 to 70) years old. Patients took an average of six (range 2 to 16) scheduled medications daily for their reported disease states (mean 4.4 range 1 to 16). Patients were hospitalized for a mean of 5 (range 2 to 12) days. This service was primarily provided via phone versus face-to-face by request of the patient. Community pharmacists identified and resolved 34 MRPs and 81 medication discrepancies after completing all aspects of the service. On average, 4.3 discrepancies and 1.8 MRPs were identified per patient. The frequency of MRPs is listed in Table 1. The most common type of MRP was underuse of medication (70.6%). Medication discrepancies were similarly distributed among the three categories (31 discrepancies between discharge paperwork and patient-self report, 25 discrepancies between discharge instructions and pharmacy dispensing profile, and 25 discrepancies between pharmacy dispensing profile and patient-self report), with a slightly higher percentage identified in the category of discrepancy between discharge instructions and patient self-report.

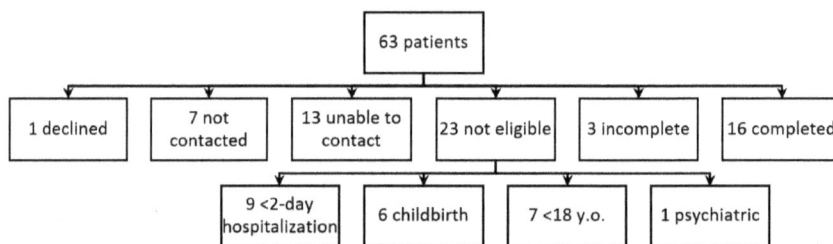

Figure 1. Flowchart of patients included and excluded from the service.

Table 1. Types of medication-related problems (MRPs) identified during service.

MRP	Frequency
Underuse of medication	24
Dose too low	2
Drug interaction	2
Dose too high	2
Inappropriate administration/technique	2
Needs additional drug therapy	1
Unnecessary drug therapy	1
Suboptimal drug	0
Adverse drug reaction	0
Overuse of medication	0

The two most commonly observed severity levels identified in the OutcomesMTM® platform were "prevented physician visit" and "prevented additional prescription order". Severity levels and frequency for each MRP are listed in Table 2. In addition to interventions that prevented additional prescription orders or physician visits, the pharmacists were able to prevent four emergency room visits and three hospital admissions. For example, during two medication reviews and consultations, the pharmacists found that the patient was prescribed a phosphodiesterase inhibitor and nitroglycerin. The pharmacist provided education to each of these patients about the risks of taking these medications concurrently and was able to resolve this issue after consulting the patient's primary care physician. OutcomesMTM® staff determined that the pharmacist's intervention in these visits prevented an emergency room visit due to the risk for significant hypotension.

Table 2. Severity levels and frequencies (verified by OutcomesMTM® staff).

Severity Level	Number of Events
Level 1: Adherence support	5
Level 2: Reduced drug costs	2
Level 3: Prevented a physician visit	10
Level 4: Prevented additional prescription order	10
Level 5: Prevented emergency room visit	4
Level 6: Prevented hospital admission	3
Level 7: Prevented a life-threatening situation	0

The OutcomesMTM Actuarial Investment Model® determined that the MRPs resolved by pharmacists over the period of 4 months provided a total estimated cost avoidance of $92,143, or $4850 per patient. If this rate of MRPs were to continue over a 12-month period, the annual cost savings related to this service would have been $276,428.

There was a statistically significant positive correlation between the number of scheduled prescription medications and the number of medications with discrepancies ($p \leq 0.01$; r = 0.825); and the number of scheduled prescription medications and the number of MRPs ($p \leq 0.01$; r = 0.697) (Table 3). In addition, statistically significant positive correlations were found between the following variables: The number of scheduled medications and the number of disease states, the number of medications with discrepancies and each of the following variables: Number of MRPs, inappropriate adherence, needing an additional drug therapy, and the number of medications with each of the following variables: Number of discrepancies, number of MRPs, and severity level determined by OutcomesMTM®. There was a strong negative correlation between patients who had a medication reconciliation completed in the hospital prior to discharge and the number of medications that were found with discrepancies after discharge ($p \leq 0.01$; r = -0.667).

Table 3. Correlations among variables.

	Number of Medications with Discrepancies	Number of MRPs
Number of scheduled prescription medications	0.825 **	0.697 **
Number of medications with discrepancies	1	0.701 **
Number of discrepancies between discharge paperwork and pharmacy dispensing profile	0.854 **	0.849 **
Number of discrepancies between discharge paperwork and pharmacy dispensing profile	0.974 **	0.610 *
Number of discrepancies between pharmacy dispensing profile and patient reported medication list	0.422	0.531 *
Number of disease states	0.823 **	0.7 **
Number of MRPs	0.701 **	1
Medication reconciliation before discharge	-0.667 **	-0.765 **

MRPs = medication-related problems. * Correlation is significant at the 0.05 level (2-tailed); ** Correlation is significant at the 0.01 level (2-tailed).

5. Discussion

BFS is a self-insured company that was interested to know whether this pilot program would reduce costs associated with transitions of care for covered employees and dependents, and whether this program should be continued. Previous research has shown positive benefits for transitions of care services from the hospital setting, but limited research has been completed in the community setting.

Our study found a strong negative correlation between patients who received prior discharge counseling in the hospital and the number of medications with discrepancies. This is consistent with previous findings. For example, an urban, academic, safety-net hospital created a reengineered discharge (RED) program that provided a package of services to decrease readmission rates [7]. This program included six nurse discharge advocates (DA) and a clinical pharmacist. Nurse discharge advocates were responsible for coordinating the discharge plan with the hospital team, creating an after-hospital care plan (AHCP), and providing discharge counseling to patients using teach-back methodology. The AHCP and discharge paperwork were faxed to the patient's primary care physician. Once a patient was discharged, a clinical pharmacist called the patient to reinforce the discharge plan, review medications with the patient, and address MRPs. If MRPs were found, they were communicated with the primary care provider or DA. Patients provided with this service had lower rates of hospital utilization when compared with usual care.

Reported MRPs per patient ranged from 0.29 to 6.0 [9,11,14–17]. Our study found a similar number of MRPs (1.8 per patient). By examining the medication discrepancies between the discharge orders, the pharmacy profile, and the patient's self-report of what they were actually taking, we discovered many sources of potential MRPs. Discrepancies associated with the discharge orders involved use of formulary medications in the same class as medications the patient had been using at home, incomplete or different use instructions, changes in medication strength, missing medications, or continuation of medications used inhouse that did not need to be continued on an outpatient basis. Discrepancies associated with the pharmacy profile involved medications that had been discontinued during the hospitalization that had not been communicated to the pharmacy, new medications that had been started during the hospitalization for which the pharmacy had not yet received a prescription, and changes in medication directions or strengths. Discrepancies associated with patient self-report included not taking medications as directed, not starting new medications, not stopping discontinued medications, and taking two medications from the same therapeutic class.

Although it is clear that community pharmacists are able to identify MRPs and discrepancies post-discharge, the impact of this service has never been quantified in terms of cost avoidance. By using the OutcomesMTM Actuarial Investment Model®, this pilot project demonstrates that the MRPs resolved by pharmacists provided a total estimated cost avoidance of $92,142 for the 19 patients who received this service, or $4850 per patient. Annualized, it is estimated that 57 BFS patients would be seen, with an annual cost avoidance of $276,450. Based on this cost avoidance and the other findings from this study, BFS has decided to continue this service for its own employees/dependents and to expand this service to any BFS patient discharged from a local regional hospital in the Kansas City area.

Previous studies have identified several barriers to efficient transitions of care, including communication between the hospital and the community pharmacist, identification of patients discharged, contact with patients, lack of time to perform medication reconciliation, incomplete/missing medication list, patient not present during consultation, patient use of multiple pharmacies, and medication reconciliation with multiple providers. The barriers we discovered were lack of discharge paperwork, lack of information about hospitalization (diagnoses), and inability to contact patients who were recently discharged from the hospital. Our pharmacists tried to obtain discharge paperwork either from the patient or requested it from the discharge hospital [6,11,16]. Many hospitals required the completion of a consent form, and it was difficult to have the patient sign and return the form in a timely manner. We also found that the insurance report for identifying patients who were discharged from the hospital did not always include the most pertinent diagnosis. For example, if the patient was admitted to the hospital with pneumonia and had deep vein thrombosis while hospitalized, only the admittance diagnosis would be listed on the report.

We utilized phone and face-to-face meetings at the pharmacy to complete this service. Although the literature has shown that face-to-face interventions are more effective than those delivered via phone [18], the majority of patients in this study preferred to complete this service via phone. The reason for selecting this mode of service was not documented, but telehealth is shown to be a preferred mode of communication for those who are unable to leave home [19]. To provide better quality care, integration of telehealth services into a transitions of care program could be considered.

One limitation of this study was the relatively small sample size. We were able to provide this service to about one half of potentially eligible patients. If this study was performed over a longer period, we would have been able to enroll more patients and obtain a larger sample size. Because this program is being continued, future research can include more patients. Another limitation is that there were two patient outliers, one patient had 12 MRPs identified and resolved, eight of these MRPs were due to adherence and an additional patient had nine MRPs, with eight resulting from non-adherence. Both patients were on nine or more scheduled medications. The literature suggests a linear relationship between the number of MRPs per patient and the number of medications that a patient is taking [20]. This relationship is seen not only in the hospital setting, but also in the ambulatory care and community settings [21–23]. In addition, we did not collect data on whether physicians accepted recommendations provided by the pharmacists, or how the pharmacists worked to resolve the MPRs. It would have been meaningful to include data on how many recommendations made to physicians/providers by pharmacists were actually implemented.

We chose residency trained pharmacists to provide this service. However, many other pharmacists should be able to address MRPs and identify discrepancies as this is part of contemporary Doctor of Pharmacy training.

Access to electronic health records would have allowed our pharmacists to address medication discrepancies and MRPs in a timelier manner and may have allowed pharmacists to recognize other MRPs that were not identified. This study shows that there is a need for health care providers to work together to achieve positive health outcomes. Future research should focus on how community pharmacists work with local health care systems to gain access to health records to provide recommendations and counseling to patients.

6. Conclusions

Community pharmacists should be a part of the transitions of care team to help prevent medication errors and discrepancies that can lead to increased health care spending. When provided with discharge paperwork, community pharmacists are able to identify and resolve MRPs and discrepancies that might not be recognized by health care providers in the hospital setting. Cost savings associated with this service are sizable. Open communication of medical conditions and discharge paperwork between health care providers is imperative in preventing rising health care costs associated with transitions of care.

Supplementary Materials: The following are available online at http://www.mdpi.com/2226-4787/7/2/51/s1, Modified CMR Worksheet and OutcomesMTM® Encounter Worksheet.

Author Contributions: Conceptualization, R.L.T. and P.G.K.; Methodology, R.L.T., Y.L., and P.G.K.; Validation, R.L.T., Y.L., and P.G.K.; Formal Analysis, Y.L.; Investigation, R.L.T., Y.L., and P.G.K.; Data Curation, R.L.T.; Writing-Original Draft Preparation, RL.T., Y.L., and P.G.K.; Writing-Review & Editing, R.L.T., Y.L., and P.G.K.; Supervision, Y.L. and P.G.K.; Project Administration, R.L.T.; Funding Acquisition, R.L.T., Y.L., and P.G.K.

Funding: This research was a Post Graduate Year 1 Community Pharmacy Residency Project at University of Missouri -Kansas City, and funded by The American Pharmacists Association Foundation Incentive Grants Program in 2014.

Pharmacy **2019**, *7*, 51

Acknowledgments: The authors would like to acknowledge the American Pharmacists Association Foundation for awarding an Incentive Grant in support of this project, and OutcomesMTM®, a Cardinal Health company, for its assistance in validating and assigning cost to the severity of MRPs identified through use of its proprietary software and information.

Conflicts of Interest: The authors declare no conflict of interest. The investigators declare no conflicts of interest, real or apparent, and no financial interests in any company, product, employment, gifts, stock holdings, or honoraria.

References

1. Martin, D.M. Medical error-the third leading cause of death in the US. The BMJ. Available online: https://www.bmj.com/content/353/bmj.i2139 (accessed on 21 September 2018).

2. Solet, D.J.; Norvell, J.M.; Rutan, G.H.; Frankel, R.M. Lost in translation: Challenges and opportunities in physician-to-physician communication during patient handoffs. *Acad. Med.* **2005**, *80*, 1094–1099. [CrossRef]

3. Hawes, E.M.; Maxwell, W.D.; White, S.F.; Mangun, J.; Lin, F.C. Impact of an outpatient pharmacist intervention on medication discrepancies and health care resource utilization in posthospitalization care transitions. *J. Primary Care Community Health* **2014**, *1*, 14–18. [CrossRef]

4. Sarangarm, P.; London, M.S.; Snowden, S.S.; Dilworth, T.J.; Koselke, L.R.; Sanchez, C.O.; D'Angio, R.; Ray, G. Impact of pharmacist discharge medication therapy counseling and disease state education: Pharmacist Assisting at Routine Medical Discharge (project PhARMD). *Am. J. Med. Qual.* **2013**, *28*, 292–300. [CrossRef] [PubMed]

5. Kern, K.A.; Kalus, J.S.; Bush, C.; Chen, D.; Szandzik, E.G.; Haque, N.Z. Variations in pharmacy-based transition-of-care activities in the United States: A national survey. *Am. J. Health-Syst. Pharm.* **2014**, *71*, 648–656. [CrossRef]

6. Sen, S.; Bowen, J.F.; Ganetsky, V.S.; Hadley, D.; Melody, K.; Otsuka, S.; Vanmali, R.; Thomas, T. Pharmacists implementing transitions of care in inpatient, ambulatory and community practice settings. *Pharm. Pract.* **2014**, *12*, 439.

7. Jack, B.W.; Chetty, V.K.; Anthony, D.; Greenwald, J.L.; Sanchez, G.M.; Johnson, A.E.; Forsythe, S.R.; O'Donnell, J.K.; Paasche-Orlow, M.K.; Manasseh, C.; et al. A reengineered hospital discharge program to decrease rehospitalization. *Ann. Internal Med.* **2009**, *150*, 178–187. [CrossRef]

8. Farley, T.M.; Shelsky, C.; Powell, S.; Farris, K.B.; Carter, B.L. Effect of clinical pharmacist intervention on medication discrepancies following hospital discharge. *Int. J. Clin. Pharm.* **2014**, *36*, 430–437. [CrossRef]

9. Snodgrass, B.; Babcock, C.K.; Teichman, A. The impact of a community pharmacist conducted comprehensive medication review (CMR) on 30-day re-admission rates and increased patient satisfaction scores: A pilot study. *Innov. Pharm.* **2013**, *4*, 1–9. [CrossRef]

10. Luder, H.R.; Frede, S.M.; Kirby, J.A.; Epplen, K.; Cavanaugh, T.; Martin-Boone, J.E.; Conrad, W.F.; Kuhlmann, D.; Heaton, P.C. TransitionRx: Impact of community pharmacy postdischarge medication therapy management on hospital readmission rate. *J. Am. Pharm. Assoc.* **2015**, *55*, 246–254. [CrossRef] [PubMed]

11. Kelling, S.E.; Bright, D.R.; Ulbrich, T.R.; Sullivan, D.L.; Gartner, J.; Cornelius, D.C. Development and implementation of a community pharmacy medication therapy management-based transition of care program in the managed Medicaid population. *Innov. Pharm.* **2013**, *4*, 137. [CrossRef]

12. OutcomesMTM®. Technology. Connect Platform. Available online: https://www.outcomesmtm.com/health-plans/technology/ (accessed on 28 February 2019).

13. Barnett, M.J.; Frank, J.; Wehring, H.; Newland, B.; VonMuenster, S.; Kumbera, P.; Halterman, T.; Perry, P.J. Analysis of Pharmacist-Provided Medication Therapy Management (MTM) Services in Community Pharmacies Over 7 Years. *J. Manag. Care Pharm.* **2009**, *15*, 18–31. [CrossRef] [PubMed]

14. Paulino, E.I.; Bouvy, M.L.; Gasterlurrutia, M.A.; Guerreiro, M.; Buurma, H.; ESCP-SIR Rejkjavik Community Pharmacy Research Group. Drug related problems identified by European community pharmacists in patients discharged from hospital. *Pharm. World Sci.* **2004**, *26*, 353–360.

15. Braund, R.; Coulter, C.V.; Bodington, A.J.; Giles, L.M.; Greig, A.M.; Heaslip, L.J.; Marshall, B.J. Drug related problems identified by community pharmacists on hospital discharge prescriptions in New Zealand. *Int. J. Clin. Pharm.* **2014**, *36*, 498–502. [CrossRef]

16. Freund, J.E.; Martin, B.A.; Kieser, M.A.; Williams, S.M.; Sutter, S.L. Transitions in Care: Medication Reconciliation in the Community Pharmacy Setting After Discharge. *Innov. Pharm.* **2013**, *4*. [CrossRef]

17. Conklin, J.R.; Togami, J.C.; Burnett, A.; Dodd, M.A.; Ray, G.M. Care transitions service: A pharmacy-driven program for medication reconciliation through the continuum of care. *Am. J. Health-Syst. Pharm.* **2014**, *71*, 802–810. [CrossRef]

18. Zomahoun, H.T.V.; Guénette, L.; Grégoire, J.P.; Lauzier, S.; Lawani, A.M.; Ferdynus, C.; Huiart, L.; Moisan, J. Effectiveness of motivational interviewing interventions on medication adherence in adults with chronic diseases: A systematic review and meta-analysis. *Int. J. Epidemiol.* **2017**, *46*, 589–602. [CrossRef]

19. Richter, K.P.; Shireman, T.I.; Ellerbeck, E.F.; Cupertino, A.P.; Catley, D.; Cox, L.S.; Preacher, K.J.; Spaulding, R.; Mussulman, L.M.; Nazir, N.; et al. Comparative and cost effectiveness of telemedicine versus telephone counseling for smoking cessation. *J. Med. Internet Res.* **2015**, *17*, e113. [CrossRef]

20. Viktil, K.K.; Blix, H.S.; Moger, T.A.; Reikvam, A. Polypharmacy as commonly defined is an indicator of limited value in the assessment of drug-related problems. *Br. J. Clin. Pharmacol.* **2007**, *63*, 187–195. [CrossRef] [PubMed]

21. Kovačević, S.V.; Miljković, B.; Ćulafić, M.; Kovačević, M.; Golubović, B.; Jovanović, M.; Vučićević, K.; de Gier, J.J. Evaluation of drug-related problems in older polypharmacy primary care patients. *J. Eval. Clin. Pract.* **2017**, *23*, 860–865. [CrossRef]

22. Willeboordse, F.; Grundeken, L.H.; van den Eijkel, L.P.; Schellevis, F.G.; Elders, P.J.; Hugtenburg, J.G. Information on actual medication use and drug-related problems in older patients: Questionnaire or interview? *Int. J. Clin. Pharm.* **2016**, *38*, 380–387. [CrossRef]

23. Peterson, C.; Gustafsson, M. Characterisation of drug-related problems and associated factors at a clinical pharmacist service-naïve hospital in northern Sweden. *Drugs Real World Outcomes* **2017**, *4*, 97–107. [CrossRef]

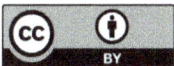

pharmacy

MDPI

Article

An Improved Comprehensive Medication Review Process to Assess Healthcare Outcomes in a Rural Independent Community Pharmacy

Geoffrey Twigg [1,*], **Tosin David** [2] **and Joshua Taylor** [2]

1   Apple Discount Drugs, Salisbury, MD 21804, USA
2   School of Pharmacy, University of Maryland Eastern Shore, Princess Anne, MD 21853, USA;
     tdavid@umes.edu (T.D.); jtaylor4@umes.edu (J.T.)
*   Correspondence: geoff@appledrugs.com

Received: 5 April 2019; Accepted: 6 June 2019; Published: 17 June 2019

check for
updates

Abstract: For years many pharmacists have been performing 'brown bag' medication reviews for patients. While most pharmacists and student pharmacists are familiar with this process, it is important to determine the value patients receive from this service. Over the course of this study the authors attempted to modernize the medication reconciliation process and collect data on patient prescription drug and over-the-counter drug use, along with quantifying the types of interventions the pharmacy's clinical staff performed for patients during this process. The pharmacy partnered with a Quality Improvement Organization to trial their Blue Bag Intervention (BBI) program. The BBI program offered several additional services to the traditional brown bag review. The BBI was instituted as a follow-up tool in the pharmacy's diabetes self-management education/training clinic to aid in patient follow-up and help the clinical staff identify medication-related events such as medication adherence issues and drug–drug interactions. The clinical staff identified approximately 2.2 events per patient with over 50% being issues that affected patient safety.

Keywords: adverse drug events; brown bag; pharmacy; medication reconciliation; pharmacy clinical services

---

1. Introduction

There are myriad potential clinical, humanistic, and pharmacoeconomic outcomes that a patient may experience as a result of medication use. Healthcare practitioners utilize medications to improve a patient's medical condition(s); however, adverse events, ranging from minor adverse drug events (ADEs) to patient death, may occur. Medication use, including both prescription and over-the-counter (OTC) drugs, are common among older patients as well as those with complex and multiple medical conditions. Polypharmacy, the concurrent use of multiple medications by the same patient at different pharmacies, can place individuals at an increased risk for ADEs [1]. Building in a mechanism for pharmacists to prevent and address these adverse events can lead to improved healthcare outcomes while decreasing healthcare expenditure.

In a recent study of hospital discharges, patients who had discrepancies in their medication reconciliation were twice as likely to experience a readmission within 30 days of discharge compared to patients who had had an accurate medication reconciliation performed. In addition, a secondary analysis of the data utilizing pharmacists' medication reviews and patient interviews showed that 89% of patients had at least one potential adverse drug event (pADE) [2]. Another study looked at the role of incorporating a non-dispensing pharmacist into general practice. This study showed the impact that a pharmacist-delivered medication reconciliation could have regarding tailored solutions for individual patients, relieving interdisciplinary tensions of overlapping tasks, and the integration of more quality metrics into medication management [3]. Within a community pharmacy, pharmacists conducted medication reviews to determine medication-related issues. However, this was not conducted in a prospective way, such as by incorporating a patient interview with the medication review [4].

One successful strategy for reducing ADEs is to engage the patient in a comprehensive medication review process with medication reconciliation, often referred to as a 'brown bag' medication review. During a 'brown bag' medication review, patients will place all their medications, prescribed and taken OTC, in a bag and bring them into a medical appointment with a healthcare professional.

Studies involving a 'brown bag' medication review have used various methodologies and designs to determine patient medications, best practices, settings, outcomes, and effectiveness measures. Many reviews included only prescription medications versus reviews that include additional OTC drugs, vitamins, and herbal supplements. Another discrepancy arises from the fact that many reviews did not define medication- or drug-related problems in the same manner [5].

It is estimated that 93% of the American population lives within 5 miles of a community pharmacy and on average a patient will see their pharmacist 35 times a year [6]. This makes the pharmacist one of the most accessible healthcare professionals available to the patient. Pharmacists, as a result of their training, are in a unique position to help patients understand their medication regimen along with the cause and effect between the medication(s) a patient takes and their intended or unintended effect(s).

The authors hypothesize that a structured, sustainable medication reconciliation program that partners patients with a pharmacist with whom they have an established relationship and features 'built-in' medication safety measures will result in improved patient health outcomes. The aim of this study was to define and classify medication therapy problems identified by a clinical pharmacist in a community pharmacy setting. Moreover, the results may enable pharmacies to show the value of their involvement to third-party insurance payers in order to justify expanding the role of pharmacist billable services.

Numerous examples showing the impact of pharmacist-driven medication reconciliation programs on improving health outcomes can be found in the literature [7–11]. The majority of studies involving medication reconciliation programs have used multiple providers and varying program settings. Previous studies tended to report the findings of ADEs in a retrospective manner, such as interventions found during a chart review [12,13]. This study aimed to show a prospective approach to medication reconciliation with pre-identified health outcome-related events during the patient's medication review. This study also sought to show the value of utilizing pharmacists practicing in a community pharmacy setting.

2. Methods/Intervention

Apple Discount Drugs is a large, independent community pharmacy that has been operating on the lower eastern shore of Maryland since 1971. Apple Discount Drugs' pharmacy group consists of four community pharmacy locations, a closed-door home infusion pharmacy, and Core Clinical Care—a separate company that houses the pharmacy's clinical programs. The pharmacy runs a diabetes center and it is accredited by the American Association of Diabetes Educators. It is the only pharmacy-based accredited diabetes center in the area and one of just a few such centers nationwide. The pharmacy also provides extensive medication therapy management (MTM) services [14].

The objective of this study was to implement a structured pharmacist-driven comprehensive medication review program and to identify both actual and potential ADEs among rural patients referred to the pharmacy for diabetes self-management education and training (DSME/T) or for comprehensive medication management. The medication-related problems that were identified by a pharmacist were then categorized according to the type and severity of the event. Medication-related problems included issues involving a possible risk to patient safety, issues surrounding medication adherence, communication errors between the patient and prescriber, and duplicate medications. This study was also designed to set a groundwork for future studies to determine the relationship between proactive pharmacist intervention and specific patient health outcomes such as effects on blood pressure and hemoglobin A1C. The pharmacy used the Blue Bag Initiative (BBI) program, developed by their Quality Improvement Organization (QIO), to provide a structured platform for the pharmacy to conduct medication reconciliation and perform comprehensive medication reviews. The BBI also assisted the pharmacy in capturing pharmacy-related outcomes related to pharmacist-led clinical services.

The BBI intervention differs from the traditional 'brown bag' interview in a number of ways. First, the BBI includes a data collection tool for pharmacists to record the number and types of ADEs, pADEs, and interventions that were identified during the medication review (Table 1). The BBI also ensures patient engagement by creating the expectation that the medication reconciliation process is an ongoing activity—for instance, a reusable, blue drawstring medication bag and a patient appointment card were provided to patients. The patient would be able to keep all medications in the medication bag for easy transport to medical appointments or for safekeeping. The BBI allows for medications that are active on the patient's regimen to be separated from expired and discontinued medications by including a separate white plastic bag.

Table 1. Blue Bag Initiative Event Classification.

Event Type
A possible risk to participant safety
Participant not taking medication as prescribed
Medication was correct, but dose was not
Participant stopped taking prescription meds without telling a clinician
Participant taking a new over-the-counter (OTC) med or supplement without telling a clinician
Drug–drug interactions could be possible
Participant failed to get medication(s) refilled
Expired medications
Participant had contraindication for one or more medications
Participant taking new prescription med (from another doctor) without telling clinician
Pill bottles brought in did not match the medication list in the patient's medical record
Duplicate medications
Stopped taking an OTC med or supplement without telling a clinician
Participant changed to cheaper medication

The study was open to patients who had been referred to the pharmacy's 10 (DSME/T), past graduates of the program, and patients that were referred to the pharmacy's MTM program for a comprehensive medication review (CMR). Patients were excluded if they were only referred to the pharmacy for a targeted medication review.

The diabetes education classes were taught by a pharmacist with a certified diabetes educator credential. The prescriber could refer the patient for group classes, or if the patient had special needs the prescriber could elect to have the classes taught one-on-one. The diabetes education cycle began with a one-on-one meeting so the pharmacist could gauge the patient's understanding of their disease, followed by 3 h classes to teach the fundamentals of managing diabetes. A patient's third-party payer benefits for follow-up upon completion varied according to the payer. Many of the commercial payers that the pharmacy contracts will allow for diabetes education follow-up on an as needed basis according to the patient's needs. Patients that have Medicare benefits are allowed 2 h of DSME/T follow-up for each subsequent year following the completion of the class cycle. This lag time in benefits, in many cases, can cause a care gap as many patients need medication management in the months following the successful completion of a DSME/T class cycle, when the patient is able to begin making lifestyle modifications.

The intervention was overseen by a pharmacist from the clinical team at Apple Discount Drugs. The clinical team consisted of two pharmacists who also held Certified Diabetes Education credentials and a licensed pharmacist completing a Community Pharmacy Residency program during their first postgraduate year.

Reviews were standardized to the BBI to maintain a uniform distribution of pharmacy care. Once the participants agreed to take part in the intervention, the pharmacist contacted their primary care provider to send an updated medication list, progress notes, and requests for intervention when necessary. Participants were instructed to put all their medications (including OTC medications, vitamins, herbal supplements, and eye drops) into the blue bag and to bring it with them to the pharmacy for their scheduled appointment. Apple Discount Drugs invited DSME/T class participants referred to the pharmacy to sign up for the BBI intervention as an extra benefit to attending the class sequence. Participants could choose to opt out of the Blue Bag comprehensive medication review with a pharmacist and still take part in the DSME/T classes.

The pharmacist reviewed the medications at the conclusion of the interview, created an updated medication list incorporating any medication changes, recorded patient outcome data into the QIO's BBI collection tool, and discussed the results with study participants. The pharmacist would also, when necessary, secure outdated, discontinued, or contraindicated medications and instruct the patient on how to safely discard medications.

3. Results

There were 110 patients who were offered the opportunity to participate and 73 patients agreed to take part in the intervention (Table 2). Patients who were referred for targeted medication reviews or patients who received telephonic MTM were excluded from participation. Over 50% of the patients in this study were Medicare beneficiaries. There was an average of 8.5 medications (prescription and OTC) per patient, with higher averages of 11 and 11.8 medications per patient in the age ranges of 86–90 years and 41–45 years, respectively. There was a similar number of medications per patient seen amongst men (average 8.4) and women (average 8.6). For patient-identified ethnic groups, there was an average of 7.6 medications per patient amongst Blacks/African-Americans and an average of 8.2 amongst Whites/Caucasians. The majority of patients seen were being treated for metabolic syndrome. Of the patients taking part, 91.8% were treated for hypertension, 87.7% were treated for diabetes, and 63% were treated for hypercholesterolemia (Table 3).

Table 2. Patient demographics.

Population	N = 73 (100%)
Sex/Gender	
Male	46 (63%)
Female	27 (37%)
Race/Ethnicity	
African American/Black	8 (11%)
Caucasian/White	46 (63%)
Patient preferred not to disclose	19 (26%)
Age (years)	
0–30	0
31–60	17 (23.3%)
61–90	50 (68.5%)
91+	1 (1.4%)
Patient preferred not to disclose	5 (6.8%)

Table 3. Conditions/disease indication by patient count.

Condition/Disease Indication	Patient Count	% of Total Patients
Hypertension	67	91.8%
Diabetes	64	87.7%
Cholesterol	46	63.0%
Pain	29	39.7%
Allergies	24	32.9%
GERD	19	26.0%
Depression	16	21.9%
Edema	10	13.7%
Anxiety	9	12.3%
Neuropathy	7	9.6%
Gout	5	6.8%

The majority of patients reported bringing all of their medications to their appointments with the pharmacist (87.7%). Participants could also state what condition their medications were prescribed for (82.2%). Less than half (49.3%) stated that any healthcare practitioner had inquired about their medication list in the past 6 months (Table 4).

Table 4. Patient medication reconciliation survey responses.

	Yes	No	No Response/Unsure
Did the participant say they brought in all their medications?	64 (87.7%)	8 (11%)	1 (1.3%)
Has anyone asked about the participant's medications in the last 6 months, not including today's discussion?	36 (49.3%)	36 (49.3%)	1 (1.3%)
Could the patient state what each medication was for?	60 (82.2%)	9 (12.3%)	4 (5.5%)

Pharmacists identified potential and actual ADEs utilizing the Blue Bag Initiative (Table 5). There was an average of 2.2 identified events per patient, with the highest number of ADEs (7 identified events) found in three patients (Figure 1). Over 50% of pADEs identified were related to a possible harm in patient safety. A 16% correlation was seen between an increased number of medications per patient and the number of identified adverse drug events. A weaker correlation of 9% was seen between the number of identified conditions per patient and the number of identified adverse drug events.

Table 5. Number of medication-related events identified.

Event Type	Patient Count	Percent
A possible risk to participant safety	41	56.20%
Participant not taking medication as prescribed	23	31.50%
Medication was correct, but dose was not	19	26.00%
Participant stopped taking prescription meds without telling a clinician	16	21.90%
Participant taking a new over-the-counter (OTC) med or supplement without telling a clinician	13	17.80%
Drug–drug interactions could be possible	12	16.40%
Participant failed to get medication(s) refilled	12	16.40%
Expired medications	11	15.10%
Participant had contraindication for one or more medications	3	4.10%
Participant taking new prescription med (from another doctor) without telling clinician	3	4.10%
Pill bottles brought in did not match the medication list in the patient's medical record	3	4.10%
Duplicate medications	2	2.70%
Stopped taking an OTC med or supplement without telling a clinician	2	2.70%
Participant changed to cheaper medication	2	2.70%

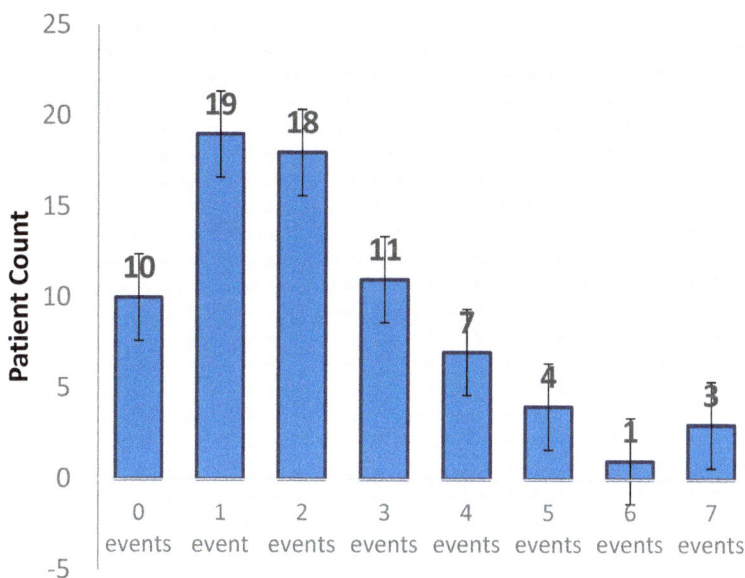

Figure 1. Events per patient.

Out of the 674 medications reviewed, 162 were over-the-counter medications (24% of the total medications reviewed). This was significant as many patients did not consider an OTC medication to be part of their medication list and many did not inform their prescribers of OTC medication use. There was a 23% correlation between patients who had OTC medications and an event occurring.

4. Limitations

This study was limited to the small number of patients that were referred to the pharmacy and agreed to participate. The pharmacists performing the medication reviews relied on the patient for an accurate accounting of medications added to the Blue Bag. The pADEs that were documented by the pharmacists were subjective, especially when considering what constitutes a risk to patient safety, which was the most common type of pADE reported. There is still a large variation in the literature as to how these events are defined. The pharmacists participating in this study determined that a risk to patient safety would include medication-related effects of the patient's regimen outside of taking one specific medication. Despite this initial training, the reporting of pADEs might have varied from reviewer to reviewer. This means that training, implementation support, and periodic data collection check-ins are recommended.

The low sample size prevented further assessment of the intervention's impact on hospital utilization, such as ED visits, admissions, readmissions, and observational stays. A systematic review published in 2017 notes the importance of measuring factors such as medication therapy management and patient-specific variables [15]. A further study investigating the effects of this intervention on the abovementioned outcomes would be a recommended expansion of this initial study.

5. Discussion

Patient empowerment helped the investigators drive this study. Patients reported a better understanding of the reasons why they were taking specific medications and how those medications worked. This allowed patients to relate side effects to a particular medication, and empowered them to become more active participants in their healthcare. Research has shown that as patient empowerment is improved there are increased levels of patient involvement and better patient behaviors such as medication adherence [16].

Polypharmacy increases with the number of chronic conditions and prescribers. As the number of medications goes up, so does the potential for medication-related problems. This is especially true in older patient populations. A recent study performed in a geriatric patient population showed that patients receiving a mean of 10 medications had the incidence of medication-related problems drop from 86.6% to 56% when a pharmacist was involved in the medication reconciliation process [17]. In this study the need for medication reconciliation was shown when surveying the individuals, as slightly less than half had not had their medications reviewed in the last 6 months. Retrospective research has shown the risk of ADEs in ambulatory settings. Patients taking multiple medications, such as non-opioid analgesics, anticoagulants, diuretics, and anti-seizure medications, have been shown to be at an increased risk [18]. This was further exacerbated by the pharmacist finding 2.2 drug-related issues per medication review. Majority of the participants that completed this study had an understanding of what their medications were for. Conversely, a third of the of patients were not taking their medications as prescribed, ranking as the second-most identified event during the medication review. The investigators also noted that many patients did not understand the associated side effects of medications. After the interview with the pharmacist utilizing the Blue Bag review, patients were able to identify the causes and effects of medication use. Cahn et al. looked at the recognition of drug-related problems before and after pharmacist intervention. There was a significant increase in identified problems seen when a pharmacist reviewed the patient's medications, resulting in increased clinical and compliance interventions [19].

There are a number of practical and innovative ways the BBI can assist in improving and quantifying pharmacy workflow processes, many of which directly impact patient safety measures. The BBI provides pharmacists with a mechanism to remove outdated and discontinued medications from a patient's medication regimen. Due to the expense of medications, often times a patient would hesitate to discard a medication once it had been discontinued. The patient would want to have the medication on hand in the event that the prescriber would restart the medication, so as to avoid an additional copayment. Having a discontinued medication stored with other medications resulted in patient confusion and a potential patient safety issue. Separating these medications from active medications proved to be a valuable intervention to patient safety.

Studies have been published on medication discrepancies during medication reconciliation and the effects of this on patients. In this study, the pharmacist found instances where the patient reported medications of which the prescriber was unaware [20]. The likelihood of this occurring became more common as the number of prescribers a patient saw increased. Each prescriber performed their version of medication reconciliation at their practice site. Quite often, there would be discrepancies among the medications a patient was prescribed from practice to practice. The BBI intervention gave the pharmacist the ability to communicate current medications and medication changes to all of the patient's prescribers as well as alert prescribers to difficulties that a patient may experience between visits.

There was a correlation between OTC medications and pADEs identified within the study; this afforded the pharmacist with an opportunity to improve patient care. Many patients felt that OTC medications were safe and effective for use without seeking treatment by a health professional. This can be complicated by a patient's use of other nonprescription and prescription medications, especially as the amount of either increases. Pharmacists have an opportunity to encounter the patient and review their medications to assess the harm of starting or stopping a nonprescription product and reporting this information to other healthcare professionals.

As patients continue managing their various condition(s), their medication dose needs to be considered for safety and efficacy. Often, medications need to be tapered up and titrated down. Pharmacist are in a unique position to interview the patient and devise an appropriate medication plan for the patient by utilizing the Pharmacists' Patient Care Process (JCPP) [21]. Pharmacists utilize evidence-based medicine and patient-specific parameters to determine an appropriate medication dose and frequency for a patient. Pharmacists play an integral role in providing patient counseling on appropriate medication administration. This encompasses education not only on a specific medication, but the patient's entire medication regimen. Pharmacist guiding patients on various interactions with supplements, herbal medications, and OTC products to avoid while taking their prescribed medication regimen can circumvent potential adverse drug events. During the interview process, many patients initially did not consider OTC and natural products to be a part of their medication regimen. It was not until the pharmacist asked pointed questions or explained how OTC products could impact a patient's overall health that many patients understood the importance of complete and accurate medication reconciliation. Several patients later reported taking their blue bags and medication cards to doctor's appointments with primary and specialty care. The BBI also helped patients to understand the importance of communication with prescribers to alert them to changes to their medication regimen.

Another area where the BBI can assist a pharmacy is in providing the pharmacy with a mechanism to quantify interventions in a systematic format in order to track and share intervention data with other healthcare professionals and insurers [22]. Many pharmacies that provide clinical services to patients perform similar types of interventions as those noted by the study investigators. A study by Tetuan et al. utilized a system where recently discharged inpatients were able to utilize the pharmacy's service in order to identify potential drug-related problems. By utilizing the BBI initiative as a marker for cost avoidance, future studies on the resolution of drug-related problems will assist pharmacies in sustaining initiatives with local health systems [23]. Without the ability to show the value of these services to third-party payers, these pharmacist interventions become value-added services. An intervention utilizing the BBI intervention showcased an average of $218 to $319 in potential savings per completed medication review [24]. When pharmacists are able to quantify and assign a value to these services, they are then able to market clinical interventions in the community pharmacy setting and, in turn, use these programs to increase pharmacy revenue [25].

6. Conclusions

This study highlighted the impact of pharmacist-driven medication reconciliation and reviews. The pharmacy's implementation of the BBI demonstrated this program to be a viable way to perform medication reconciliation and identify pADEs so as to improve health outcomes for patients. By collecting specific data points from the patient and highlighting areas of correlation, pharmacists will be equipped to display where their skills lie in medication management. Patients embraced the interactive nature of the BBI and seemed to be willing to take a more active role in their healthcare as a result.

Apple Discount Drugs is also expanding the use of the BBI to try to determine the cost savings associated with the prevention of ADEs, and to use the outcomes from the BBI to expand the number of billable services offered to pharmacies in coordination with third-party payers. The expansion of the availability of this medication reconciliation program could have a great impact on the care afforded to patients and could strengthen the implementation and data collection support offered to healthcare providers. Additional studies on healthcare outcomes and control group comparisons are recommended for future impact analyses of pharmacist-driven medication reconciliation in the community pharmacy setting.

Author Contributions: Conceptualization, G.T. and T.D.; methodology, G.T. and T.D.; validation, T.D.; formal analysis, G.T. and T.D.; investigation, G.T. and T.D.; resources, T.D.; data curation, T.D.; writing—original draft preparation, G.T., T.D., and J.T.; writing—review and editing, G.T., T.D., and J.T.; visualization, T.D.; supervision, G.T.; project administration, T.D.

Funding: This research received no external funding in the completion of this project.

Acknowledgments: The analytics were prepared by Health Quality Innovators (HQI), the Medicare Quality Innovation Network-Quality Improvement Organization for Maryland and Virginia, under contract with the Centers for Medicare and Medicaid Services (CMS), an agency of the US Department of Health and Human Services. The contents of this manuscript do not necessarily reflect CMS policy.

Conflicts of Interest: The authors declare no conflict of interest.

References

1. Golchin, N.; Frank, S.; Vince, A.; Isham, L.; Neropol, S. Polypharmacy in the elderly. *J. Res. Pharm. Pract.* **2015**, *4*, 85–88. [CrossRef] [PubMed]

2. Agency of Healthcare Research and Quality. Medication Discrepancies and Potential Adverse Drug Events During Transfer of Care from Hospital to Home. Content Last Reviewed August 2017. Agency for Healthcare Research and Quality: Rockville, MD, USA. Available online: https://www.ahrq.gov/professionals/quality-patient-safety/patient-safety-resources/resources/liability/advances-in-patient-safety-medical-liability/neumiller.html (accessed on 30 May 2018).

3. Hazen, A.C.; de Bont, A.A.; Leendertse, A.J.; Zwart, D.L.; de Wit, N.J.; de Gier, J.J.; Bouvy, M.L. How Clinical Integration of Pharmacists in General Practice has Impact on Medication Therapy Management: A Theory-oriented Evaluation. *Int. J. Integr. Care* **2019**, *19*, 1. [CrossRef] [PubMed]

4. Goedken, A.M.; Huang, S.; Mcdonough, R.P.; Deninger, M.J.; Doucette, W.R. Medication-Related Problems Identified Through Continuous Medication Monitoring. *Pharmacy (Basel)* **2018**, *6*, 86. [CrossRef] [PubMed]

5. McGalliard, B.; Shane, R.; Rosen, S. A Pill Organizing Plight. Published September 2016. Available online: https://psnet.ahrq.gov/webmm/case/383/A-Pill-Organizing-Plight (accessed on 10 May 2019).

6. National Association of Chain Drug Stores. *2011–2012 Chain Pharmacy Industry Profile*; National Association of Chain Drug Stores: Alexandria, VA, USA, 2011.

7. American College of Clinical Pharmacy; Kirwin, J.; Canales, A.E.; Bentley, M.L.; Bungay, K.; Chan, T.; Dobson, E.; Holder, R.M.; Johnson, D.; Lilliston, A.; et al. Process indicators of quality clinical pharmacy services during transitions of care. *Pharmacotherapy* **2012**, *32*, e338–e347. [PubMed]

8. Daliri, S.; Hugtenburg, J.G.; ter Riet, G.; van den Bemt, B.J.; Buurman, B.M.; op Reimer, W.J.S.; van Buul-Gast, M.C.; Karapinar-Çarkit, F. The effect of a pharmacy-led transitional care program on medication-related problems post-discharge: A before-After prospective study. *PLoS ONE* **2019**, *14*, e0213593. [CrossRef] [PubMed]

9. Lehnbom, E.C.; Stewart, M.J.; Manias, E.; Westbrook, J.I. Impact of medication reconciliation and review on clinical outcomes. *Ann. Pharmacother.* **2014**, *48*, 1298–1312. [CrossRef] [PubMed]

10. Sen, S.; Bowen, J.F.; Ganetsky, V.S.; Hadley, D.; Melody, K.; Otsuka, S.; Vanmali, R.; Thomas, T. Pharmacists implementing transitions of care in inpatient, ambulatory and community practice settings. *Pharm. Pract.* **2014**, *12*, 439.

11. Sarzynski, E.; Luz, C.; Zhou, S.; Rios-Bedoya, C. Medication Reconciliation in an Outpatient Geriatric Clinic: Does Accuracy Improve if Patients "Brown Bag" their Medications for Appointments. *J. Am. Geriatrics Soc.* **2014**, *62*, 567–569. [CrossRef] [PubMed]

12. Johnson, C.M.; Marcy, T.R.; Harrison, D.L.; Young, R.E.; Stevens, E.L.; Shadid, J. Medication reconciliation in a community pharmacy setting. *J. Am. Pharm. Assoc.* **2010**, *50*, 523–526. [CrossRef] [PubMed]

13. Shaver, A.; Morano, M.; Pogodzinski, J.; Fredrick, S.; Essi, D.; Slazak, E. Impact of a community pharmacy transitions-of-care program on 30-day readmission. *J. Am. Pharm. Assoc.* **2019**, *59*, 202–209. [CrossRef] [PubMed]

14. Home. Apple Discount Drugs. Available online: https://www.appledrugs.com/ (accessed on 10 May 2019).

15. Huiskes, V.J.; Burger, D.M.; Van den ende, C.H.; Van den bemt, B.J. Effectiveness of medication review: A systematic review and meta-analysis of randomized controlled trials. *BMC Fam. Pract.* **2017**, *18*, 5. [CrossRef] [PubMed]

16. Náfrádi, L.; Nakamoto, K.; Schulz, P.J. Is patient empowerment the key to promote adherence? A systematic review of the relationship between self-efficacy, health locus of control and medication adherence. *PLoS ONE* **2017**, *12*, e0186458. [CrossRef] [PubMed]

17. Nachtigall, A.; Heppner, H.J.; Thürmann, P.A. Influence of pharmacist intervention on drug safety of geriatric inpatients: A prospective, controlled trial. *Ther. Adv. Drug Saf.* **2019**, *10*. [CrossRef] [PubMed]

18. Field, T.S.; Gurwitz, J.H.; Harrold, L.R.; Rothschild, J.; DeBellis, K.R.; Seger, A.C.; Auger, J.C.; Garber, L.A.; Cadoret, C.; Fish, L.S.; et al. Risk factors for adverse drug events among older adults in the ambulatory setting. *J. Am. Geriatr Soc.* **2004**, *52*, 1349–1354. [CrossRef] [PubMed]

19. Chan, W.W.T.; Dahri, K.; Partovi, N.; Egan, G.; Yousefi, V. Evaluation of Collaborative Medication Reviews for High-Risk Older Adults. *Can. J. Hosp. Pharm.* **2018**, *71*, 356–363. [CrossRef] [PubMed]

20. Llinan, S.; O'mahony, D.; Byrne, S. Application of the structured history taking of medication use tool to optimise prescribing for older patients and reduce adverse events. *Int. J. Clin. Pharm.* **2016**, *38*, 374–379.

21. Joint Commission of Pharmacy Practitioners. Pharmacists' Patient Care Process. 29 May 2014. Available online: https://jcpp.net/wp-content/uploads/2016/03/PatientCareProcess-with-supporting-organizations.pdf (accessed on 30 March 2019).

22. Morimoto, T.; Gandhi, T.K.; Seger, A.C.; Hsieh, T.C.; Bates, D.W. Adverse drug events and medication errors: Detection and classification methods. *Qual. Saf. Health Care* **2004**, *13*, 306–314. [CrossRef] [PubMed]

23. Tetuan, C.E.; Guthrie, K.D.; Stoner, S.C.; May, J.R.; Hartwig, D.M.; Liu, Y. Impact of community pharmacist-performed post-discharge medication reviews in transitions of care. *J. Am. Pharm. Assoc.* **2018**, *58*, 659–666. [CrossRef] [PubMed]

24. Fernández, E.V.; Warriner, C.L.; David, T.N.; Gordon, E.A.; Jackson, S.; Twigg, G.; Carroll, N.V. Potential Cost Savings by Prevention of Adverse Drug Events with A Novel Medication Review Program. *Value Health* **2018**, *21*, S320. [CrossRef]

25. Twigg, G.; Motsko, J.; Sherr, J.; El-Baff, S. Interprofessional Approach to Increase Billable Care-Events in a Rural Community. *Innov. Pharm.* **2017**, *8*, 1–8. [CrossRef]

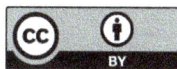

pharmacy

MDPI

Article

Clinical Results of Comprehensive Medication Management Services in Primary Care in Belo Horizonte

Carina de Morais Neves [1], Mariana Martins Gonzaga do Nascimento [2],
Daniela Álvares Machado Silva [1] and Djenane Ramalho-de-Oliveira [1,*]

[1]   Center for Pharmaceutical Care Studies, College of Pharmacy, Universidade Federal de Minas Gerais, Belo Horizonte, MG 31270-901, Brazil; carinamneves@gmail.com (C.d.M.N.); dalvaresms@gmail.com (D.Á.M.S.)

[2]   Department of Pharmaceutical Sciences, College of Pharmacy, Universidade Federal de Minas Gerais, Belo Horizonte, MG 31270-901, Brazil; marianamgn@yahoo.com.br

*   Correspondence: djenane.oliveira@gmail.com.br or droliveira@ufmg.br; Tel.: +55-31-98329-0528

check for updates

Received: 28 April 2019; Accepted: 6 June 2019; Published: 12 June 2019

Abstract: The high prevalence of chronic diseases and use of multiple medications identified in Primary Health Care (PHC) suggest the need for the implementation of Comprehensive Medication Management (CMM) services. This study aimed to evaluate the clinical results of CMM services in a Brazilian PHC setting. A quasi-experimental study was performed with patients followed-up for two years ($n = 90$). Factors associated with the detection of four drug therapy problems (DTP) or more in the initial assessment were evaluated (univariate and multivariate analyses), as well as the clinical impact observed in laboratory parameters (HbA1c, Blood Pressure, LDL- and HDL-covariance analysis). A predominance of women (61.1%), a mean age of 65.5 years, and a prevalence of polypharmacy (87.8%)—use of five or more drugs—were observed. A total of 441 DTP was identified, 252 required interventions with the prescriber, 67.9% of which were accepted and 59.6% were solved. The main DTP were 'non-adherence' (28.1%), 'need for additional drug therapy' (21.8%), and 'low dose' (19.5%). Hypertension was positively associated with the identification of four DTP or more. A statistically significant reduction was detected in all assessed laboratory parameters ($p < 0.05$). CMM services contributed to the resolution of DTP and improved clinical outcomes.

Keywords: Comprehensive Medication Management; pharmaceutical care; primary health care; chronic diseases; clinical results

1. Introduction

Primary Health Care (PHC) is the patient's gateway to the public health system and has significant participation in the management of chronic diseases and prevention of adverse health outcomes through the integration of preventive and curative actions [1]. In Brazil, its organizational axis is the Family Health Strategy (eSF—Equipe Saúde da Família), which, in turn, is supported by the Family Health Support Team (NASF—Núcleo de Apoio à Saúde da Família). The NASF was established in 2008 by the Ministry of Health and consists of multidisciplinary teams (composed of pharmacists, nutritionists, physical therapists, social workers, and others) that provide support to the work of the eSF (composed mainly of a primary care physician and a nurse) [2]. The demands for a multidisciplinary approach in primary health care is increasing, since a large part of the population followed in this scenario has multiple health conditions, uses many medications, and is now composed of older adults, representing about 12.6% of the Brazilian population [3].

Patients treated in the PHC have a high prevalence of chronic diseases, such as diabetes mellitus (DM), hypertension, and dyslipidemia and consequently use multiple medications. Therefore, adequate drug therapy management becomes necessary, considering the complex drug therapy of this population. Thus, the provision of Comprehensive Medication Management (CMM) services by a competent clinical pharmacist inserted in the NASF can be an important strategy to enhance health outcomes and the operationalization of PHC [4].

CMM is a clinical service grounded in the theoretical framework of Pharmaceutical Care Practice that aims at the responsible provision of drug therapy to achieve tangible results that improve the quality of life of the patients [5]. Thus, in CMM services, the pharmacist checks whether the medicines used by the patient are the most appropriate, if they are effective, safe, and convenient for use in daily living in order to optimize their drug therapy. Thus, when he/she detects a drug therapy problem (DTP), defined as an event or circumstance linked to drug therapy that may actually or potentially interfere with the expected treatment results, pharmacists intervene with the patient or the team to solve it. It is worth emphasizing that patients are central to this practice and in partnership with the pharmacist and other professionals define the best way to reach their therapeutic goals [6].

Studies have shown that CMM has a considerable impact on the enhancement of the treatment of chronic diseases and contributes significantly to improve patients' clinical results [7–10]. However, few studies have shown the clinical impact of a CMM service in the Brazilian PHC and provided directly by a NASF pharmacist. Therefore, this study aims to describe a CMM service in the primary care of the Brazilian city of Belo Horizonte (MG) and to evaluate its clinical impact.

2. Materials and Methods

This study has a quasi-experimental longitudinal design, with a single group of patients that received the CMM service. It should be emphasized that the World Health Organization encourages the evaluation of the impact of the implementation of services through a quasi-experimental design, and accordingly this study reflects this recommendation, which consists of a baseline and post-intervention evaluation (uncontrolled before–after study type) [11,12].

2.1. Setting

The CMM service in question was provided by a single pharmacist in two community primary care clinics of the municipality of Belo Horizonte, Minas Gerais. The populations assigned to these two units were at the time of the study 22,000 and 15,023 users and were attended by, respectively, six and four eSFs.

The pharmacist has a weekly workload of 40 h divided into 20 h for technical and managerial activities (e.g., medicines inventory control and coordination of the drug dispensing activities) and 20 weekly hours for patient care activities (provision of CMM services, health education, and scheduled meetings for discussion of cases referred to NASF professionals).

2.2. The Patient Care Process

CMM services as its theoretical underpinnings the practice of pharmaceutical care, whose patient care process involves the use of a rational decision-making process called Pharmacotherapy Workup (PW), as proposed by Cipolle et al. [13,14] Thus, the care process utilized in these services includes the pharmacist's assessment of all of a patient's drug therapy, including over-the-counter, supplements and prescribed medications, in order to identify, prevent, and resolve DTP that might be preventing the patient to achieve his or her goals of therapy. Care plans are developed for each medical condition and follow-up evaluations are carried out to determine actual outcomes.

2.3. Study Design and Data Collection

In order to assess the impact of the CMM service, the documentation of the CMM encounters were analyzed retrospectively for the total number of patients ($n = 90$) followed-up by the pharmacist at the clinics over the two-year period (February 2015–February 2017). The following data were collected: age (full years at the first visit), gender, place of care at the initial assessment (at home or at the health service unit), number of health problems, number of medications used (prescribed and non-prescribed), number of interventions (with the prescriber or the patient) and their acceptability (intervention with the physician—accepted or not accepted), number of DTP identified and resolved, as well as their types.

DTP were categorized according to the PW process meaning they were classified according to an evaluation of the indication, effectiveness, safety, and convenience of each medication the patient was taking [5,6]. DTP associated with the indication of a drug product include unnecessary drug therapy (DTP1) or the need for additional drug therapy (DTP2). DTP related to effectiveness include ineffective drug product (DTP3) or a dosage too low to be effective (DTP4). In the safety category, the patient can have an adverse drug reaction (DTP5) or a dosage too high (DTP6). After evaluating the first three categories, the pharmacist will assess the convenience of the drug product for that specific patient, which might lead to the identification of a DTP of non-adherence (DTP7).

The Charlson Comorbidity Index (CCI) [15] was calculated for each patient enrolled in the service and the following initial (detected at the first or second CMM visit) and final (detected at the last visit) laboratory parameters were collected: glycosylated hemoglobin (HbA1c, in percentage), systolic blood pressure (SBP, in mmHg), diastolic blood pressure (DBP, in mmHg), low-density lipoprotein-cholesterol (LDLc, in mg/dL) and high-density lipoprotein-cholesterol (HDLc, in mg/dL).

2.4. Study Variables and Data Analysis

The data were first analyzed descriptively, measuring the absolute and relative frequencies of the qualitative variables and the mean and standard deviation (SD) of the quantitative variables. Then, univariate and multivariate analyses were performed to identify factors associated with the identification of multiple DTP in the initial assessment (first and second consultations), and, therefore, patients that should be prioritized to receive CMM services. For such purpose, the variable "number of initial DTP" was dichotomized (0–3 DTP, ≥4 DTP) and the dependent variable, therefore, was defined as the identification of four DTP or more. The independent variables defined were: age (22–69; ≥70 years), gender, number of health problems (0–2; ≥3), number of medications used (0–7; ≥8), the presence of hypertension and DM. The quantitative variables (age, CCI, number of medications, and number of DTP) were dichotomized according to their median.

Univariate analyses were performed using the Pearson's chi-square test or Fisher's exact test when the expected value for one or more cells was equal to or less than five. Independent variables with $p < 0.20$ in the univariate analysis were included in the multivariate model calculated by logistic regression. A probability test was used to compare the models and the Hosmer–Lemeshow test was run to evaluate the model's quality of fit. Univariate and multivariate analyses were based on the odds ratio (OR) and their respective 95% confidence intervals estimated by logistic regression. A level of statistical significance of 5% was adopted to identify the characteristics independently associated with the dependent variable.

The clinical impact of the CMM service was assessed by comparing the initial and final clinical/laboratory parameters (HbA1c, SBP, DBP, LDLc, and HDLc). Only patients with more than one visit (68 patients) were considered, and among these, only those with a measurement of the specific clinical parameter at the initial and final visit. First, the normal distribution of the clinical variables was verified with the Shapiro–Wilk test. As all variables had a normal distribution, the difference between their initial and final values was assessed through covariance analysis with repeated measures (ANCOVA) adjusted by the following covariates in their continuous format: CCI, age, number of health problems, and number of medicines. Repeated measure designs facilitate the measurement of the impact of the treatment on each subject rather than just comparing the means between two groups. In this case, each subject serves as their control and the variability between subjects can be isolated. Also, the ANCOVA analysis enables us to control the difference between the two measures by other covariates, increasing the test's sensitivity. All statistical analyses were performed by the Stata® statistical program, version 12.

2.5. Ethical Aspects

This study was approved by the ethics committee of the Federal University of Minas Gerais, Report No. 25780314.4.0000.0149. Anonymity of the participants and confidentiality of the information were guaranteed.

3. Results

A female majority ($n = 55, 61.1\%$), with a mean age of 66.5 ± 13.4 years (minimum: 22, maximum: 89) was observed among the patients followed up, revealing a predominance of elderly individuals with 60 years or more ($n = 68; 75.6\%$). Table 1 shows the demographic, health and medication use profile of the patients enrolled in the CMM service.

Table 1. Demographic, health and medication profile of patients enrolled in the Comprehensive Medication Management (CMM) service ($n = 90$). Belo Horizonte. 2015–2017.

Characteristic	n (%)
Gender	
Female	55 (61.1)
Male	35 (38.9)
Age (full years)	
22–68	50 (55.6)
≥69	40 (44.4)
Number of health problems in the initial assessment *	
0–2	28 (31.1)
≥3	62 (68.9)
Charlson Comorbidity Index	
0–3	41 (45.6)
≥2	49 (54.4)
Number of drugs in initial assessment *	
0–7	47 (52.2)
≥8	43 (47.8)
Number of DTP identified in initial visits *	
0–3	45 (50.0)
≥4	45 (50.0)

* Initial assessment = 1st and 2nd CMM visits.

A total of 251 consultations was performed by the pharmacist (mean ± SD = 2.8 ± 1.6). In the initial assessment, most patients were using five or more medications ($n = 79; 87.8\%$), setting a mean of 7.6 ± 2.7 medications (minimum: 2, maximum: 18). The patients had a mean of 3.23 ± 1.4 health problems (minimum: 1, maximum: 7), with a mean CCI of 4.1 ± 0.2 (minimum = 0; maximum = 12). The most prevalent diseases were hypertension ($n = 74; 82.2\%$), dyslipidemia ($n = 69; 76.6\%$) and diabetes ($n = 58; 64.4\%$).

A total of 346 DTP were identified in the initial assessment (mean = 3.8 ± 2.4; minimum = 0; maximum = 10; median = 3.5), and 441 DTP in all consultations, and the most prevalent were related to: 'non-adherence' (DTP 7—$n = 124; 28.1\%$); 'need for additional drug therapy' (DTP 2—$n = 96; 21.8\%$); and 'low dose' (DTP 4—$n = 86; 19.5\%$). Table 2 describes the number of stratified DTP by type.

Table 2. Absolute (*n*) and relative (%) frequency of drug-related problems (DTP) by category.

DTP Category	*n* (%)
1. Unnecessary medication	42 (9.5)
2. Need for additional drug therapy	96 (21.8)
3. Ineffective medication	19 (4.3)
4. Low dose	86 (19.5)
5. Adverse drug reaction	40 (9.1)
6. High dose	34 (7.7)
7. Non-adherence	124 (28.1)
Total	441 (100.0)

The main drugs associated with 'non-adherence' DTP were aspirin (*n* = 13; 10.5%) and simvastatin (*n* = 12; 9.7%). The drug cholecalciferol—vitamin D (*n* = 14; 14.6%) was the main drug requiring inclusion in drug therapy ('need for additional therapy' DTP). Regarding 'low-dose' DTP, the main drug involved was NPH insulin (*n* = 32; 37.2%). Of the total DTP, 59.6% (*n* = 263) were resolved (*n* = 263), 57.1% (*n* = 252) required interventions with the prescriber for resolution, and 67.9% (*n* = 171) of these interventions were accepted. Also, 364 interventions were performed directly with the patient (interventions performed vs. 82.5% of total DTP).

Table 3 shows the results of the univariate and multivariate analyses, which indicate that the presence of hypertension was independently and positively associated with the dependent variable, which was the identification of four DTP or more in the initial assessment, in a statistically significant way (*p* = 0.031).

Table 3. Univariate and multivariate analysis of the characteristics associated with the dependent variable—identification of four or more drug-related problems in the initial assessment. Belo Horizonte. 2015–2017.

Variables	Univariate Analysis		Multivariate Analysis	
	OR (95% CI) **	*p*-Value ***	OR (95% CI) **	*p*-Value ****
Age (full years)				
22–69	1.0			
≥70	1.20 (0.52–2.75)	0.067	0.99 (0.41–2.44)	0.991
Gender				
Female	1.0			
Male	0.75 (0.32–1.77)	0.517		
Number of health problems				
0–2	1.0		1.00	
≥3	2.47 (1.16–5.29)	0.020	1.67 (0.63–4.41)	0.300
Number of drugs				
0–7	1.00		1.00	
≥8	1.88 (0.76–4.66)	0.172	2.27 (0.93–5.55)	0.071
Hypertension				
No	1.00		1.00	
Yes	5.69 (1.49–21.66)	0.006	4.56 (1.14–18.19)	0.031
Diabetes Mellitus				
No	1.00			
Yes	1.48 (0.62–3.52)	0.378		

Note: Number of DTP identified during the first and second visit; ** Odds ratio (95% CI) estimated by logistic regression; *** Pearson's chi-square; included in the multivariate model when *p* < 0.20; **** Logistic regression; significant when *p* < 0.05.

After multiple adjustments, a statistically significant difference was detected between the initial and final values of HbA1c, SBP, DBP, LDLc, and HDLc (Table 4).

Table 4. Comparison of initial and final values of defined clinical and laboratory parameters.

Parameter (Unit/Number of Evaluated Patients)	Median Initial Visit	Median Final Visit	*p*-Value **
HbA1c (%; *n* = 31)	8.4	7.8	<0.001
SBP (mmHg; *n* = 54)	136.5	132.2	0.020
DBP (mmHg; *n* = 54)	82.8	79.7	0.002
LDLc (mg/dL; *n* = 29)	119.7	109.1	<0.001
HDLc (mg/dL; *n* = 28)	45.3	50.4	<0.001

Note: HbA1c = glycosilated hemoglobin; SBP = Systolic blood pressure; DBP = Diastolic blood pressure; LDLc = Low-density lipoprotein cholesterol; HDLc = High-density lipoprotein cholesterol; ** Estimated by covariance analysis with repeated measures (ANCOVA) adjusted by the Charlson Comorbidity Index (ICC), age, number of health problems, and number of drugs.

4. Discussion

The elderly majority among the patients assisted (75.6%) tended to increase the complexity of the service described in this study. This population has a high number of chronic diseases, as a consequence uses the health system more frequently, and usually consists of multiple-medication users [16], as indicated by the high mean number of health problems (3.2 ± 1.4) and drugs used by patients enrolled in the CMM service (7.6 ± 2.7). These findings reinforce the need to develop drug therapy qualification strategies such as the implementation of CMM services since the use of drugs in the elderly is generally associated with the occurrence of a more significant number of DTP [17].

With demographic and epidemiological transition, chronic and degenerative diseases have begun to gain greater representativity [18]. This was reflected in the results of this study, where a high prevalence of hypertension, DM, and dyslipidemia was detected, with a high number of patients with three concomitant diseases (*n* = 44; 49.0%—a result not previously described). Such complexity evidences the required action of the clinical pharmacist who is in charge of the drug therapy of these patients.

Hypertension was the most prevalent (82.2%) chronic condition and was positively and independently associated with the identification of four or more DTP in the initial assessment. This result may be related to the fact that the PHC pharmacist has greater mastery and experience for decision-making and identification of DTP related to hypertension since it is a chronic condition of high national prevalence. Also, patients with cardiovascular diseases, such as hypertension, often prompt the clinical pharmacist to evaluate the presence of DTP related to indication or appropriateness of drug therapy that might lead to the inclusion of medications for adequate cardiovascular prevention [14]. This type of DTP was the second most frequently identified in the initial assessment of this study (22.3%—results not described).

In a study that evaluated the clinical, economic, and humanistic outcomes of CMM services provided over a ten-year period in the health system of Minnesota [19], the authors pointed out the need for additional medication (accounting for 28.1% of total DTP), the use of low dose (26.1%), and non-adherence to drug therapy (16.5%) as the most frequent DTP identified. This result is comparable to the DTP frequency of this study. However, the reversed incidence was observed among DTP. In the present study, the most frequent DTP was non-adherence (28.12%), followed by the need for additional drug therapy (21.77%) and lastly the low dose, representing 19.50% of the total DTP. Another study [20] with a sample of patients from South Australia also found that the most frequent DTP were non-adherence to drug therapy (31.7%), followed by the need of additional medication (15.9%), and then drug ineffectiveness (15.7%).

The leading causes of non-adherence DTP were forgetfulness and failing to understand the instructions, which is consistent with the study population of mostly elderly, and therefore being more susceptible to cognitive impairments. The high frequency of this type of DTP can contribute adversely to the clinical outcomes of this population since the understanding, acceptability, and continuity of medication use are necessary conditions for the adequate management of chronic diseases. Thus, interventions with the patient are essential in resolving these DTP and showed high frequency in this study (performed to solve 82.5% of DTP). It should be noted that this type of intervention is deeply rooted in the philosophy of pharmaceutical care practice, which aims for shared-decision making between pharmacists and patients and to empower patients to get closely involved in the management of their own care [13].

Patients' non-adherence to drug therapy, especially among patients with chronic diseases and with more complex treatments remains a challenge for health services [2]. Considering preventive pharmacological measures, the difficulty of patients to understand the need for a medication may be the main reason that aspirin and simvastatin were the most frequent drugs involved in the non-adherence DTP. In Brazil, a study carried out in the city of Araucária-Paraná found that, among hypertensive patients, non-adherence can reach 60% of users, and among the factors that contribute most are schooling, failing to understand the disease, family history of cardiovascular disease, and the type of drug combination used [21]. In Santa Catarina, a study showed that, among users of lipid-lowering drugs, non-adherence increased in an average period of 19 months, after the onset of treatment [22]. Among diabetic patients, the low adherence to treatment was estimated at 50%, leading to poor glycemic control [23]. Furthermore, among the elderly, self-reported rates of 62.9% of non-adherence to treatment were found, and polypharmacy (use of five or more medications) is related to this problem [24].

The second most prevalent DTP, the need for additional drug therapy, reinforces the need for an expanded view of the pharmacist, who should focus not only on the drug therapy already in place but also on the screening and identification of untreated health conditions. The drug that was most frequently associated with this type of DTP, namely, Cholecalciferol (Vitamin D), is used against hypovitaminosis, prevalent in the world, that has an even more significant representativeness and risk among the elderly, who were the majority of the patients attended in this study [25,26].

For this reason, the Brazilian Society of Endocrinology and Metabology recommends supplementation for individuals who are at risk of vitamin D deficiency, such as the elderly, patients with osteoporosis, and those with a history of falls and fractures [25]. Thus, it is common practice for the pharmacist to request the screening exam in the initial CMM assessment, since a high percentage of the population is elderly. When a deficiency is detected, the propaedeutic procedure is to start therapy and communicate the eSF during the matrix-based strategy meetings to guarantee continuity of care.

The third most prevalent DTP was too low a dosage, due to a sub-therapeutic dose, incorrect administration, or use at inappropriate intervals, while NPH insulin was the primary drug associated with this DTP. Several factors are considered as impediments in the treatment of DM, influencing the achievement of patients' therapeutic goals and increasing the frequency of DTP. This condition requires complex treatment and involves the need for self-monitoring and frequent adjustments of insulin dose in a large number of patients [27]. Besides, DM changes the life of the patient and is in continuous clinical progression. The patients' daily routine and non-pharmacological measures also influence the effectiveness of insulin treatment. Thus, health professionals must be specifically trained to care for patients in insulin therapy, as the therapeutic goals should be individualized according to the characteristics of the patient and the stage of the disease [28].

In this study, most of the interventions were accepted by the prescribers (67.9%; $n = 171$), in a proportion higher than that found in CMM services provided to patients with COPD (55.2% of the accepted interventions) [8], with cancer (59.6%) [29], and with hypertension (42.7%) [30]. This may have influenced the high number of DTP resolved (59.6%). This result reflects the strengthening of the working relationship between the pharmacist and physicians, with a growing confidence in the pharmacist's clinical competence due to her participation in the workflows of the healthcare units. By allowing discussions of patient cases directly with prescribers on a regular basis, the matrix-based strategies (within or outside the fixed schedule) seem to favor the reassessment of the therapeutic goals by the healthcare team and the shared construction of care plans. The necessary communication between professionals rarely occurred through letters or phone calls, which were used only when the pharmacist needed to contact professionals working outside her healthcare network.

A statistically significant decline was observed in all clinical and laboratory parameters (HbA1c, SBP, DBP, LDL, and HDL) of the CMM patients at the end of the follow-up period. A quasi-experimental longitudinal study conducted by Bunting (2008) [31] in Asheville also evaluated the clinical outcomes of a CMM service. The service was provided to patients with hypertension and dyslipidemia for six years, and the results also showed reduced SBP parameters (137.3–126.3 mmHg; $p < 0.001$); DBP (82.6–77.8 mmHg; $p < 0.001$); LDL (127.2–108.3 mg/dL; $p < 0.001$); TC (211.4–184.3 mg/dL; $p < 0.001$) and TG (192.8–154.4 mg/dL; $p < 0.001$).

Some limitations were found in this study. First, there was a single pharmacist providing CMM who was still a novice at the implementation stage of the service. The pharmacist was still in the process of learning the practice, the method of documentation, and all that is involved in the process of transformation from a traditional pharmacist to a pharmaceutical care practitioner. The lack of training and the fact that the service was provided by only one professional could have reduced the quality and completeness of the documentation and, in consequence, hindered the evaluation of the clinical impact in the present study. The process of documentation becomes perfected over time and requires professional mastery and experience and, as highlighted by Ramalho de Oliveira (2011), it directly affects the quality of the data collected, the care provided, and consequently the obtained and evaluated results [6].

Another limitation was the difficulty of the other members of the health team to understand the service provided, due to its non-institutionalization at the workplace pointed out by Machado-Silva et al. (2018) in a study developed in the same health care unit [32]. In the Brazilian context, the professional pharmacist acts with some constraints regarding drug therapy change when he/she deems it necessary, always depending on the prescriber to accept and implement the suggested changes [32,33]. Physicians generally do not expect pharmacists to have a clinical role in proposing interventions [32,33]. Also, professional turnover requires that physicians always be updated regarding the inclusion of a service that is new and, therefore, unknown, hampering the establishment of partnerships [32]. This may be one of the factors explaining interventions that were not accepted ($n = 80$; 31.8%).

We should also consider some factors such as the qualification of referrals. Many of the patients were referred to the pharmacist because of problems of non-adherence. The pharmacist could only make interventions or recommendations after receiving an update of the requested tests by the eSF, and this caused some delay in the establishment of clinical conducts. As reported by Cipolle (2012) [13], it is inconsistent to promote drug adherence without the evaluation of the indication, effectiveness, and safety parameters. Also, the CMM service requires that pharmacists be trained and updated in their clinical training to provide a quality and safe service for patients.

In addition, even though the present study demonstrated the significant impact that CMM services had in the improvement of clinical parameters of non-communicable diseases, the reduced number of patients limited these results to this particular setting and may not be applicable to a different patient population or other primary health care setting. However, we highlight the importance of studies such as the one hereby presented, since research describing and evaluating CMM services in the Brazilian PHC, which is the gateway for the largest universal public health care system, is still scarce.

5. Conclusions

This study showed that the CMM service had a significant impact on the clinical outcomes of patients. The clinical pharmacist was able to identify and propose interventions to solve and prevent DTP. As a result, the streamlining of drug therapy improved the control of the most prevalent chronic health conditions and proved to be a useful service in primary care. Thus, its incorporation into the

PHC of the Brazilian health system should be considered a priority strategy for the control of prevalent chronic diseases.

Author Contributions: M.M.G.d.N., D.R.-d.-O.: Conceptualization; Methodology; Data analysis; Validation; and supervision. C.M.N., M.M.G.d.N., D.Á.M.S., D.R.-d.-O.: Data collection; Data curation; Writing—original draft preparation; Writing—review and Editing.

Funding: This research received no external funding.

Conflicts of Interest: The authors declare no conflict of interest.

References

1. Matta, G.C.; Morosini, M.V.G. Atenção Primária à Saúde: Dicionário da Educação Profissional em Saúde, 2009, 23–28. Available online: http://www.midias.epsjv.fiocruz.br/upload/d/Atencao_Primaria_a_Saude_-_recortado.pdf (accessed on 28 May 2019).
2. Brasil. Ministério da Saúde. Secretaria de Atenção à Saúde. Departamento de Atenção Básica. Ferramentas para a Gestão e para o Trabalho Cotidiano: Núcleo de Apoio Saúde da Família. Brasília, 2014, 116p. Available online: http://bvsms.saude.gov.br/bvs/publicacoes/nucleo_apoio_saude_familia_cab39.pdf (accessed on 28 May 2019).
3. IBGE. Instituto Brasileiro de Geografia e Estatística: Síntese de Indicadores Sociais: Uma Análise das Condições de vida da População Brasileira, 2013. Available online: https://biblioteca.ibge.gov.br/visualizacao/livros/liv66777.pdf (accessed on 28 May 2019).
4. Brasil. Secretaria de Atenção à Saúde. Departamento de Atenção Básica. Práticas Farmacêuticas no Núcleo de Apoio à Saúde da Família (Nasf). Brasília: Ministério da Saúde, 2017. Available online: http://www.saude.goiania.go.gov.br/docs/divulgacao/NASF_praticas_farmaceuticas_nasf_2017.pdf (accessed on 28 May 2019).
5. Hepler, C.D.; Strand, L.M. Opportunities and responsibilities in pharmaceutical care. *Am. J. Hospital. Pharm.* **1990**, *47*, 533–543. [CrossRef]
6. Ramalho de Oliveira, D. *Atenção Farmacêutica: Da Filosofia ao Gerenciamento da Terapia Medicamentosa*; RCN Editora: São Paulo, Brazil, 2011; 328p.
7. Mendonça, S.A.M.; Melo, A.C.; Pereira, G.C.C.; Santos, D.M.D.S.D.; Grossi, E.B.; Sousa, M.D.C.V.B.; de Ramalho de Oliveira, D.; Soares, A.C. Clinical outcomes of medication therapy management services in primary health care. *Braz. J. Pharm. Sci.* **2016**, *52*, 365–373. [CrossRef]
8. Detoni, K.B.; Oliveira, I.V.; Nascimento, M.M.; Caux, T.R.; Alves, M.R.; Ramalho-de-Oliveira, D. Impact of a medication therapy management service on the clinical status of patients with chronic obstructive pulmonary disease. *Int. J. Clin. Pharm.* **2016**, *39*, 1–9. [CrossRef]
9. Obreli-neto, P.R.; Marusic, S.; Guidoni, C.M.; Baldoni Ade, O.; Renovato, R.D.; Pilger, D.; Cuman, R.K.; Pereira, L.R. Economic evaluation of a pharmaceutical care program for elderly diabetic and hypertensive patients in primary health care: A 36-month randomized controlled clinical trial. *J. Manag. Care Spec. Pharm.* **2015**, *21*, 66–75. [CrossRef] [PubMed]
10. Cid, A.S. Avaliação da Efetividade da Atenção Farmacêutica no Controle da Hipertensão Arterial. Master's Thesis, Universidade Federal de Ouro Preto, Minas Gerais, Brazil, 2008.
11. Peter, D.H.; Tran, N.T.; Adam, T. *Implementation Research in Health: A Practical Guide*; Alliance for Health Policy and System Research; World Health Organization: Geneva, Switzerland, 2013.
12. Grimshaw, J.; Campbell, M.; Eccles, M.; Steen, N. Experimental and quasi-experimental designs for evaluating guideline implementation strategies. *Fam. Pract.* **2000**, *17*, 11–16. [CrossRef] [PubMed]
13. Cipolle, R.J.; Strand, L.M.; Morley, P.C. *Pharmaceutical Care Practice: The Patient Centered Approach to Medication Management*, 3rd ed.; McGraw-Hill: New York, NY, USA, 2012.
14. Cipolle, R.J.; Strand, L.M.; Morley, P.C. *Pharmaceutical Care Practice: The Clinician's Guide*, 2nd ed.; McGraw-Hill: New York, NY, USA, 2004.
15. Charlson, M.E.; Pompei, P.; Ales, K.L.; MacKenzie, C.R. A new method of classifying prognostic comorbidity in longitudinal studies: Development and validation. *J. Chron. Dis.* **1987**, *40*, 373–383. [CrossRef]

16. Veras, R. Envelhecimento populacional contemporâneo: Demandas, desafios e inovações—Populationagingtoday: Demands, challengesandinnovations. *Rev. Saúde Pública* **2009**, *43*, 548–554. [CrossRef] [PubMed]

17. Jansen, P.A.; Brouwers, J.R. Clinical Pharmacology in Old Persons. *Scientifica* **2012**, *2012*, 723678. [CrossRef] [PubMed]

18. Monteiro, M. As transições demográfica e epidemiológica no Brasil. *Acta Paul. Enferm.* **2000**, *13*, 65–76.

19. Isetts, B.J.; Schondelmeyer, S.W.; Artz, M.B.; Lenarz, L.A.; Heaton, A.H.; Wadd, W.B.; Brown, L.M.; Cipolle, R.J. Clinical and economic outcomes of medication therapy management services: The Minnesota experience. *J. Am. Pharm. Assoc.* **2008**, *48*, 203–211. [CrossRef] [PubMed]

20. Rao, D.; Gilbert, A.; Strand, L.M.; Cipolle, R.J. Drug therapy problems found in ambulatory patient populations in Minnesota and South Australia. *Pharm. World Sci.* **2007**, *29*, 647–654. [CrossRef] [PubMed]

21. Melchiors, A.C. Hipertensão Arterial: Análise dos Fatores Relacionados com o Controle Pressórico e a Qualidade de Vida. Master's Thesis, Universidade Federal do Paraná, Curitiba, Brazil, 2008.

22. Cunico, C. Dislipidemia e Efetividade do Uso de Hipolipemiantes em População do Extremo Oeste do Estado de Santa Catarina. Master's Thesis, Universidade Federal do Paraná, Curitiba, Brazil, 2011.

23. Souza, R.A.P.; Correr, C.; Melchiors, A. Determinants of glycemic control and quality of life in type 2 diabetic patients. *Lat. Am. J. Pharm.* **2011**, *30*, 860–867.

24. Rocha, C.H. Medication adherence of elderly in Porto Alegre, RS. *Ciênc Saúde Coletiva* **2008**, *13*, 703–710. [CrossRef]

25. Maeda, S.S. Recomendações da Sociedade Brasileira de Endocrinologia e Metabologia (SBEM) para o diagnóstico e tratamento da hipovitaminose D. *Arq. Bras. Endocrinol. Metab.* **2014**, *55*, 91–105. [CrossRef]

26. Bandeira, F.; Griz, L.; Dreyer, P.; Eufrazino, C.; Bandeira, C.; Freese, E. Vitamin D deficiency: A global perspective. *Arq. Bras. Endocrinol. Metab.* **2006**, *50*, 640–646. [CrossRef]

27. Sociedade Brasileira de Diabetes. *Diretrizes da Sociedade Brasileira de Diabetes (2015–2016)*; A.C. Farmacêutica: São Paulo, Brazil, 2016.

28. Chatterjee, S.; Davies, M.J. Current management of diabetes mellitus and future directions in care. *Postgrad. Med. J.* **2015**, *91*, 612–621. [CrossRef]

29. Bremberg, E.R.; Hising, C.; Nylén, U.; Ehrsson, H.; Eksborg, S. An evaluation of pharmacist contribution to an oncology ward in a Swedish hospital. *J. Oncol. Pharm. Pract.* **2006**, *12*, 75–81. [CrossRef]

30. Sookaneknum, P.; Richards, R.M.; Sanguansermsri, J.; Teerasut, C. Pharmacist involvement in primary care improves hypertensive patient clinical outcomes. *Ann. Pharmacother.* **2004**, *38*, 2023–2028. [CrossRef]

31. Bunting, B.A.; Smith, B.H.; Sutherland, S.E. The Asheville Project: Clinical and economic outcomes of a community-based long-term medication therapy management program for hypertension and dyslipidemia. *J. Am. Pharm Assoc.* **2008**, *48*, 23–31. [CrossRef]

32. Machado-Silva, D.A.; Medina, S.D.; Ramalho de Oliveira, D. Clinical practice of pharmacists in family health Support team. *Trab. Educ Saúde* **2018**, *16*, 659–682.

33. Machado-Silva, D.A.; Mendonça, S.A.M.; O´Dougherty, M.; Ramalho de Oliveira, D.; Chemello, C. Autoethnography as an Instrument for Professional (Trans) Formation in Pharmaceutical Care Practice. *Qualit. Rep.* **2017**, *22*, 2926–2942.

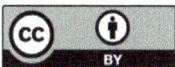

pharmacy

MDPI

Article

Using the Theory of Planned Behavior to Understand Factors Influencing South Asian Consumers' Intention to Seek Pharmacist-Provided Medication Therapy Management Services

Shaquib Al Hasan *, Jagannath Mohan Muzumdar, Rajesh Nayak and Wenchen Kenneth Wu

Department of Pharmacy Administration and Public Health, College of Pharmacy and Health Sciences, St. John's University, 8000 Utopia Parkway, Jamaica, NY 11439, USA
* Correspondence: shaquib.hasan111@gmail.com

Received: 31 May 2019; Accepted: 9 July 2019; Published: 11 July 2019

check for updates

Abstract: The study purpose was to use the theory of planned behavior to understand factors influencing South Asian consumers' intention to seek pharmacist-provided medication therapy management services (MTMS). Specific objectives were to assess effects of attitude, subjective norm (SN), perceived behavioral control (PBC), and socio-demographics on South Asian consumers' intention to seek MTMS. Participants who were ≥18 years of age, of South Asian origin, with a previous visit to a pharmacy in the US for a health-related reason, and with ability to read and comprehend English were recruited from independent pharmacies in New York City. Responses were obtained through a self-administered survey. Descriptive statistics were performed, and multiple linear regression analysis was conducted to assess the study objective. SPSS was used for data analyses. Out of 140 responses, 133 were usable. Mean scores (standard deviation) were 4.04 (0.97) for attitude, 3.77 (0.91) for SN, 3.75 (0.93) for PBC, and 3.96 (0.94) for intention. The model explains 80.8% of variance and is a significant predictor of intention, $F_{(14,118)} = 35.488$, $p < 0.05$. While attitude ($\beta = 0.723$, $p < 0.05$) and PBC ($\beta = 0.148$, $p < 0.05$) were significant predictors of intention, SN ($\beta = 0.064$, $p = 0.395$) was not. None of the socio-demographics were significant predictors of intention. Strategies to make South Asians seek MTMS should focus on creating positive attitudes and removing barriers in seeking MTMS.

Keywords: intention; medication therapy management; pharmacy services; South Asian; theory of planned behavior.

---

1. Introduction

Drug-related problems (DRPs), such as adverse drug reactions, drug interactions, poor adherence etc., significantly affect morbidity and mortality rates and contribute to rising health care expenditures [1,2]. As healthcare professionals, pharmacists can identify, prevent, and resolve DRPs by helping patients understand and self-manage their medications [3,4]. Emphasizing these professional roles of pharmacists, the Centers for Medicare and Medicaid Services (CMS) recognized medication therapy management services (MTMS) under the Medicare Modernization Act of 2003 [5,6]. Medication therapy management (MTM) has been defined as a "distinct service or group of services that optimize therapeutic outcomes for individual patients" [7]. MTM services (MTMS) typically include collecting medical and drug histories from patients, patient education, comprehensive medication review, medication monitoring, and provider outreach to convey recommendations for adjustments to drug therapy when necessary [8–10]. Pharmacist-provided MTMS helped improve clinical outcomes such as blood pressure, HbA1c, LDL cholesterol [11]; humanistic outcomes such as medication adherence, patient knowledge, patient satisfaction [11,12]; and economic outcomes such as positive return on investment from MTMS [12].

Previous studies on MTMS mostly focused on healthcare professionals [13,14] and patients [13,15–26]. In the literature reviewed, patient-focused studies regarding pharmacist-provided MTMS explored patients' awareness about MTM [15], attitude toward MTMS [16], perceptions and expectations about MTMS [17], perception about pharmacists' role [15], perceived medication-related needs [22], patient perceived benefits/values [18], interest or willingness to receive MTMS [20], willingness to pay for MTMS [18], satisfaction with MTMS [21], barriers in receiving MTMS [22], effective strategies for marketing MTM [22], and impact of promotional strategies on patient acceptance of MTMS [24].

However, these patient-focused studies also had their own set of limitations, such as limited sample size [15,21,24], lack of generalizability of study findings [15,17,18,22], low response rate [17,24], and selection bias [21]. In addition, two major limitations are demographics of study participants and lack of theoretical approach in study design. Respondents in previous patient-focused studies were predominantly white [15,18,20]. Their responses might not truly represent opinions of the non-white population, particularly the South Asian population. The South Asian population (people from India, Pakistan, Bangladesh, Nepal, Sri Lanka, Bhutan, and the Maldives) is one of the fastest growing immigrant communities in the United States (US). Members of this racial group have their own social and cultural characteristics, such as language, religion, family ties etc., that may influence their health behavior and healthcare decision making [27,28]. It has been reported that South Asians in the US face various barriers including language, communication, and cultural barriers in accessing health care services [28]. Effective delivery of culturally and linguistically appropriate services can help pharmacists provide better services to this group. In order to design and deliver pharmacy services such as MTMS in a culturally competent way, it is important to understand what influences the intention of South Asians in the US to seek specialized pharmacy services like MTMS. The second major limitation in past literature was the absence of a theoretical framework to explain factors influencing the intention of patients to seek or receive MTMS. Understanding behavior change theories and using them skillfully in research and practice can help design better interventions for patients [29]. This study used the theory of planned behavior (TPB) as a theoretical framework which has been used extensively to explain and predict behavioral intentions and health behaviors including health services utilization [30]. The purpose of this study was to use the theory of planned behavior (TPB) to understand factors influencing intention of South Asian consumers to seek pharmacist-provided medication therapy management (MTM) services. Based on the TPB model, specific study objectives were to assess the influence of South Asian consumers' (1) attitude on their intention to seek pharmacist-provided MTM services, (2) subjective norm on their intention to seek pharmacist-provided MTM services, (3) perceived behavioral control on their intention to seek pharmacist-provided MTM services, and (4) external variables such as age, gender, income, education, number of medications etc. on their intention to seek pharmacist-provided MTM services.

2. Background Literature and Theoretical Framework

The theory of planned behavior is an individual level health behavior theory which hypothesizes that intention is a precursor of actual behavior. According to TPB, intention is influenced by attitude towards performing a behavior, subjective norm associated with the behavior, and perceived control over the behavior [30].

Attitude has been defined as an individual's positive or negative feelings about performing a behavior [31]. Past application of TPB found that attitude was a significant predictor of pharmacists' intent to provide MTMS [31], community pharmacists' intention to utilize a prescription drug monitoring program [32], pharmacists' intention to report serious adverse drug events (ADEs) to the Food and Drug Administration (FDA) [33], and medical students' intention to improve oral hygiene [34]. Based on the research cited above, it was hypothesized that

Hypothesis 1 (H1). *South Asian consumers' attitude toward seeking MTM services would be a significant predictor of their intention to seek MTM services.*

Subjective norm is an individual's perception of whether people important to the individual think the behavior should be performed [31]. Past TPB research found that subjective norm was a significant predictor of intention in both pharmacists and consumers. Previous research on pharmacists found that subjective norm was a significant predictor of pharmacists' intention to provide MTMS [31], intention to utilize a prescription drug monitoring program [32], and intention to report serious ADEs to the FDA [33]. Previous research on consumers found that subjective norm was a significant predictor of consumers' intention to adopt Pharmacy Value Added Services (PVAS) [35]. Based on the research cited above, the corresponding hypothesis was

Hypothesis 2 (H2). *South Asian consumers' subjective norm associated with seeking MTM services would be a significant predictor of their intention to seek MTM services.*

Perceived behavioral control reflects a person's beliefs as to how easy or difficult it will be to perform the behavior [36]. Like subjective norm, perceived behavioral control was also found to be a significant predictor of intention in both pharmacists and consumers. Perceived behavioral control was found to be a significant predictor of pharmacists' intent to provide MTMS [31], pharmacists' intention to utilize a prescription drug monitoring program [32], as well as consumers' intention to adopt Pharmacy Value Added Services (PVAS) [35]. In the study by Tan et al., perceived behavioral control was found to be the most influential predictor among all TPB constructs in building intent of consumers to adopt PVAS [35]. Based on the research cited above, it was hypothesized that

Hypothesis 3 (H3). *South Asian consumers' perceived behavioral control in seeking MTM services would be a significant predictor of their intention to seek MTM services.*

As per TPB, other external variables such as age, gender, type of disease etc., can influence attitude, subjective norm, and perceived behavioral control, and in turn can influence intention to perform certain behavior [30]. In a previous study, age and type of health problems were correlated with willingness to pay for MTMS [18]; gender, income, education, number of health problems, and previous work experience in the healthcare profession were associated with willingness to accept pharmacist-provided MTMS [20]. Among individuals from different cultural groups, length of time in the United States and socio-economic status influenced their beliefs about health, disease, and treatment [37]. Previous research found that gender, education level, and race were significant predictors of the use of family, friends, and co-workers as a source of health information by US adults [38]. Based on this literature, it was hypothesized that

Hypothesis 4 (H4). *South Asian consumers' socio-demographic characteristics and other external variables would be significant predictors of their intention to seek MTM services.*

A summary of these hypotheses has been presented in Figure 1.

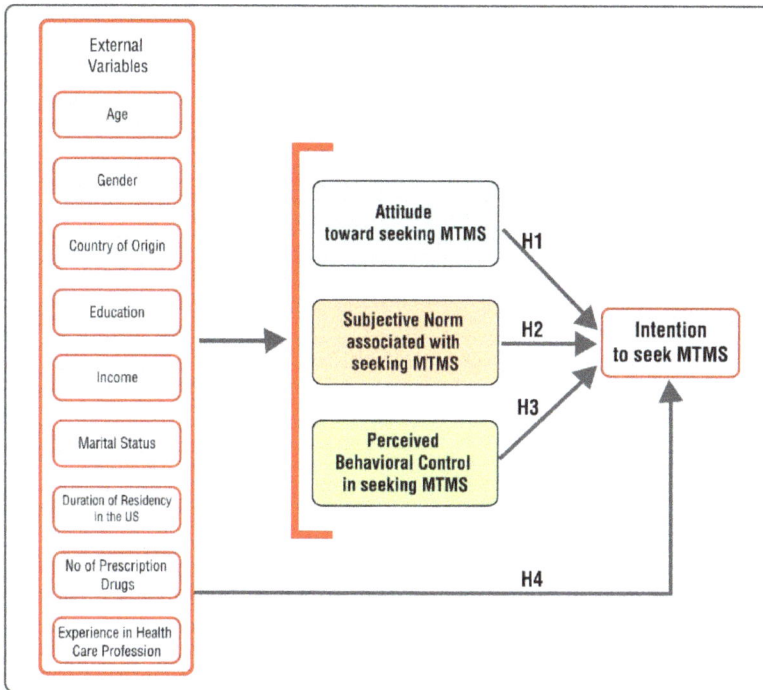

Figure 1. Proposed model of the theory of planned behavior in predicting intention to seek medication therapy management services (MTMS). *Source: Modified from K. Glanz, B. K. Rimer, and K. Viswanath, Health Behavior and Health Education: Theory, Research, and Practice. John Wiley & Sons, pp. 70, 2008.*

3. Methods

3.1. Study Design

A cross-sectional, non-experimental, quantitative research design with a self-administered survey approach was used in order to achieve the study objectives.

3.2. Target Population and Participant Recruitment

Study participants for survey research were recruited from neighborhoods in New York City. New York City is one of the most diverse cities in the US with a population of different racial backgrounds including South Asians [39]. Moreover, New York State has the second largest concentration of South Asians in the US following California [28]. About 72% of South Asians in New York State resides in New York City [28]. Participants were recruited from New York City neighborhoods of Jamaica Hills and Jackson Heights in Queens, and Ozone Park in Brooklyn where the South Asian population was the most prevalent during the study period. A non-probability convenient sampling was followed for convenience and ease of access to participants. Upon approval from the human subjects review committee, pharmacists in independent pharmacies located in Jackson Heights-Elmhurst, Jamaica Hills, and Ozone Park in New York City were contacted by the primary researcher to inform them about the study purpose and study design, and to seek permission to use their pharmacy premises as the study setting for data collection. Three out of seven pharmacies which were contacted allowed the researcher to use their premises as the study setting and for conducting surveys among consumers visiting their pharmacies. Permissions from the interested pharmacies were taken through signed consent letters.

Study participants were South Asian consumers visiting these three pharmacies. Participants were included in the study if they were of South Asian origin, were at least 18 years of age, had previously visited a pharmacy in the United States for a health related issue, and were able to read and comprehend English. The target sample size calculated for this study was 154 participants. This target sample size was determined from past literature describing methods for sample size calculations required for data analysis techniques (multiple linear regression and factor analysis) used in this study [40–42].

3.3. Survey Development and Administration

A 28-item survey was developed for data collection. Survey items were developed to measure attitude (five items), subjective norm (four items), perceived behavioral control (five items), and intention (five items). These items were scored on a 5-point Likert scale with possible answers being strongly disagree, disagree, neutral, agree, and strongly agree. Items related to socio-demographic characteristics—age, gender, country of origin, highest level of education, annual household income, marital status, duration of residency in the US, number of medications being taken, and work experience as a health care professional (9 items)—were also included. No personal identifying information of participants was collected to ensure anonymity of participants.

Items assessing attitude and intention were based on the core elements of MTMS (medication therapy review, medication-related action plan, intervention and/or referral, and follow-up) as jointly reported by the American Pharmacists Association (APhA) and the National Association of Chain Drug Stores (NACDS) Foundation [7]. Items from a previous TPB study on pharmacist intention to provide MTMS were modified to develop items assessing subjective norm in this study [31]. Items to assess the perceived behavioral control were developed using past literature on TPB questionnaire construction by Ajzen [43]. Patient-reported barriers to receive MTMS, such as inability to fix appointments due to patients' busy schedule; inaccessibility to pharmacist (location, parking) and time of day/week reported in past literature were considered while developing items to assess perceived behavioral control [13,22].

Face validity of the survey instrument was done with the help of graduate students and three faculty members having expertise in research methods, survey methodology, and medication therapy management services (MTMS). The survey was approved by the institutional review board.

Upon approval from the human subjects review committee, the survey was pilot tested on a convenience sample of consumers visiting the selected pharmacies between October 2018 and November 2018. The primary researcher approached consumers visiting respective pharmacies and requested for their voluntary participation in the study. The study purpose, procedure of the study, and voluntary nature of participation were explained to the consumers. Interested participants provided their voluntary consent through a participant invitation letter and informed consent form. Consumers who agreed to participate in the study were provided the study survey. A total of 30 surveys were completed in the pilot study as recommended by Viechtbauer et al. [44]. It took approximately 6–10 min for each participant to complete the survey.

Necessary changes were made to the original survey based on the findings from the pilot study. After the pilot study, two items on the intention scale were merged into one item and one item from demographic information was deleted to keep the survey concise. Items asking for previous work experience in the health care profession were moved towards the end of the survey so that participants who did not work in the health care profession did not feel offended in the middle of completing the survey. Moreover, wording for some of the items was changed and examples were provided for some items in the survey to make sure that participants understood the survey items easily. The revised survey was submitted to the human subjects review committee as an amendment to the original Institutional Review Board (IRB) application.

Upon getting the approval for the final survey from the human subjects review committee, data was collected for the main study from mid November 2018 to the end of February 2019. It took approximately 4–8 min for each participant to respond to the survey questionnaire in the main study. The response time for each participant for the main study (4–8 min) was less compared to the pilot study (6–10 min) as the survey instrument for the main study was more easily understandable to participants due to the reduction of the number of items, changes in wording, and addition of examples in the revised survey instrument. To reduce the selection bias, every alternative consumer was requested for participation in the study. A total of 140 consumers participated in this study.

3.4. Data Analysis

Prior to data analysis, completeness of survey responses was checked. Any missing data for study variables of a respondent was replaced with an average score of other available items' responses of the scale within that respondent [45]. Construct validity for survey items was confirmed through factor analysis using principal component analysis with varimax rotation. Items with factor loadings less than 0.60 were considered for deletion. Following the factor analysis, the internal consistency of measures was tested using Cronbach's alpha. As suggested in the literature, a Cronbach's alpha of 0.70 or higher was considered as an acceptable reliability coefficient [46].

Socio-demographic characteristics of the study sample were analyzed using descriptive statistical methods. Multiple linear regression analysis was used to assess the influence of independent variables on the dependent variable [47]. In multiple linear regression, attitude, subjective norm, perceived behavioral, and socio-demographic variables were independent variables. Intention was the dependent variable. Before running multiple regression, all of the socio-demographic variables were recoded as dichotomous variables. If the *p*-value was <0.05, the independent variable(s) was considered significant predictor(s) of the intention to seek MTMS. All statistical analyses were performed using IBM SPSS Statistics Version 23.0 (IBM Corp., New York, NY, USA, 2015).

4. Results

Out of 140 surveys received, 133 surveys were usable for the study. Seven surveys were not used as six of them had incomplete response to items related to TPB constructs and one did not have demographic information.

4.1. Socio-Demographic Characteristics

The majority of the participants were male (71.4%), were 18–45 years old (72.9%), were married or in a domestic relationship (62.4%), had a bachelor's degree or higher (51.1%), had an annual income less than $35,000 (54.9%), were living in the US for at least 5 years (63.9%), and had no experience in the health care profession (88.0%), as shown in Table 1.

4.2. Validity and Reliability of Survey Items

Based on the findings from factor analysis, two items from the initial five items assessing attitude and one item from the initial four items assessing subjective norm were deleted. One of the items for the subjective norm scale was retained in spite of having a factor loading less than 0.60 (0.48) as it is recommended to keep at least three items for each component [48]. No item was deleted from the set of items assessing perceived behavioral control and intention. Finally, data analysis was done on three items for the attitude scale, three items for the subjective norm scale, five items for the perceived behavioral control scale, and five items for the intention scale, as shown in Table 2.

Cronbach's alpha for the entire survey (excluding sociodemographic variables) was 0.96. Cronbach's alpha values for attitude, subjective norm, perceived behavioral control, and intention were found to be 0.88, 0.88, 0.93, and 0.93, respectively, as shown in Table 2. Cronbach's alpha values greater than 0.70 for all of the constructs indicate attitude, subjective norm, perceived behavioral control, and intention scales to be reliable multi-item measures.

Table 1. Socio-demographic characteristics of the study sample (N = 133).

Characteristic	Number	Percent
Age		
Between 18 and 30 years	51	38.3
Between 31 and 45 years	46	34.6
Between 46 and 65 years	27	20.3
65 years or more	9	6.8
Gender		
Male	95	71.4
Female	38	28.6
Country of Origin		
Bangladesh	102	76.7
India	11	8.3
Nepal	12	9.0
Pakistan	8	6.0
Education		
Less than high school	13	9.8
High school or equivalent	33	24.8
Some college, no degree	10	7.5
Associate degree	9	6.8
Bachelor's degree	29	21.8
Graduate degree	39	29.3
Household income		
Less than $20,000	42	31.6
$20,000 to $34,999	31	23.3
$35,000 to $49,999	23	17.3
$50,000 to $74,999	14	10.5
$75,000 to $99,999	14	10.5
$100,000 or more	9	6.8
Marital status		
Single (never married)	46	34.6
Married, or in a domestic partnership	83	62.4
Widowed	2	1.5
Divorced	1	0.8
Separated	1	0.8
Duration of residency in the US		
Less than 1 year	2	1.5
1 to 3 years	22	16.5
3 to 5 years	24	18.0
5 to 10 years	43	32.3
10 years or more	42	31.6
No. of daily prescription drug		
0	51	38.3
1	30	22.6
2	21	15.8
3	6	4.5
4 or more	25	18.8
Experience in health care profession		
Yes	16	12.0
No	117	88.0

Table 2. Theory of planned behavior scale constructs used to measure intention to seek MTMS (N = 133).

Construct	No. of Items Retained (No. of Initial Items)	Mean [a]	Standard Deviation [a]	Lowest Individual Score	Highest Individual Score	Cronbach's Alpha
Attitude	3 (5)	4.04	0.97	1.00	5.00	0.88
Subjective norm	3 (4)	3.77	0.91	1.00	5.00	0.88
Perceived behavioral control	5 (5)	3.75	0.93	1.00	5.00	0.93
Intention	5 (5)	3.96	0.94	1.00	5.00	0.93

[a] Individual items were measured on a Likert scale (1 = strongly disagree through 5 = strongly agree). Higher scores signify more positive attitudes, more favorable subjective norm, more perceived behavioral control and stronger intention to seek MTMS.

4.3. Descriptive Statistics for TPB Constructs

Descriptive statistics for TPB constructs have been presented in Table 2. Participants had a mean attitude score of 4.04 with a standard deviation of 0.97. A mean score of 3.77 was found for subjective norm with a standard deviation of 0.91. The lowest mean score of 3.75 with a standard deviation of 0.93 was found for perceived behavioral control based on three items. Finally, a mean score of 3.96 with a standard deviation of 0.94 was found for intention. These mean scores were computed on a Likert scale of 1 to 5 with 1 representing "strongly disagree" and 5 representing "strongly agree".

4.4. Item-Wise Descriptive Statistics for TPB Constructs

Descriptive statistics for individual items including the percentage of respondents having a positive response (either agree or strongly agree), neutral response, and negative response (disagree or strongly disagree) for each statement have been presented in Table 3.

Table 3. Survey statements and descriptive statistics by construct (N = 133).

Construct	Statement	Mean (SD) [a]	Percent Agree [b]	Percent Neutral	Percent Disagree [c]
Attitude	If pharmacist advises me on how to avoid medicine-related problems such as possible adverse effects or side effects, allergy due to medicine; it will be helpful for me.	3.99 (1.14)	82.0	4.5	13.5
	If pharmacist guides me on how to handle my medicines by myself (such as taking appropriate action if the dose is missed, using a pill reminder chart for taking medicines timely), it will be helpful for me.	4.11 (1.03)	88.0	3.0	9.0
	If pharmacist communicates with me to ensure that I am taking my medicines according to doctor's prescription, it will be good for me.	4.02 (1.06)	83.5	4.5	11.3
Subjective Norm	If I want to take pharmacy services, my family members will support me.	3.90 (0.92)	79.7	9.0	11.3
	If I want to take pharmacy services, my friends will support me.	3.75 (1.05)	68.4	20.3	11.3
	People important to me in my community will support me to take pharmacy services.	3.65 (1.05)	69.2	17.3	13.5
Perceived Behavioral Control	I can easily meet my pharmacist to take his/her services.	3.76 (0.99)	72.9	11.3	15.0
	I am confident that I shall be able to take pharmacy services.	3.92 (0.97)	79.7	10.5	9.8
	I shall be able to take pharmacy services without any difficulty.	3.74 (1.06)	72.2	13.5	14.3
	I have enough time for taking services provided by pharmacist.	3.55 (1.16)	63.2	18.8	18.0
	Taking pharmacy services is entirely within my control.	3.77 (1.10)	72.9	12.0	13.5
Intention	I am willing to take the service in which my pharmacist … … will evaluate my medicines and tell me how to avoid medicine-related problems such as possible adverse effects or side effects, allergy due to medicine etc.	3.95 (1.05)	81.2	7.5	11.3
	… will educate me so that I can handle my medicines by myself (such as taking appropriate action if the dose is missed, using pill reminder chart for taking medicines timely).	3.95 (1.08)	83.5	3.8	12.8
	… will educate me on diet, physical activity, smoking, drinking etc. so that I can manage diseases such as diabetes.	3.96 (1.05)	82.0	6.8	11.3
	… will recommend my doctor to change the medicine where there is more effective or safe medicine.	3.86 (1.09)	77.4	8.3	14.3
	… will contact me and give advice to make sure that I am continuing medicines according to my doctor's prescription.	4.05 (1.04)	86.5	3.8	9.8

SD = standard deviation. [a] Coded as 1 = strongly disagree, 2 = disagree, 3 = neutral, 4 = agree, 5 = strongly agree. [b] Percent stating they agreed or strongly agreed. [c] Percent stating they disagreed or strongly disagreed.

In terms of attitudes toward seeking MTMS, consumers mostly had positive responses to the items measuring attitude towards seeking MTMS. More than 80% of respondents agreed that pharmacists' advice on how to avoid medication-related problems would be helpful for them, pharmacists' guidance on self-management of medications would be helpful for them, and pharmacists' follow-up to ensure patients' adherence to medications would be good for them. Participants had the most positive attitude towards pharmacists' guidance on self-management of medications. A total of 88% of the respondents agreed that pharmacists' guidance on self-management of medications would be helpful for them. On the other hand, respondents had the maximum disagreement with pharmacists' guidance on avoiding medication-related problems. A total of 14% of the respondents disagreed to the statement that pharmacists' advice on how to avoid medication-related problems would be useful for them. A total of 84% of the respondents agreed to the statement that pharmacists' follow-up to ensure patients' adherence to medications would be good for them.

For subjective norm, more consumers (80%) agreed that family members would support them in taking MTM services than agreed that friends and people important in community would support them in taking MTM services. However, 68% of respondents still agreed that friends would encourage them and 69% of respondents agreed that people important in community would support them in seeking MTM services.

In terms of perceived behavioral control, 80% of respondents believed that they were confident that they would be able to take MTM services. At least 70% of respondents believed that they could easily meet their pharmacist to take his/her services, they should be able to take MTM services without any difficulty, and taking pharmacy services was entirely within their control. However, this percentage was lower in the case of having enough time for taking MTM services. More than one third (37%) of the respondents did not feel (18% disagreed and 19% were neutral) that they had enough time for taking pharmacist-provided MTM services.

Most of the respondents had positive intention toward seeking MTM services. More than 80% of respondents had positive intention to take pharmacists' follow-up service to ensure adherence to medications. More than 80% of respondents had positive intention to take services in which their pharmacists would review medicines and advise on how to avoid medication-related problems, would educate them on self-management of medications, and educate them on lifestyle changes to help them self-manage their diseases. On the contrary, respondents had the least positive intention to seek service of pharmacists' recommendations to physicians about medications. A total of 22% of respondents did not feel (14% disagreed and 8% were neutral) that they had intention to seek services where pharmacists would recommend physicians for better medications. Nevertheless, 77% of respondents had positive intention to seek services where pharmacists would recommend physicians for better medications.

4.5. Multiple Linear Regression Predicting Intention

Hypothesis testing was done by multiple linear regression. Hierarchical multiple regression was used for the study variables to find out the relative contribution of socio-demographic variables versus other TPB constructs (attitude, subjective norm, and perceived behavioral control) in predicting intention. In step 1, attitude, subjective norm, and perceived behavioral control were included as predictor variables (Model 1). In step 2, along with TPB constructs (attitude, subjective norm, and perceived behavioral control), socio-demographic variables were entered as predictors of intention (Model 2). Table 4 presents model summary for Model 1 and Model 2.

Table 4. Model summary of multiple linear regression analysis predicting intention.

Model [a]	R	R^2	Adjusted R^2	Standard Error of Estimate	R^2 Change	F Change	df1	df2	Sig. F Change
1	0.889 [b]	0.791	0.786	0.43605	0.791	162.655	3	129	0.000
2	0.899 [c]	0.808	0.785	0.43680	0.017	0.959	11	118	0.487

[a.] Dependent variable: intention. [b.] Predictors (constant): attitude, subjective norm, perceived behavioral control. [c.] Predictors (constant): attitude, subjective norm, perceived behavioral control, age more than 45 years, male gender, married or in a domestic relationship, Bangladeshi origin, Nepali origin, Indian origin, bachelor's degree or higher, income more than $35,000, duration of residency in the US, daily prescription drug quantity, experience in health care profession.

Model 1 had an R^2 value equal to 0.791 and Model 2 had an R^2 value equal to 0.808. It means that 79.1% of the variance in intention was explained by the independent variables in Model 1 and 80.8% of the variance in intention was explained by the independent variables in Model 2. Entry of socio-demographic variables (Model 2) resulted in a change in R^2 of 0.017. This means that entry of socio-demographic variables increased the explained variance in intention by only 1.7% to a total of 80.8%. This increase was not statistically significant by the F change test, F $(11,118) = 0.959, p = 0.487$. These findings suggest that the first set of predictor variables other than socio-demographic variables (attitude, subjective norm, and perceived behavioral control) were a more powerful set of predictors than socio-demographic variables and inclusion of socio-demographic variables did not increase explanatory power significantly.

4.5.1. Influence of Attitude on Intention

The first specific objective of the study was to assess the influence of South Asian consumers' attitude toward seeking MTMS on their intention to seek MTMS. The regression analysis for Model 1 found that attitude was a statistically significant predictor of intention, $\beta = 0.732, t = 11.258, p < 0.05$, as shown in Table 5. The regression analysis for Model 2 also found that attitude was a statistically significant predictor of intention, $\beta = 0.723, t = 10.303, p < 0.05$, as shown in Table 5. This means attitude was a significant predictor of intention ($p < 0.05$) for both models.

Table 5. Parameter estimates from multiple linear regression analysis predicting intention to seek medication therapy management services (N = 133).

Model	Variable	Unstandardized Coefficients		Standardized Coefficients	t Statistic	P Value
		B	Standard Error	Beta		
	Constant	0.274	0.177		1.550	0.124
	Attitude	0.711	0.063	0.732	11.258	0.000 *
1 [a]	Subjective norm	0.043	0.074	0.042	0.587	0.558
	Perceived behavioral control	0.171	0.063	0.169	2.738	0.007 *
	Constant	0.444	0.239		1.860	0.065
	Attitude	0.703	0.068	0.723	10.303	0.000 *
	Subjective norm	0.067	0.078	0.064	0.854	0.395
	Perceived behavioral control	0.150	0.067	0.148	2.224	0.028 *
	Age	−0.100	0.109	−0.047	−0.918	0.361
	Gender	−0.014	0.099	−0.007	−0.143	0.887
	Bangladeshi Origin	0.042	0.168	0.019	0.251	0.802
2 [a,b]	Nepali Origin	−0.065	0.209	−0.020	−0.311	0.756
	Indian Origin	0.112	0.214	0.033	0.522	0.602
	Education	−0.031	0.083	−0.016	−0.368	0.714
	Income	0.011	0.092	0.006	0.123	0.902
	Marital Status	−0.138	0.091	−0.071	−1.511	0.133
	Duration of Residency in the US	−0.142	0.092	−0.072	−1.540	0.126
	No of Daily Rx Drug	0.147	0.114	0.066	1.286	0.201
	HCP Experience	0.092	0.123	0.032	0.748	0.456

* Significant predictor of intention at a level of significance of 0.05. [a] Dependent variable: intention. [b] Age was coded as 1 = more than 45 years, 0 = 18 to 45 years; gender was coded as 1 = male, 0 = female; Bangladeshi origin was coded as 1 = Bangladeshi origin, 0 = non- Bangladeshi origin; Nepali origin was coded as 1 = Nepali origin, 0 = non- Nepali origin; Indian origin; Indian origin was coded as 1 = Indian origin, 0 = non-Indian origin; education was coded as 1 = bachelor's and above, 0 = Less than bachelor's; income was coded as 1 = $35,000 and above, 0 = up to $34,999; marital status was coded as 1 = married or in a domestic relationship, 0 = other; duration of residency in the US was coded as 1 = more than 5 years, 0 = up to 5 years; daily prescription drug quantity was coded as 1 = 3 or more, 0 = less than 3; health care profession (HCP) experience was coded as 1 = previous experience in health care profession, 0 = no experience in health care profession.

4.5.2. Influence of Subjective Norm on Intention

The second study objective was to assess the influence of South Asian consumers' subjective norm associated with seeking MTM services on their intention to seek MTMS. The regression analysis for Model 1 found that subjective norm was not a statistically significant predictor of intention, $\beta = 0.042$, t = 0.587, p = 0.558, as shown in Table 5. The regression analysis for Model 2 also found that subjective norm was not a statistically significant predictor of intention, β = 0.064, t = 0.854, p = 0.395, as shown in Table 5. This means subjective norm was not a significant predictor of intention (p < 0.05) for both models.

4.5.3. Influence of Perceived Behavioral Control on Intention

The third study objective was to assess the influence of South Asian consumers' perceived behavioral control in seeking MTM services on their intention to seek MTMS. The regression analysis for Model 1 found that perceived behavioral control was a statistically significant predictor of intention, β = 0.169, t = 2.738, p < 0.05, as shown in Table 5. The regression analysis for Model 2 found that perceived behavioral control was a statistically significant predictor of intention, β = 0.148, t = 2.224, p < 0.05, as shown in Table 5. This means perceived behavioral control was a significant predictor of intention (p < 0.05) for both models.

4.5.4. Influence of Socio-Demographic Characteristics on Intention

The fourth specific study objective was to assess the influence of South Asian consumers' socio-demographic characteristics on their intention to seek MTMS. Prediction by none of these socio-demographic variables was found to be significant at a level of significance of 0.05, as shown in Table 5.

5. Discussion

To the researcher's knowledge, this is the first consumer/patient focused study regarding MTMS that used TPB. However, the results found in this study may be influenced by the demographics of study participants. The study group was quite skewed toward younger people, with only 6.8% of participants having an age of 65 years or more, whereas 16% of the total US population are 65 years or older [49]. A total of 51 out of 133 respondents (38.3%) reported no prescription medications taken daily and these respondents may not perceive a need for MTM at all. While 53% of the total South Asian population in the US are male [28], 71.4% of study participants in this study were male. This gender skewing (95 males to 38 females) could also have influenced responses. The educational data showed 51.1% with bachelor or higher degrees while this percentage for South Asians in the entire US is 59% [28]. These data indicate that findings from this study may not be generalizable to the entire US population. Due to skewness in demographics of study participants, results may slightly vary from opinions of the total South Asian population in the US.

The purpose of this study was to use the theory of planned behavior (TPB) to understand factors influencing intention of South Asian consumers to seek pharmacist-provided medication therapy management (MTM) services. The study results found that the overall attitude, subjective norm, perceived behavioral control, and intention of South Asian consumers to seek MTMS was positive. This is consistent with findings from previous studies regarding MTMS where patients had a positive attitude towards receiving MTMS, were willing to take MTMS, and recognized pharmacists as potential providers of MTMS [18]. The majority of respondents had positive intention to seek each component of MTMS, as shown in Table 3. However, respondents had the least agreement with the statement that they would be willing to take MTM services where pharmacists will recommend physicians for safer or more effective medication. This finding is consistent with findings from the study by Brown et al. [20] where consumers were not favoring services that involve contacting their physicians for recommending safer or more effective medications.

The study findings indicate that South Asian consumers' intention to seek MTMS was driven by attitude and perceived behavioral control. This finding is consistent with previous research regarding applications of TPB in health-related behaviors [32–34,50,51]. However, considering the influence of subjective norm, this finding is slightly different from TPB research assessing intention to receive pharmacy services [35]. Details on the influence of attitude, subjective norm, perceived behavioral control, and socio-demographic characteristics on intention have been described below:

5.1. Influence of Attitude on Intention

South Asian consumers' attitude towards seeking MTM services was found to be a significant and strongest predictor of their intention to seek MTM services. This finding is consistent with previous TPB research assessing pharmacists' intent to provide MTMS [31], community pharmacists' intention to utilize a prescription drug monitoring program [32], pharmacists' intention to report serious ADEs to the FDA [33], patients' intention to participate in physical exercise [52], and medical students' intention to improve oral hygiene [34].

More than 80% of respondents had a positive attitude toward seeking each component of MTMS, as shown in Table 3. This finding is consistent with previous findings from the study by Schultz et al., aimed at determining patient-perceived value of MTMS. Schultz et al. found that MTMS was considered to be valuable, satisfactory, and financially beneficial to patients [19]. In this current study, respondents were the most positive with services involving the pharmacist's educating self-management of medications and were the least positive with services involving the pharmacist's guidance on managing drug-related problems (DRPs). Similar results were also evident in past research [16]. Like this current study, in a study by Doucette et al., services involving explaining how to use medications had the highest mean score [23].

To strengthen South Asian consumers' intention to seek MTM services, pharmacists should focus on creating and maintaining positive attitude toward MTM services. Previous research found that participants had a positive attitude toward pharmacists in terms of pharmacists' knowledge and problem solving capability [22] and pharmacists were believed to be good candidates to provide MTM services [15]. Patients receiving MTM services also identified their MTM pharmacist as a supporter, advocate, confidant, resource for education, and coordinator of medications [19]. However, perception of pharmacists revolved around the medication dispensing function [15] and patients were skeptical about pharmacists' interaction with patients [22]. This perception may have a negative influence on attitudes towards seeking pharmacist-provided services. It is a matter of further investigation of which factors influence South Asian consumers' attitude toward seeking pharmacist-provided services. To create a positive attitude toward seeking pharmacist-provided MTMS, pharmacists have to create a perception of providing personalized information about medications and advising South Asian patients on medications through interaction with South Asian patients beyond traditional dispensing. During this current study, it has been found that pharmacy technicians have the opportunity to interact with patients. Along with pharmacists, pharmacy technicians may also contribute to creating a positive attitude towards pharmacy and pharmacy services though positive interactions with South Asian patients. A previous study found that the perceived importance of pharmacist-provided comprehensive medication reviews was more in patients experiencing comprehensive medication reviews than in patients not experiencing comprehensive medication reviews from pharmacists [23]. In order to increase perceived importance of MTMS, pharmacists can provide MTMS for free or a reduced/discounted price for a short time (like a trial version) to have South Asian patients experience the flavor of MTMS and then for an extended period (like a full version) once South Asian patients have experienced MTMS.

5.2. Influence of Subjective Norm on Intention

Subjective norm was not a statistically significant predictor of intention. This finding differs with findings from previous applications of TPB where subjective norm was a significant predictor of pharmacists' intent to provide MTMS [31], intention to utilize a prescription drug monitoring program [32], and intention to report serious ADEs to the FDA [33]. This may due to the fact that pharmacists felt the competitiveness to provide MTMS seeing other pharmacists providing MTMS.

On the other hand, consumers might intend to seek MTMS when they experience certain health conditions or medications.

However, this finding also differs with the result from a consumer-focused study done by Tan et al. using TPB. Malaysian consumers' subjective norm was found to be a significant predictor of intention to adopt Pharmacy Value Added Services (PVAS) introduced by Malaysia's Ministry of Health [35]. As described by Fishbein, the degree of influence of attitude, subjective norm, and perceived behavioral control on intention may vary depending on behavior and the population being considered [53]. The difference in population (South Asians in the US vs. Malaysians in Malaysia) and behavior (seeking MTMS vs. adopting PVAS) may explain different degrees of influence of subjective norm on intention.

Considering South Asian consumers typically get their health care related information primarily from family members and physicians, this finding was particularly interesting [27]. This finding also conflicts with previous research where influence of family members was found an important factor for South Asian patients' health behavior, such as medication adherence among South Asian patients with cardiac diseases [54]. Further studies would be needed to explore why subjective norm did not significantly predict intention of South Asian consumers to seek MTMS.

5.3. Influence of Perceived Behavioral Control on Intention

In this study, perceived behavioral control was found to be a statistically significant predictor of intention. This finding is consistent with the results from previous research on pharmacists and consumers where perceived behavioral control was found to be a significant predictor of pharmacists' intent to provide MTMS [31], pharmacists' intention to utilize a prescription drug monitoring program [32], as well as consumers' intention to adopt Pharmacy Value Added Services (PVAS) [35].

In order to increase South Asian consumers' intention to seek MTMS, focus should be given to minimizing their perceived barriers in seeking MTMS. In this study's findings, most respondents were confident that they can take pharmacist-provided services. However, a total of 37% of respondents did not feel (18% disagreed and 19% were neutral) that they had enough time for taking pharmacist-provided services, as shown in Table 3. This finding is also consistent with findings from previous studies on patient-reported barriers to receive MTMS [19,22]. This indicates that matching the patient's convenient time with the MTM pharmacist's available time would be an important consideration in facilitating the patient's taking of MTM services. Although inability to fix times with MTM pharmacists due to patients' busy schedules is a common problem found in previous studies; Moczygemba et al. found that patients were satisfied with pharmacist-provided telephone-based MTM care [21]. In telephone-based MTM care, patients viewed pharmacists as easily accessible and responsive to patients' problems [21]. In order to match the timing between pharmacists and South Asian patients, pharmacists can consider providing telephone-based MTM care as an alternative option for South Asian patients.

In the previous literature, patient-reported barriers to receive MTMS were patients' lack of knowledge of MTMS; lack of perceived need for MTMS; out-of-pocket cost; lack of availability of the MTM pharmacist at patients' convenient time; inability to fix appointments due to patients' busy schedule; inaccessibility to pharmacist MTM practice due to the location, parking, time of day/week; and fear of obtaining recommendations conflicting with their physician's plan of care [13,19,22]. Pharmacists can check if these barriers are also South Asian consumers' barriers to receive MTMS. Pharmacists should keep any such barriers as low as possible so that patients are willing to seek MTMS. Pharmacists should also observe and resolve any cultural barriers (such as language barriers) specifically faced by South Asian consumers in order to strengthen South Asian patients' intention to seek MTMS.

5.4. Influence of Socio-Demographic Characteristics on Intention

In this study, none of the socio-demographic characteristics was found to be statistically significant predictors of intention.

Age was expected to be an important factor influencing intention to seek MTMS. Since elderly people are more prone to have chronic diseases and use multiple medications, they are supposed to need help in managing their medications. Moreover, previous research found a correlation of age with willingness to pay for MTMS [18]. Unexpectedly, age was not a significant predictor of intention to seek MTMS in the South Asian group.

In previous studies, the willingness to accept pharmacist-provided MTMS differed in terms of gender [20]. In the current study, intention to seek MTMS differed in terms of gender. Although the survey was anonymous, a number of females, because of their conservative cultural background, did not respond to the survey during the study. A common response from female consumers for their non-participation in the survey was "I cannot fill up any survey without my husband's permission". This non-response has resulted in a decreased proportion of female participants compared to male participants. However, gender was not found to be a significant predictor of intention to seek MTMS.

In previous studies, the willingness to accept pharmacist-provided MTMS differed in terms of education level and income [20]. In the current study, intention to seek MTMS also differed in terms of education and income. Nonetheless, none of the variables were found to be significant predictors of intention to seek MTMS in this particular group. Although married consumers had a mean intention score less than unmarried ones, marital status was not found to be a significant predictor of intention to seek MTMS.

Duration of residency in the US was included as a socio-demographic predictor variable as consumers may get acquainted with the US health care system and be more aware of health services with the increasing duration of residency in the US. Country of origin was included as socio-demographic variable as culture in different countries can influence health behavior. Neither duration of residency in the US nor country of origin was found to be a significant predictor of intention to seek MTMS.

In past research, consumers' work experience in the healthcare profession was found associated with their willingness to accept MTM services [20]. It was expected that South Asian consumers' work experience in the healthcare profession would influence their intention to seek MTMS. Unexpectedly, experience in the healthcare profession had no influence on South Asian consumers' intention to seek MTMS.

The noteworthy unexpected finding was that number of medications had no statistically significant impact on intention to seek MTMS. It was expected that the more medications one takes, the more would be the need for managing medications and thus, intention to seek MTMS. It is possible that patients are taking medications on an on-demand basis and not on a regular basis, or they are already familiar with medications. That is why they probably did not feel the need for MTMS and had no intention to seek such services. More than one-third (38.3%) of the respondents were taking no prescription drugs. It may be due to the fact that many non-patient consumers visited pharmacies to get medications for their family members.

6. Limitations and Future Research

Like any other research, this study has some limitations, too. Firstly, most of the respondents (76.7%) were of Bangladeshi origin. Demographically, the selected sample as a whole may not represent South Asian consumers in the US. Although the South Asian community is diverse in languages and religious practices, there are many shared social and cultural characteristics among South Asians [28]. Thus, although most of the respondents were of Bangladeshi origin, they still represent South Asians holding those social and cultural characteristics. Secondly, the target sample size could not be reached due to the limited duration of the study period and non-response from South Asian consumers, particularly from females. However, a sample size of 133 used in this study is sufficient for factor analysis for both Model 1 and Model 2 [40,41] and also adequate for multiple linear regression analysis for Model 1 [42]. Only for multiple linear regression analysis in Model 2, a sample size of 133 is less than the recommended sample size of 154 [42]. Thirdly, this study did not consider the actual behavior of consumers, an important construct of TPB, which may vary from intention measured in the study.

Fourthly, this study assessed degree of influence of attitude, subjective norm, and perceived behavioral control on intention but did not find out the reasons for such influence. A qualitative study would complement quantitative research in finding out specific reasons for such influence. Finally, although previous research found that disease state, number of health problems, familiarity with medications, and insurance status had correlations with either willing to receive MTMS or willingness to pay for MTMS, these variables were not included in this study. Future research can include these variables.

Future research opportunities include conducting qualitative research to find out the reasons behind the influence of factors such as attitude, subjective norm, and perceived behavioral control on intention to seek pharmacist-provided MTMS. Previous research showed that not all respondents willing to receive MTMS are willing to pay for MTMS [18] and most of the respondents think that insurance companies should cover cognitive pharmacy services [55]. South Asian consumers' willingness to pay for MTMS can also be studied to assess how payment influences their intention and actual performance of behavior, that is, receiving pharmacist-provided MTM services.

7. Conclusions

Overall, South Asian consumers showed a positive attitude, favorable subjective norm, favorable perceived behavioral control, and positive intention to seek MTM services. The TPB was revealed to be a good model to measure and predict South Asian consumers' intention to seek MTM services. Multiple linear regression analysis showed that attitude and perceived behavioral control were significant predictors of intention ($p < 0.05$), but subjective norm was not a significant predictor of intention. Socio-demographic characteristics did not have a significant effect on intention.

Strategies to make South Asian consumers seek MTM services should focus on enhancing and maintaining positive attitudes by showing expertise in medicines through interactions with South Asian patients, identifying and promoting factors (e.g., pharmacists' knowledge) responsible for positive attitudes among South Asian patients, promoting perceived facilitators (e.g., easy access) in seeking MTMS, and resolving possible barriers (e.g., timing, language) perceived by South Asian patients in seeking MTMS.

Author Contributions: Conceptualization, J.M.M. and S.A.H.; formal analysis, S.A.H.; investigation, S.A.H.; methodology, S.A.H., J.M.M. and R.N.; software, S.A.H. and J.M.M.; supervision, J.M.M.; validation, J.M.M., R.N. and W.K.W.; writing—original draft preparation, S.A.H.; writing—review and editing, S.A.H., J.M.M., R.N. and W.K.W.

Funding: This research received no external funding.

Acknowledgments: The authors would like to thank and acknowledge Jon C. Schommer, MS, PhD, R.Ph., for advising on participant recruitment and research methods; Somnath Pal, MBA, PhD, for advising on survey administration and statistical analyses. The authors would like to thank and acknowledge all of the participants who participated in the study and pharmacies where study was conducted.

Conflicts of Interest: The authors declare no conflict of interest.

References

1. Ernst, F.R.; Grizzle, A.J. Drug-related morbidity and mortality: updating the cost-of-illness model. *J. Am. Pharm. Assoc.* **2001**, *41*, 192–199. [CrossRef]
2. Johnson, J.A.; Bootman, J.L. Drug-related morbidity and mortality. A cost-of-illness model. *Arch. Intern. Med.* **1995**, *155*, 1949–1956. [CrossRef] [PubMed]
3. Viktil, K.K.; Blix, H.S. The impact of clinical pharmacists on drug-related problems and clinical outcomes. *Basic Clin. Pharmacol. Toxicol.* **2008**, *102*, 275–280. [CrossRef] [PubMed]
4. Ramanath, K.; Nedumballi, S. Assessment of Medication-Related Problems in Geriatric Patients of a Rural Tertiary Care Hospital. *J. Young Pharm. JYP* **2012**, *4*, 273–278. [CrossRef] [PubMed]
5. Pellegrino, A.N.; Martin, M.T.; Tilton, J.J.; Touchette, D.R. Medication therapy management services: definitions and outcomes. *Drugs* **2009**, *69*, 393–406. [CrossRef] [PubMed]

6. Stuart, B.; Loh, F.E.; Roberto, P.; Miller, L.M. Increasing Medicare part D enrollment in medication therapy management could improve health and lower costs. *Health Aff. Proj. Hope* **2013**, *32*, 1212–1220. [CrossRef] [PubMed]

7. American Pharmacists Association. National Association of Chain Drug Stores Foundation Medication therapy management in pharmacy practice: Core elements of an MTM service model (version 2.0). *J. Am. Pharm. Assoc. JAPhA* **2008**, *48*, 341–353. [CrossRef]

8. Avalere Health LLC. *Exploring Pharmacists' Role in a Changing Healthcare Environment*; Avalere Health LLC: Washington, DC, USA, 2014; pp. 1–30.

9. McGivney, M.S.; Meyer, S.M.; Duncan–Hewitt, W.; Hall, D.L.; Goode, J.-V.R.; Smith, R.B. Medication therapy management: Its relationship to patient counseling, disease management, and pharmaceutical care. *J. Am. Pharm. Assoc.* **2007**, *47*, 620–628. [CrossRef]

10. McCarthy, R.L.; Schafermeyer, K.W.; Plake, K.S. The Pharmacist and the Pharmacy Profession. In *Introduction to Health Care Delivery*; Jones & Bartlett Publishers: Burlington, MA, USA, 2012; pp. 81–110. ISBN 978-1-4496-7557-8.

11. Chisholm-Burns, M.A.; Kim Lee, J.; Spivey, C.A.; Slack, M.; Herrier, R.N.; Hall-Lipsy, E.; Graff Zivin, J.; Abraham, I.; Palmer, J.; Martin, J.R.; et al. US pharmacists' effect as team members on patient care: systematic review and meta-analyses. *Med. Care* **2010**, *48*, 923–933. [CrossRef]

12. Ramalho de Oliveira, D.; Brummel, A.R.; Miller, D.B. Medication therapy management: 10 years of experience in a large integrated health care system. *J. Manag. Care Pharm. JMCP* **2010**, *16*, 185–195. [CrossRef] [PubMed]

13. Oladapo, A.O.; Rascati, K.L. Review of survey articles regarding medication therapy management (MTM) services/programs in the United States. *J. Pharm. Pract.* **2012**, *25*, 457–470. [CrossRef] [PubMed]

14. Westberg, S.M.; Reidt, S.L.; Sorensen, T.D. Chapter 4. Medication Therapy Management. In *Community and Clinical Pharmacy Services: A Step-by-Step Approach*; Ellis, A.W., Sherman, J.J., Eds.; The McGraw-Hill Companies: New York, NY, USA, 2013.

15. Law, A.V.; Qkamoto, M.P.; Brock, K. Perceptions of Medicare Part D enrollees about pharmacists and their role as providers of medication therapy management. *J. Am. Pharm. Assoc.* **2008**, *48*, 648–653. [CrossRef] [PubMed]

16. Doucette, W.R.; Witry, M.J.; Alkhateeb, F.; Farris, K.B.; Urmie, J.M. Attitudes of Medicare beneficiaries toward pharmacist-provided medication therapy management activities as part of the Medicare Part D benefit. *J. Am. Pharm. Assoc. JAPhA* **2007**, *47*, 758–762. [CrossRef] [PubMed]

17. Truong, H.-A.; Layson-Wolf, C.; de Bittner, M.R.; Owen, J.A.; Haupt, S. Perceptions of patients on Medicare Part D medication therapy management services. *J. Am. Pharm. Assoc.* **2009**, *49*, 392–398. [CrossRef] [PubMed]

18. Friedrich, M.; Zgarrick, D.; Masood, A.; Montuoro, J. Patients' needs and interests in a self-pay medication therapy management service. *J. Am. Pharm. Assoc.* **2010**, *50*, 72–77. [CrossRef] [PubMed]

19. Schultz, H.; Westberg, S.M.; de Oliveira, D.R.; Brummel, A. Patient-perceived value of Medication Therapy Management (MTM) services: A series of focus groups. *INNOVATIONS Pharm.* **2012**, *3*. [CrossRef]

20. Brown, L.M.; Rashrash, M.E.; Schommer, J.C. The certainty in consumers' willingness to accept pharmacist-provided medication therapy management services. *J. Am. Pharm. Assoc. JAPhA* **2017**, *57*, 211–216. [CrossRef]

21. Moczygemba, L.R.; Barner, J.C.; Brown, C.M.; Lawson, K.A.; Gabrillo, E.R.; Godley, P.; Johnsrud, M. Patient satisfaction with a pharmacist-provided telephone medication therapy management program. *Res. Soc. Adm. Pharm. RSAP* **2010**, *6*, 143–154. [CrossRef]

22. Garcia, G.M.; Snyder, M.E.; McGrath, S.H.; Smith, R.B.; McGivney, M.S. Generating demand for pharmacist-provided medication therapy management: Identifying patient-preferred marketing strategies. *J. Am. Pharm. Assoc.* **2009**, *49*, 611–616. [CrossRef]

23. Doucette, W.R.; Zhang, Y.; Chrischilles, E.A.; Pendergast, J.F.; Newland, B.A.; Farris, K.B.; Frank, J. Factors affecting Medicare Part D beneficiaries' decision to receive comprehensive medication reviews. *J. Am. Pharm. Assoc. JAPhA* **2013**, *53*, 482–487. [CrossRef] [PubMed]

24. Huet, A.L.; Frail, C.K.; Lake, L.M.; Snyder, M.E. Impact of passive and active promotional strategies on patient acceptance of medication therapy management services. *J. Am. Pharm. Assoc.* **2015**, *55*, 178–181. [CrossRef] [PubMed]

25. Nau, D.P.; Pacholski, A.M. Impact of pharmacy care services on patients' perceptions of health care quality for diabetes. *J. Am. Pharm. Assoc.* **2007**, *47*, 358–365. [CrossRef] [PubMed]

26. Garcia-Cardenas, V.; Perez-Escamilla, B.; Fernandez-Llimos, F.; Benrimoj, S.I. The complexity of implementation factors in professional pharmacy services. *Res. Soc. Adm. Pharm.* **2017**, *14*, 498–500. [CrossRef] [PubMed]

27. Bangladeshi CHRNA (Community Health Resources and Needs Assessment). Available online: https://med.nyu.edu/asian-health/sites/default/files/asian-health2/Bangladeshi%20Community%20Report_FINAL.pdf (accessed on 13 June 2017).

28. Cao, A.; Ahmed, T.; Islam, N. *Community Health Needs & Resource Assessment: An Exploratory Study of South Asians in NYC*; Community Health Needs & Resource Assessment; NYU Center for the Study of Asian American Health: New York, NY, USA, 2007; pp. 1–34.

29. Glanz, K.; Rimer, B.K.; Viswanath, K. Theory, Research, and Practice in Health Behavior and Health education. In *Health Behavior and Health Education: Theory, Research, and Practice*; John Wiley & Sons: San Fransisco, CA, USA, 2008; pp. 23–40. ISBN 978-0-470-43248-8.

30. Glanz, K.; Rimer, B.K.; Viswanath, K. Theory of Reasoned Action, Theory of Planned Behavior, and the Integrated Behavior Model. In *Health Behavior and Health Education: Theory, Research, and Practice*; John Wiley & Sons: San Fransisco, CA, USA, 2008; pp. 67–96. ISBN 978-0-470-43248-8.

31. Herbert, K.E.; Urmie, J.M.; Newland, B.A.; Farris, K.B. Prediction of pharmacist intention to provide Medicare medication therapy management services using the theory of planned behavior. *Res. Soc. Adm. Pharm. RSAP* **2006**, *2*, 299–314. [CrossRef]

32. Gavaza, P.; Fleming, M.; Barner, J.C. Examination of psychosocial predictors of Virginia pharmacists' intention to utilize a prescription drug monitoring program using the theory of planned behavior. *Res. Soc. Adm. Pharm.* **2014**, *10*, 448–458. [CrossRef]

33. Gavaza, P.; Brown, C.M.; Lawson, K.A.; Rascati, K.L.; Wilson, J.P.; Steinhardt, M. Examination of pharmacists' intention to report serious adverse drug events (ADEs) to the FDA using the theory of planned behavior. *Res. Soc. Adm. Pharm.* **2011**, *7*, 369–382. [CrossRef]

34. Dumitrescu, A.L.; Wagle, M.; Dogaru, B.C.; Manolescu, B. Modeling the theory of planned behavior for intention to improve oral health behaviors: the impact of attitudes, knowledge, and current behavior. *J. Oral Sci.* **2011**, *53*, 369–377. [CrossRef]

35. Tan, C.L.; Gan, V.B.; Saleem, F.; Hassali, M.A. Building intentions with the Theory of Planned Behaviour: the mediating role of knowledge and expectations in implementing new pharmaceutical services in Malaysia. *Pharm. Pract.* **2016**, *14*, 850. [CrossRef]

36. Peters, R.M.; Aroian, K.J.; Flack, J.M. African American Culture and Hypertension Prevention. *West. J. Nurs. Res.* **2006**, *28*, 831–863. [CrossRef]

37. Congress, E.P.; Lyons, B.P. Cultural Differences in Health Beliefs. *Soc. Work Health Care* **1992**, *17*, 81–96. [CrossRef] [PubMed]

38. Jacobs, W.; Amuta, A.O.; Jeon, K.C. Health information seeking in the digital age: An analysis of health information seeking behavior among US adults. *Cogent Soc. Sci.* **2017**, *3*, 1302785. [CrossRef]

39. Walker, A. New York leads America's Major Cities in Diversity and Income Disparity. Available online: https://ny.curbed.com/2017/5/8/15584428/new-york-city-diversity-income-disparity (accessed on 14 July 2018).

40. Mundfrom, D.J.; Shaw, D.G.; Ke, T.L. Minimum Sample Size Recommendations for Conducting Factor Analyses. *Int. J. Test.* **2005**, *5*, 159–168. [CrossRef]

41. Comrey, A.L.; Lee, H.B. *A First Course in Factor Analysis*, 2nd ed.; Lawrence Erlbaum Associates, Inc.: Hillsdale, NJ, USA, 1992.

42. Green, S.B. How Many Subjects Does It Take To Do A Regression Analysis. *Multivar. Behav. Res.* **1991**, *26*, 499–510. [CrossRef] [PubMed]

43. Ajzen, I. *Constructing a TpB Questionnaire: Conceptual and Methodological Considerations*; Semantic Scholar- The Allen Institute for Artificial Intelligence: Seattle, WA, USA, 2006; pp. 1–14.

44. Viechtbauer, W.; Smits, L.; Kotz, D.; Budé, L.; Spigt, M.; Serroyen, J.; Crutzen, R. A simple formula for the calculation of sample size in pilot studies. *J. Clin. Epidemiol.* **2015**, *68*, 1375–1379. [CrossRef] [PubMed]

45. Siddiqui, O.I. Methods for Computing Missing Item Response in Psychometric Scale Construction. *Am. J. Biostat.* **2015**, *5*, 1–6. [CrossRef]

46. Nunnally, J.C. *Psychometric Theory*, 2nd ed.; McGraw-Hill: New York, NY, USA, 1978; ISBN 978-1-4625-2477-8.

47. Trochim, W.M.; Donnelly, J.P.; Arora, K. Inferential Analysis. In *Research Methods The Essential Knowledge Base*; Cengage Learning: Boston, MA, USA, 2014; pp. 305–326. ISBN 978-1-133-95477-4.

48. O'Rourke, N.; Hatcher, L. Principal Component Analysis. In *A Step-by-Step Approach to Using SAS for Factor Analysis and Structural Equation Modeling*, 2nd ed.; SAS Institute: Cary, NC, USA, 2013; pp. 1–41. ISBN 978-1-62959-244-2.

49. U.S. Census Bureau QuickFacts: United States. Available online: https://www.census.gov/quickfacts/fact/table/US/PST045218 (accessed on 28 April 2019).

50. Godin, G.; Kok, G. The theory of planned behavior: a review of its applications to health-related behaviors. *Am. J. Health Promot. AJHP* **1996**, *11*, 87–98. [CrossRef]

51. Fleming, M.L.; Barner, J.C.; Brown, C.M.; Shepherd, M.D.; Strassels, S.; Novak, S. Using the theory of planned behavior to examine pharmacists' intention to utilize a prescription drug monitoring program database. *Res. Soc. Adm. Pharm.* **2014**, *10*, 285–296. [CrossRef]

52. Rhodes, R.E.; Courneya, K.S. Investigating multiple components of attitude, subjective norm, and perceived control: an examination of the theory of planned behaviour in the exercise domain. *Br. J. Soc. Psychol.* **2003**, *42*, 129–146. [CrossRef]

53. Fishbein, M. A Reasoned Action Approach to Health Promotion. *Med. Decis. Mak. Int. J. Soc. Med. Decis. Mak.* **2008**, *28*, 834–844. [CrossRef]

54. Ens, T.A.; Seneviratne, C.C.; Jones, C.; King-Shier, K.M. Factors influencing medication adherence in South Asian people with cardiac disorders: An ethnographic study. *Int. J. Nurs. Stud.* **2014**, *51*, 1472–1481. [CrossRef] [PubMed]

55. Daftary, M.N.; Lee, E.; Dutta, A.P.; Olagundoye, A.; Xue, Z. (Eric) Patients' Willingness to Pay for Cognitive Pharmacy Services in Ambulatory Care Settings in the USA. *J. Pharm. Pract. Res.* **2003**, *33*, 265–267. [CrossRef]

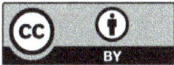

pharmacy

MDPI

Article

Development, Testing and Results of a Patient Medication Experience Documentation Tool for Use in Comprehensive Medication Management Services

Stephanie Redmond [1], Nicole Paterson [2], Sarah J. Shoemaker-Hunt [3] and Djenane Ramalho-de-Oliveira [4,*

[1] Ridgeview Medical Center, Waconia, MN 55387, USA; Stephanie.Redmond@ridgeviewmedical.org
[2] Fairview Pharmacy Services, Medication Therapy Management Services, Minneapolis, MN 55414, USA; npaterson@fairview.org
[3] Abt Associates, Cambridge, MA 02138-1168, USA; Sarah_Shoemaker@abtassoc.com
[4] Center for Pharmaceutical Studies, College of Pharmacy, Universidade Federal de Minas Gerais, Belo Horizonte 31.270-901, Brazil
* Correspondence: droliveira@ufmg.br; Tel.: +55-31-98329-0528

Received: 1 May 2019; Accepted: 15 June 2019; Published: 20 June 2019

check for
updates

Abstract: The medication experience is an individual's subjective experience of taking a medication in daily life and can be at the root of drug therapy problems. It is recommended that the patient-centered approach to comprehensive medication management (CMM) starts with an understanding of the patient's medication experience. This study aims to develop a medication experience documentation tool for use in CMM services, and to understand the usefulness and challenges of using the tool in practice. The tool was developed based on previous research on patients' medication experiences. It was tested in two rounds by ten CMM pharmacists utilizing the tool as they provided care to patients. Focus groups were conducted to revise the tool after each round and to understand pharmacists' experiences. The tool was tested for 15 weeks in 407 patient encounters. There was at least one medication experience documented in the electronic medical record 62% of the time. Pharmacists found the tool helpful in raising awareness of the medication experience and motivational interviewing strategies, planning for follow-up visits, as a teaching tool, and making pharmacists realize the fluidity of the medication experience. The tool offered pharmacists a better way to recognize and address medication experiences affecting medication taking behaviors.

Keywords: comprehensive medication management services; medication experience; pharmaceutical care practice; documentation; focus groups

---

1. Introduction

The profession of pharmacy continues to shift from the traditional dispensing role to a more patient-focused practice revolving around the provision of Comprehensive Medication Management (CMM) services. Several studies have shown the value of CMM in the care of patients with chronic conditions through the resolution of drug therapy problems [1–4]. It should be noted that there are different approaches to medication management services emerging in practice: the prescription-focused and the patient-centered approach. The first one is related to activities performed at the time of dispensing a drug to a patient. The patient-centered approach delivers the service on an appointment basis applying specific standards of care to each patient encounter [4].

In providing a patient-focused service, CMM pharmacists have been challenged with using evidence-based medication guidelines, while understanding the patient's unique medication experience to improve patient outcomes [5–7]. The medication experience is an individual's subjective experience of taking a medication in daily life and includes the patient's preferences, feelings, concerns, beliefs, and behaviors associated with medications [5]. Patients often have perceptions and beliefs about medications based on their own experiences or the experiences of others, which may influence or even prevent them from taking medications as recommended [5]. Patients might adjust doses to minimize unwanted effects and make the regimen more acceptable, or they can weigh risks against benefits, as a response to perceptions that go from gratitude that medicines exist to fear and uncertainty about adverse effects, or they can consider two or more medications being used for the same condition as unnecessary, or they might even completely deny their illness [8]. Other concerns that patients may have include fear of the actual administration of medicine or drug dependence. These concerns are often due to insufficient knowledge of the medication [8]. In this context, understanding the meanings that medications have for patients may help pharmacists to positively impact their medication-taking behavior [5].

Previous research has shown that pharmacists have used the patient's medication experience to guide the education provided to patients starting new medications to prevent the development of drug therapy problems (DTP), as well as to tailor their interventions to resolve drug therapy problems [6]. Ultimately, research findings indicate that there are many examples of drug therapy problems for which the medication experience is at the root cause [7].

In order to improve these experiences or change patients' perceptions of their medications, different strategies can be utilized in practice. Some studies show that strategies to overcome a negative medication experience are focused around influencing a perception, an attitude or a behavior change [8–10]. This is not always as simple as resolving a DTP, where a dose can be adjusted or a new medication started, if another one was not effective. Motivational Interviewing (MI) has been found to be an effective intervention to promote behavioral changes. It is a form of collaborative conversation between provider and patient directed towards strengthening a patient's own motivation and commitment to change. MI strategies are particularly useful for those who are reluctant or ambivalent about changing a behavior [11–13]. Also, some research has indicated that CMM pharmacists have successfully used MI strategies to affect patients' medication experiences [6,7].

It is recommended that the patient-centered approach to comprehensive medication management starts with an understanding of the patient's medication experience [4,14]. However, documenting the patient's medication experience and intentionally using this knowledge to make decisions about strategies to resolve DTPs and meet patients' medication-related needs is still not a common habit in practice.

The purpose of this research was to develop a medication experience documentation tool for use in CMM services, test the tool in practice with experienced CMM pharmacists, and understand the usefulness and challenges of having pharmacists use the tool in practice.

2. Materials and Methods

The tool was iteratively developed and refined based on two rounds of testing in practice and focus groups with CMM pharmacists. The methods are described by tool development, testing, and focus groups, as seen in Figure 1.

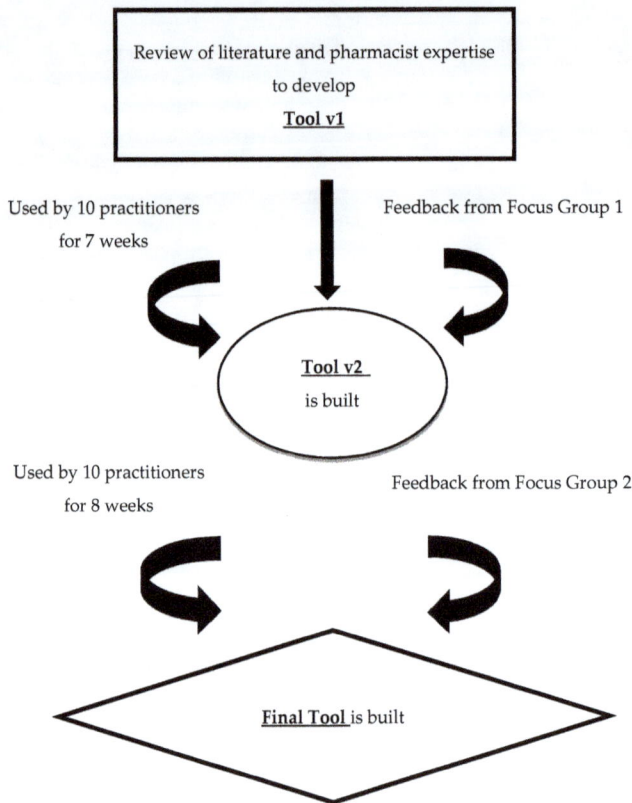

Figure 1. Approach to Developing and Testing the Medication Experience Documentation Tool.

2.1. Tool Development

The aim of the medication experience documentation tool was to facilitate the documentation of a patient's medication experiences perceived to be at the root of drug therapy problems (DTPs) by CMM pharmacists, as they conducted an assessment of a patient's medication-related needs. The tool also allows pharmacists to indicate the motivational interviewing strategies used to address the identified medication experience and associated DTPs.

The initial version of the medication experience assessment tool (Tool v1) was developed based on previously published research on patients' medication experiences and pharmacists' perspectives encountering patients' medication experiences in their practice [3–7,14] and motivational interviewing strategies [11–13]. The tool was built in the electronic medical record (EMR), where CMM pharmacists routinely document the care they provide. The tool included two drop-down lists from which to select: (1) the patient's medication experience and (2) the motivational interviewing strategies used to address that specific medication experience. There was also a write-in option for any experience or strategy not reflected in the list and a 'none' option if no experience was identified at that specific visit. The tool was located at the end of the assessment section of the EMR documentation. The pharmacists were instructed to use the tool during every patient encounter, though only medication experiences that negatively impacted a patient's medication-taking behavior were deemed to require an intervention and thus be documented with the tool. Multiple medication experiences could be identified during a single visit, thus the drop-down boxes allowed for multiple options to be selected. However, the pharmacist would document only the experiences he or she attempted to affect during that specific encounter.

2.2. Tool Testing

2.2.1. Setting

The tool was tested with pharmacists in a large health care system consisting of 7 hospitals and 38 ambulatory clinics. CMM services have been provided in this health system for over 15 years. Participating pharmacists had a range of experience practicing CMM spanning from 4 months to 15 years and were all practicing in ambulatory primary care clinics. CMM pharmacists document their progress notes in the electronic medical record in the form of a SOAP note (subjective/objective/assessment/plan). All of the CMM pharmacists participating in this study had previously undergone training on how to use the medication experience tool and on motivational interviewing. In practice, the pharmacists identified medication experiences through the pharmaceutical care assessment process by asking open-ended questions and listening for conversation clues. Then, motivational interviewing techniques were used to affect those experiences that were perceived by the pharmacist as negatively impacting the patient's medication taking behavior. They were instructed to use the documentation tool during the time that they conducted the assessment of each patient.

2.2.2. Testing Period

All 20 CMM pharmacists practicing in the health care system were invited to contribute to this research and 10 agreed to participate. The participating ten pharmacists utilized the first version of the tool (Tool v1) for seven weeks as part of their practice providing comprehensive patient-centered medication management (CMM) services to patients in the primary care setting. The same 10 pharmacists used the second version of the tool (Tool v2) for eight (8) weeks.

2.2.3. Tool Results

The EMR of all patients cared for by the 10 participating pharmacists during the studied period were analyzed to identify the type and the number of experiences documented as well as the strategies utilized to address those experiences in all patient encounters. All data were documented in an excel spreadsheet and the frequencies of the identified medication experiences and the utilized strategies were calculated.

2.3. Focus Groups with Pharmacists

Two focus groups were conducted with all participating ten pharmacists using the techniques proposed by Krueger and Casey [15]. The aims of the focus groups were to understand pharmacists' experiences using the documentation tool in practice, in terms of usefulness and challenges.

A focus group was conducted after each testing period with Tool v1 and Tool v2. The information revealed in the focus groups informed revisions to the tool. The focus groups were two hours in length. A focus group discussion guide did not used any specific framework, but it was developed with the purpose of stimulating discussion to elucidate pharmacists' experiences, reactions, and expectations related to the medication experience and motivational interviewing strategies in the tool. See Table 1 for a list of questions used in the focus groups.

Table 1. Focus Group Discussion Questions.

Focus Group 1	Focus Group 2
• What was it like for you to document your patients' medication experiences?	
○ Has it been helpful to you to document these experiences, how and why?	
• What medication experiences or strategies should stay, should not be there, what are missing?	
• How do you see this being useful tool for other practitioners, new practitioners, students?	
• Has documenting the medication experience been useful for follow-up visits?	
• What do you think of the tool? What was it like to use the tool?	• Is the revised tool easier to use? What would make it easier and/or more helpful?
• Can the tool be used in patients with no medication experiences?	• Is this tool important enough to incorporate as a requirement in our documentation notes?
	• Is the placement of the tool in the "assessment" section appropriate?
	• Does documenting and having a more in-depth awareness of patient's medication experience help with or change your therapy decisions?
	• Has this helped you in developing your motivational interviewing skills? How?
	• Are you noticing the medication experience can change over time?
	• In your experience with documenting these patients' experiences, how do they connect to drug therapy problems?

All focus groups were audio-recorded and then professionally transcribed verbatim. All researchers independently coded the data to identify significant sections about pharmacists' perspectives on the tool. Then, they met to form a consensus about the common themes of pharmacists' experiences and perspectives on utilizing the documentation tool. The final themes are described below.

Human Subjects Protection

Pharmacists were assured confidentiality that any information provided could not be traced to them or to individual patients. This study was approved by the Institutional Review Board at the University of Minnesota.

3. Results

3.1. Tool Development

After the completion of testing Tool v1 and the first focus group, several changes were incorporated into Tool v2, see Table 2. After the completion of testing Tool v2 and the second focus group, changes were also incorporated into the final tool, see Table 2. The final tool can be found in Appendix A.

Table 2. The Medication Experience Documentation Tool: Overview of Testing Rounds, Use and Changes.

	Round 1	Round 2
Tool Version	Tool v1	Tool v2
Testing Duration	7 weeks	8 weeks
Pharmacists	10 RPhs	10 RPhs (same as Round1)
Pharmacists'MTM experience	4 months–15 years	4 months–15 years
# of Patient encounters	620	649
# (%) Patient encounters pharmacists used Tool	180 (29%)	227 (35%)
Changes to the Tool		
Changes to the Medication Experiences	- Condensed and reordered the tool into subcategories for ease of use - One medication experience deleted: "positive medication experience, does not want to use alternative non-drug therapy or lifestyle changes" - Four medication experiences added: "does not want to use because they are too reliant on Rx medication (s)", "feelings of burden and being overwhelmed", "fear of side effects from personal history", and "fear about history of addiction" - One medication experienced revised: economic value question changed to "cannot reconcile value of medication over cost"	- Shortened verbiage in tool - Moved some subcategories back into major categories - Added and removed one medication experience each - Combined one medication experience
Changes to Strategies	- Removed empathy and listening	- Added referral to care team member

3.2. Tool Utilization and Results

A summary of the tool testing approach, utilization and results is provided in Table 2. In round 1, pharmacists utilized the tool 29% of the time in 180 of 620 patient encounters in the 7-week testing period. In round 2, pharmacists utilized the tool 35% of the time in 227 of 649 patient encounters in the 8-week testing period. The tool was used 32% of the time in a total of 407 patient encounters.

When the tool was used in 407 patient encounters, it was observed that patients had a documented medication experience 62% of the time. Specifically, in round 2, no medication experience was selected in 29%, 86 out of 292 total medication experiences. Table 3 shows round 2, the most common medication experiences identified and the most common strategies utilized by the pharmacists to address each medication experience; presented in decreasing order of frequency. Definitions used for the strategies can be found in the Appendix B.

Table 3. Most Common Medication Experiences Encountered and Motivational Interviewing (MI) Strategies Used for Round 2.

Most Common Medication Experiences (Med Exp)	Medication Experiences N (%)	MI Strategies Used (% for each Med Exp)					
		Raise Concern, Educate or Inform	Collaboration/SDM	Open-Ended Question	Support Autonomy	Roll With Resistance	Negotiate
Self-adjusts medication regimen (increases, decrease, or skips doses)	31 (15%)	87%	77%	77%	52%	19%	19%
Feelings of burden and being overwhelmed (e.g., pill burden)	27 (13%)	93%	78%	67%	56%	41%	37%
Fears/concerns about side effects: History of personal side effects.	23 (11%)	91%	87%	70%	35%	30%	26%
Fears/concerns about side effects: Current personal side effects.	17 (8%)	76%	82%	76%	65%	18%	35%
Prefers alternative non-drug therapy or lifestyle changes.	16 (8%)	81%	88%	88%	44%	6%	6%
Fear of not having medication(s)/(security).	10 (5%)	80%	90%	70%	60%	40%	20%
Does not want to take medications: Does not like to take them (cultural background, other).	10 (5%)	90%	80%	70%	50%	40%	20%
Other Experiences.	72 (35%)						
Total	206 (100%)						

Note: SDM: shared decision-making.

3.3. Pharmacist Focus Groups

The major themes that emerged from the focus groups are described below in terms of the usefulness and challenges of using the medication experience documentation tool. The findings reflect the experiences of the 10 CMM pharmacists that utilized the tool and participated in both focus groups.

3.3.1. Usefulness of the Tool

Participants expressed the usefulness of the tool as the following themes: the tool makes CMM pharmacists more aware of the medication experience and more reflexive; using the tool makes pharmacists realize the fluidity of the medication experience; the tool assists with teaching; and the tool helps with future care plans.

The Tool Makes CMM Pharmacists More Aware of the Medication Experience and More Reflexive

The group of 10 CMM pharmacists expressed feelings that the tool led them to document more details of the visit in relation to the medication experience and the reasoning behind a patient's medication taking behaviors. Some of them asserted that usually they use the tool as an afterthought. They also expressed that the documentation process changed their practices, as they felt more conscious of and more likely to address and explore a patient's medication experience to help patients to better understand the need for their medications and what to expect from them.

"The fact that I had to think about the experience and what strategies I would use, it changed my practice. I put it into an important piece of my every day work. . . . and then I started thinking I should really use this strategy the next time I talk to a patient about this type of thing" (Pharmacist 3).

Awareness was created and the pharmacists felt more able to truly identify what the patient wants out of the visit.

"I feel more aware and I am thinking about it more. Before it was more subconscious" (Pharmacist 1).

Using the tool and documenting the medication experience helped CMM pharmacists to become more reflexive. As the pharmacist in the last quote emphasized, it was felt that documenting the medication experience helped them to be more aware of patients' experiences and what they could do to improve those experiences.

Since the tool was embedded into note templates, during the CMM visit, pharmacists could see it on the computer screen. It was agreed that simply seeing the tool during the visit was a good reminder and created consciousness of MI strategies that could be used during the consultation to motivate the patient.

"When I see it [the tool] there in the visit, it causes me to think about it with the patient and make sure I get to the bottom of it" (Pharmacist 8).

Using the Tool Makes Pharmacists Realize the Fluidity of the Medication Experience

As participants documented the medication experience at each visit, it became more evident how fluid and dynamic these experiences can be.

"The same patient can have different experiences associated with different medications" (Pharmacist 4).

"The experience can change from one visit to the next. So, we really need to pay attention to the patients' expressions at each visit. We cannot predict what is happening today based on our last visit" (Pharmacist 1).

To understand the changeability of the medication experience was an important result of utilizing the tool. These experiences are subjective and impacted by different factors meaning that the pharmacist needs to carefully listen at each visit and use the appropriate strategies to address them when needed.

The Tool Assists with Teaching

Participants in the focus group agreed that one of the most useful aspects of the documentation tool was for teaching purposes—for both students and new CMM pharmacists. It helps to frame concepts that CMM pharmacists are naturally evaluating, but are not necessarily able to explain or discuss aloud with students or novice pharmacists.

"When I am with a student, the tool pushes me to express what is inside my head, the connections I am making to take a certain decision" (Pharmacist 10).

"The medication experience is a difficult concept to teach because people tend to think that is too philosophical, too abstract. But it is definitely not! The tool helps to bring the medication experience to a more practical level when I am teaching" (Pharmacist 2).

Several pharmacists emphasized how using the tool helped students to pay more attention to the subjective aspects of taking medications, which is usually a type of knowledge neglected in pharmacy curricula.

"By using it [the tool] students start to become more attentive to what kinds of factors impact patients' decisions and behaviors regarding their meds" (Pharmacist 5).

The Tool Helps with Future Care Plans

Documenting the medication experience was found to be helpful for deciding a course of action for the next patient's visit.

"It was helpful for follow-up visits to know how to approach that patient next time if you knew how they were feeling and how they responded to certain strategies . . . It helps me know what avenue to go down to or to avoid based on previous visits." (Pharmacist 4)

"I tell my student, after looking at a previous note [with an experience documented in it], that we have to frame our next conversation with the patient considering this information" (Pharmacist 9).

3.3.2. Challenges of Using the Tool

Participants revealed the challenges of the tool as the following themes: being reflexive can be burdensome and unearthing the difference between the medication experience and a drug therapy problem.

Being Reflexive Can Be Burdensome

The CMM pharmacists felt they were already subconsciously identifying and addressing the medication experience during their routine assessment of a patient, so to have to stop and document forced them to reflect, which was described at times as "burdensome". It was often difficult to categorize experiences since this is a component of the assessment that the group was not used to documenting.

"I think it is just hard to stop and reflect on how patients' feelings and previous experiences with medications can impact their attitudes and decisions. I know this is there, it's everywhere, but to document it forces me to rethink over and over again" (Pharmacist 1).

"It takes time. So, it can be challenging" (Pharmacist 6).

It should be noted that this setting includes a group of experienced CMM pharmacists—all with experience in MI and having prior understanding and exposure to the medication experience concept.

"The tool may be more redundant for us at times because our group does this innately, but it would probably be even more helpful for other groups" (Pharmacist 10).

Unearthing the Difference between the Medication Experience and a Drug Therapy Problem

For pharmacists, one of the most important challenges in using this tool was to understand the difference between a medication experience and a DTP, since at times they seem to overlap. It was agreed that the medication experience is completely subjective and usually emotional—typically revolving around a strong feeling or fear. It describes the patient's relationship with medications and provides the background on how it changes their views on medications, and often times their behaviors. It is not present in all patients.

For several participants in the study, using the documentation tool multiple times with many different patients triggered them to perceive the difference between a DTP and a medication experience.

"Before I started using the tool I never really stopped to think about how the medication experience is the same or different from a DTP. I felt there was a connection, but now I know they are related but different concepts" (Pharmacist 5).

The group ultimately defined a negative medication experience as "when an experience can get in the way of a patient getting the most benefit from a medication and can lead to a drug therapy problem".

"To me, the medication experience is associated with feelings or attitudes toward taking medications that is getting in the way of doing what I think is best for them" (Pharmacist 7).

A patient could have multiple DTPs that are not necessarily associated with a medication experience. On the other hand, a patient might have a medication experience, but no DTP identified at that point in time.

4. Discussion

The results showed that using the tool has utility for the practice of patient-centered comprehensive medication management services. Even though it can be "overwhelming" or burdensome to document one more aspect of the patient care process, the course of documenting the patient's medication experience makes the CMM pharmacist more reflexive. Reflexivity has been shown to be an important trait of a patient-centered practitioner [16,17]. Reflexivity assists pharmacists to become more present at consultations, more attentive to patients' needs and more open to patients' unique perspectives and experiences. In addition, reflexivity may help pharmacists to look more critically at themselves as professionals and human beings, which creates space for a broader awareness regarding their way of relating to patients and other health care providers [18].

Almost all of the participating pharmacists reported using the documentation tool as an after-thought. Yet some used it to stimulate ideas of motivational interviewing during the encounter, so having it embedded into the note template was fundamental in making it useful. Interestingly, most of the strategies listed in Table 3 are the same regardless of the medication experience identified. This may suggest that some strategies are more effective in general or possibly easier to use. On the other hand, it may reflect that pharmacists may not be familiar with certain MI strategies and implies that further work is needed to learn and implement new interventions in practice. Similarly, in adherence studies that utilized motivational interviewing, no one intervention consistently enhanced adherence for all patients alike because many variables affect a patient's decision-making process. Typically, a combination of interventions is needed to best address a patient's needs [19]. As MI has outperformed traditional advice given for a broad range of behavioral problems and diseases, having pharmacists refine these skills may be a useful way to impact patient health outcomes [20].

For the participants in this study, using the tool helped them to emphasize to students the importance of the medication experience in patients' decision-making and, therefore, in the delivery of CMM services. Students often do not realize that many patients do not take their medications without resistance and naturally tend to focus much more on their knowledge of pharmacotherapy versus understanding their patients' experiences and goals. Using the tool to document the medication experience helps bring a broader understanding to that concept. The pharmacists remarked that they had seen it shape their students' approach to patients' visits and create attentiveness to what types of factors impact patients' decisions and behaviors regarding medications. In other words, the documentation tool might have encouraged pharmacists and students to become more patient-centered. As indicated by previous research, incorporating patients' medication experiences into clinical decision-making is not an easy task, thus, it is paramount to teach pharmacy students and novice pharmacists how to identify and use this information in daily clinical practice [6,7,20–22].

Another important outcome of using the tool to document patients' medication experience was a better understanding of the difference between a drug therapy problem and a medication experience. For instance, consider the DTP that a patient needs additional drug therapy. There is no need to have a patient experience involved with it unless there is resistance to starting the medication, which would need to be further explored by the pharmacist. An example of a DTP not correlated with a medication experience would be when a dose adjustment is needed, and the patient's perceptions or feelings are not associated with this. A caveat to this would be if the patient refuses to increase the dose because he or she fears side effects or if they equate taking a higher dose with worsening health status or personal failure, which reflects a medication experience. The CMM pharmacists agreed that a DTP may or may not be linked to an experience or attitude towards taking a medication. However, when that is the case, it is the CMM responsibility to address this experience with the goal to improve it or include the patient's perspective into the decision-making process [20].

Several situations emerged with utilizing the medication experience documentation tool. The medication experience was found to be dynamic and often changed from visit to visit. Therefore, the CMM pharmacists agreed they should be intentional in assessing and documenting the presence of a medication experiences at every single visit. The CMM pharmacists also expressed that it was ultimately important to document if, at a particular visit, a patient did *not* have a medication experience that was affecting medication taking or patient outcomes—hence, the creation of the 'none' option for medication experience. It was agreed that the most meaningful way to use the tool was to limit the selection of strategies to a maximum of the one or two that were the most effective that day. This helped them to avoid becoming "desensitized", as it was hard to interpret which strategies were most effective when preparing for a follow-up visit if several strategies were listed.

The research recently conducted by Nascimento et al. corroborates the results of this study as it exposed the complexity of the medication experience. It emphasized the fact that the same individual can simultaneously experience daily medication use in diverse ways, depending on the medical condition and the medication used. In that study, patients experienced daily medication use in four general ways: resolution, adversity ambiguity, or irrelevance. These ways are related to the manner the medication affects the patient´s personal world, which means that taking a medication is much more than purely a mechanical action. Medications can disturb the patient´s relationship with his body, her perception of herself, or his relationship with others [22].

Certain logistics of the tool were challenging with regard to placement of the tool in a documentation note, understanding when to use the tool, and keeping the documentation brief and simple enough for convenience and ease of use. The group could not troubleshoot how to prevent from misinterpreting that a medication experience applies to all medications a patient is taking versus just one. The tool was not linked to certain conditions or medications. The experience can change based on the medication and can be different for each visit, so the challenge moving forward is understanding how to link the documented experience to a specific medication without making the tool too lengthy and cumbersome to use.

It should be noted that this setting includes a group of experienced CMM pharmacists—all with experience in MI and having some prior understanding and exposure to the medication experience concept. As suggested by other studies, educational programs would likely be needed to teach how to identify patients' medication experiences and documenting them with the tool and how to apply MI strategies to their practice [21,22].

It is important to state that the use of the documentation tool in the patient's assessment has become the standard of practice for CMM pharmacists in the studied health care system. There needs to be an expansion of available strategies to understand the best way to improve a patient's medication experience. Evaluating positive medication experiences may also provide insight on effective methods and strategies to use with patients. Limited published information shows the use of the pharmacist applying MI as a strategy to address the medication experience. There are studies that show trends of improved medication adherence when MI is used as an intervention by nurses, physicians, and therapists in patients with chronic conditions [23]. Improved therapy adherence is associated with lowered healthcare cost and increase in workplace productivity [24]. Our study looked much further than adherence, as the medication experience can impact all categories of drug therapy problems (indication, effectiveness, safety, and adherence) [6,20,21]. More studies should measure how intervening on the medication experience affects specific drug therapy problems and patient outcomes.

Limitations

This study should be interpreted in light of its limitations. The initial tool was developed based on studies that aimed for a patient-centered understanding of patients' medication experiences and pharmacists' experiences encountering these experiences in practice.

During the testing time period, there was a substantial gap between the total number of patient encounters and the encounters in which the tool was used resulting in selection bias. Possible reasons for this could be that the pharmacists simply forgot, were too busy to use the tool in their documentation, or did not recognize a medication experience important enough to document. It took time for pharmacists to incorporate the documentation tool into their existing practices. While MI has been shown to outperform traditional advice giving in the treatment of a broad range of behavioral problems, no new strategies were identified during the focus group and the group of pharmacists using the tool struggled with utilizing the listed strategies [20]. Additionally, the design of the documentation tool did not identify if a strategy was effective or not. It documented that a certain strategy was used during the visit, but the effectiveness of the strategy was not followed up on at the subsequent visit to determine true effectiveness of the intervention. Only negative medication experiences were assessed with this tool, as we assumed these to be the most meaningful to impact and require intervention for improved outcomes.

The results originated from a group of CMM pharmacists within one health system, and can not necessarily be extrapolated or generalized to other practices.

5. Conclusions

CMM pharmacists commonly encounter patients' medication experiences in their practices. The documentation tool was developed and tested to assist pharmacists to better recognize patients´ medication experiences and elect associated strategies to improve medication outcomes. Pharmacists' acknowledged that awareness of the medication experience and a toolbox of strategies to affect it helped improve patient-centered care in their practices. Continued reflection and documentation of the medication experience is essential in continuing to advance CMM and pharmacist patient-centered practice.

Author Contributions: Conceptualization, N.P. and D.R.-d.-O.; Methodology, S.J.S.-H. and D.R.-d.-O.; Validation, S.R., N.P., S.J.S.-H. and D.R.-d.-O.; Formal Analysis, N.P. and D.R.-d.-O.; Investigation, S.R.; Resources, D.R.-d.-O.; Data Curation, S.R. and D.R.-d.-O.; Writing-Original Draft Preparation, S.R., N.P.; Writing-Review & Editing, N.P., S.J.S.-H. and D.R.-d.-O.; Supervision, D.R.-d.-O.; Project Administration, S.R. and D.R.-d.-O.

Funding: This research received no external funding.

Acknowledgments: The authors would like to acknowledge and thank the CMM pharmacists at the studied health care system for using the tool in their practices and for their participation in the focus groups. Also, we thank the managers of the CMM department for their support in the development of this research project.

Conflicts of Interest: The authors declare no conflict of interest.

Appendix A The Medication Experience Documentation Tool

MEDICATION EXPERIENCE AFFECTING MEDICATION OUTCOMES FOR TODAY'S VISIT
(select one or more and then select associated overall strategies):

None

Feelings of burden and being overwhelmed (ex: pill burden)

Does not want to take medications because:

    Doesn't like to take (cultural background, other)
    Doubts the need
    Doesn't feel the benefits
    Can't reconcile value of medication(s) over cost
    Associates with a "stigma" and is ashamed/embarrassed to use it
    Does not like administration (swallow, infusion, injection) process

---

Fears/concerns about side effects:

    Current personal side effects
    History of personal side effects
    Observing friend or family member experience
    Media

Fears/concerns about becoming dependent on a medication

Fears/concerns medication (ex: generic) will not be effective

---

Self adjusts medication regimen (increases, decrease, or skips doses)

Increasing medication(s) or increasing medication dose(s) means:

    Personal failure
    Worsening health status

Prefers alternative non-drug therapy or lifestyle changes

Fear of not having medication(s)/too reliant on Rx medication(s) (security)

*** (write-in)

STRATEGIES USED TODAY THAT EFFECTIVELY IMPROVED MEDICATION RELATED OUTCOMES:

Open ended questions

Collaboration/Shared Decision Making

Negotiate

Evocation/Empower

Support autonomy /Emphasizing personal choice and control

Ask permission

Raise concern, educate, or inform

Reframe/ Reflection

Roll with resistance

Using a rating scale, on scale of 1-10, Importance *** Confidence ***

Elicit change talk

Encourage non-drug therapy or lifestyle changes

Referral to care team member

*** (write-in)

Appendix B Motivational Interviewing Strategy Definitions (11–13)

1. **Open ended questions:** Using stems such as "what" and "how" that can elicit unlimited answers from a patient and invite them to talk.
2. **Collaboration/Shared Decision Making:** Co-developing goals with the patient to make sure they are involved in creating a plan that will indeed work for the patient.
3. **Negotiate:** Meeting the patient "in the middle". Perhaps the plan does not exactly match what you want as the practitioner, but is a smaller more reasonable goal is agreed upon that acts as a stepping stone to reach the ultimate goal.
4. **Evocation/Empower:**

    a. Helping your patient explore how they can make a difference in their own health by utilizing their own ideas and resources.
    b. Facilitating the patient in bringing their own expertise to the discussion on how best to accomplish change.
    c. Drawing out the patient's own motivation to change.

5. **Support autonomy/Emphasizing personal choice and control:**

    a. Acknowledge to the patient that they are ultimately responsible for change and as the practitioner we separate ourselves from the outcome.
    b. Communicating respect and dignity of the patient through unconditional positive regard.

6. **Ask permission:** Informing or advising only after the patient has given you permission to do so. Forms of permission would include a patient asking for advice or asking the patient for permission to inform (like knocking on a door before entering). Examples are; "May I make a suggestion?" or prefacing advice with "You can tell me what you think of this idea … .".
7. **Raise concern, educate, or inform**: The actual act of providing patient with information and advice.
8. **Reframe/Reflection:**

    a. Captures and returns to patients something about what they have just said (rephrasing one or two ideas)
    b. They do not have to be accurate (could be amplified or exaggerated) and may or may not introduce new meaning.
    c. Different types of complex reflections: adding content or meaning, amplification, double-sided, reframing, verbalizing unspoken emotion, emphasizing one side

9. **Roll with resistance:** When patients display signs of resistance, such as blaming or minimizing, the practitioner lets the resistance flow rather than use oppositional tactics, such as telling the person he is wrong.
10. **Using a rating scale, one a scale of 1–10, Importance***Confidence***** Using a numerical rating scale or other ruler to assess the patient's attitude toward importance and confidence behind changing a certain behavior. Typically asked as: "Could you tell me, on a scale from 1 to 10, how important it is for you to _____? Why did you give yourself a score of __ and not 1?" The same style question can be asked about confidence. Could follow up with a question such as "How can I help you move higher up the scale?" These types of questions will help support self-efficacy.
11. **Elicit change talk:**

    a. Explore how their current behavior is inconsistent with their values.
    b. Selectively asking and identifying when patients state desire, ability, reasons for, and the need to change and responding to this by evoking, affirming, and reflecting these back to them.

Encourage non-drug therapy or lifestyle changes: Supporting non-prescription therapy to help patient reach goals and outcomes.

References

1. Ramalho de Oliveira, D.; Brummel, A.R.; Miller, D.B. Medication Therapy Management: 10 years of experience in a large integrated health care system. *J. Manag. Care Pharm.* **2010**, *16*, 185–195. [CrossRef] [PubMed]
2. Isetts, B.J.; Schondelmeyer, S.W.; Artz, M.B.; Lenarz, L.A.; Heaton, A.H.; Wadd, W.B.; Brown, L.M.; Cipolle, R.J. Clinical and economic outcomes of medication therapy management services: The Minnesota experience. *J. Am. Pharm. Assoc.* **2008**, *48*, 203–211. [CrossRef] [PubMed]
3. Cipolle, R.J.; Strand, L.M.; Morley, P.C. *Pharmaceutical Care Practice: The Clinician's Guide*, 2nd ed.; McGraw-Hill: New York, NY, USA, 2004.
4. Cipolle, R.J.; Strand, L.M.; Morley, P.C. *Pharmaceutical Care Practice: The Patient-Centered Approach to Medication Management*, 3rd ed.; McGraw-Hill: New York, NY, USA, 2012.
5. Shoemaker, S.J.; Ramalho de Oliveira, D. Understanding the meaning of medications for patients: The medication experience. *Pharm. World Sci.* **2008**, *30*, 86–91. [CrossRef] [PubMed]
6. Shoemaker, S.J.; Ramalho de Oliveira, D.; Alves, M.; Ekstrand, M. The medication experience: Preliminary evidence of its value for patient education and counseling on chronic medications. *Patient Educ. Couns.* **2011**, *83*, 443–450. [CrossRef]
7. Ramalho de Oliveira, D.; Shoemaker, S.J.; Ekstrand, M.; Alves, M.R. Preventing and resolving drug therapy problems by understanding patients' medication experiences. *J. Am. Pharm. Assoc.* **2012**, *52*, 71–80. [CrossRef] [PubMed]
8. Moen, J.; Bohm, A.; Tillenius, T.; Antonov, K.; Nilsson, J.L.; Ring, L. "I don't know how many of these [medicines] are necessary."—A focus group study among elderly users of multiple medicines. *Patient Educ. Couns.* **2009**, *74*, 135–141. [CrossRef] [PubMed]
9. Alfano, G. The older adult and drug therapy: Part two. Meaning of the medication: Clue to acceptance or rejection. *Geriatr. Nurs.* **1982**, *3*, 28–30. [CrossRef]
10. Seale, C.; Champlin, R.; Lelliot, P.; Quirk, A. Antipsychotic medication, sedation and mental clouding: An observational study of psychiatric consultations. *Soc. Sci. Med.* **2007**, *65*, 698–711. [CrossRef] [PubMed]
11. Sim, M.G.; Wain, T.; Khong, E. Influencing behavior change in general practice; Part 1 brief intervention and motivational interviewing. *Aust. Fam. Physician* **2009**, *38*, 885–888. [PubMed]
12. Rollnick, S.; Miller, W.; Butler, C. *Motivational Interviewing in Health Care*; Helping Patients Change Behavior; The Guilford Press: New York, NY, USA, 2008.
13. Sim, M.G.; Wain, T.; Khong, E. Influencing behavior change in general practice; Part 2 motivational interviewing approaches. *Aust. Fam. Physician* **2009**, *38*, 986–989. [PubMed]
14. PCPCC Medication Management Task Force. *The Patient-Centered Medical Home: Integrating Comprehensive Medication Management to Optimize Patient Outcomes*, 2nd ed.; Patient-Centered Primary Care Collaborative: Washington, DC, USA, 2012.
15. Krueger, R.A.; Casey, M.A. *Focus Groups: A Practical Guide for Applied Research*; SAGE: Thousand Oaks, CA, USA, 2009.
16. Droege, M. The role of reflective practice in pharmacy. *Educ. Health* **2003**, *1*, 68–74. [CrossRef] [PubMed]
17. Ramalho de Oliveira, D.; Shoemaker, S.J. Achieving patient centeredness in pharmacy practice: Openness and the pharmacist's natural attitude. *J. Am. Pharm. Assoc.* **2006**, *46*, 56–66. [CrossRef]
18. Ramalho-de-Oliveira, D. Autoethnography—Overview and its Prospect to Advance Pharmacy Education and Practice. *Am. J. Pharm. Educ.* **2019**. [CrossRef]
19. Possidente, C.J.; Bucci, K.K.; McClain, W.J. Motivational interviewing: A tool to improve medication adherence? *Am. J. Health Syst. Pharm.* **2005**, *62*, 1311–1314. [CrossRef] [PubMed]
20. Rubak, S.; Sandbaek, A.; Lauritzen, T.; Christensen, B. Motivational interviewing: A systematic review and meta-analysis. *Br. J. Gen. Pract.* **2005**, *55*, 305–312. [PubMed]
21. Oliveira, I.V.; Freitas, E.L.; Detoni, K.B.; Ramalho-de-Oliveira, D. Use of the patient's medication experience in pharmacists' decision making process. *Int. J. Pharm.* **2017**, *7*, 1–8.

22. Nascimento, Y.d.A.; Silva, L.D.; Ramalho-de-Oliveira, D. Experiences with the daily use of medications among chronic hepatitis c patients. *Res. Soc. Adm. Pharm.* **2019**, in press. [CrossRef] [PubMed]
23. Levensky, E.R.; Forcehimes, A.; O'Donohue, W.T.; Beitz, K. Motivational interviewing; An evidence-based approach to counseling helps patients follow treatment recommendations. *Am. J. Nurs.* **2007**, *107*, 50–58. [CrossRef] [PubMed]
24. Behner, P.; Klink, A.; Visser, S.; Böcken, J.; Etgeton, S. *Unleashing the Potential of Therapy Adherence; High Leverage Changes in Patient Behavior for Improved Health and Productivity*; Booz & Company: Amsterdam, The Netherlands, 2012.

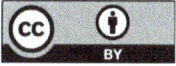

pharmacy

MDPI

Article

Reducing Medication Therapy Problems in the Transition from Hospital to Home: A Pre- & Post-Discharge Pharmacist Collaboration

Anne Schullo-Feulner [1,2,*] [iD], Lisa Krohn [1] and Alison Knutson [1]

1   Park Nicollet Health Services, St. Louis Park, MN 55426, USA
2   Pharmaceutical Care & Health Systems, University of Minnesota College of Pharmacy, Minneapolis, MN 55455, USA
*   Correspondence: anne.schullo_feulner@parknicollet.com

Received: 20 May 2019; Accepted: 4 July 2019; Published: 9 July 2019

Abstract: Background: With 30-day Medicare readmission rates reaching 20%, a heightened focus has been placed on improving the transition process from hospital to home. For many institutions, this charge has identified medication-use safety as an area where pharmacists are well-positioned to improve outcomes by reducing medication therapy problems (MTPs). Methods: This system-wide (425 bed community hospital plus 18 primary care clinics) prospective study recruited inpatient and ambulatory pharmacists to provide comprehensive medication management before and after hospital discharge. The results analyzed were the success rate and timing of the inpatient to ambulatory pharmacist handoff, as well as the number, type, and severity of MTPs resolved in both settings. Results: Of the 105 eligible patients who received a pharmacist evaluation before discharge, 61 (58%) received follow-up with an ambulatory pharmacist an average of 2.88 days after discharge (range 1–8 days). An average of 5 and 1.4 MTPs per patient were identified and resolved in the inpatient vs. ambulatory setting, respectively. Although average MTP severity ratings were higher in the inpatient setting, the highest severity rating was seen most frequently in the ambulatory setting. Conclusions: In the transition from hospital to home, pharmacist evaluation in both the inpatient and ambulatory settings are necessary to resolve medication therapy problems.

Keywords: transitions in care; pharmacist; medication therapy problems; medication safety; comprehensive medication management; readmissions

---

1. Introduction

In the era of accountable care, organizations are charged with reaching quality metrics to optimize reimbursement. For some, this charge identified medication-use safety during transitions from hospital to home as an area for quality improvement [1–3]. Pharmacists in both inpatient and ambulatory settings have the potential to work together to improve medication-use safety by reducing medication therapy problems (MTPs) during the transition process [2–4]. One method to achieve this vision may be found in strategic alliances and collaboration across the care system to develop and evaluate a new model of pharmacy service.

With nearly one-fifth of hospitalized Medicare fee-for-service patients readmitted within 30 days, a heightened focus has been placed on improving the quality of the transition process to reduce costs and improve patient care [5]. Previous studies have demonstrated significant medication-related problems at the time of discharge, including mediation discrepancies that doubled readmission rates [6], as well as a lack of patient understanding, where 50% of patients were unable to state the name and purpose of their medications at the time of discharge [7]. One study found that over 50% of medication-related admissions were preventable, while another determined that these preventable admissions resulted in significantly longer hospital stays [8,9]. The Agency for Healthcare Research and Quality (AHRQ) recommends medication reconciliation, defined as the "comparison of the patient's current medication regimen against the physician's admission, transfer, and/or discharge orders to identify discrepancies," as a beginning to improving medication safety [10]. Although this is necessary and provides the value of an accurate and complete medication list, it does not create a clinical assessment to ensure: (1) appropriate indication, (2) effectiveness, (3) safety, and (4) convenience/adherence for each medication. These four components provide the framework for the Patient-Centered Primary Care Collaborative model for comprehensive medication management (CMM) [11]. Through this assessment, pharmacists are able to identify, prevent, and/or resolve mediation therapy problems (MTPs). MTPs are defined as an event or circumstance involving drug treatment (pharmacotherapy) that interferes with the optimal provision of medical care [12]. Pharmacists are specifically trained to provide this comprehensive service, yet they remain underutilized during the transition process [13]. Previous scholarship substantiates pharmacist benefit, demonstrating that patients who met with a pharmacist either at the time of discharge or shortly after returning home have consistently lower readmission rates through the identification and resolution of MTPs [14–20]. The current study sought to build on this body of knowledge by evaluating a coordinated pharmacy service (CMM delivered by an inpatient pharmacist prior to discharge and an ambulatory pharmacist post-discharge) across the hospital to home transition of care.

This paper describes the implementation and evaluation of a pharmacist-driven care transitions model in a large health care system. The specific objectives were to evaluate: (1) the success rate and timing of transferring patients from an inpatient to an ambulatory pharmacist, (2) the number and types of MTPs identified in the inpatient and ambulatory setting, and (3) the difference in MTP severity ratings (inpatient vs. ambulatory) for patients with a successful transfer of care.

2. Materials and Methods

This pharmacy-based care transition model was developed and conducted in a 425-bed community hospital and 18 primary care clinics within the Park Nicollet Health Services system in the Minneapolis-St Paul, Minnesota, United States of America (USA) metropolitan area. All pharmacists were employed by the health system, had full access to the electronic medical record, and were embedded in the care teams of their respective settings. Patients who received CMM from an inpatient pharmacist, ambulatory pharmacist, or both between August 2013 and November 2013 were included. Patients discharged to a skilled nursing facility or under hospice care were excluded from an ambulatory pharmacist evaluation but were still eligible to receive an inpatient pharmacist evaluation.

2.1. Care Transition Model Logistics

Although discharging physicians were at liberty to request that any patient be included in the study, patients admitted with acute myocardial infarction, pneumonia, chronic obstructive pulmonary disease, and heart failure (i.e., U.S. Medicare Measures) were prioritized. Inpatient pharmacists completed a comprehensive medication management visit with the patient, as well as any caregivers present prior to discharge. The pharmacist discussed subsequent recommendations with the physician prior to the discharge medication ordering process. The pharmacy intervention was documented in the electronic medical record and sent with a referral for ambulatory pharmacy services to follow-up post discharge. As an integrated component of Park Nicollet's medical home model, clinical ambulatory pharmacists are geographically dispersed around the region served. The post-discharge intervention consisted of an ambulatory CMM evaluation identical to that performed while the patient was hospitalized. This follow-up was performed either in person or by phone to reinforce inpatient recommendations, as well as identify and address any new MTPs that developed following discharge. See Figure 1 for a pictorial representation of the care transition process.

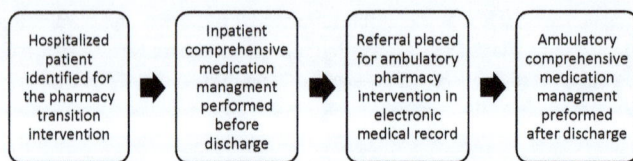

Figure 1. Care Transition Process.

2.2. Clinical Services Provided

Pharmacists in both settings collaborated with the care team (patient, nurse, physician, social work, etc.) to resolve MTPs and prepare a revised medication list. The inpatient care team helped to identify appropriate patients, as well as their anticipated date of discharge and discharge disposition. The team also provided additional information about the patient and current medical concerns. The revised medication list was created through calling pharmacies to review refill records, chart review, patient and/or family interview, and healthcare team collaboration. During the pharmacist visit, whether inpatient or ambulatory, a focus was placed on:

1. *Comprehensive Medication Management (CMM)*: Creating a medication list that is accurate across the transition, as well as ensuring each medication is indicated, effective, safe, and convenient with complete administration directions.
2. *Patient Centered Care*: Educating patients on a medication list developed in collaboration with patient needs and preferences.
3. *Medication Access*: Ensuring that patients have access to all medications and that each discharge prescription is sent to the correct pharmacy and/or location.

2.3. Data Collection/Research Methods

This study was given exemption status by Park Nicollet Health Services IRB and the University of Minnesota IRB. A total of 12 pharmacists, four inpatient and eight ambulatory, were trained to participate. Inpatient pharmacist documentation included both immediate resolution of MTPs and recommendations for consideration in the ambulatory setting. Ambulatory pharmacist documentation addressed inpatient recommendations, identified new MTPs since discharge, and provided a plan for continued ambulatory follow-up. In both settings, identified MTPs were categorized into eight types, consisting of: "medication inaccuracy," "adverse drug reaction," "non-adherence," "lack of understanding," "dose too high," "lack of needed drug" (addition of a drug), "dose too low," and "unnecessary medication" (unnecessary or duplicate medication). After an MTP was identified and typed, each one was given a severity rating from 1 (lowest) to 3 (highest/life-threatening) based on the potential for patient harm had the MTP not been resolved. Severity ratings for each intervention were documented based on reporting standards for skilled nursing facilities from the Department of Health and Human Services [21]; see Table 1 for detailed descriptions. Severity ratings were documented in real-time by the pharmacist but were also verified by three independent pharmacist raters via blind review after the study was completed. All raters were standardized using an inter-rater reliability test. When no MTP was identified, a severity rating of 0 was recorded.

Table 1. Potential Medication Therapy Problem Severity Rating.

Severity Rating	Description
1	If no intervention, potential for minimal (would require patient self-management) or no harm
2	If no intervention, potential for moderate harm (would require healthcare professional intervention or hospitalization to resolve)
3	If no intervention, potential for severe harm (permanent disability or death)

Note: Adapted from Medicare Nursing Home Levels of Harm categories.

2.4. Statistical Methods

A generalized estimating equation (GEE) was chosen as a marginal model in order to account for the correlation of multiple measurements within some patients. An exchangeable correlation structure was specified, and a Gaussian distribution was chosen in order to compare the mean difference between the maximum severity ratings at ambulatory and inpatient evaluations. Additionally, paired t-tests comparing the inpatient and ambulatory severity ratings for only those patients with both interventions (i.e., successful transfer) were analyzed and the results were compared to those from the GEE analysis. Both models were implemented for the primary (overall severity) and secondary (individual MTPs rated for severity) analyses, with an α level of 0.05 considered significant.

3. Results

All 12 trained pharmacists (four inpatient and eight ambulatory) participated. Patients were categorized based on having either a successful inpatient-to-ambulatory pharmacist transfer (n = 61) or having an inpatient evaluation only (n = 73). Baseline Characteristics (Table 2) between the two groups were well balanced with the following two exceptions. Patients who followed up with an ambulatory evaluation had shorter lengths of stay in the hospital (3.4 days compared to 5.1 days, p-value ≤ 0.001) and were more likely to discharge to home rather than a skilled nursing facility (p-value < 0.001). The average age, gender, marital status, number of chronic conditions, number of medications, and reason for evaluation were not found to be significantly different between the two groups.

Table 2. Baseline Characteristics.

Characteristic	Inpatient Intervention Only (n = 73)		Inpatient and Ambulatory Intervention (n = 61)		*p*-Value
Mean Age (years)	75.5		73.0		0.277
Sex					
Female	36	(49.3%)	38	(62.3%)	0.183
Male	37	(50.7%)	23	(37.7%)	
Marital Status					
Single	17	(23.3%)	15	(24.6%)	
Married	26	(35.6%)	29	(47.5%)	0.249
Divorced	2	(2.7%)	3	(4.9%)	
Widowed	28	(38.4%)	14	(23.0%)	
Mean Length of Stay (days)	5.1		3.4		<0.001
Mean Chronic Conditions (n)	9.2		10.6		0.076
Mean Chronic Medications (n)	12.5		13.5		0.290
Discharge Disposition					
Home	40	(54.8%)	56	(91.8%)	
Home (With Care)	4	(5.5%)	5	(8.2%)	<0.001
Skilled Nursing Facility	29	(39.7%)	0	(0%)	
Insurance					
Private	5	(6.8%)	6	(9.8%)	
Medicare	62	(84.9%)	50	(82.0%)	0.456
Medicaid	5	(6.8%)	2	(3.3%)	
None	1	(1.4%)	3	(4.9%)	
Reason for Evaluation *					
COPD	17		11		
MI	4		2		
Pneumonia	8		11		0.498
CHF	13		16		
Other	36		26		

* Patients could contribute to multiple categories.

3.1. Success Rate of the Care Transition Model

Prior to discharge from the hospital, 134 patients received an inpatient pharmacist intervention. Of these 134 patients, 29 were discharged to a skilled nursing facility, excluding them from ambulatory follow-up. Of the patients eligible for an ambulatory intervention (n = 105), the transfer of care from the inpatient to the ambulatory setting was successful in 61 (58%) patients. In total, 44 eligible patients were lost to ambulatory follow-up due to: Inpatient pharmacist failure to place a transfer in the electronic system (44%); ambulatory pharmacist failure to act on a new patient transfer (31%); ambulatory pharmacist failure to reach the patient for follow-up (16%); patient readmission prior to ambulatory follow-up (7%); and lastly, patient declined ambulatory visit (2%). Excluding one outlier with a follow-up of 16 days, the average time to follow-up with an ambulatory pharmacist was 2.88 days (range 1–8 days).

3.2. Number and Types of Medication Therapy Problems Identified

An average of five MTPs per patient were identified and resolved in the inpatient setting prior to discharge. The most common types of MTP found in the inpatient setting were: "lack of needed drug" (identified in 60% of patients), "lack of understanding" (45% of patients), and "medication inaccuracy" (42% of patients). During the ambulatory follow-up, an average of 1.4 MTPs per patient were identified and resolved. In 75% of the patients who received both an inpatient and ambulatory intervention, the ambulatory pharmacist identified the presence of at least one MTP. During the ambulatory CMM intervention, medication "non-adherence" and "lack of needed drug" were the most common MTPs identified and resolved (each identified in 25% of patients), followed by "lack of understanding" (19.7% of patients) and "adverse drug reaction" (18.0% of patients).

3.3. Severity Rating Comparison of Medication Therapy Problems Identified

Table 3 depicts the mean difference in maximum severity rating between the inpatient and ambulatory settings for patients with a successful transfer of care (i.e., the "inpatient and ambulatory CMM intervention cohort" n = 61). In terms of capacity to cause patient harm, all of the MTP types identified by pharmacists demonstrate a trend toward being less severe in the ambulatory vs. inpatient setting. When looked at as a whole, the mean difference in "overall MTP severity" decreased by 0.25 (CI: (−0.58, 0.08), p-value = 0.141) in the ambulatory setting, however, this difference did not reach significance. Four of the eight MTP types showed a similar nonstatistical trend toward reduced severity in the ambulatory setting. The other four MTP types (i.e., "medication inaccuracy," "adverse drug reaction," "dose too high," and "lack of needed drug"), all demonstrated a statistically significant reduction in severity in the ambulatory vs. inpatient setting.

Table 3. Medication Therapy Problem Severity Comparison for the Inpatient and Ambulatory CMM Intervention Cohort (n = 61) *.

MTP Severity Rating	Mean Difference in Inpatient vs. Ambulatory Maximum Severity	95% CI	*p*-Value
Overall Severity	−0.25	(−0.58, 0.08)	0.141
Medication Inaccuracy	−0.34	(−0.58, −0.11)	0.004
Adverse Drug Reaction	−0.33	(−0.63, −0.02)	0.036
Non-Adherence	−0.20	(−0.47, 0.08)	0.159
Lack of Understanding	−0.23	(−0.53, 0.07)	0.137
Dose Too High	−0.34	(−0.55, −0.14)	0.001
Lack of Needed Drug	−0.46	(−0.75, −0.17)	0.002
Dose Too Low	−0.07	(−0.32, 0.19)	0.610
Unnecessary Medication	−0.18	(−0.38, 0.02)	0.070

* Represents only patients receiving both an inpatient and ambulatory pharmacist evaluation (n = 61).

Table 4 depicts the frequency of each severity rating (0–3) for all patients in either the inpatient (n = 134) or ambulatory (n= 61) setting. There were a greater percentage of patients with no MTPs (identified as having a severity rating of "0") in the ambulatory (26%) vs. inpatient setting (4%). Correspondingly, MTPs with severity ratings of 1 or 2 were seen more frequently in the inpatient setting. However, when it came to the highest severity rating (a rating of 3 indicating the potential for "permanent disability or death"), it was found more often in the ambulatory setting (found in 10% of patients in the ambulatory vs. 6% in the inpatient setting).

Table 4. Frequency of Severity Ratings.

Severity Rating	Inpatient (n = 134)		Ambulatory (n = 61)	
0	5	(3.7%)	16	(26.2%)
1	29	(21.6%)	7	(11.5%)
2	92	(68.7%)	32	(52.5%)
3	8	(6.0%)	6	(9.8%)

4. Discussion

Previous scholarship provides insight into the potential of pharmacists to improve medication safety via medication reconciliation in either the inpatient or ambulatory setting [2,3]. This study demonstrates a care model that created a successful direct handoff from inpatient pharmacists prior to discharge to ambulatory pharmacists' post-discharge in 58% of eligible patients. The two most common reasons for failure (i.e., failure of inpatient pharmacist to place the transfer and failure of ambulatory pharmacist to follow-up on the transfer) primarily represented electronic and personnel system inefficiencies that have since been rectified. The inpatient process to initiate an ambulatory CMM intervention for a patient has been simplified down to three clicks in the electronic medical chart and can now be performed without a physician order by student pharmacists at the behest of a licensed pharmacist preceptor. On the ambulatory side, one FTE (full-time equivalent) of administrative personnel has been added to coordinate patient outreach in setting up either phone or in person visits for the health system wide ambulatory pharmacist group.

An average of five MTPs per patient were found in our inpatient cohort, while patients who received ambulatory follow-up only three days after discharge still had an average of 1.4 MTPs identified by this second CMM intervention. The benefit of comprehensive medication management both at the time of and directly after discharge has been demonstrated before [22,23]. One study found that two-thirds of patients discharged from an emergency department did not comprehend home care instructions, follow-up instructions, medications, and/or discharge diagnoses [23]. The current study supports this finding showing that despite receiving CMM just prior to discharge, nearly 75% of patients had at least one MTP at the ambulatory intervention. The presence of newly identified MTPs post-discharge demonstrates the need for comprehensive medication management at each transition in order to minimize medication related MTPs.

Although not statistically significant for all MTP types, this study demonstrated a reduction in overall MTP severity from the inpatient to ambulatory setting. This could be expected due to the acute illness of hospitalized patients. Perhaps more interesting is that while hospitalized patients had more severe MTPs, a greater percentage of severity level 3 (potential for severe harm) MTPs were found in the ambulatory setting. One possible explanation is that the level 3 MTPs identified in the ambulatory setting involved a lack of adherence to high-risk medications such as a hypoglycemic, opioid, or antithrombotic medication. Most commonly, non-adherence resulted from the patient preferring not to take, forgetting to take, an inability to afford the medications, and/or a lack of information retention post-discharge. Overall, data from this study shows that while more MTPs are found and resolved in the inpatient setting, those that persist and/or present themselves early in the ambulatory setting are of a more severe nature, emphasizing the importance of pharmacist intervention at both of these critical times during transitions in care.

There are several limitations to this study. Twelve pharmacists identified and classified MTPs. Although the pharmacy team underwent a norming process, there is still the potential for inter-rater variability. Similarly, MTP severity ratings were adjudicated by three separate normed judges. Further, the severity rating tool utilized was developed for use in long-term skilled nursing facilities, rather than hospitalized inpatients. This U.S. Department of Health and Human Services-based rating tool was selected by the health system's Quality, Innovation, and Population Health Services department to align with other system-wide medication safety initiatives. Severity classification scales rating medication safety concerns in the inpatient [24,25] and outpatient [25] setting should be noted. There were limits on the discharge disposition type the ambulatory pharmacists were able to reach, as patients going to a skilled nursing facility were not seen across the transition. Due to the complexity of these patients' medication regimens, follow-up with this population warrants further evaluation and is planned for the future. Also, due to the small sample size, this study was unable to show if pharmacy-based CMM reduced readmission rates.

5. Conclusions

This study demonstrates a transition of care model for the transfer of patient care from an inpatient to an ambulatory pharmacist before and after discharge. This transition was successful in 58% of patients an average of 2.88 days after discharge. The two most common reasons for failure were failure of inpatient pharmacist to place the transfer and failure of ambulatory pharmacist to follow-up on the transfer. An average of five MTPs per patient were found in the inpatient cohort, and patients who received ambulatory follow-up roughly three days after discharge still had an average of 1.4 MTPs. Although overall MTP severity ratings were higher in the inpatient setting, MTPs that persisted and/or presented themselves early after discharge in the ambulatory setting were the most likely to lead to serious patient harm.

Author Contributions: Conceptualization and methodology, A.S.-F. and A.K.; investigation, A.K. and L.K.; formal analysis, writing—original draft preparation, and writing—review and editing, A.S.-F., A.K. and L.K.

Funding: This research received no external funding.

Acknowledgments: Thanks for contributions of Reilly E. Hourigan, M.S., Kelsey E. Brown, M.S. and Mark Desjardins, Pharm.D.

Conflicts of Interest: The authors declare no conflict of interest.

References

1. Johansen, J.S.; Havnes, K.; Halvorsen, K.H.; Haustreis, S.; Skaue, L.W.; Kamycheva, E.; Mathiesen, L.; Viktil, K.K.; Granås, A.G.; Garcia, B.H. Interdisciplinary collaboration across secondary and primary care to improve medication safety in the elderly (IMMENSE study): Study protocol for a randomized controlled trial. *BMJ Open* **2018**, *8*, e020106. [CrossRef] [PubMed]
2. Hohl, C.M.; Partovi, N.; Ghement, I.; Wickham, M.E.; McGrail, K.; Reddekopp, L.N.; Sobolev, B. Impact of early in-hospital medication review by clinical pharmacists on health services utilization. *PLoS ONE* **2017**, *2*, e0170495. [CrossRef] [PubMed]
3. Martin, P.; Tamblyn, R.; Benedetti, A.; Ahmed, S.; Tannenbaum, C. Effect of a Pharmacist-Led Educational Intervention on Inappropriate Medication Prescriptions in Older Adults: The D-PRESCRIBE Randomized Clinical Trial. *JAMA* **2018**, *18*, 1889–1898. [CrossRef]
4. Dudas, V.; Bookwalter, T.; Kerr, K.; Pantilat, S. The impact of follow-up telephone calls to patients after hospitalization. *Am. J. Med.* **2001**, *111*, 26–30. [CrossRef]
5. Unruh, M.A.; Jung, H.Y.; Vest, J.R.; Casalino, L.P.; Kaushal, R. Meaningful Use of Electronic Health Records by Outpatient Physicians and Readmissions of Medicare Fee-for-Service Beneficiaries. *Med. Care* **2017**, *55*, 493–499. [CrossRef]
6. Coleman, E.A.; Smith, J.D.; Raha, D.; Min, S.J. Posthospital medication discrepancies: Prevalence and contributing factors. *Arch. Intern. Med.* **2005**, *165*, 1842–1847. [CrossRef]

7.	Makaryus, A.N.; Friedman, E.A. Patients understanding of their treatment plans and diagnosis at discharge. *Mayo Clin. Proc.* **2005**, *80*, 991–994. [CrossRef]

8.	Winterstein, A.G.; Sauer, B.C.; Hepler, C.D.; Poole, C. Preventable drug-related hospital admissions. *Ann. Pharm.* **2002**, *36*, 1238–1248. [CrossRef]

9.	Dormann, H.; Neubert, A.; Criegee-Rieck, M.; Egger, T.; Radespiel-Tröger, M.; Azaz-Livshits, T.; Hahn, E.G. Readmissions and adverse drug reactions in internal medicine: The economic impact. *J. Intern. Med.* **2004**, *255*, 653–663. [CrossRef]

10.	Agency for Healthcare Research and Quality (AHRQ): Medications at Transitions and Clinical Handoffs (MATCH) Toolkit for Medication Reconciliation. Available online: http://www.ahrq.gov/qual/match/ (accessed on 11 June 2019).

11.	Patient-Centered Primary Care Collaborative Resource Guide: The Patient-Centered Medical Home: Integrating Comprehensive Medication Management to Optimize Patient outcomes. Available online: http://www.pcpcc.org/sites/default/files/media/medmanagement.pdf (accessed on 11 June 2019).

12.	Strand, L.M.; Morley, P.C.; Cipolle, R.J.; Ramsey, R.; Lamsam, G.D. Drug-related problems: Their structure and function. *DICP Ann. Pharmacother.* **1990**, *24*, 1093–1097. [CrossRef]

13.	Kern, K.A.; Kalus, J.S.; Bush, C.; Chen, D.; Szandzik, E.G.; Haque, N.Z. Variations in pharmacy-based transition-of-care activities in the United States: A national survey. *Am. J. Health Syst. Pharm.* **2014**, *71*, 648–656. [CrossRef] [PubMed]

14.	Bellone, J.M.; Barner, J.C.; Lopez, D.A. Postdischarge interventions by pharmacists and impact on hospital readmission rates. *J. Am. Pharm. Assoc.* **2012**, *52*, 358–362. [CrossRef] [PubMed]

15.	Conklin, J.R.; Togami, J.C.; Burnett, A.; Dodd, M.A.; Ray, G.M. Care transitions service: A pharmacy-driven program for medication reconciliation through the continuum of care. *Am. J. Health Syst. Pharm.* **2014**, *71*, 802–810. [CrossRef] [PubMed]

16.	Monika, G.; Mikaitis, D.; Gayle, S.; Johnson, T.; Sims, S. Impact of a combined pharmacist and social worker program to reduce hospital readmissions. *J. Manag. Care Pharm.* **2013**, *19*, 558–563.

17.	Kilcup, M.; Schultz, D.; Carlson, J.; Wilson, B. Postdischarge pharmacist medication reconciliation: Impact on readmission rates and financial savings. *J. Am. Pharm. Assoc.* **2013**, *53*, 78–84. [CrossRef]

18.	Kripalani, S.; Roumie, C.L.; Dalal, A.K.; Cawthon, C.; Businger, A.; Eden, S.K.; Huang, R.L. Effect of a pharmacist intervention on clinically important medication errors after hospital discharge: A randomized trial. *Ann. Intern. Med.* **2012**, *157*, 1–10. [CrossRef] [PubMed]

19.	Pal, A.; Babbott, S.; Wilkinson, S.T. Can the targeted use of a discharge pharmacist significantly decrease 30-day readmissions? *Hosp. Pharm.* **2013**, *48*, 380–388. [CrossRef]

20.	Mekonnen, A.B.; McLachlan, A.J.; Brien, J.A. Effectiveness of pharmacist-led medication reconciliation programmes on clinical outcomes at hospital transitions: A systematic review and meta-analysis. *BMJ Open* **2016**, *6*, e010003. [CrossRef]

21.	Medicare.gov. Medicare Nursing Home Levels of Harm Categories. Available online: Http://www.medicare.gov/NHCompare/static/related/incdrawlevelofharm.asp?language=English&version=default (accessed on 11 June 2019).

22.	Phatak, A.; Prusi, R.; Ward, B.; Hansen, L.O.; Williams, M.V.; Vetter, E.; Chapman, N.; Postelnick, M. Impact of pharmacist involvement in the transitional care of high-risk patients through medication reconciliation, medication education, and postdischarge call-backs (IPITCH Study). *J. Hosp. Med.* **2016**, *11*, 39–44. [CrossRef]

23.	Engel, K.G.; Buckley, B.A.; Forth, V.E.; McCarthy, D.M.; Ellison, E.P.; Schmidt, M.J.; Adams, J.G. Patient understanding of emergency department discharge instructions: Where are knowledge deficits greatest? *Acad. Emerg. Med.* **2012**, *19*, E1035–E1044. [CrossRef]

24.	Hartwig, S.C.; Siegel, J.; Schneider, P.J. Preventability and severity assessment in reporting adverse drug reactions. *Am. J. Hosp. Pharm.* **1992**, *49*, 2229–2232. [CrossRef] [PubMed]

25.	National Coordinating Council for Medication Error Reporting and Prevention (NCC MERP) Taxonomy of Medication Errors. Available online: http://www.NCCMERP.org (accessed on 28 June 2019).

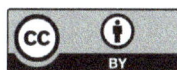

pharmacy

MDPI

Article

Community Pharmacist-Provided Wellness and Monitoring Services in an Employee Wellness Program: A Four-Year Summary

Yifei Liu [1], Kendall D. Guthrie [1,*], Justin R. May [2] and Kristen L. DiDonato [3]

[1] Division of Pharmacy Practice and Administration, School of Pharmacy, University of Missouri-Kansas City, Kansas City, MO 64108, USA
[2] Bothwell Regional Health Center, Sedalia, MO 65301, USA
[3] The Kroger Co. Columbus Division, Kroger Pharmacy, Toledo, OH 43615, USA
* Correspondence: guthriekd@umkc.edu

Received: 27 April 2019; Accepted: 28 June 2019; Published: 2 July 2019

check for updates

Abstract: Objective: To assess the clinical outcomes of participants of an employee wellness program during four years of service implementation. **Methods:** A prospective cohort study was conducted at 15 independent community pharmacy chain locations in northwest and central Missouri. A total of 200 participants were enrolled in an employee wellness program, and the program included five monitoring groups—cholesterol, blood pressure, blood glucose, weight, and healthy participant groups. Participants selected a pharmacist wellness coordinator and wellness appointments were conducted, consisting of education, goal-setting, and monitoring through physical assessment and point of care testing. The primary outcome measures were total cholesterol (TC), triglycerides (TG), high-density lipoprotein cholesterol (HDL-C), low-density lipoprotein cholesterol (LDL-C), systolic blood pressure (SBP), diastolic blood pressure (DBP), fasting blood glucose (FBG), body mass index (BMI), and waist circumference (WC). The secondary outcome measures were the proportion of patients who achieved the clinical value goals at baseline versus 48 months. The primary outcome measures among data collection time points were compared using one-way analysis of variance (ANOVA) tests, and the secondary outcomes were compared between baseline and 48 months by Chi-square or Fisher's exact tests. One-way ANOVA post hoc tests were also performed using least significant difference, to further identify which time points differed from each other. **Results:** At baseline, there were 134 patients in the cholesterol monitoring group, 129 in the weight monitoring group, 117 in the blood pressure monitoring group, 46 in the blood glucose monitoring group, and 26 in the healthy participant monitoring group. For patients in the blood pressure monitoring group, compared with baseline, there was a significant decrease in DBP at months 12, 24, 36, and 48, and a significant increase in the proportion of patients achieving blood pressure goals at 48 months. For patients in the blood glucose monitoring group, compared with baseline, there was a significant decrease in FBG at months 12, 24, 36, and 48, and a significant increase in the proportion of patients achieving blood glucose goals at 48 months. **Conclusions:** Pharmacist-led wellness visits provided to employee wellness patients in a community pharmacy may lead to improvements in BP and FBG values.

Keywords: community pharmacy; pharmacist services; wellness programs

---

1. Introduction

According to the Centers for Disease Control and Prevention, sixty percent of adults in the United States (U.S.) are living with a chronic condition. In addition, forty percent of American adults have been diagnosed with two or more chronic conditions [1]. These chronic conditions significantly contribute to healthcare spending. A report published by the Agency for Healthcare Research and Quality shows eighty-six percent of the total healthcare expenditures was attributed to individuals with one or more chronic conditions. Furthermore, the agency states that seventy-one cents of every healthcare dollar are spent on individuals with multiple chronic conditions [2].

In the U.S., employers cover fifty-eight percent of employee medical costs [3]. Employees with chronic conditions not only incur higher medical costs, but also have more missed workdays and show less productivity [3]. To address these issues, many employers have incorporated wellness initiatives into their benefits programs as a cost-containment strategy. A wide range of employer-sponsored wellness services have been implemented including worksite wellness clinics, web-based programs, activity challenges, medication therapy management services, and disease state management programs [4–22].

Community pharmacists are highly accessible and in an optimal position to provide these services. As the role of the pharmacist shifts from dispensing to service provision, studies have demonstrated the values of pharmacist-provided services [23,24]. In particular, health coaching principles can be utilized by community pharmacists to help patients better manage their chronic conditions or overall health status. Health coaching involves helping an individual take actionable steps towards their health and wellness goals. Health coaches take on many different roles including enhancing wellbeing, providing social support, instruction, and skill development [25].

DiDonato et al. demonstrated that a one-year employee wellness program (EWP) provided by pharmacists significantly lowered patients' cardiovascular risk [26]. This EWP was implemented in an independent community pharmacy chain, and the participants were employees of the company and their spouses. This study is a follow-up to the study of DiDonato et al., and documents the full results during four years of EWP implementation. We intend to build on previous research efforts and further promote pharmacist involvement in wellness initiatives for patients and employer groups. In addition, the complete results of four years would reveal if further clinical improvements were made or if patients reverted to their previous lifestyles.

2. Objective

The objective of this study was to assess the clinical outcomes of participants during four years of EWP implementation. At the time of the study, the EWP was implemented at fifteen rural independent community pharmacy chain locations in northwest and central Missouri. This family-owned chain pharmacy was self-insured.

3. Methods

3.1. Study Design

The study details the full results of the EWP implemented. Of note, the first year's results of 81 patients were previously reported [26]. The inclusion criteria were as follows: 18 years and older, non-pregnant, and employees of the self-insured pharmacy chain or their spouses. All company employees could enroll in the EWP, but those who were not insured with the company's health insurance benefit were excluded from analysis. EWP participants received a discounted rate on their health insurance premium. A study protocol was designed and approved by the University of Missouri-Kansas City Adult Health Sciences Institutional Review Board. Each pharmacy participating in the study obtained a Clinical Laboratory Improvement Amendments certificate of waiver to conduct point-of-care testing. According to this waiver, manufacturer recommendations for using the point-of-care testing equipment were followed and quality control procedures were conducted on all equipment utilized.

3.2. Intervention

At the time of enrollment and annually, participants completed a personal health assessment questionnaire; cardiovascular disease and diabetes risk assessment; and a pharmacist-conducted screening for total cholesterol (TC), serum triglycerides (TG), high-density lipoprotein cholesterol (HDL-C), low-density lipoprotein cholesterol (LDL-C), systolic blood pressure (SBP), diastolic blood pressure (DBP), fasting blood glucose (FBG), weight, body mass index (BMI), and waist circumference (WC).

All wellness coordinators in the program were pharmacists. Participants had the option of personally selecting a pharmacist wellness coordinator or, if no preference, a pharmacist coordinator was assigned to them. Patients were placed into one or more of four monitoring groups (i.e., cholesterol, blood pressure, blood glucose, and weight monitoring groups) if they were identified through screenings to be outside of target ranges or to have a diagnosis of a related chronic condition (established hyperlipidemia, hypertension, and/or diabetes) [26]. The clinical value goals were decided according to the clinical guidelines available at the time of the study [27–30]. Upon enrollment, patients were assigned a TC goal of less than 200 mg/dL; an HDL-C goal of greater than 40 mg/dL (men) and greater than 50 mg/dL (women); and an LDL-C goal of less than 100 mg/dL (coronary heart disease and its risk equivalents), less than 130 mg/dL (multiple risk factors), or less than 160 mg/dL (0–1 risk factor) [27]. Patients without a diagnosis of hypertension or a compelling indication (such as coronary artery disease, heart failure, and diabetes) were assigned a blood pressure goal of less than 120/80 mm Hg. A goal of less than 140/90 mm Hg was assigned to those diagnosed with hypertension. A goal of less than 130/80 mm Hg was assigned to those diagnosed with renal disease, diabetes, or established cardiovascular disease [28]. Participants with diabetes at baseline were assigned a goal of 70–130 mg/dL for fasting blood glucose and a goal of less than 180 mg/dL for postprandial blood glucose. For those without a diagnosis of diabetes, the target FBG was set as less than 100 mg/dL [29]. For all patients, the target BMI was less than 25 kg/m^2. In addition, a waist circumference less than 35 inches for females and less than 40 inches for males was considered as the goal [30].

Individuals could be in more than one patient monitoring group. Otherwise, if none of the above criteria was met, participants were placed into a healthy participant monitoring group. The placement of study subjects into monitoring groups helped guide the education provided by wellness coordinators. Patients in the cholesterol, blood pressure, blood glucose, and weight monitoring groups were encouraged to meet with their wellness coordinator every one to two months, especially for the first year. Participants in the healthy participant monitoring group were encouraged to meet with their wellness coordinator every three months, especially for the first year.

3.3. Practice Innovation

A total of 34 pharmacist wellness coordinators were selected on a voluntary basis. The study took place before the National Consortium for Credentialing Health and Wellness Coaches offered a national certification for health and wellness coaches [31]. While no formal health coach training occurred during the study period, many roles taken on by pharmacists involved in the conduction of study procedures were very similar to the roles of a health coach. Each coordinator received training on the point-of-care testing equipment and physical assessment to ensure appropriate techniques and performance consistency. Additionally, each coordinator was provided with an electronic file package including program policies and procedures, enrollment paperwork, screening documentation forms, assessment tools, physician communication forms, quality assurance forms, and the most current clinical guidelines. These documents were reviewed and updated annually. Furthermore, coordinators were provided with disease-specific monitoring tool kits that contained hardcopies of disease-specific SOAP (subjective, objective, assessment, and plan) note templates, patient report cards, and patient education handouts. Throughout the program, materials were developed by pharmacists and pharmacy students for the following disease states: dyslipidemia, hypertension, diabetes, overweight/obesity, asthma, depression, gastroesophageal reflux disease, menopause, osteoporosis, sleep disorders, smoking cessation, and contraception. These materials served as a resource for coordinators to use during patient encounters. Disease states that were not related to four monitoring groups were more of a focus for those in the healthy participant monitoring group.

Each wellness visit consisted of discussion, disease-specific education, goal setting, and physical assessment, which lasted up to 60 min. The education was structured and delivered face to face. The progress was assessed by comparing results with the previous visits. The visits occurred in a semi-private counseling area during normal work hours and were free of charge. If needed, following a wellness visit, the patient's primary care provider was contacted to notify him/her of the screening results and/or make recommendations regarding medication therapy as warranted.

3.4. Evaluation

To examine the impact of pharmacist wellness and monitoring services, for each group, the primary outcome measures were the clinical values of TC, TG, HDL-C, LDL-C, SBP, DBP, FBG, BMI, and WC at baseline, 12, 24, 36, and 48 months. The secondary outcome measures were the proportion of participants who achieved the clinical value goals at baseline versus 48 months. Data were collected at baseline (i.e., time of enrollment), 12, 24, 36 and 48 months. Participant recruitment was open during the four-year period, but the study ended in year 4. For example, if an individual was enrolled in year 2 and did not drop out, he/she would have data at baseline, 12, 24, and 36 months. Descriptive statistics were calculated for participants' demographics. The primary outcome measures among data collection time points were compared using one-way ANOVA tests. In addition, one-way ANOVA post hoc tests were performed using least significant difference, to further identify which time points differed from each other. The secondary outcomes were compared between baseline and 48 months by Chi-square tests, or Fisher's exact tests if expected values were less than 5. We also performed the same analyses to compare primary and secondary measures after excluding those who withdrew from the program. A *p*-value of <0.05 was considered statistically significant.

The physician communication forms were primarily used to communicate screening results to each patient's primary care provider. This was done to ensure continuity of care and alert the provider of out-of-range results, but these recommendations were not tracked. In addition, this program's savings for the employer were requested, but not all information was made available by the pharmacy administration as a result of barriers to compiling the data. Therefore, pharmacists' recommendations and the program's savings were not assessed in the study.

4. Results

For the first year, 169 patients were eligible and 90 were enrolled, with a response rate of 53.3% [26]. At the end of year 1, 48 participants withdrew from the program; at the end of year 2, 17 withdrew from the program; at the end of year 3, 16 withdrew from the program; and at the end of year 4, 4 withdrew from the program. In total, 85 withdrew from the program. Additionally, 10 of them withdrew before baseline data collection, and were excluded from the study.

A total of 200 participants regardless of start and end date were included in the analyses. For example, if an individual was enrolled but dropped out 12 months later, he/she would be included in analysis at baseline and 12 months. At baseline, there were 134 patients in the cholesterol monitoring group, 129 in the weight monitoring group, 117 in the blood pressure monitoring group, 46 in the blood glucose monitoring group, and 26 in the healthy participant monitoring group (Table 1). For the 200 participants, the average age was 38 years old. Most participants were female and Caucasian with at least some college education. When comparing the patient monitoring groups, the healthy participant group was younger than the other four groups.

Table 1. Participants' demographics in employee wellness program monitoring groups at baseline.

Characteristic	Healthy Group	Cholesterol Monitoring Group	Blood Pressure Monitoring Group	Blood Glucose Monitoring Group	Weight Monitoring Group	All Participants
N	26	134	117	46	129	200
Age, years						
Mean ± SD	30.7 ± 11.8	40.3 ± 13.4	42.3 ± 13.1	46.2 ± 11.7	39.9 ± 12.9	38.4 ± 13.2
(Range)	(19–55)	(19–69)	(21–69)	(19–69)	(19–69)	(19–69)
Gender, n (%)						
Male	4 (15.4%)	30 (22.4%)	32 (27.4%)	14 (30.4%)	30 (23.3%)	44 (22.0%)
Female	22 (84.6%)	104 (77.6%)	85 (72.6%)	32 (69.6%)	99 (76.7%)	156 (78.0%)
Race, n (%)						
Caucasian	25 (96.2%)	128 (95.5%)	110 (94.0%)	43 (93.5%)	122 (94.6%)	190 (95.0%)
African Amer.	0 (0.0%)	2 (1.5%)	4 (3.4%)	2 (4.3%)	2 (1.6%)	4 (2.0%)
Hispanic/Latino	1 (3.8%)	2 (1.5%)	1 (0.9%)	0 (0.0%)	2 (1.6%)	3 (1.5%)
Amer. Indian or Alaskan Native	0 (0.0%)	1 (0.7%)	1 (0.9%)	0 (0.0%)	1 (0.8%)	1 (0.5%)
Not Specified	0 (0.0%)	1 (0.7%)	1 (0.9%)	1 (2.2%)	2 (1.6%)	2 (1.0%)
Education, n (%)						
High school or less	5 (19.2%)	33 (24.6%)	26 (22.2%)	14 (30.5%)	27 (21.0%)	42 (21.0%)
Some college	4 (15.4%)	43 (32.1%)	35 (29.9%)	13 (28.3%)	41 (31.8%)	61 (30.5%)
College grad	6 (23.1%)	26 (19.4%)	26 (22.2%)	8 (17.4%)	27 (20.9%)	40 (20.0%)
Post-grad/ Professional	11 (42.3%)	30 (22.4%)	28 (23.9%)	11 (23.9%)	31 (24.0%)	53 (26.5%)
Not Specified	0 (0.0%)	2 (1.5%)	2 (1.7%)	0 (0.0%)	3 (2.3%)	4 (2.0%)

Note: A patient could be enrolled in multiple monitoring groups at any given time.

Figure 1 displays changes in mean clinical values among the four patient monitoring groups, and Figure 2 compares the proportion of patients achieving clinical value goals between baseline and 48 months. In these figures, the cholesterol monitoring group was associated with clinical values of TC, TG, LDL-C, and HDL-C; the blood pressure monitoring group was associated with SBP and DBP; the blood glucose monitoring group was associated with FBG; and the weight monitoring group was associated with BMI and WC. Clinical values were only reported and compared for the associated monitoring group. For example, clinical values of TC, TG, LDL-C, and HDL-C were only analyzed and reported for the cholesterol monitoring group.

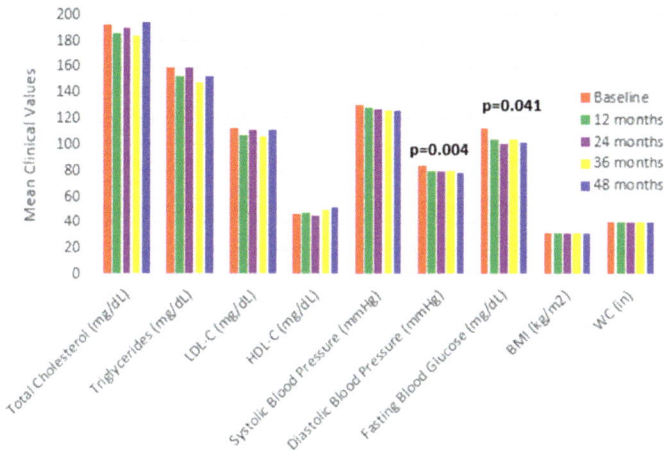

Notes:

Total cholesterol, triglycerides, LDL-C, and HDL-C were reported for the cholesterol monitoring group.

Systolic blood pressure and diastolic blood pressure were reported for the blood pressure monitoring group.

Fasting blood glucose was reported for the blood glucose monitoring group.

BMI and WC were reported for the weight monitoring group.

P-values were only indicated for statistically significant results (p < 0.05).

Figure 1. Changes in mean clinical values among four patient monitoring groups from baseline to 48 months.

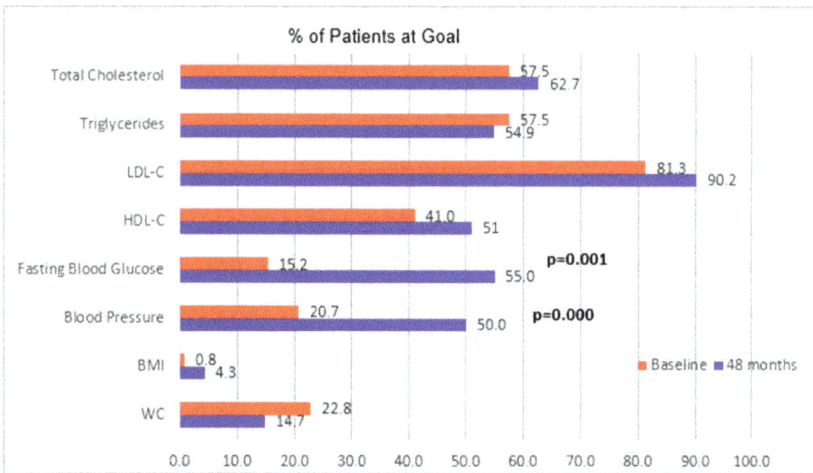

Notes:

Total cholesterol, triglycerides, LDL-C, and HDL-C were reported for the cholesterol monitoring group.

Blood pressure was reported for the blood pressure monitoring group.

Fasting blood glucose was reported for the blood glucose monitoring group.

BMI and WC were reported for the weight monitoring group.

P-values were only indicated for statistically significant results (p < 0.05).

Figure 2. Proportion of patients achieving goals of clinical values among four patient monitoring groups from baseline to 48 months.

The two figures reveal two significant findings. First, for patients in the blood pressure monitoring group, compared with baseline, there was a significant decrease in DBP (Figure 1), and a significant increase in the proportion of patients achieving blood pressure goals at 48 months (Figure 2). Second, for patients in the blood glucose monitoring group, compared with baseline, there was a significant decrease in FBG (Figure 1), and a significant increase in the proportion of patients achieving blood glucose goals at 48 months (Figure 2).

In one-way ANOVA post hoc tests, for DBP, the value at baseline (84.2 mm HG, $n = 117$) was significantly higher than at 12 months (80.2 mm HG, $n = 88$), 24 months (80.3 mm Hg, $n = 68$), 36 months (80.2 mm Hg, $n = 55$), and 48 months (79.0 mm HG, $n = 44$); and the comparisons between any other pairs of time points were not significant. For FBG, the value at baseline (113.2 mg/dL, $n = 45$) was significantly higher than at 12 months (103.7 mg/dl, $n = 37$), 24 months (101.3 mg/dL, $n = 28$), 36 months (103.5 mg/DL, $n = 26$), and 48 months (101.6 mg/dL, $n = 20$); and the comparisons between any other pairs of time points were not significant.

For individuals in the healthy participant monitoring group, no significant findings were found in one-way ANOVA and Chi-square tests (or Fisher's exact tests) for all clinical variables. Regarding potential confounding variables, we assessed smoking (yes/no), alcohol use (yes/no), and exercises (a categorical variable) at baseline. Chi-square tests were used to compare these variables for those in each of the five groups versus not. The results were not significant, so the confounding effects of the three variables could be ruled out.

Furthermore, we reanalyzed the data after excluding 75 participants who withdrew the program, but at least completed baseline data collection. Figure 3 displays changes in mean clinical values among the four patient monitoring groups, and Figure 4 compares the proportion of patients achieving clinical value goals between baseline and 48 months. These results were consistent with the results for all participants. In addition, for patients in the blood pressure monitoring group, compared with baseline, there was also a significant decrease in SBP (Figure 3).

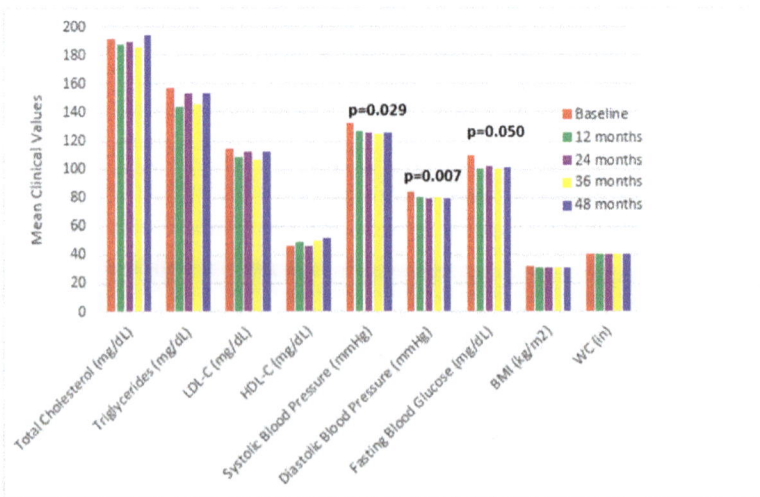

Notes:

Total cholesterol, triglycerides, LDL-C, and HDL-C were reported for the cholesterol monitoring group.

Systolic blood pressure and diastolic blood pressure were reported for the blood pressure monitoring group.

Fasting blood glucose was reported for the blood glucose monitoring group.

BMI and WC were reported for the weight monitoring group.

P-values were only indicated for statistically significant results (p < 0.05).

Figure 3. Changes in mean clinical values among four patient monitoring groups from baseline to 48 months after excluding patients who withdrew from the program.

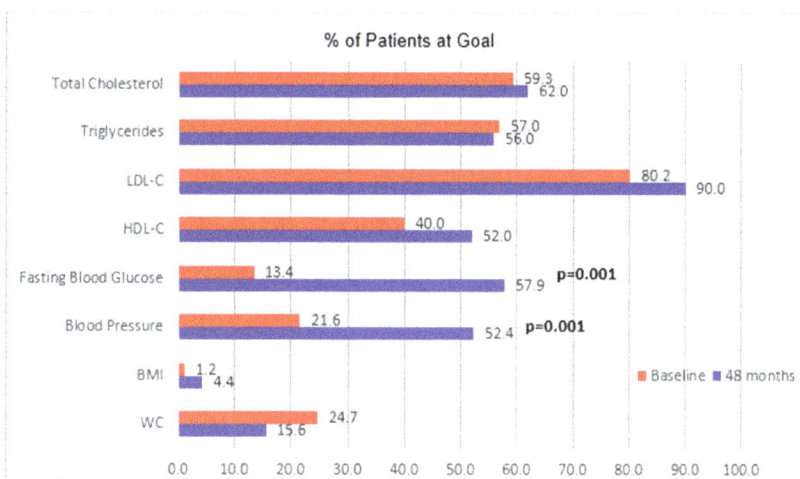

% of Patients at Goal

Notes:

Total cholesterol, triglycerides, LDL-C, and HDL-C were reported for the cholesterol monitoring group.

Blood pressure was reported for the blood pressure monitoring group.

Fasting blood glucose was reported for the blood glucose monitoring group.

BMI and WC were reported for the weight monitoring group.

P-values were only indicated for statistically significant results (p < 0.05).

Figure 4. Proportion of patients achieving goals of clinical values among four patient monitoring groups from baseline to 48 months after excluding patients who withdrew from the program.

5. Discussion

The results of this study show that community pharmacist-led wellness services improved DBP and FBG values in an EWP. In addition, a 2014 systematic review revealed that patients in EWPs have improved quality of life [32]. For an employer, an EWP has been shown to bring $3.48 in return for each dollar spent on the program [33]. Therefore, an EWP offers a great opportunity for pharmacist wellness coordinators to demonstrate their value to both patients and employers.

For both all participants and those who did not withdraw from the program, we found a significant improvement of DBP in the blood pressure monitoring group compared with baseline. However, a significant improvement of SBP was only identified in those who did not drop out. The Seventh Report of the Joint National Committee on Prevention, Detection, Evaluation, and Treatment of High Blood Pressure (JNC-7), the governing blood pressure guideline at the time of study conduction, states there are higher control rates of DBP than SBP. According to the guideline, many primary care physicians were trained to emphasize DBP control more than SBP [27]. In 2017, the American College of Cardiology and the American Heart Association released new guidelines for blood pressure management [34]. The new guidelines classify a blood pressure of 130/80 mm Hg as Stage I hypertension, rather than 140/90 mm Hg in JNC-7. There may be participants who met their blood pressure goal under JNC-7, but would not be at the goal under the new guidelines.

Although DiDonato et al. found significant improvements in cholesterol levels (TC, LDL-C, and HDL-C) for the first year, these improvements were not sustained over the next three years of the program [26]. Similar to the results of DiDonato et al., no significant changes in BMI or WC were observed in the weight monitoring group at 48 months. Of note, the baseline averages of LDL-C, SBP, DBP, and FBG were lower in our study population than in comparable studies, suggesting a healthier baseline patient population [26,35,36]. In addition, following study closure, new cholesterol practice guidelines were published [37]. This new guidance removes the previous goal-driven treatment methodology and supports using maximally tolerated statin therapy. With this new guidance, we might have seen different results in the cholesterol monitoring group, with more participants reaching the "goal" of being on the appropriate statin intensity. Furthermore, we believe that as the program progressed, some patients regressed to previous unhealthy habits.

In this study, FBG rather than HbA1c was evaluated because of four reasons. First of all, when the EWP was developed and implemented, diabetes guidelines recommending HbA1c as a method of diagnosis [38] were not available. Secondly, although some participants did receive HbA1c point-of-care testing, the manufacturer discontinued production of the device for a period of time during the study. Therefore, HbA1c results were not consistently monitored and reported. Thirdly, FBG was a more cost-effective approach as this measurement was included in the cholesterol panel the participants were already receiving. Lastly, most participants in the diabetes monitoring group were not diagnosed with diabetes. As co-morbidity becomes more and more common [1], the number of chronic conditions or out-of-range clinical values could be useful to target and monitor the combination of disease states in an EWP. This raises a question of whether patients who have multiple interventions would have improved health outcomes when compared with those who have a single intervention. In this study, only 39 patients were enrolled in one of the four patient monitoring groups (i.e., they had one disease state and one intervention for that disease state). Because the majority of patients ($n = 136$) were enrolled in more than one patient monitoring group, and most clinical variables had no significant change over a four-year period, it is implied that the impact of multiple inventions was limited in this study.

Despite the encouraged regular meetings between participants and pharmacist wellness coordinators, a study limitation was the decline of participants each year. This could be because of fatigue from regular follow-ups with the coordinators. At each visit, participants were held accountable for the goals set at previous visits. If goals were not being met, this could have led to some patients feeling discouraged or frustrated with the process. As mentioned earlier, another reason could be that participants tended to revert to their previous lifestyles.

Recently, Jones et al. reported that there is little evidence to support the positive impact of employee wellness programs, and most existing studies utilize observational comparisons between a study group and a control group [39]. In a randomized control trial, they identified a strong pattern of selection that program participants were already healthier than non-participants. A response rate of 53.3% for the first year may indicate a potential selection bias that healthier participants were enrolled. In addition, despite having a healthy participant monitoring group, this study did not employ a control group, which was another limitation. Perhaps if we had included a control group, we would have found that individuals in the control group had significant increases in these clinical variables.

There were also two other limitations. First, we did not collect information for all potential confounding variables, such as medication adherence and healthy eating. Second, given the observational study design and the fact that the employees might know each other well, we were unable to control for externalities (e.g., passive smoking or drinking alcohol in some social occasions).

For future EWPs, the training for pharmacist wellness coordinators should include how to conduct participant follow-ups to ensure participants feel the value of the service. We believe that regular and effective follow-ups could not only have prevented participants from dropping out of the EWP, but also from reverting to unhealthy behaviors. In addition, future EWPs could consider applying additional incentives, as feasible, to encourage participation and motivate participants to reach their goals. To encourage participation in the EWP, participants received a discounted health insurance premium of $50, pedometers, and water bottles. However, incentives directly associated with outcomes, such as a cash reward for meeting goals, may have been more motivating to individuals versus a cost-savings incentive structure. In a study conducted by Schramm et al., a financially incentivized weight loss challenge led to significant weight loss in the study population [22]. Interestingly, Jones et al. revealed a diminishing effect on participation when the incentive was increased from $100 to $200 [39]. Including incentives focused on achievement of goals in addition to incentives for participation may have led to improved outcomes.

6. Conclusions

Pharmacist-led wellness visits provided to employee wellness patients in a community pharmacy may lead to improvements in BP and FBG values. Significant improvements were seen in cholesterol outcome measures after one year of the program, but were not sustained over the next three years, suggesting participants may have reverted to their previous habits.

Author Contributions: Conceptualization, J.R.M. and K.L.D.; Methodology, Y.L., J.R.M., and K.L.D.; Validation, Y.L. and K.L.D.; Formal Analysis, Y.L.; Investigation, Y.L., K.D.G., J.R.M., and K.L.D.; Data Curation, K.L.D.; Writing—Original Draft Preparation, Y.L., K.D.G., and K.L.D.; Writing—Review & Editing, Y.L., K.D.G., J.R.M., and K.L.D.; Project Administration, K.D.G., J.R.M., and K.L.D.

Funding: This research received no external funding.

Conflicts of Interest: The authors declare no conflict of interest.

References

1. National Center for Chronic Disease Prevention and Health Promotion (NCCDPHP); Centers for Disease Control and Prevention. About Chronic Diseases. 2018. Available online: https://www.cdc.gov/chronicdisease/about/index.htm (accessed on 1 March 2019).

2. Department of Health and Human Services; Agency for Healthcare Quality and Research. Multiple Chronic Conditions Chartbook. 2014. Available online: https://www.ahrq.gov/sites/default/files/wysiwyg/professionals/prevention-chronic-care/decision/mcc/mccchartbook.pdf (accessed on 1 March 2019).

3. Asay, G.R.B.; Roy, K.; Lang, J.E.; Payne, R.L.; Howard, D.H. Absenteeism and employer costs associated with chronic diseases and health risk factors in the US workforce. *Prev Chronic Dis.* **2016**, *13*, E141. [CrossRef] [PubMed]

4. Bright, D.R.; Terrell, S.L.; Rush, M.J.; Kroustos, K.R.; Stockert, A.L.; Swanson, S.C.; DiPietro, N.A. Employee Attitudes Toward Participation in a Work Site-Based Health and Wellness Clinic. *J. Pharm. Pract.* **2012**, *25*, 530–536. [CrossRef] [PubMed]

5. Dalal, K.; Khoury, A.; Nyce, S. Demonstrating high performance at an on-site corporate health center. *Benefits Q.* **2014**, *30*, 55–67. [PubMed]

6. Berdine, H.J.; O'Neil, C.K. Development and implementation of a pharmacist-managed university-based wellness center. *J. Am. Pharm. Assoc.* **2007**, *47*, 390–397. [CrossRef] [PubMed]

7. Borah, B.J.; Egginton, J.S.; Shah, N.D.; Wagie, A.E.; Olsen, K.D.; Yao, X.; Lopez-Jimenez, F. Association of Worksite Wellness Center Attendance with Weight Loss and Health Care Cost Savings. *J. Occup. Environ. Med.* **2015**, *57*, 229–234. [CrossRef] [PubMed]

8. Fanous, A.M.; Kier, K.L.; Rush, M.J.; Terrell, S. Impact of a 12-week, pharmacist-directed walking program in an established employee preventive care clinic. *Am. J. Health Pharm.* **2014**, *71*, 1219–1225. [CrossRef]

9. Williams, L.C.; Day, B.T. Medical Cost Savings for Web-Based Wellness Program Participants from Employers Engaged in Health Promotion Activities. *Am. J. Health Promot.* **2011**, *25*, 272–280. [CrossRef]

10. Nishita, C.; Cardazone, G.; Uehara, D.L.; Tom, T. Empowered diabetes management: Life coaching and pharmacist counseling for employed adults with diabetes. *Health Educ. Behav.* **2012**, *40*, 581–591. [CrossRef]

11. Johnson, C.L.; Nicholas, A.; Divine, H.; Perrier, D.G.; Blumenschein, K.; Steinke, D.T. Outcomes from DiabetesCARE: A pharmacist-provided diabetes management service. *J. Am. Pharm. Assoc.* **2008**, *48*, 722–730. [CrossRef]

12. Wilson, J.B.; Osterhaus, M.C.; Farris, K.B.; Doucette, W.R.; Currie, J.D.; Bullock, T.; Kumbera, P. Financial Analysis of Cardiovascular Wellness Program Provided to Self-Insured Company from Pharmaceutical Care Provider's Perspective. *J. Am. Pharm. Assoc.* **2005**, *45*, 588–592. [CrossRef]

13. Yoder, V.G.; Dixon, D.L.; Barnette, D.J.; Beardsley, J.R.; Pawloski, P.; Cusick, D.; Amborn, L. Short-term outcomes of an employer-sponsored diabetes management program at an ambulatory care pharmacy clinic. *Am. J. Health Pharm.* **2012**, *69*, 69–73. [CrossRef] [PubMed]

14. Pinto, S.L.; Bechtol, R.A.; Partha, G. Evaluation of outcomes of a medication therapy management program for patients with diabetes. *J. Am. Pharm. Assoc.* **2012**, *52*, 519–523. [CrossRef] [PubMed]

15. Divine, H.; Nicholas, A.; Johnson, C.L.; Perrier, D.G.; Steinke, D.T.; Blumenschein, K. PharmacistCARE: Description of a pharmacist care service and lessons learned along the way. *J. Am. Pharm. Assoc.* **2008**, *48*, 793–802. [CrossRef] [PubMed]

16. Kraemer, D.F.; Kradjan, W.A.; Bianco, T.M.; Low, J.A. A randomized study to assess the impact of pharmacist counseling of employer-based health plan beneficiaries with diabetes: The EMPOWER study. *J Pharm. Pract.* **2012**, *25*, 169–179. [CrossRef] [PubMed]

17. Iyer, R.; Coderre, P.; McKelvey, T.; Cooper, J.; Berger, J.; Moore, E.; Kushner, M. An employer-based, pharmacist intervention model for patients with type 2 diabetes. *Am. J. Health Pharm.* **2010**, *67*, 312–316. [CrossRef] [PubMed]

18. Shimp, L.A.; Kucukarslan, S.N.; Elder, J.; Remington, T.; Wells, T.; Choe, H.M.; Lewis, N.J.; Kirking, D.M. Employer-based patient-centered medication therapy management program: Evidence and recommendations for future programs. *J. Am. Pharm. Assoc.* **2012**, *52*, 768–776. [CrossRef] [PubMed]

19. Johannigman, M.J.; Leifheit, M.; Bellman, N.; Pierce, T.; Marriott, A.; Bishop, C.; Johannigmn, M.J. Medication therapy management and condition care services in a community-based employer setting. *Am. J. Health Pharm.* **2010**, *67*, 1362–1367. [CrossRef]

20. Theising, K.M.; Fritschle, T.L.; Scholfield, A.M.; Hicks, E.L.; Schymik, M.L. Implementation and Clinical Outcomes of an Employer-Sponsored, Pharmacist-Provided Medication Therapy Management Program. *Pharmacother. J. Hum. Pharmacol. Drug Ther.* **2015**, *35*, e159–e163. [CrossRef]

21. Wittayanukorn, S.; Westrick, S.C.; Hansen, R.A.; Billor, N.; Braxton-Lloyd, K.; Fox, B.I.; Garza, K.B. Evaluation of Medication Therapy Management Services for Patients with Cardiovascular Disease in a Self-Insured Employer Health Plan. *J. Manag. Care Pharm.* **2013**, *19*, 385–395. [CrossRef]

22. Schramm, A.M.; DiDonato, K.L.; May, J.R.; Hartwig, D.M. Implementation of a financially incentivized weight loss competition into an already established employee wellness program. *Innov. Pharm.* **2014**, *5*. [CrossRef]

23. Cranor, C.; Bunting, B.; Christensen, D.B. The Asheville Project: Long-term clinical and economic outcomes of a community pharmacy diabetes care program. *J. Am. Pharm. Assoc.* **2009**, *49*, 164–170. [CrossRef]

24. Fera, T.; Bluml, B.M.; Ellis, W.M. Diabetes Ten City Challenge: Final economic and clinical results. *J. Am. Pharm. Assoc.* **2009**, *49*, 383–391. [CrossRef]

25. May, C.S.; Russell, C.S. Health Coaching: Adding Value in Healthcare Reform. *Glob. Adv. Health Med.* **2013**, *2*, 92–94. [CrossRef] [PubMed]

26. DiDonato, K.L.; May, J.R.; Lindsey, C.C. Impact of wellness coaching and monitoring services provided in a community pharmacy. *J. Am. Pharm. Assoc.* **2013**, *53*, 14–21. [CrossRef] [PubMed]

27. Expert Panel on Detection, Evaluation, and Treatment of High Blood Cholesterol in Adults. Executive summary of the Third Report of the National Cholesterol Education Program (NCEP) Expert Panel on Detection, Evaluation, and Treatment of High Blood Cholesterol in Adults (Adult Treatment Panel III). *JAMA* **2001**, *285*, 2486–2497. [CrossRef] [PubMed]

28. Chobanian, A.V.; Bakris, G.L.; Black, H.R.; Cushman, W.C.; Green, L.A.; Izzo, J.L., Jr.; Jones, D.W.; Materson, B.J.; Oparil, S.; Wright, J.T., Jr.; et al. The seventh report of the Joint National Committee on Prevention, Detection, Evaluation, and Treatment of High Blood Pressure: The JNC 7 (Express) Report. *JAMA* **2003**, *289*, 2560–2572. [CrossRef]

29. American Diabetes Association. Standards of Medical Care in Diabetes 2010. *Diabetes Care* **2010**, *33*, S11–S61. [CrossRef] [PubMed]

30. NHLBI Obesity Education Initiative Expert Panel on the Identification, Evaluation, and Treatment of Overweight and Obesity in Adults. *Clinical Guidelines on the Identification, Evaluation, and Treatment of Overweight and Obesity in Adults*; Publication No. 98-4083; National Institutes of Health: Bethesda, MD, USA, 1998.

31. Stelter, N.; DiDonato, K.L. Health Coaching. In *Pharmacotherapy Self-Assessment Program (PSAP) Book 2 (CNS/Pharmacy Practice)*, 8th ed.; American College of Clinical Pharmacy: Lenexa, KS, USA, 2015.

32. Kivelä, K.S.; Elo, S.; Kyngäs, H.; Kääriäinen, M. The effects of health coaching on adult patients with chronic diseases: A systematic review. *Patient Educ. Couns.* **2014**, *97*, 147–157. [CrossRef]

33. Keller, P.A.; Lehmann, D.R.; Milligan, K.J. Effectiveness of Corporate Well-Being Programs. *J. Macromark.* **2009**, *29*, 279–302. [CrossRef]

34. Whelton, P.K.; Carey, R.M.; Aronow, W.S.; Casey, D.E.; Collins, K.J.; Himmelfarb, C.D.; DePalma, S.M.; Gidding, S.; Jamerson, K.A.; Jones, D.W.; et al. 2017 ACC/AHA/AAPA/ABC/ACPM/AGS/APhA/ASH/ASPC/NMA/PCNA Guideline for the Prevention, Detection, Evaluation, and Management of High Blood Pressure in Adults: A Report of the American College of Cardiology/American Heart Association Task Force on Clinical Practice Guidelines. *Hypertension* **2017**, *71*, e13–e115.

35. Bluml, B.M.; McKenney, J.M.; Cziraky, M.J. Pharmaceutical Care Services and Results in Project ImPACT: Hyperlipidemia. *J. Am. Pharm. Assoc. (1996)* **2000**, *40*, 157–165. [CrossRef]

36. Bunting, B.A.; Smith, B.H.; Sutherland, S.E. The Asheville Project: Clinical and economic outcomes of a community-based long-term medication therapy management program for hypertension and dyslipidemia. *J. Am. Pharm. Assoc.* **2008**, *48*, 23–31. [CrossRef] [PubMed]

37. Grundy, S.M.; Stone, N.J.; Bailey, A.L.; Beam, C.; Birtcher, K.K.; Blumenthal, R.S.; Braun, L.T.; de Ferranti, S.; Faiella-Tommasino, J.; Forman, D.E.; et al. 2018 AHA/ACC/AACVPR/AAPA/ABC/ACPM/ADA/AGS/APhA/ASPC/NLA/PCNA Guideline on the Management of Blood Cholesterol: A Report of the American College of Cardiology/American Heart Association Task Force on Clinical Practice Guidelines. *J. Am. Coll. Cardiol.* **2019**, *73*, 3168–3209. [CrossRef] [PubMed]

38. American Diabetes Association. 2. Classification and Diagnosis of Diabetes: Standards of Medical Care in Diabetes-2018. *Diabetes Care* **2018**, *41* (Suppl. 1), S13–S27. [CrossRef] [PubMed]

39. Jones, D.; Molitor, D.; Reif, J. *What Do Workplace Wellness Programs Do? Evidence from the Illinois Workplace Wellness Study.* NBER Working Paper #24229. 2018. Available online: https://www.nber.org/papers/w24229 (accessed on 1 July 2019).

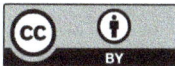

pharmacy

MDPI

Article

"It Made a Difference to Me": A Comparative Case Study of Community Pharmacists' Care Planning Services in Primary Health Care

Theresa J. Schindel[iD]**, Rene R. Breault and Christine A. Hughes ***

Faculty of Pharmacy and Pharmaceutical Sciences, University of Alberta, 3-171 Edmonton Clinic Health Academy, 11405 87 Avenue NW, Edmonton, AB T6G 1C9, Canada
* Correspondence: christine.hughes@ualberta.ca; Tel.: +1-780-492-5903

Received: 28 May 2019; Accepted: 7 July 2019; Published: 11 July 2019

check for
updates

Abstract: In some jurisdictions, governments and the public look to community pharmacies to provide expanded primary health care services, including care plans with follow-up. Care planning services, covered by the Compensation Plan in Alberta, Canada, require pharmacists to assess an eligible patient's health history, medication history, and drug-related problems to establish goals of treatment, interventions, and monitoring plan. Follow-up assessments are also covered by the Compensation Plan. A comparative case study method facilitated an in-depth investigation of care planning services provided by four community pharmacy sites. Data from 77 interviews, 61 site-specific documents, and 94 h of observation collected over 20 months were analyzed using an iterative constant comparative approach. Using a sociomaterial theoretical framework, the perceived value of care planning services was examined through an investigation of the relationships and interactions between people and information. Patients perceived the value of care planning as related to waiting time to access care and co-creating individualized plans. Physicians and other health care professionals valued collaboration, information sharing, and different perspectives on patient care. Pharmacists valued collaboration with patients and other health care professionals, which renewed their sense of responsibility, increased satisfaction, and gave meaning to their role.

Keywords: pharmacist services; community pharmacy; care plan; compensation; primary health care; information sharing; qualitative research; comparative case study; value

1. Introduction

Primary health care is based on the principles of equity, collaboration, and community participation [1]. It has been defined as the first place individuals go to receive health care services [2]. Attributes of primary health care include patient and family centeredness, continuity of relationships, and information continuity and management [3]. The delivery of primary health care involves teams of health care providers; the exact composition of these teams depends on patients' needs. As team members, pharmacists do their part to meet patients' needs and provide essential drugs. In many parts of the world, pharmacists are becoming increasingly involved in the delivery of primary health care, contributing to chronic disease management and providing immunization services [4,5] and the community pharmacy is a place that the public would go to receive some primary health care services [6,7]. Describing community pharmacists as "primary care pharmacists" recognizes not only their accessibility to patients, but also their contributions as team members delivering primary health care services including management of chronic conditions such as hypertension, treatment of minor ailments, administration of vaccinations, and triaging and referring patients with acute conditions to emergency departments or family physicians [8,9]. Governments, such as those in Canada and

Alberta, and the public therefore look to community pharmacists as providers of primary health care services [2,10].

Research examining pharmacists' preferences for existing and potential roles indicates a preference to provide more patient-centered services [11] and to contribute more to meeting primary health care needs in their communities through teamwork [12]. Pharmacists are now involved in providing enhanced services that support primary health care such as comprehensive medication reviews, immunizations, adherence packaging, and development of comprehensive care plans with follow-up [13].

A care plan is an essential component of the patient care process [14] and refers to a detailed document prepared by a pharmacist that outlines the pharmacist's and patient's responsibilities to resolve drug therapy problems or health needs to achieve the patient's health goals, and to prevent potential drug therapy problems. Care plans are developed with input and participation of the patient and can be developed collaboratively with other health care providers involved in the patient's care [15]. Documented care plans are fundamental to delivery of pharmaceutical care services [14,16], quality care, and communication with team members [17]. For example, care plans for chronic disease management can improve information sharing, enhance patients' engagement in self-management, and promote collaboration among health care professionals [18]. Involvement in care planning services has the potential to increase the engagement of pharmacists in primary health care [19] and increase recognition of the value of pharmacists' contributions to patient care.

Demonstrating value in primary health care addresses the triple aim of health systems to improve patient health outcomes, improve patient experience of care, and reduce health care costs [20,21]. Other approaches to show value acknowledge the role of care planning, along with access to care, continuity of care, relationships, evidence-based therapy, and patient engagement in the process [22]. Parameters that may be useful to demonstrate the value of care planning include patients' experienced health, increased accessibility, building of trust, improved communication with care providers, relationship continuity of patients and care providers over time, information management [23,24], and experiences of health care providers including conditions that support health care providers to find meaning in their work [25].

Although care plans communicate value from perspectives of the effectiveness and cost-effectiveness of pharmacy services [26] and provide documentation that supports bi-directional communication of health care providers [27], very little research has been conducted regarding the perceived value of pharmacists' care planning services. This study addresses this gap from the perspectives of patients and health care providers who have experience with care planning services. The overall objectives of this study are to explore how care pharmacists' planning services covered by the Compensation Plan in Alberta were implemented and the perceived value of the care planning services. This paper aims to contribute to what is known about the perceived value of care planning services provided by pharmacists through community pharmacies.

2. Materials and Methods

2.1. Context

The setting for this research is the western-Canadian province of Alberta. Since 2006, pharmacists can access patient information including laboratory tests and records of dispensed medications through a provincial electronic health record known as Netcare [28]. The scope of practice for Albertan pharmacists enables them to order laboratory tests, administer drugs by injection, and prescribe drugs. Prescribing authority involves 3 types of prescribing: emergency prescribing, adapting prescriptions, and independent prescribing [29]. All pharmacists can prescribe in an emergency when patients cannot access other health services and all have authority to adapt a prescription initiated by another prescriber. When pharmacists prescribe by adapting a prescription, they may modify a prescription to extend therapy, change a dose or formulation. Pharmacists who have successfully applied for Additional

Prescribing Authorization (APA) may also prescribe to initiate new drug therapy [29]. The APA application process involves peer review of a prescribing portfolio that includes narrative description of the pharmacists' practice, documentation of patient care cases, and self-assessment of prescribing competencies [30]. Documentation of prescribing decisions is required along with communication with any other health professional whose care of a patient may be affected by the pharmacist's prescribing decision [31]. At the time of this study, Alberta had a population of 4.2 million [32]. There were 5363 practicing pharmacists including 1658 with APA, 1377 registered pharmacy technicians, and 1232 licensed pharmacies [33]. Community pharmacy practice in Alberta varies from pharmacist to pharmacist within the scope of practice and their roles are continually evolving [34,35].

The Compensation Plan for Pharmacy Services, approved by the Government of Alberta and implemented in 2012, supports the scope of practice for pharmacists in Alberta by offering one of the most comprehensive fee schedules available for remuneration of pharmacy services in Canada [36]. It allows for payment to community pharmacies for a range of pharmacy services provided by pharmacists such as prescription renewals, administration of drugs and vaccines by injection, and care planning services, including follow-up assessments [37]. Since implementation, the number of compensated services increased from 30,000 per month (July 2012) to 170,000 per month (March 2016) and Comprehensive Annual Care Plans (CACP) and CACP follow-up assessments were among the top 8 services claimed by community pharmacies [36]. Similar to medication therapy management (MTM) services provided by pharmacists under the Medicare Modernization Act (2003) in the United States (US) [38], Albertan pharmacists involved in care planning services must assess a patient's health and medication history, establish goals of treatment, suggest interventions, and implement a monitoring plan. To be eligible for a CACP covered under the Compensation Plan, patients must meet certain criteria; for example, they must have specific chronic diseases (e.g., diabetes) or have certain risk factors (e.g., tobacco use).

CACP is defined as "a plan that is prepared and documented by a Clinical Pharmacist that documents the required elements" (see Table 1) [39]. The components of the plan are consistent with the patient care processes outlined by the National Association of Pharmacy Regulatory Authorities in Canada [15] and National Association of Joint Commission of Pharmacy Practitioners in the US [14]. Different from MTM services in the US, the CACP service criteria are fixed and the Alberta government pays pharmacies for the service as long as patients are covered by the provincial health care system (i.e., have an Alberta health care number). CACPs are developed by pharmacists in collaboration with the patient, after which all interactions are documented and shared with other health care professionals involved in the patient's care [36]. Community pharmacies and pharmacists developed customized CACP templates as there are no prescribed care plan documentation templates. Patients must sign that they have reviewed and discussed their CACP with the pharmacist who prepared it as well as received a summary of the CACP [39]. Pharmacists with appropriate authorizations, including APA or injections, may implement interventions such as adjusting doses of chronic medications, prescribing smoking cessation therapy, or administering vaccines. Pharmacists may choose to suggest or discuss interventions with the patient's physician or refer to other health care providers.

2.2. Theoretical Framework

The theoretical framework for this study draws on sociomaterial theory [40] and document theory [41], allowing us to explore the value of care planning services (Figure 1). A sociomaterial approach recognizes the importance of the social (i.e., relational) and material (i.e., care plans) aspects of everyday activities and their influence on our understanding of reality. A care plan, as a physical (material) document, combined with human (social) endeavors, serves to include, exclude and regulate actions [42]. Document theory considers a care plan as a source of information existing in 3 dimensions: material, social, and mental [41]. Thus, research based on document theory explores how these dimensions interact in different environments in which documentation takes place; in this study, document theory is applied in the context of care planning services associated with primary health care.

In pharmacy practice, care plan documents themselves may be in the background when contemplating primary health care services. By acknowledging the role of these documents, this study brings care plans to the foreground of scholarly thinking, making them visible and asserting their value as part of the care planning services provided by pharmacists.

Table 1. Summary of patient eligibility criteria, information, and fees associated with Comprehensive Annual Care Plan (CACP) services [37,39].

	CACP [1]	CACP Follow-up
Patient eligibility criteria	Two or more of the following chronic conditions: Hypertension Diabetes Chronic obstructive pulmonary disorder Asthma Heart failure Angina pectoris Ischemic heart disease Mental health disorder OR One of the above conditions plus 1 risk factor: Tobacco Obesity Addiction	CACP must have been completed. CACP Follow-up may be provided if a referral from a physician or hospital admission/discharge within 14 days of the CACP service OR A pharmacist determines that follow-up is needed.
Information gathered and recorded	Demographics Allergies and intolerances Health conditions Symptoms or signs to be treated Pregnancy or lactation status Medication use history/review (Best Possible Medication History—BPMH) Other health care products or devices Lifestyle factors—weight, tobacco use, illicit drug use, alcohol use, exercise Laboratory values Care plan—agreed goals of medication therapy, drug therapy problems, identification of possible interventions, plans for monitoring, and follow-up assessment	
Fees [2]	$100 [3]	$20 [4]

[1] CACPs—Comprehensive Annual Care Plans; [2] Canadian dollars; [3] Limit of 1 CACP per year; [4] Limit of 12 CACP Follow-up per year.

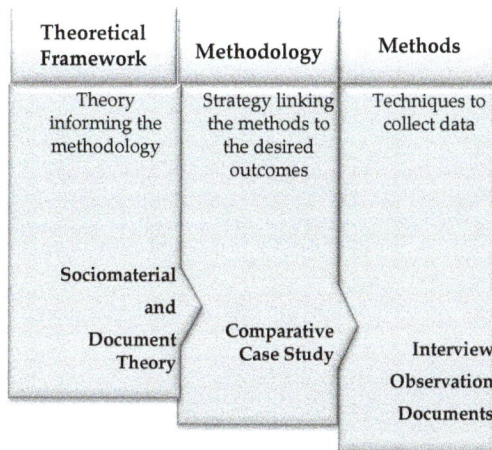

Figure 1. Elements of research used in this study.

2.3. Methodology—Comparative Case Study

A comparative case study approach was used in order to gain an in-depth understanding of compensated care planning services within the real-world context of patient care in community pharmacy practice in Alberta [43,44]. The unit of study, or the case, was the CACP [45]. Case study research is ideal for exploring "how" and "why" research questions [45]. As part of larger study, the case study method was chosen to explore how pharmacists implemented care planning services and why services are perceived as valuable. Case study research may involve a single case or multiple case design [43]. This comparative case study was designed to include 4 different community pharmacy sites, or cases, a priori. The more sites included in a comparative case study, the greater the range of variation, thus the greater the contribution to what is known about care planning services in different contexts [43].

2.4. Methods

Three methods of data collection were used in this study: interviews, observation, and documents. Interviews were semi-structured, consisted of open-ended questions, were conducted by members of the research team, were approximately 30–60 min in length, and were conversational in style (Appendix A, Table A1). One research team member was assigned to each site. The lead team member coordinated the site visit with the research assistant and both were involved in data collection. The research assistants were trained by the co-principal investigators. Most interviews were conducted in person at the sites. Some interviews with patients and physicians were conducted over the telephone following site visits. Interviews were audio recorded and transcribed verbatim. The second method of data collection, direct observation of the provision of patient care services, permitted the study of care planning within its natural setting or real-world context [45]. Researchers observed individuals involved in care planning services (pharmacists, pharmacy technicians, pharmacy staff, other health care providers, and patients), took field notes, and wrote a narrative description based on what was seen, heard, or sensed on site [44]. Observational data were collected at the time of the site visits using a pre-prepared form to guide documentation of observations and support reflexive research practices (Appendix A, Table A2). The research team developed the observation form to address the research questions. Observations focused on care planning interactions between pharmacists and patients, pharmacists and pharmacy staff, as well as development, storing and sharing of the care plan document. The researcher documented observations in a notebook, using the observation form as a guide. After the interaction concluded, the researcher transcribed notes to an electronic version of the observation form. A summary of interview questions related to observations were noted. Site-specific documents related to CACP services such as care plan templates and communication templates were also collected at site visits (Appendix A, Table A3). Data collected from observation and documents were incorporated into the interview process to invite materiality into interviews (Figure 2) [46].

2.5. Recruitment

The researchers identified types of community pharmacy sites where services covered by the Compensation Plan for Pharmacy Services were provided. Sites were selected by the research team using a purposive sampling technique [47] based on pre-defined variables [44]. The study included 4 community pharmacy sites where CACP services were provided, selected based on the following information: type of pharmacy (independent, franchise, corporate), population size (population centre) [48], volume of CACP services (number of reported CACPs provided per month), and provision of other compensated services (pharmacists with APA and injections authorization). A list of pharmacies and prescribing pharmacists provided by the Alberta College of Pharmacy and guidance from the Research Advisory Committee members were used to identify community pharmacy sites that represented pre-defined variables and likely to be engaged in care planning services under the Compensation Plan for Pharmacy Services.

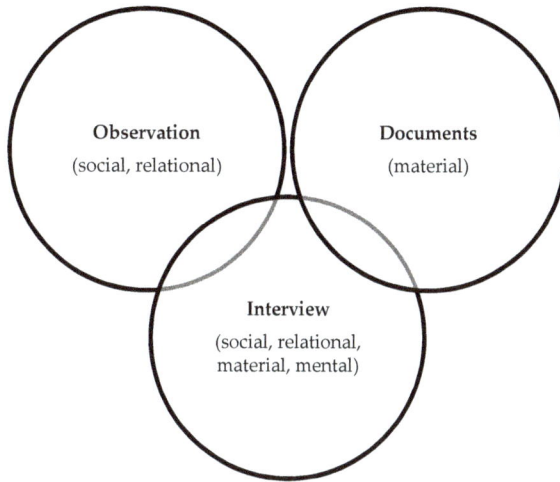

Figure 2. Methods of data collection used in this study. Interviews incorporated data from observation and documents.

Pharmacy managers were initially approached by a member of the research team to discuss their pharmacy as a potential site for the case study. A total of 5 sites were recruited. One site withdrew from the study prior to the start of data collection due to unexpected staffing changes. All 4 cases involved community pharmacies and extended beyond the physical space to include patients, physicians, and other health care professionals involved in care planning services. Participants were recruited on site (patients, pharmacists, pharmacy technicians, pharmacy students, and staff) and in the local community (other health care providers involved with the pharmacist in the care planning process) [49]. Other health care providers included nurses, nurse practitioners, and physicians. Information posters about the study were displayed at the community pharmacies to indicate that researchers were on site and invited patients to approach researchers if they were interested in the study. Physicians associated with the community pharmacies and involved with care planning services were identified by the community pharmacists or patients and subsequently invited to participate in the study by the researchers. All participants provided informed consent. This research study was approved by the University of Alberta Health Research Ethics Board (Pro00059814).

2.6. Data Analysis

Data from interviews, observations, and documents collected at the sites were analyzed using an inductive constant comparative approach based on constructivist grounded theory [47]. Following transcription of the interviews, a member of the research team reviewed each transcript for accuracy and removed identifying information such as names of individuals, pharmacies, and towns or cities. The initial analysis entailed line-by-line coding of each phrase or portion of data from the various data sources by 1 research team member. All team members reviewed codes, emerging concepts, and supporting data following each site visit and at monthly research meetings to reach consensus. In keeping with the grounded theory approach, interview questions were adjusted to ensure an in-depth understanding of concepts (see Appendix A, Table A1). Separate analysis of data from each site permitted comparison of the data in terms of perceived value of care planning services. NVivo 12 software was used for storing data, coding, and analysis.

2.7. Rigour

The case study method is a rigorous qualitative research approach that ensures the trustworthiness of the results of research [50]. Elements of trustworthiness include credibility, dependability, confirmability, and transferability; these are parallel concepts to internal validity, reliability–reproducibility, objectivity, and generalizability, all concepts associated with the quality of quantitative research [51]. Trustworthiness was achieved through use of a combination of data sources (credibility), in-depth presentation of data and analysis (dependability), detailed documentation at all research stages, and sharing of research results with participants (confirmability). Based on this description of the study setting, readers can judge for themselves about the transferability of its results to other contexts.

2.8. Reflexivity

The roles and views of research team members were discussed throughout the research process: personal views and positions on the Compensation Plan for Pharmacy Services, the effect of care planning services on the pharmacy sites included in this study, the influence of archival documents and the media reports of compensated pharmacy services by the public and other audiences [52]. The research team addressed these issues reflexively at monthly research meetings held throughout the planning, data collection, analysis, and reporting phases of the project. In addition, reflexivity was incorporated in the form used to document observational data (Appendix A, Table A2). All members of the research team are associated with the pharmacy profession, 2 as practicing pharmacists (C.A.H., R.R.B.), but not involved in provision of compensated CACP services in community pharmacy practice.

3. Results

3.1. Sites

The four sites recruited for this study represented different practice contexts associated with CACP services. These included two independent pharmacies, a franchise pharmacy, and a large corporate chain pharmacy, all from population centers ranging widely in size [48,53]. Site 1 served a small population center as well as rural communities within 100 km of the community pharmacy. Site 2 served patients in an inner-city neighborhood in a large population center. Site 3 was located in a suburban area and routinely involved pharmacy students from the University of Alberta in care planning services. Site 4 provided CACPs for patients in care facilities outside of the pharmacy and worked closely with family physicians in primary care practices. At all sites, pharmacists integrated CACP services within their established practices. Sites 1, 2, and 3 developed approximately 20 CACPs each month, whereas Site 4 developed over 100 CACPs per month. Details of the sites are summarized in Table 2.

Table 2. Details of sites included in this study.

Description	Site 1	Site 2	Site 3	Site 4
Pharmacy type [53]	Independent	Franchise	Corporate	Independent
Population center [48]	Small [1]	Large [2]	Medium [3]	Large [2]
Pharmacists (with APA [4], injections authorization)	3 (3,3)	3 (1,3)	3 (1,3)	5 (4,5)
Registered technicians	1	-	1	2
Assistants	3	3	2	6
Pharmacy students	-	Periodically	Regularly	-
CACPs [5] completed per month	<20	<20	<20	>100

[1] Population between 1000 and 29,999; [2] Population of 100,000 and over; [3] Population between 30,000 and 99,999; [4] APA—Additional Prescribing Authorization; [5] CACPs—Comprehensive Annual Care Plans.

3.2. Data Collected

Data were collected over a period of 20 months between May 2016 and January 2018. Each site was visited three times over the course of a year, typically at 6 and 12 months following the initial visit. The data set included 77 interviews, 94 h of observation, and 61 site-specific documents. Table 3 summarizes the numbers of interviews and observation hours. Researchers collected document templates developed by each site to facilitate information gathering (e.g., care plan, patient assessment, medication history) and sharing (e.g., letters to physicians, medication lists, patient action plans). Types of documents collected are listed in Appendix A, Table A3.

Table 3. Interviews and observation hours.

Data	Site 1	Site 2	Site 3	Site 4	Total
Total number of interviews	27	15	16	19	77
Patient	11	5	8	5	29
Physician	2	2	-	2	6
Nurse	2	-	-	3	5
Pharmacy staff	4	4	2	3	13
Pharmacy student	-	-	2	-	2
Pharmacist [1]	8	4	4	6	22
Hours of observation	24	28.5	26	15.5 [2]	94

[1] The number of pharmacist interviews exceeds the number of pharmacists participating in the study due to the fact that multiple interviews were conducted over the 12-month data collection period at each site. Some pharmacists were interviewed more than once; [2] The number of observation hours required at site 4 was less than other sites due to the higher number of care planning services observed.

3.3. Value of Care Planning Services

The value of care planning services was evident in the interactions between people and information. Six areas of value were identified: reinforcing patient-centered care, reducing waiting time for care, co-creating individualized plans with patients, collaborating with physicians and other health care providers, revealing possibilities for pharmacists' contributions to primary health care, and making sense of pharmacists' roles in primary health care. Results are presented in the sections below. They reflect a sociomaterial exploration of value, which emphasizes the importance of the social and material aspects of care planning services and how they are related to action in practice. Representative quotes from interview data are provided in Appendix A, Table A4.

3.3.1. Reinforcing Patient-Centered Care

"I like the structure and deliberateness ... [it] is a remarkable way to connect with people and to help them manage their health. It's been really good that way to make that a deliberate process" (Site 2, Pharmacy Manager)

The care plan document focused pharmacists' and pharmacy technicians' work to support the patient care processes. Value was associated with the changes made to work arrangements in everyday practice so that pharmacists could "sit down in the room", "connect with patients", and complete the "whole care plan process". To accomplish this, pharmacists physically excused themselves from dispensing and other duties to prioritize care plan development and follow-up. Other pharmacists and pharmacy technicians or assistants at the sites adjusted their work to accommodate. At Site 4, pharmacists were specifically assigned to provide care planning services exclusively. Modifications to the duties of the pharmacy technician at Site 1 included identification of patients who presented to the pharmacy with questions about their care plans or patients who were eligible for care planning services based on the Compensation Plan (i.e., the CACP).

Pharmacists used care plan templates to structure care planning services. These templates guided the processes of gathering information, identifying drug-related problems, obtaining information to support drug-therapy decisions, preparing documents for physicians and patients, scheduling follow-up interviews or monitoring, and updating patient information systems. Information gathering from the patient's electronic health records and pharmacy system was usually completed prior to the care plan meeting with patients and documented on the CACP template. The time required for the CACP varied from pharmacist to pharmacist, sometimes taking up to 4 h to complete the process. Care plan documents were valued for their ability to guide changes in work and reinforce the focus of the work on patient care services

3.3.2. Reducing Waiting Time for Care

"I waited actually over 15 months to see a specialist . . . The pharmacist in five minutes told me more than that specialist did, and there was no waiting period." (Site 3, Patient 1)

Patients valued care planning services, which saved time and increased convenience. Patients associated the CACP with timely access to care. Access to care at the pharmacy was more convenient than scheduling appointments at physicians' offices. Patients compared their prior experiences in both environments, noting lengthy waiting times to see their physicians, less comfortable medical office environments, and greater formality than at the pharmacy. Access to care was not only easier; the community pharmacy environment was more conducive to conversations about health and concerns. Patients noted that their CACP interviews with pharmacists were less formal than physician interviews. Speaking to their pharmacists was like speaking to "family". Reduced waiting time to see a pharmacist led patients to seek advice and answers to questions previously directed to their physicians. For example, they might ask a pharmacist to determine if a visit to a physician or hospital emergency room was required. They also sought information about their health conditions, looking to pharmacists for education about various medical issues. The value of the care plan for patients was thus associated with reduced waiting time and convenient access to care.

3.3.3. Co-Creating Individualized Plans with Patients

"It made a difference to me. I mean, I appreciate it. I appreciate the chance to go over my meds and things that bother me at the time or what we could do about one thing or another." (Site 1, Patient 4)

The initial development of the CACP promoted relationship building between patients and pharmacists. Subsequent patient–pharmacist interactions arising from CACP monitoring plans and scheduled follow-up reinforced previously established relationships and improved rapport. Some patients initiated follow-up with pharmacists as new information or questions arose. Through frequent and continuous conversations, individualized plans were created with patients' willing participation in the process. These interactions frequently involved the patient and pharmacist both interacting with others, such as the patient's family members or caregivers, physicians, or nurse practitioners. In developing CACPs, pharmacists and patients also interacted with information and other material objects such as weigh scales, blood pressure monitors, insulin pumps, and electronic resources. Following the CACP interview, patients were provided with a current list of medications. Patients who left with an understanding of their goals and action items associated with the CACP were motivated to engage further in their care. However, not all patients left the CACP experience with a CACP document and a clear understanding of their goals and action plan. Through involvement in the care planning, patients' engagement with their care was enhanced. Patients valued the time spent with pharmacists, noting that pharmacists took "time to listen", and valued knowing more about their care and a sense of their responsibilities for action.

The CACP was more than a document that recorded important information about patients and their goals. It caused things to happen and made a difference in patients' experiences with health care services. Patients valued care planning services for emotional reasons as well as practical ones. Patients valued the CACP for the "peace of mind" and "secure feeling" they got after using the services.

Value was therefore derived from patients and pharmacists working together to create care plans and patients' experiences of care provided by pharmacists.

3.3.4. Collaborating with Physicians and Other Health Care Providers

"It's a wonderful adjunct to my practice. It makes my practice better . . . It makes me think about things in a different way." (Site 4, Physician 2)

Information sharing is essential to the collaboration associated with care planning services. Information was gathered from patient records at the pharmacy, from patients' electronic health records, and from other health care professionals such as nurses and physicians. At Sites 1 and 4, pharmacists accessed physicians' medical care plans. Pharmacists at Site 1 routinely requested medical care plans directly from physicians' offices. Some pharmacists at Site 4 were co-located with physicians at practice sites outside the community pharmacy. Pharmacists and physicians at Site 4 worked closely, sometimes meeting with patients together and co-developing care plan documents.

Methods of information sharing between pharmacists and physicians varied. The most frequent method involved pharmacists sharing a copy of the CACP with physicians after the care planning documentation was completed. To do this, they transmitted a facsimile of either the entire CACP document or a summary of the action items or issues outlined in the CACP. Transmission of information (faxing care plans to physicians) is required by the Compensation Plan. Physicians at Site 1 adjusted their office procedures to store the CACP within their information systems. Establishing processes for information sharing facilitated the building of relationships and supported care planning services. When pharmacists and physicians knew each other, the process worked more efficiently. For care planning services at the urban Site 2 and suburban Site 3, where pharmacists and physicians in the community did not have working relationships, frustration arose around information sharing. Other information sharing methods involved direct communication with physicians through telephone conversations, text messages, or face-to-face conversations.

The timing of information sharing was important. Most information sharing activities occurred after the care plan was completed. However, information sharing that occurred before completion of the care plan or through face-to-face communications was highly valued because clarifications could occur or more information gathered in those interactions. Some physicians valued information sharing at the time of development of care plans rather than receiving information after the fact. For example, a physician at Site 1 routinely contacted pharmacists to proactively share information and update documentation. Some physicians expressed frustration with pharmacist-developed care plans, citing instances of incomplete information, differences in opinions regarding drug therapy or prescribing decisions, or confusing documentation. Pharmacists and physicians that communicated directly about these frustrations worked together to improve information-sharing practices. Some adjustments resulted in tailored documentation to meet patient needs; for example, care plan summary templates were created to expedite the information sharing process. Care plans co-developed by pharmacists and physicians at Site 4 were valued by the physicians for their tendency to make them "think about things in a different way".

Once patients were familiar with care planning services, they came to expect information sharing and collaboration from their pharmacists and physicians. Patients valued knowing that pharmacists and physicians shared information and communicated about their care. The value of care planning services was therefore associated with "interaction" and being "connected".

3.3.5. Revealing Possibilities for Pharmacists' Contributions to Primary Health Care

"I didn't know that [the pharmacist] would talk to me about it. I thought I would just walk in, get my prescription and walk out, right? That's the way I thought it was." (Site 4, Patient 1)

Patients were generally unaware of the existence of care planning services prior to being approached by their pharmacist. Through interactions between patients and health care providers and increased familiarity with care plan documents, patients gained knowledge of community pharmacy services, for example, prescribing, that extended beyond the boundaries of traditional preparing and providing medications. Patients and physicians were long familiar with pharmacists' dispensing services. However, expectations of the CACP were initially unclear. After gaining some experience with care planning services, one patient referred to the pharmacist as a "secret doctor" indicating that the abilities and expertise of the pharmacists were kept a secret until revealed through the CACP experience. Patients began to see pharmacists as primary health care providers who could do more than "fill prescriptions"; they began to appreciate the benefits they derived from the CACP, particularly receiving information about their medications and conditions. Providing care planning services revealed pharmacists' drug therapy expertise and increased their interactions and information sharing with patients and other health care providers. Nurses and physicians viewed pharmacists as "an integral part" of primary health care teams. Physicians gained more respect for pharmacists' roles and abilities. Despite their increased awareness of care planning services and pharmacists' roles, patients did not refer to the CACP as a care plan, but rather as a "medication review". The value of care planning services stemmed from having first-hand knowledge of and experience with pharmacists, revealing possibilities for their future contributions to primary health care.

3.3.6. Meaning of Pharmacists' Roles in Primary Health Care

"I like what I do better, because it feels like I'm contributing more and I know I'm contributing more. And I appreciate being compensated for it. I've come to value it more appropriately as well ... Now that we do have compensation for some of the clinical skills that we're using all of the time, it makes it far more satisfying." (Site 2, Pharmacy Manager)

As discussed earlier, pharmacists changed the focus of their work to provide care planning services, enabling them to co-create CACPs with patients and collaborate with other health care professionals. They spent time working with the CACP document template to gather information before meeting with the patient and to expedite the care planning and documentation processes. Increased interactions with people and their information fostered a sense of "doing more" for patients. As pharmacists gained experience with care planning services, they accepted more responsibility for patient care. While these activities (patient assessment, care planning, and documentation) were established as part of pharmaceutical care practice and gradually became embedded in their everyday work, there was a perceptible change in how they experienced their role. For some, the role felt "heavy" and "like I made a difference". These changes were observed in association with the increased time pharmacists spent with patients, with the CACP document, and in activities related to information sharing. As well as feeling more connected to patients, pharmacists felt the CACP represented an investment because of the effort contributed to future encounters with patients; through involvement in the care planning process, pharmacists were positioned to support patients better through "rough times". Pharmacists derived greater satisfaction with their work, felt that they were "contributing more" to patient care and primary health care, that they were staying "more current", and that they enjoyed having "people depend on [them]". These realizations, along with the material compensation associated with care planning services, changed how pharmacists experienced their role: with a renewed sense of responsibility, satisfaction, and meaning.

4. Discussion

This study employed a novel theoretical approach to explore the perceived value of compensated care planning services provided by pharmacists. This approach placed the care plan document in the foreground. It also examined interactions between information and people. This study found that care plans provided material information, influenced everyday practice, linked people together, and mediated meaning-making. Care planning services were valued for their role in reinforcing patient-centered care, reducing waiting time for care, co-creating individualized plans with patients, collaborating with physicians and other health care providers, and revealing possibilities for pharmacists' roles. This study also highlights pharmacists' renewed sense of responsibility, satisfaction, and understanding of their role and potential contributions to primary health care.

Through involvement with care planning services, everyday work by pharmacists and pharmacy staff changed in that more attention was focused on patients' needs. Results echoed areas of value associated with primary health care services, namely accessibility, patient centredness, patient engagement, and experiences of health care providers [3,22–25]. These areas of value were also noted in prior research on care plans [19,54,55]. Similar to this current study, Council et al. [55] employed a prospective case study design to explore care planning by a group family practice at a community hospital in the US. In their setting, physicians, nurses, residents, and medical assistants all contributed to care planning. In that study, increased patient centredness, and patient involvement in the care plan were reported [55]. Thus, care plans bring value when patients are engaged in their development with primary care providers.

Through their participation in care planning services, patients valued having time and opportunity to talk with pharmacists about their medications and health concerns. Patients felt cared for and listened to. This experience represented a departure from patients' past experiences. The difference was attributed to care planning. Brown et al. [54] summarized the essence of care planning as having a "better conversation". The initial CACP interview became an ongoing conversation through various follow-up appointments at the pharmacy or telephone calls with patients; the conversation was often expanded to include physicians and others involved in the patient's care. From patients' perspectives, the conversation with pharmacists was less formal than speaking with physicians, like speaking with family members. This reflects the trust and confidence in the relationships built between patients and the pharmacists in this study. The results of this current study pointed to the unique conversation brought about by care planning services.

Previous research by Hindi et al. [19] found that care plans help to integrate community pharmacists into primary health care teams. Shared care plans, those co-developed by pharmacists and physicians, may further integrate community pharmacy in primary health care as well as address issues such as duplication of work and improve teamwork, which was seen in our study. Brown et al. [54] asserted the value of delivering a single coherent message to a patient in a shared care plan, describing how these plans support patients to engage in their own care and implement changes to their lifestyle. Experiences developing shared care plans in this current study were valued by patients, pharmacists, and physicians. Physicians valued the different perspectives and expertise brought by pharmacists as well as the efficiency of shared care plans.

Information sharing is recognized as a significant part of care planning services [54]. In the current study, care plans facilitated coordination of information and patient care activities. Care plan documents, themselves, contribute patient information. With pharmacists contributing more and more to patient care in the primary health care system, care plan documents will become even more important for information sharing. However, lack of access to or incomplete patient information presents challenges for pharmacists providing care planning services. In Alberta, pharmacists have had access to provincial electronic health records, including laboratory tests and records of dispensed medications, since 2006 [28]. In the current study, complete information shared through documents or in conversation was highly valued and necessary to ensure accuracy and informed decision-making. Information systems, like NetCare in Alberta, are needed to support care planning services. Enhancements to the NetCare system that allow pharmacists to upload care plan documents to patients' records will support easier information sharing between health care providers. Some pharmacists in this study lacked access to patients' medical care plans. Having information from different perspectives of physicians and nurses would support pharmacists' care planning services. In addition, information sharing mechanisms that support conversations between patients, physicians, pharmacists and other health care providers will bring further value to patients. Other research draws attention to the value of information sharing. Hindi et al. [19] conducted focus groups of patients, pharmacists, and general practitioners to identify how community pharmacy services may be better integrated within the primary care pathway for people with chronic conditions. Their results emphasized the need for robust information systems that included two-way flow of information. Council et al. [55] found that patient-centered care plans increased efficiency and the validity of information was enhanced as multiple team members and the patients were involved in construction of information. Methods to support information sharing contribute to collaboration and quality of primary health care services. Brown et al. [54] reviewed studies that evaluated care planning to develop a theoretically informed framework for how care planning works best. These investigators noted that sharing of written care plans within and across teams for patients with multimorbidity ensures consistency of messages. Attention to the quality of the care plan, along with completeness of information and consistency in presentation [19,56], may further enhance the value of information sharing associated with pharmacist care planning services and improve patient care.

Collaboration in the form of information sharing occurred in different ways at the sites included in this study depending on the individuals involved in care planning and the particular practice setting and location. Research by Talja [57] describes types and levels of collaborative information sharing related to documents. Talja's 4 classifications relate to different goals and contexts and highlight the social aspects of information sharing including to: (1) provide information; (2) maximize efficiency; (3) form or strengthen relationships; and (4) develop novel approaches. In the context of the current study, information sharing by physicians and pharmacists at Site 4 produced shared care plans. This arrangement is an example of a novel information sharing strategy through which the relationships between pharmacists and physicians may be enhanced, and actions associated with care planning services in primary health care may be improved. Other strategies may also provide opportunities to expand information sharing strategies that support care planning services in primary health care.

In the current study, care planning services were associated with gaining enhanced knowledge of community pharmacy services and identifying potential contributions to primary health care. Patients, physicians, and other health care providers initially had little knowledge of the nature and potential of care planning services. Moving forward, pharmacists' involvement in care planning could add more value to the system if more individuals were aware of its intended aims and benefits. Latif et al. [58] reported that patients in the United Kingdom had poor awareness of the New Medicines Service provided by pharmacists. In their study, physicians were also unaware of the benefits of this service. Strategies are needed to educate patients about the value of the service to improve mutual understanding of policy among laypeople and professionals [58]. Expectations must be outlined for how the service is to be delivered, information shared, and anticipated outcomes. Providing patients with care plans may enhance patient experiences, improve knowledge of care planning services [59,60], and support goal setting, shared decision-making, and self-management [54].

The findings regarding pharmacists' perceptions of the time required for care planning services were unexpected. Pharmacists in this study needed to spend significant time to develop a CACP, yet most regarded benefits of the care planning service as worthwhile for the patient and for themselves. In other research, the time and resources required to implement care planning services in community pharmacies represents a concern for pharmacists implementing similar services [61]. In contrast, pharmacists derived value from spending time to collaborate with patients and other health care professionals; involvement in care planning services sparked a renewed sense of responsibility, increased satisfaction, and gave meaning to their role. Despite the challenges associated with implementing care planning services, especially the time required for information sharing and documentation, pharmacists participating in this study reported high levels of satisfaction with their experiences. They also observed the value of CACPs in terms of compensation, interactions with patients, and engagement with others involved in the service. In addition, pharmacists perceived their role differently; they gained a greater sense of responsibility for patient care and their contributions to primary health care services.

Given their access to information and prescribing authorization, the practice environment in Alberta supports changes in pharmacists' roles and provides opportunities for them to contribute more to primary health care [35]. While pharmacists were well positioned to take on expanded roles in primary health care before the introduction of the Compensation Plan, care planning services were not prominent. Remuneration has been previously identified as a barrier to changing practice, implementing new services, and integrating pharmacists in primary health care [62–65]. Compensation directed towards valued patient care services may represent the final shift required for pharmacists to engage fully in patient care [66].

The strengths and limitations of this research must be considered when interpreting its results. Strengths of this research included the use of a longitudinal case study method that compared 4 sites, and combined multiple methods of data collection, materials, and perspectives. However, this study is limited in that it focuses on the practice environment in Alberta. Community pharmacy practice is diverse; thus, it is difficult to represent the entire range of experiences with care planning services. In Alberta, pharmacist involvement in care planning services has been fairly recently implemented and is still evolving. The number of care plans per month, which in this study was used as the variable representing experience with care plans, was self-reported and low at most sites. Finally, physician experiences and perspectives are integral to the question of value. Physician participation in the study was low; those that did respond may have had more favorable experiences with pharmacist involvement in care planning services. This selection bias should be addressed in future research confirming the results of this study.

In this study, an analytical focus on the social and material aspects of care planning services afforded an opportunity to explore the perceived value of compensated pharmacist care planning services, deepening our understanding of how care plans "made a difference" to patients, pharmacists, and other health care providers. The results of this study present implications for practice, policy, and research. Pharmacists may benefit from an understanding of how care plans make a difference to patients, the importance of the care plan document itself, possibilities for shared care plans, the importance of providing patients with copies of care plans, and how to align information sharing strategies with desired outcomes. Policy makers may consider providing compensation for care planning services that are most valued by stakeholders in order to derive the most benefit in primary health care. Including compensation for shared care plans and proactive and real-time information sharing, such as remuneration for phone calls, may be considered [19,55]. In the age of greater pharmacist engagement in primary health care, introducing compensation for new services may aid in timely and effective service delivery. Future research is needed to clarify the impact of compensation, level of reimbursement required to offset provision of care planning services, the processes and outcomes of shared care plans, how to provide patients with care plans, and various care plan documentation approaches [54,56].

Author Contributions: Conceptualization, T.J.S. and C.A.H.; Data curation, T.J.S. and C.A.H.; Formal analysis, T.J.S., R.R.B. and C.A.H.; Funding acquisition, T.J.S., R.R.B. and C.A.H.; Investigation, T.J.S., R.R.B. and C.A.H.; Methodology, T.J.S., R.R.B. and C.A.H.; Project administration, T.J.S. and C.A.H.; Resources, C.A.H.; Supervision, C.A.H.; Writing—original draft, T.J.S.; Writing—review & editing, T.J.S., R.R.B. and C.A.H.

Funding: This study was supported by grants from the Canadian Foundation for Pharmacy and the Alberta Pharmacists' Association.

Acknowledgments: The authors gratefully acknowledge the study participants and the community pharmacy sites for allowing us to observe their practices, Deborah Hicks, Amy Semaka, and Iryna Hurava for assisting with the data collection, and Stuart Drozd, Cathryn Gunn, as well as the anonymous peer reviewers for reviewing the manuscript.

Conflicts of Interest: The authors declare no conflict of interest. The sponsors had no role in the design, execution, interpretation, or writing of the study.

Appendix A

Table A1. Interview Topic Guide.

Participant	Topics
Patient	History with the pharmacy Experiences with care planning (CACP) services Perceptions and explanations of the value of care planning (CACP) services Added for site visit 3: Do you talk about your care plan goals? Do you have an action plan after a care plan has been developed for you?
Physician, Other Health Care Professional	History of the practice Experiences with the pharmacy Experiences with care planning (CACP) services provided by pharmacists How is the CACP stored? Perceptions and explanations of the value of care planning (CACP) services
Pharmacist, Pharmacy Technician, and Pharmacy Staff	History with the pharmacy Description of patient care services Experiences with care planning (CACP) services Implementation of care planning services Support provided/required to provide patient care services Benefits/challenges associated with provision of patient care services Changes, if any, to the professional role or activities of the pharmacy staff since the implementation of the Compensation Plan for Pharmacy Services Learning and professional development related to provision of patient care services Perceptions and explanations of the value of care planning (CACP) services Added for site visit 3: What information sources do you use for care planning (CACP) services? Do you have access to the medical care plan? What kind of feedback have you received on your care plans? How do you know if the care plan makes a difference? What professional development was helpful?

Table A2. Observation Form Topics.

Observational Data—Comprehensive Annual Care Plan (CACP) Services
Observations
Pre-CACP activities Pharmacist–staff interactions Patient–staff interactions Patient–pharmacist interactions Patient involvement in CACP development Information seeking and use Documents/forms/tools used "Take away" documentation provided to the patient Physician (or other) communication CACP documentation sharing, storing Post-patient interaction activities Time spent on the activity
Clarifications
Questions to ask in interviews
Description of the setting
Location of staff in the setting, including changes over the course of the observation Physical description of the setting
Researcher reflexivity
What changes to the observation process should be made for the next time? How does the researcher feel about the day's occurrences? How do the observed actions compare to the findings from the document analysis? Do the key messages found there affect/influence/contradict the observations? Did the researcher(s) have any apparent influence on the activities?

Table A3. Site-Specific Documents.

Site 1	Site 2	Site 3	Site 4
Care Plan Template (Example)	Care Plan Template	Care Plan Template	Care Plan Template
Initial Assessment with APA Template	Smoking Cessation Template	Smoking Assessment Template	Initial Assessment Template
Medication Sheet (Example)	Follow up Progress Notes (Example)	Adult Vaccination Assessment Template	Medication History Template
Alberta Health Services	Summary of Care Plan to a physician (Example)	Specific Disease-based Templates	Pharmacy Balance Care Plan Template
Care Plan Summary Template		Asthma Action Plan Template	Pharmacy Balance Patient Goal and Plan Template
Continuing Care Template			Letter to a physician (Example)
Alberta College of Pharmacy Documentation Templates			Pharmacist Prescribing Adaptation (Example)

Table A4. Value of Care Planning Services and Representative Quotes.

Value	Representative Quotes
Reinforcing patient-centered care	
	The value of it is a connection. The start of the connection. Before, you kind of got a connection with a patient sometimes if you listened to them over the counter and they told you their story … But now it seems like a given if you get the opportunity to sit down in the room with that patient. (Site 1, Pharmacy Manager)
	I feel like this … allowed [pharmacists] to prioritize what was important … I feel like I've been supported more. (Site 3, Pharmacy Manager)
	I like the structure and deliberateness. … [it] is a remarkable way to connect with people and to help them manage their health. It's been really good that way to make that a deliberate process. (Site 2, Pharmacy Manager)
	This whole care plan process has made our pharmacists here do more for the patients. Like, we're doing more—I'm not saying we weren't doing the work before, but I feel like this, the whole care plan process has [compelled] us to really make sure that we're following up with our patients with regards to a lot of medical conditions and medications that they start, you know, whereas we didn't necessarily do that before. (Site 3, Pharmacy Manager)
	We build a relationship … That's the foundation of my process of care … . So, instead of having my fulfillment come from any sort of outcome, it's definitely attached to the process. (Site 4, Pharmacist 2)
	It's [making] you close to patients—feel you're close and patient. They phone and ask for [us] by names … they feel more comfortable talking to me or to [other pharmacists]. And you have more relationship with the patient. (Site 3, Pharmacist 1)
Reducing waiting time for care	
	I waited actually over 15 months to see a specialist with all my diabetes. The pharmacist in five minutes told me more than that specialist did, and there was no waiting period. (Site 3, Patient 1)
	You just felt more comfortable. With the doctor it's more professional or, like I said, these [pharmacists] feel like family, you know. They're easier to talk to. (Site 1, Patient 5)
	Sometimes you don't have to go to the doctor's appointment, you think, because [the pharmacist] helped you figure it out without doing that (Site 1, Patient 1)

Table A4. *Cont.*

Value	Representative Quotes
	The doctor at the pain clinic was very busy all the time and you can't get in to see him. You have to make an appointment a month or two ahead. And so it was easier for me to come and talk to the pharmacist who was talking back and forth with me at that time. [There was time] for him to sit down and tell me what exactly the situation [was]. (Site 4, Patient 1)
	There has been times when I have reacted to a medication, usually an antibiotic, on a weekend where I ... was too sick to get to a doctor. And [the pharmacist] would advise me on what to do to get to the point where I could go to a doctor. (Site 2, Patient 5)
	[The pharmacist] takes the time to explain stuff to you. So I really appreciate that, because there's not much of that anymore. (Site 4, Patient 5)
Co-creating individualized plans with patients	
	It made a difference to me. I mean, I appreciate it. I appreciate the chance, to go over my meds and things that bother me at the time or what we could do about one thing or another. (Site 1, Patient 4)
	When I call her regarding something, it's very important. She always takes some time to listen. (Site 2, Patient 5)
	They listen to my concerns. Like, if I have any concerns about my medication somebody always takes the time to answer my questions. (Site 3, Patient 7)
	They're not just your pharmacist, you know. They're concerned about you too, you know. So that's a good thing. ... rather than just giving you pills like they used to. (Site 1, Patient 5)
	Well, my goals are to get my blood sugar down to an acceptable level because I'm Type 2 diabetes, and my blood sugar was way up in the 26 range. And with the help of [named pharmacist] and my family doctor, it is now down roughly about 6. (Site 3, Patient 7)
	Before, I abused myself. I didn't care, right? And now, you know, this [success] is a result of just trying a few healthy things that [the pharmacist] has expressed interest that maybe I should think about doing. [It] has changed my life. Really. (Site 2, Patient 4)
Collaborating with physicians and other health care providers	
	Before, you had your doctor. Then this. Now it seems like they're, you know, all connected. So it's more interaction. Everybody isn't out in the dark, you know. It seems like it's better that way now. [Better] than it was before. (Site 1, Patient 5)
	It's a wonderful adjunct to my practice. It makes my practice better ... It makes me think about things in a different way. (Site 4, Physician 2)
	I know that with both [pharmacist and physician] they have my best interests at heart. They are working together to do the things that I need to have done. In fact, my doctor was saying the other day that the relationship I have with her, and she has with [the pharmacist], allows her to do and follow up on things that she normally wouldn't have the chance to do. (Site 2, Patient 5)
	I talked to my doctor about my pharmacist and they said, "that's good, we'll talk back and forth". It started out with the pharmacist talking with my doctor ... back and forth, about my care. (Site 4, Patient 1)
	The value of someone's follow-ups is unbelievable when you have different pharmacists rotating ... I'll even look back and it will be an interaction [with] the other pharmacist had in May ... I'm dealing with the problem in September. I'll understand how that went. (Site 1, Pharmacy Manager)

Table A4. *Cont.*

Value	Representative Quotes
	The piece about talking to people and gathering information from them … to document that properly, really follow that up properly, and share the information properly so that other professionals I work with can be in on the story as well and can be part of that follow-up. (Site 2, Pharmacy Manager)
	The physician will outline a care plan for this patient … specific goals for therapy which I can then pull in to my care plans. I'm fortunate to be able to have access to those charts. (Site 4, Pharmacist 5)
	[The care plans] gets scanned into our EMR [electronic medical record] so that I can refer back to it at any point and also because we all share the same patients. Information is really important. (Site 1, Physician 2)
	We're starting to get more of their care plans faxed to us. And because they're doing [care plans, we are] getting more patients coming back to us with questions. And some of that's very good because it seems we hadn't realized he'd fallen by the way. And sometimes it's a little bit of a nuisance because there's a good reason why this patient isn't on a statin and now we have to have this conversation all over again. (Site 2, Physician 1)
Revealing possibilities for pharmacists' contributions to primary health care	
	I didn't know that [the pharmacist] would talk to me about it. I thought I would just walk in, get my prescription and walk out, right? That's the way I thought it was. (Site 4, Patient 1)
	Well, it was interesting. I've never done that [care plan] before, you know. The ones that give you the prescriptions are the doctors, and it seems like the pharmacy doesn't know anything about it. But I found that I could get more information from [the pharmacist] than I could from a doctor. (Site 2, Patient 2)
	I don't know if you are aware of this [pharmacist] but he's a kind of a diabetes specialist … he gets my blood reports … he's monitoring them … You've heard of a secret Santa? He's kind of a secret doctor, you know. (Site 3, Patient 1)
	I think pharmacies are changing … I didn't know that that [care planning] service was available, to tell you the truth. I always thought that, you know, pharmacists were just there to fill out the prescription, right? I didn't think they really knew that much about what was going on. (Site 2, Patient 4)
	I have more respect for pharmacists now. Let's be honest about it. I always thought they were just dispensing meds and whatever. (Site 4, Physician 2)
	I find that they are, have just become, an extension of my health care colleagues. (Site 4, Nurse Practitioner)
	This [care planning service] is a resource in limited situations like [this town]. It's nice. We know we're never going to have enough physicians to look after everybody properly like we should. So, it's nice that the pharmacist can take some of that load. (Site 1, Physician 1)
Meaning of pharmacists' roles in primary care	
	I like what I do better, because it feels like I'm contributing more and I know I'm contributing more. And I appreciate being compensated for it. I've come to value it more appropriately as well. … Now that we do have compensation for some of the clinical skills that we're using all of the time, it makes it far more satisfying. (Site 2, Pharmacy Manager)
	I feel like even compared to a few years ago … I've noticed people depend on [me]—they come in more. They call you for more clinical questions. (Site 1, Pharmacist 2)

Table A4. *Cont.*

Value	Representative Quotes
	It's just like little light bulbs going off all throughout the day, it's like I feel so good. I helped that person. I can't believe what I just did. (Site 1, Pharmacy Manager)
	I'm more responsible. I feel more responsible for things than I ever did before. (Site 2, Pharmacy Manager)
	Being able to do at least a little bit of tracking [follow-up] to make me feel like I made a difference. (Site 4, Pharmacist 5)
	I honestly feel like the system [framework] that's in place has allowed me to continue to stay more and more current because, you're just looking at all the clinical stuff on a daily basis instead of just dispensing the medication … I think it definitely increased my knowledge and allowed me to stay a little bit more on top of the changes that occur. (Site 3, Pharmacy Manager)
	I have a responsibility to be good and to give [patients] quality and to continue to give good service. So, that kind of holds on you. It's kind of heavy. (Site 4, Pharmacist 2)

References

1. World Health Organization. Primary Health Care. Available online: https://apps.who.int/iris/bitstream/handle/10665/39228/9241800011.pdf?sequence=1&isAllowed=y (accessed on 21 May 2019).
2. Alberta Health. Alberta's Primary Health Care Strategy. Available online: https://open.alberta.ca/dataset/1cac62b5-a383-4959-8187-1b2a6798d0ac/resource/2ff5246a-bdd9-428a-ab04-62e5475c90ed/download/6849603-2014-albertas-primary-health-care-strategy-2014-01.pdf (accessed on 10 May 2019).
3. Haggerty, J.; Burge, F.; Lévesque, J.; Gass, D.; Pineault, R.; Beaulieu, M.; Santor, D. Operational definitions of attributes of primary health care: Consensus among Canadian experts. *Ann. Fam. Med.* **2007**, *5*, 336–344. [CrossRef] [PubMed]
4. Manolakis, P.; Skelton, J. Pharmacists' contributions to primary care in the United States collaborating to address unmet patient care needs: The emerging role for pharmacists to address the shortage of primary care providers. *Am. J. Pharm. Educ.* **2010**, *74*. [CrossRef] [PubMed]
5. Mossialos, E.; Courtin, E.; Naci, H.; Benrimoj, S.; Bouvy, M.; Farris, K.; Noyce, P.; Sketris, I. From "retailers" to health care providers: Transforming the role of community pharmacists in chronic disease management. *Health Policy* **2015**, *119*, 628–639. [CrossRef] [PubMed]
6. Feehan, M.; Walsh, M.; Godin, J.; Sundwall, D.; Munger, M.A. Patient preferences for healthcare delivery through community pharmacy settings in the USA: A discrete choice study. *J. Clin. Pharm Ther.* **2017**, *42*, 38–49. [CrossRef] [PubMed]
7. Policarpo, V.; Romano, S.; António, J.H.C.; Correia, T.S.; Costa, S. A new model for pharmacies? Insights from a quantitative study regarding the public's perceptions. *BMC Health Serv. Res.* **2019**, *19*, 186. [CrossRef] [PubMed]
8. Tsuyuki, R.T. The primary care pharmacist. *Can. Pharm. J.* **2016**, *149*, 61–63. [CrossRef] [PubMed]
9. Munger, M.A. Primary care pharmacists: Provision of clinical-decision services in healthcare. *Am. J. Pharm. Educ.* **2014**, *78*. [CrossRef] [PubMed]
10. Romanow, R.L. Building on Values: The Future of Health Care in CANADA. November 2002. Available online: http://publications.gc.ca/collections/Collection/CP32-85-2002E.pdf (accessed on 26 June 2019).
11. Grindrod, K.A.; Marra, C.A.; Colley, L.; Tsuyuki, R.T.; Lynd, L.D. Pharmacists' preferences for providing patient-centered services: A discrete choice experiment to guide health policy. *Ann. Pharmacother.* **2010**, *44*, 1554–1564. [CrossRef] [PubMed]
12. Scott, A.; Bond, C.; Inch, J.; Grant, A. Preferences of community pharmacists for extended roles in primary care: A survey and discrete choice experiment. *Pharmacoeconomics* **2007**, *25*, 783–792. [CrossRef] [PubMed]
13. Fay, A.E.; Ferreri, S.P.; Shepherd, G.; Lundeen, K.; Tong, G.L.; Pfeiffenberger, T. Care team perspectives on community pharmacy enhanced services. *J. Am. Pharm. Assoc.* **2018**, *58*, S83–S88. [CrossRef] [PubMed]

14. Joint Commission of Pharmacy Practitioners. Pharmacists' Patient Care Process. 29 May 2014. Available online: https://jcpp.net/wp-content/uploads/2016/03/PatientCareProcess-with-supporting-organizations.pdf (accessed on 26 June 2019).

15. National Association of Pharmacy Regulatory Authorities. Professional Competencies for Canadian Pharmacists at Entry to Practice. 2014. Available online: https://napra.ca/pharmacists/professional-competencies-canadian-pharmacists-entry-practice-2014 (accessed on 29 June 2019).

16. Strand, L.M.; Cipolle, R.J.; Morley, P.C. Documenting the clinical pharmacist's activities: Back to basics. *Drug Intell. Clin. Pharm.* **1988**, *22*, 63–67. [CrossRef] [PubMed]

17. Drummond, C.; Simpson, A. 'Who's actually gonna read this?' An evaluation of staff experiences of the value of information contained in written care plans in supporting care in three different dementia care settings. *J. Psychiatr. Ment. Health Nurs.* **2017**, *24*, 377–386. [CrossRef] [PubMed]

18. Lawn, S.; Delany, T.; Sweet, L.; Battersby, M.; Skinner, T. Barriers and enablers to good communication and information-sharing practices in care planning for chronic condition management. *Aust. J. Prim. Health* **2015**, *21*, 84–89. [CrossRef] [PubMed]

19. Hindi, A.M.K.; Schafheutle, E.I.; Jacobs, S. Community pharmacy integration within the primary care pathway for people with long-term conditions: A focus group study of patients', pharmacists' and GPs' experiences and expectations. *BMC Fam. Pract.* **2019**, *20*. [CrossRef] [PubMed]

20. Berwick, D.M.; Nolan, T.W.; Whittington, J. The Triple Aim: Care, Health and Cost. *Health Aff.* **2008**, *27*, 759–769. [CrossRef] [PubMed]

21. Porter, M.E. What is value in health care? *N. Engl. J. Med.* **2010**, *363*, 2477–2481. [CrossRef] [PubMed]

22. Rollow, W.; Cucchiara, P. Achieving value in primary care: The primary care value model. *Ann. Fam. Med.* **2016**, *14*, 159–165. [CrossRef]

23. Nordgren, L. Value creation in health care services—Developing service productivity: Experiences from Sweden. *Int. J. Public Sect. Manag.* **2009**, *22*, 114–127. [CrossRef]

24. Bodenheimer, T.; Sinsky, C. From triple to quadruple aim: Care of the patient requires care of the provider. *Ann. Fam. Med.* **2014**, *12*, 573–576. [CrossRef]

25. Sikka, R.; Morath, J.M.; Leape, L. The quadruple aim: Care, health, cost and meaning in work. *BMJ Qual. Saf.* **2015**, *24*, 608–610. [CrossRef]

26. Twigg, M.J.; Wright, D.; Barton, G.; Kirkdale, C.L.; Thornley, T. The pharmacy care plan service: Evaluation and estimate of cost-effectiveness. *Res. Soc. Adm. Pharm.* **2019**, *15*, 84–92. [CrossRef] [PubMed]

27. Nguyen, E.; Holmes, J.T. Pharmacist-provided services: Barriers to demonstrating value. *J. Am. Pharm. Assoc.* **2019**, *59*, 117–120. [CrossRef] [PubMed]

28. Hughes, C.A.; Guirguis, L.M.; Wong, T.; Ng, K.; Ing, L.; Fisher, K. Influence of pharmacy practice on community pharmacists' integration of medication and lab value information from electronic health records. *J. Am. Pharm. Assoc.* **2011**, *51*, 591–598. [CrossRef] [PubMed]

29. Yuksel, N.; Eberhart, G.; Bungard, T.J. Prescribing by pharmacists in Alberta. *Am. J. Health-Syst. Pharm.* **2008**, *65*, 2126–2132. [CrossRef] [PubMed]

30. Charrois, T.; Rosenthal, M.; Tsuyuki, R.T. Stories from the trenches: Experiences of Alberta pharmacists in obtaining additional prescribing authority. *Can. Pharm. J.* **2012**, *145*, 30–34. [CrossRef]

31. Alberta College of Pharmacy. Appendix A: Patient Record Requirements. 2011. Standards of Practice for Pharmacists and Pharmacy Technicians. Available online: https://abpharmacy.ca/sites/default/files/StandardsOfPractice_May2014_v2.pdf (accessed on 29 June 2019).

32. Statistics Canada. Population by Year, by Province and Territory. Available online: http://www.statcan.gc.ca/tables-tableaux/sum-som/l01/cst01/demo02a-eng.htm (accessed on 21 May 2019).

33. Alberta College of Pharmacy. Ripples of Change in the Care of ALBERTANS. *2016-107 Annual Report*. Available online: https://abpharmacy.ca/sites/default/files/ACP_AR2016_FinalWeb_0.pdf (accessed on 10 May 2019).

34. Guirguis, L.M.; Hughes, C.A.; Makowsky, M.J.; Sadowski, C.A.; Schindel, T.J.; Yuksel, N. Survey of pharmacist prescribing practices in Alberta. *Am. J. Health-Syst. Pharm.* **2017**, *74*, 62–69. [CrossRef]

35. Schindel, T.J.; Yuksel, N.; Breault, R.; Daniels, J.; Varnhagen, S.; Hughes, C.A. Perceptions of pharmacists' roles in the era of expanding scopes of practice. *Res. Soc. Adm. Pharm.* **2017**, *13*, 148–161. [CrossRef]

36. Breault, R.; Whissell, J.; Hughes, C.A.; Schindel, T.J. Development and implementation of the compensation plan for pharmacy services in Alberta, Canada. *J. Am. Pharm. Assoc.* **2017**, *57*, 532–541. [CrossRef]

37. Breault, R.; Schindel, T.J.; Whissell, J.; Hughes, C.A. Updates to the compensation plan for pharmacy services in Alberta, Canada. *J. Am. Pharm. Assoc.* **2018**, *58*, 597–598. [CrossRef]

38. Gruber, J. Medication therapy management: A challenge for pharmacists. *Consult. Pharm.* **2012**, *11*, 782–796. [CrossRef]

39. Government of Alberta. Compensation Plan for Pharmacy Services. Ministerial Order 614/2018. 2018. Available online: https://open.alberta.ca/dataset/0e5f556a-2ac0-40a6-8fbc-d46fb92b0ee1/resource/a6c00fcd-58db-4b45-b368-df9992111739/download/mo-614-2018-pharmacycompensation.pdf (accessed on 29 June 2019).

40. Fenwick, T. Sociomateriality in medical practice and learning: Attuning to what matters. *Med. Educ.* **2014**, *48*, 44–52. [CrossRef] [PubMed]

41. Lund, N.W.; Skare, R. Document theory. In *Encyclopedia of Library and Information Sciences*, 3rd ed.; Bates, M.J., Maack, M.N., Eds.; CRC Press: Boca Raton, FL, USA, 2010; pp. 1632–1639.

42. Fenwick, T.; Nerland, M.; Jensen, K. Sociomaterial approaches to conceptualising professional learning and practice. *J. Educ. Work* **2012**, *25*, 1–13. [CrossRef]

43. Merriam, S.B. Qualitative case study research. In *Qualitative Research: A Guide to Design and Implementation*, 3rd ed.; Merriam, S.B., Ed.; Jossey-Bass: Hoboken, NJ, USA, 2014; pp. 39–54.

44. Yin, R.K. *Applications of Case Study Research*; Sage: Thousand Oaks, CA, USA, 2012.

45. Merriam, S.B. *Case Study Research in Education: A Qualitative Approach*; Jossey-Bass: San Francisco, CA, USA, 1988.

46. Hultin, L. On becoming a sociomaterial researcher: Exploring epistemological practices grounded in a relational, performative ontology. *Inf. Organ.* **2019**, *29*, 91–104. [CrossRef]

47. Charmaz, K. *Constructing Grounded Theory: A Practical Guide Through Qualitative Analysis*; Sage: London, UK, 2006.

48. Statistics Canada. Population Centre and Rural Area Classification. Available online: https://www.statcan.gc.ca/eng/subjects/standard/pcrac/2016/introduction (accessed on 21 May 2019).

49. Kaae, S.; Søndergaard, B.; Haugbølle, L.S.; Traulsen, J.M. Development of a qualitative exploratory case study research method to explore sustained delivery of cognitive services. *Pharm. World Sci.* **2010**, *32*, 36. [CrossRef] [PubMed]

50. Denzin, N.K.; Lincoln, Y.S. Introduction: The discipline and practice of qualitative research. In *The Sage Handbook of Qualitative Research*, 4th ed.; Denzin, N.K., Lincoln, Y.S., Eds.; Sage Publications: Thousand Oaks, CA, USA, 2011; pp. 1–19.

51. Given, L.M.; Saumure, K. Trustworthiness. In *The SAGE Encyclopedia of Qualitative Research Methods*; Given, L.M., Ed.; Sage Publications: Thousand Oaks, CA, USA, 2008; pp. 895–896.

52. Hughes, C.A.; Breault, R.R.; Hicks, D.; Schindel, T.J. Positioning pharmacists' roles in primary health care: A discourse analysis of the compensation plan in Alberta, Canada. *BMC Health Serv. Res.* **2017**, *17*, 770. [CrossRef]

53. Perepelkin, J.; Dobson, R.T. Influence of ownership type on role orientation, role affinity, and role conflict among community pharmacy managers and owners in Canada. *Res. Soc. Adm. Pharm.* **2010**, *6*, 280–292. [CrossRef]

54. Brown, S.; Lhussier, M.; Dalkin, S.M.; Eaton, S. Care planning: What works, for whom, and in what circumstances? A rapid realist review. *Qual. Health Res.* **2018**, *28*, 2250–2266. [CrossRef]

55. Council, L.; Geffken, D.; Valeras, A.; Orzano, A.; Rechisky, A.; Anderson, S. A medical home: Changing the way patients and teams relate through patient-centered care plans. *Fam. Syst. Health* **2012**, *30*, 90–98. [CrossRef]

56. Van Dongen, J.J.J.; Van Bokhoven, M.A.; Daniëls, R.; Van Der Weijden, T.; Emonts, W.W.G.P.; Beurskens, A. Developing interprofessional care plans in chronic care: A scoping review. *BMC Fam. Pract.* **2016**, *17*. [CrossRef]

57. Talja, S. Information Sharing in Academic Communities: Types and Levels of Collaboration in Information Seeking and Use. *New Rev. Inf. Behav. Res.* **2002**, *3*, 143–160. Available online: https://www.researchgate.net/publication/228999169_Information_sharing_in_academic_communities_Types_and_levels_of_collaboration_in_information_seeking_and_use (accessed on 21 May 2019).

58. Latif, A.; Waring, J.; Watmough, D.; Boyd, M.J.; Elliott, R.A. 'I expected just to walk in, get my tablets and then walk out': On framing new community pharmacy services in the English healthcare system. *Sociol. Health Illn.* **2018**, *40*, 1019–1036. [CrossRef] [PubMed]

59. Dolovich, L.; Austin, Z.; Waite, N.; Chang, F.; Farrell, B.; Grindrod, K.; Houle, S.; McCarthy, L.; MacCallum, L.; Sproule, B. Pharmacy in the 21st century: Enhancing the impact of the profession of pharmacy on people's lives in the context of health care trends, evidence and policies. *Can. Pharm. J.* **2019**, *152*, 45–53. [CrossRef] [PubMed]

60. Newbould, J.; Burt, J.; Bower, P.; Blakeman, T.; Kennedy, A.; Rogers, A.; Roland, M. Experiences of care planning in England: Interviews with patients with long term conditions. *BMC Fam. Pract.* **2012**, *13*. [CrossRef] [PubMed]

61. Twigg, M.J.; Wright, D.; Kirkdale, C.L.; Desborough, J.A.; Thornley, T. The UK pharmacy care plan service: Description, recruitment and initial views on a new community pharmacy intervention. *PLoS ONE* **2017**, *12*, e0174500. [CrossRef] [PubMed]

62. Roberts, A.S.; Benrimoj, S.I.; Chen, T.F.; Williams, K.A.; Aslani, P. Practice change in community pharmacy: Quantification of facilitators. *Ann. Pharmacother.* **2008**, *42*, 861–868. [CrossRef] [PubMed]

63. Wang, J.; Hong, S.H.; Meng, S.; Brown, L.M. Pharmacists' acceptable levels of compensation for MTM services: A conjoint analysis. *Res. Soc. Adm. Pharm.* **2011**, *7*, 383–395. [CrossRef] [PubMed]

64. Freeman, C.; Cottrell, W.N.; Kyle, G.; Williams, I.; Nissen, L. Integrating a pharmacist into the general practice environment: Opinions of pharmacists, general practitioners, health care consumers, and practice managers. *BMC Health Serv. Res.* **2012**, *12*. [CrossRef]

65. McMillan, S.S.; Wheeler, A.J.; Sav, A.; King, M.A.; Whitty, J.A.; Kendall, E.; Kelly, F. Community pharmacy in Australia: A health hub destination of the future. *Res. Soc. Adm. Pharm.* **2013**, *9*, 863–875. [CrossRef]

66. Tsuyuki, R.T.; Schindel, T.J. Changing pharmacy practice: The leadership challenge. *Can. Pharm. J.* **2008**, *141*, 174–180. [CrossRef]

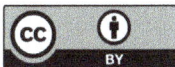

MDPI

St. Alban-Anlage 66

4052 Basel

Switzerland

Tel. +41 61 683 77 34

Fax +41 61 302 89 18

www.mdpi.com

Pharmacy Editorial Office

E-mail: pharmacy@mdpi.com

www.mdpi.com/journal/pharmacy